T0195352

NETTER'S ORTHOPAEDIC CLINICAL EXAMINATION

AN EVIDENCE-BASED APPROACH

NOTE TO INSTRUCTORS

Contact your Elsevier Sales Representative for teaching resources for this title—including image collections—or request these supporting materials at http://evolve.elsevier.com/Cleland/Netter/orthopaedic/

4TH EDITION

NETTER'S ORTHOPAEDIC CLINICAL EXAMINATION

AN EVIDENCE-BASED APPROACH

Joshua A. Cleland, PT, PhD, FAPTA
Professor
Director of Research and Faculty Development
Doctor of Physical Therapy Program
Department of Public Health and Community Medicine
School of Medicine
Tufts University
Boston, Massachusetts

Shane Koppenhaver, PT, PhD
Clinical Professor
Doctoral Physical Therapy Program
Baylor University
Waco, Texas

Jonathan Su, PT, DPT, LMT
Sports/Orthopaedic Physical Therapy Clinician
San Francisco Bay Area, California

Illustrations by **Frank H. Netter, MD**

Contributing Illustrators
Carlos A. G. Machado, MD
John A. Craig, MD

ELSEVIER

Elsevier
1600 John F. Kennedy Blvd.
Ste 1800
Philadelphia, PA 19103-2899

NETTER'S ORTHOPAEDIC CLINICAL EXAMINATION: AN EVIDENCE-BASED
APPROACH, FOURTH EDITION   ISBN: 978-0-323-69533-6

Copyright © 2022 by Elsevier, Inc. All rights reserved.

No part of this publication may be reproduced or transmitted in any form or by any means, electronic or
mechanical, including photocopying, recording, or any information storage and retrieval system, without
permission in writing from the publisher. Details on how to seek permission, further information about the
Publisher's permissions policies and our arrangements with organizations such as the Copyright Clearance
Center and the Copyright Licensing Agency, can be found at our website: www.elsevier.com/permissions.

This book and the individual contributions contained in it are protected under copyright by the Publisher
(other than as may be noted herein).

Permission to use Netter Art figures may be sought through the website *NetterImages.com* or by emailing
Elsevier's Licensing Department at H.Licensing@elsevier.com.

Notice

Practitioners and researchers must always rely on their own experience and knowledge in evaluating
and using any information, methods, compounds or experiments described herein. Because of rapid
advances in the medical sciences, in particular, independent verification of diagnoses and drug dosages
should be made. To the fullest extent of the law, no responsibility is assumed by Elsevier, authors, editors
or contributors for any injury and/or damage to persons or property as a matter of products liability,
negligence or otherwise, or from any use or operation of any methods, products, instructions, or ideas
contained in the material herein.

Previous editions copyrighted 2016, 2011, and 2005.

Library of Congress Control Number: 2020947127

Senior Content Strategist: Elyse O'Grady
Content Development Specialist: Meredith Madeira
Publishing Services Manager: Catherine Jackson
Senior Project Manager: Daniel Fitzgerald
Designer: Patrick Ferguson

Printed in India.

Last digit is the print number: 9   8   7   6   5   4   3

Working together
to grow libraries in
developing countries

www.elsevier.com • www.bookaid.org

*To our incredible mentors and colleagues
who have fostered our passion for
evidence-based practice and orthopaedics.*

*To our photography models (Jessica Palmer, Nicole Koppenhaver,
and Farah Faize) and photographers (Sara Randall, Lindsey Browne,
Jeff Hebert, and Patrick Moon) for spending more hours
and retakes than we'd like to admit.*

*To Dr. Frank Netter and the Elsevier editorial staff
who turned our ideas into a fantastic literary guide.*

*And, most important, to our wonderful families,
whose sacrifices and support
made this considerable endeavor possible.*

About the Authors

Joshua A. Cleland, PT, PhD, FAPTA

Dr. Cleland earned a Master of Physical Therapy degree from Notre Dame College in 2000 and a Doctor of Physical Therapy degree from Creighton University in 2001. In February of 2006 he received a PhD from Nova Southeastern University. He received board certification from the American Physical Therapy Association as an Orthopaedic Clinical Specialist in 2002 and completed a fellowship in manual therapy through Regis University in Denver in 2005. Josh is presently Director of Research and Faculty Development and Doctor of Physical Therapy Program in the Department of Public Health and Community Medicine and School of Medicine at Tufts University. Dr. Cleland is actively involved in numerous clinical research studies investigating the effectiveness of manual physical therapy and exercise in the management of spine and extremities disorders. He has published over 250 manuscripts in peer-reviewed journals and is an Editorial Review Board Member for the Journal of Orthopaedic and Sports Physical Therapy. He is currently an author/editor on four textbooks. Dr. Cleland is a well-known speaker both nationally and internationally. Additionally, he has received numerous awards for his teaching and research efforts.

Shane Koppenhaver, PT, PhD

Dr. Koppenhaver received his Master of Physical Therapy degree from the U.S. Army–Baylor University Graduate Program in 1998 and a PhD in Exercise Science from the University of Utah in 2009. He became board certified in Orthopedic Physical Therapy in 2001 and completed a fellowship in manual therapy through Regis University in 2009. Dr. Koppenhaver currently serves as a Clinical Professor and Director of Research and Faculty Development in the Doctoral Physical Therapy Program at Baylor University, where he teaches Evidence-Based Practice, Anatomy and Musculoskeletal Interventions. His research primarily focuses on physiologic and clinical outcomes associated with complementary and alternative therapies in patients with neuromusculoskeletal conditions, which has resulted in approximately $2.7 million in grant funding, 70 scientific papers in peer-reviewed journals, and multiple research awards.

Jonathan Su, PT, DPT, LMT

Dr. Su earned a Doctor of Physical Therapy degree from U.S. Army–Baylor University in 2013. He received board certification from the American Physical Therapy Association as a Sports Clinical Specialist in 2015 and as an Orthopaedic Clinical Specialist in 2016. Dr. Su is a former Captain in the U.S. Army who served at the Sports Medicine/Physical Therapy Clinic at U.S. Military Academy West Point. He also served as the subject matter expert on human performance optimization, rehabilitation/reconditioning, and injury prevention for the 25th Infantry Division. Dr. Su is currently a busy clinician and consultant in the San Francisco Bay Area integrating the latest research into clinical practice. He is passionate about delivering high-quality patient-centered care for neuromusculoskeletal conditions.

About the Artists

Frank H. Netter, MD

Frank H. Netter was born in 1906 in New York City. He studied art at the Art Students League and the National Academy of Design before entering medical school at New York University, where he received his medical degree in 1931. During his student years, Dr. Netter's notebook sketches attracted the attention of the medical faculty and other physicians, allowing him to augment his income by illustrating articles and textbooks. He continued illustrating as a sideline after establishing a surgical practice in 1933, but he ultimately opted to give up his practice in favor of a full-time commitment to art. After service in the United States Army during World War II, Dr. Netter began his long collaboration with the CIBA Pharmaceutical Company (now Novartis Pharmaceuticals). This 45-year partnership resulted in the production of the extraordinary collection of medical art so familiar to physicians and other medical professionals worldwide.

In 2005, Elsevier, Inc. purchased the Netter Collection and all publications from Icon Learning Systems. More than 50 publications feature the art of Dr. Netter and are available through Elsevier, Inc. (in the US: https://www.us.elsevierhealth.com/ and outside the US: www.elsevierhealth.com).

Dr. Netter's works are among the finest examples of the use of illustration in the teaching of medical concepts. The 13-book *Netter Collection of Medical Illustrations*, which includes the greater part of the more than 20,000 paintings created by Dr. Netter, became and remains one of the most famous medical works ever published. The Netter *Atlas of Human Anatomy*, first published in 1989, presents the anatomical paintings from the Netter Collection. Now translated into 16 languages, it is the anatomy atlas of choice among medical and health professions students the world over.

The Netter illustrations are appreciated not only for their aesthetic qualities, but, more important, for their intellectual content. As Dr. Netter wrote in 1949, ". . . clarification of a subject is the aim and goal of illustration. No matter how beautifully painted, how delicately and subtly rendered a subject may be, it is of little value as a medical illustration if it does not serve to make clear some medical point." Dr. Netter's planning, conception, point of view, and approach are what inform his paintings and what makes them so intellectually valuable.

Frank H. Netter, MD, physician and artist, died in 1991.

Learn more about the physician-artist whose work has inspired the Netter Reference collection: https://netterimages.com/artist-frank-h-netter.html.

Carlos A. G. Machado, MD

Carlos Machado was chosen by Novartis to be Dr. Netter's successor. He continues to be the main artist who contributes to the Netter collection of medical illustrations.

Self-taught in medical illustration, cardiologist Carlos Machado has contributed meticulous updates to some of Dr. Netter's original plates and has created many paintings of his own in the style of Netter as an extension of the Netter collection. Dr. Machado's photorealistic expertise and his keen insight into the physician/patient relationship inform his vivid and unforgettable visual style. His dedication to researching each topic and subject he paints places him among the premier medical illustrators at work today.

Learn more about his background and see more of his art at: https://netterimages.com/artist-carlos-a-g-machado.html.

Foreword

Appropriate treatment decisions depend on an in-depth understanding of anatomy and an accurate diagnosis. This book is unique in that it combines the extensive library of classic Netter anatomical drawings with high-quality photos and now even video in this edition demonstrating special tests. The authors should be applauded for including quality ratings for 269 studies investigating a test's reliability using the 11-item "Quality Appraisal of Diagnostic Reliability Checklist." This edition includes 84 new studies, 34 new photos, and 25 new videos demonstrating special tests. As a PT/ATC and director of a PT sports medicine doctoral program, I see great utility for this reference from the entry level student athletic trainer and physical therapist to ortho/sports residency and fellowship training PTs and MDs. The book is extremely user-friendly and well organized as it walks the reader through the anatomy, clinical exam, and then critically reviews all literature for given diagnostic tests. As we constantly strive for better evidence-based medicine, new and old clinicians would be well served by such a powerful book detailing the utility of diagnostic tests and even evaluating evidence for treatment modalities when available.

Thank you for this extremely helpful tool.

Don Goss, PT, PhD
Associate Professor
Doctor of Physical Therapy Program
High Point University

If we can make the correct diagnosis, the healing can begin.

A. Weil

As an occupational therapist and certified hand therapist, I naturally gravitate toward the chapters on the upper limb. These chapters are exceptional! This is a must-have text for therapists at all levels of experience. The up-to-date tables that provide quality ratings on research facilitate evidence-based practice. The photos demonstrating special tests are invaluable for new learners, as are the supplemental videos included in this fourth edition. This book signifies a clear intent of the authors to provide a critical resource for therapists. It also shows commitment to education, a desire to translate research into advanced clinical practice, and a vision to advance rehabilitation science through accurate diagnostic evaluation. As I staff upper limb orthopedic cases of my students in training, this book is in my hands and on my clinic exam table as an open-book, go-to reference. It's an educator's dream to have all this valuable information in one text!

Kathleen Yancosek, OT, PhD
Director
Upward Call Rehabilitation, Inc.
Adjunct Faculty
Gannon University

Preface

Over the past several years evidence-based practice has become the standard in the medical and healthcare professions. As described by Sackett and colleagues (*Evidence-Based Medicine: How to Practice and Teach EBM*, 2nd ed, London, 2000, Harcourt Publishers Limited), evidence-based practice is a combination of three elements: the best available evidence, clinical experience, and patient values. Sackett has further reported that "when these three elements are integrated, clinicians and patients form a diagnostic and therapeutic alliance which optimizes clinical outcomes and quality of life." Each element contributes significantly to the clinical reasoning process by helping to identify a diagnosis or prognosis or establish an effective and efficient plan of care. Unfortunately, the evidence-based approach confronts a number of barriers that may limit the clinician's ability to use the best available evidence to guide decisions about patient care, most significantly a lack of time and resources. Given the increasing prevalence of new clinical tests in the orthopaedic setting and the frequent omission from textbooks of information about their diagnostic utility, the need was clear for a quick reference guide for students and busy clinicians that would enhance their ability to incorporate evidence into clinical decision making.

The purpose of *Netter's Orthopaedic Clinical Examination: An Evidence-Based Approach* is twofold: to serve as a textbook for musculoskeletal evaluation courses in an academic setting and to provide a quick, user-friendly guide and reference for clinicians who want to locate the evidence related to the diagnostic utility of commonly utilized tests and measures.

The first chapter is intended to introduce the reader to the essential concepts underlying evidence-based practice, including the statistical methods it employs and the critical analysis of research articles. The remainder of the book consists of chapters devoted to individual body regions. Each chapter begins with a review of the relevant osteology, arthrology, myology, and neurology and is liberally illustrated with images by the well-known medical artist Frank H. Netter, MD. The second portion of each chapter provides information related to patient complaints and physical examination findings. Reliability and diagnostic utility estimates (sensitivity, specificity, and likelihood ratios) are presented for each patient complaint and physical examination finding and are accompanied by quick access interpretation guides. Test descriptions and definitions of positive test findings are included as reported by the original study authors, both to minimize any alteration of information and to provide readers insight into difference values reported by different studies. At the end of each chapter are tables listing information on commonly used outcome measures.

We hope that clinicians will find *Netter's Orthopaedic Clinical Examination* a user-friendly clinical resource for determining the relevance of findings from the orthopaedic examination. We also hope that students and educators will find this a valuable guide to incorporate into courses related to musculoskeletal evaluation and treatment.

Joshua A. Cleland
Shane Koppenhaver
Jonathan Su

Contents

Diagnostic and Reliability Interpretation Keys

Diagnostic Interpretation Key

+ LR	Interpretation	−LR
≥10	Large	<.1
5.0-10.0	Moderate	.1-.2
2.0-5.0	Small	.2-.5
1.0-2.0	Rarely important	.5-1.0

Reliability Interpretation Key

ICC or κ	Interpretation
.81-1.0	Substantial agreement
.61-.80	Moderate agreement
.41-.60	Fair agreement
.11-.40	Slight agreement
.0-.10	No agreement

Video Contents

NETTER'S ORTHOPAEDIC CLINICAL EXAMINATION

AN EVIDENCE-BASED APPROACH

The Reliability and Diagnostic Utility of the Orthopaedic Clinical Examination

1

Reliability

The health sciences and medical professions continue to focus on evidence-based practice defined as the integration of the best available research evidence and clinical expertise with the patient's values.[1,2] Evidence should be incorporated into all aspects of physical therapy patient and client management, including the examination, evaluation, diagnosis, prognosis, and intervention. Perhaps the most crucial component is a careful, succinct clinical examination that can lead to an accurate diagnosis, the selection of appropriate interventions, and the determination of a prognosis. Thus, it is of utmost importance to incorporate evidence of how well clinical tests and measures can distinguish between patients who present with specific musculoskeletal disorders and patients who do not.[1,2]

The diagnostic process entails obtaining a patient history, developing a working hypothesis, and selecting specific tests and measures to confirm or refute the formulated hypothesis. The clinician must determine the pretest (before the evaluation) probability that the patient has a particular disorder. Based on this information the clinician selects appropriate tests and measures that will help determine the posttest (after the evaluation) probability of the patient having the disorder, until a degree of certainty has been reached such that patient management can begin (the *treatment threshold*). The purpose of clinical tests is not to obtain diagnostic certainty but rather to reduce the level of uncertainty until the treatment threshold is reached.[2] The concepts of pretest and posttest probability and treatment threshold are elaborated later in this chapter.

As the number of reported clinical tests and measures continues to grow, it is essential to thoroughly evaluate a test's diagnostic properties before incorporating the test into clinical practice.[3] Integrating the best evidence available for the diagnostic utility of each clinical test is essential in determining an accurate diagnosis and implementing effective, efficient treatment. It seems only sensible for clinicians and students to be aware of the diagnostic properties of tests and measures and to know which have clinical utility. This text assists clinicians and students in selecting tests and measures to ensure the appropriate classification of patients and to allow for quick implementation of effective management strategies.

The assessment of diagnostic tests involves examining several properties, including reliability and diagnostic accuracy. A test is considered *reliable* if it produces precise and reproducible information. A test is considered to have *diagnostic accuracy* if it can discriminate between patients who have a specific disorder and patients who do not have it.[4] Scientific evaluation of the clinical utility of physical therapy tests and measures involves comparing the examination results with reference standards such as radiographic studies (which represent the closest measure of the truth). Using statistical methods from the field of epidemiology, the diagnostic accuracy of the test, that is, its ability to determine which patients have a disorder and which do not, is then calculated. This chapter focuses on the characteristics that define the reliability and diagnostic accuracy of specific tests and measures. The chapter concludes with a discussion of the quality assessment of studies investigating reliability and diagnostic utility.

Reliability

For a clinical test to provide information that can be used to guide clinical decision making, it must have acceptable reliability. *Reliability* is the degree of consistency with which an instrument or rater measures a particular attribute.[5] When we investigate the reliability of a measurement, we are determining the proportion of that measurement that is a true representation and the proportion that is the result of measurement error.[6]

When discussing the clinical examination process, it is important to consider two forms of reliability: intraexaminer and interexaminer reliability. *Intraexaminer reliability* is the ability of a single rater to obtain identical measurements during separate performances of the same test. *Interexaminer reliability* is a measure of the ability of two or more raters to obtain identical results with the same test.

The kappa coefficient (κ) is a measure of the proportion of potential agreement after chance is removed[1,5,7]; it is the reliability coefficient most often used for categorical data (positive or negative).[5] The correlation coefficient commonly used to determine the reliability of data that are continuous in nature (e.g., range-of-motion data) is the intraclass correlation coefficient (ICC).[7]

Although interpretations of reliability vary, coefficients are often evaluated by the criteria described by Shrout,[8] with values less than 0.10 indicating no reliability, values between 0.11 and 0.40 indicating slight reliability, values between 0.41 and 0.60 indicating fair reliability, values between 0.61 and 0.80 indicating moderate reliability, and values greater than 0.81 indicating substantial reliability. "Acceptable reliability" must be decided by the clinician using the specific test or measure[9] and should be based on the variable being tested, the reason a particular test is important, and the patient on whom the test will be used.[6] For example, a 5% measurement error may be very acceptable when measuring joint range of motion but is not nearly as acceptable when measuring pediatric core body temperature.

Diagnostic Accuracy

Clinical tests and measures can never absolutely confirm or exclude the presence of a specific disease.[10] However, clinical tests can be used to alter the clinician's estimate of the probability that a patient has a specific musculoskeletal disorder. The accuracy of a test is determined by the measure of agreement between the clinical test and a reference standard.[11,12] A reference standard is the criterion considered the closest representation of the truth of a disorder being present.[1] The results obtained with the reference standard are compared with the results obtained with the test under investigation to determine the percentage of people correctly diagnosed or the diagnostic accuracy.[13] Because the diagnostic utility statistics are completely dependent on both the reference standard used and the population studied, we have specifically listed these within this text to provide information to consider when selecting the tests and measures reported. Diagnostic accuracy is often expressed in terms of positive and negative predictive values (PPVs and NPVs), sensitivity and specificity, and likelihood ratios (LRs).[1,14]

2×2 Contingency Table

To determine the clinical utility of a test or measure, the results of the reference standard are compared with the results of the test under investigation in a 2×2 contingency table, which provides a direct comparison between the reference standard and the test under investigation.[15] It allows for the calculation of the values associated with diagnostic accuracy to assist with determining the utility of the clinical test under investigation (Table 1-1).

The 2×2 contingency table is divided into four cells (a, b, c, d) for the determination of the test's ability to correctly identify true positives (cell a) and rule out true negatives (cell d). Cell b represents the false-positive findings wherein the diagnostic test was found to be positive yet the reference standard obtained a negative result. Cell c represents the false-negative findings wherein the diagnostic test was found to be negative yet the reference standard obtained a positive result.

Once a study investigating the diagnostic utility of a clinical test has been completed and the comparison with the reference standard has been performed in the 2×2 contingency table, determination of the clinical utility in terms of overall accuracy, PPVs and NPVs, sensitivity and specificity, and LRs can be calculated. These statistics are useful in determining whether a diagnostic test is useful for either ruling in or ruling out a disorder.

Table 1-1 2×2 Contingency Table Used to Compare the Results of the Reference Standard with Those of the Test under Investigation

	Reference Standard Positive	**Reference Standard Negative**
Clinical Test Positive	True-positive results a	False-positive results b
Clinical Test Negative	False-negative results c	True-negative results d

Table 1-2 2×2 Contingency Table Showing the Calculation of Positive Predictive Values (PPVs) and Negative Predictive Values (NPVs) Horizontally and Sensitivity and Specificity Vertically

	Reference Standard Positive	Reference Standard Negative	
Clinical Test Positive	True positives a	False positives b	$PPV = a/(a+b)$
Clinical Test Negative	c False negatives	d True negatives	$NPV = d/(c+d)$
	Sensitivity $= a/(a+c)$	Specificity $= d/(b+d)$	

Overall Accuracy

The overall accuracy of a diagnostic test is determined by dividing the correct responses (true positives and true negatives) by the total number of patients.[16] Using the 2×2 contingency table, the overall accuracy is determined by the following equation:

$$\text{Overall accuracy} = 100\% \times (a+d)/(a+b+c+d) \tag{1-1}$$

A perfect test would exhibit an overall accuracy of 100%. This is most likely unobtainable in that no clinical test is perfect, and each will always exhibit at least a small degree of uncertainty. The accuracy of a diagnostic test should not be used to determine the clinical utility of the test, because the overall accuracy can be a bit misleading. The accuracy of a test can be significantly influenced by the prevalence of a disease, or the total instances of the disease in the population at a given time.[5,6]

Positive and Negative Predictive Values

PPVs estimate the likelihood that a patient with a positive test actually has a disease.[5,6,17] PPVs are calculated horizontally in the 2×2 contingency table (Table 1-2) and indicate the percentage of patients accurately identified as having the disorder (true positive) divided by all the positive results of the test under investigation. A high PPV indicates that a positive result is a strong predictor that the patient has the disorder.[5,6] The formula for the PPV is:

$$PPV = 100\% \times a/(a+b) \tag{1-2}$$

NPVs estimate the likelihood that a patient with a negative test does not have the disorder.[5,6] NPVs are also calculated horizontally in the 2×2 contingency table (see Table 1-2) and indicate the percentage of patients accurately identified as not having the disorder (true negative) divided by all the negative results of the test under investigation.[11] The formula for the NPV is as follows:

$$NPV = 100\% \times d/(c+d) \tag{1-3}$$

The predictive values are significantly influenced by the prevalence of the condition.[11] Hence, we have not specifically reported these in this text.

Sensitivity

The *sensitivity* of a diagnostic test indicates the test's ability to detect those patients who actually have a disorder as indicated by the reference standard. This is also referred to as the *true-positive rate*.[1] Tests with high sensitivity are good for ruling out a particular disorder. The acronym *SnNout* can be used to remember that a test with high *Sensitivity* and a *Negative* result is good for ruling *out* the disorder.[1]

Consider, for example, a clinical test that, compared with the reference standard, exhibits a high sensitivity for detecting lumbar spinal stenosis. Considering the rule above, if the test is negative it assists with ruling out lumbar spinal stenosis. If the test is positive, it is likely to accurately identify a high percentage of patients presenting with stenosis. However, it also may identify as positive

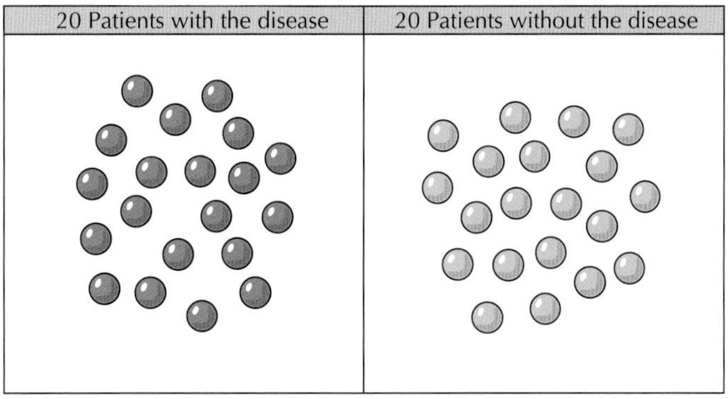

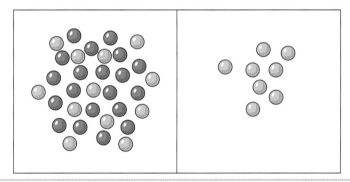

20 Patients with the disease	20 Patients without the disease

Figure 1-1
Sensitivity and specificity example. Twenty patients with and 20 patients without the disorder.

Figure 1-2
100% Sensitivity. One hundred percent sensitivity infers that if the test is positive, all those with the disease will be captured. However, although this test captured all those with the disease, it also captured many without it. Yet if the test result is negative, we are confident that the disorder can be ruled out (SnNout).

many of those without the disorder (false positives). Thus, although a negative result can be relied on, a positive test result does not allow us to draw any conclusions (Figs. 1-1 and 1-2).

The sensitivity of a test also can be calculated from the 2×2 contingency tables. However, it is calculated vertically (see Table 1-2). The formula for calculating a test's sensitivity is as follows:

$$\text{Sensitivity} = 100\% \times a/(a+c) \tag{1-4}$$

Specificity

The *specificity* of a diagnostic test simply indicates the test's ability to detect those patients who actually do not have the disorder as indicated by the reference standard. This is also referred to as the *true-negative rate*.[1] Tests with high specificity are good for ruling in a disorder. The acronym *SpPin* can be used to remember that a test with high *Sp*ecificity and a *P*ositive result is good for ruling *in* the disorder.[16,18,19]

Consider a test with high specificity. It would demonstrate a strong ability to accurately identify all patients who do not have a disorder. If a highly specific clinical test is negative, it is likely to identify a high percentage of those patients who do not have the disorder. However, it is also possible that the highly specific test with a negative result will identify a number of patients who actually have the disease as being negative (false negative). Therefore, we can be fairly confident that a highly specific test with a positive finding indicates that the disorder is present (Fig. 1-3).

The formula for calculating test specificity is as follows:

$$\text{Specificity} = 100\% \times d/(b+d) \tag{1-5}$$

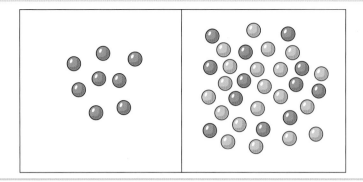

Figure 1-3
100% Specificity. One hundred percent specificity infers that if the test is negative, all those without the disease will be captured. However, although this test captured all those without the disease, it also captured many with it. Yet if the test is positive, we are confident that the patient has the disorder (SpPin).

Sensitivity and specificity have been used for decades to determine a test's diagnostic utility; however, they possess a few clinical limitations.[11] Although sensitivity and specificity can be useful in assisting clinicians in selecting tests that are good for ruling in or out a particular disorder, few clinical tests demonstrate both high sensitivity and high specificity.[11] Also the sensitivity and specificity do not provide information regarding a change in the probability of a patient having a disorder if the test results are positive or negative.[18,20] Instead, LRs have been advocated as the optimal statistics for determining a shift in pretest probability that a patient has a specific disorder.

Likelihood Ratios

A test's result is valuable only if it alters the pretest probability of a patient having a disorder.[21] LRs combine a test's sensitivity and specificity to develop an indication in the shift of probability given the specific test result and are valuable in guiding clinical decision making.[20] LRs are a powerful measure that can significantly increase or reduce the probability of a patient having a disease.[22]

LRs can be either positive or negative. A positive LR indicates a shift in probability favoring the existence of a disorder, whereas a negative LR indicates a shift in probability favoring the absence of a disorder. Although LRs are often not reported in studies investigating the diagnostic utility of the clinical examination, they can be calculated easily if a test's sensitivity and specificity are available. Throughout this text, for studies that did not report LRs but did document a test's sensitivity and specificity, the LRs were calculated by the authors.

The formula used to determine a positive LR is as follows:

$$LR = Sensitivity / (1 - Specificity) \tag{1-6}$$

The formula used to determine a negative LR is as follows:

$$LR = (1 - Sensitivity) / Specificity \tag{1-7}$$

A guide to interpreting test results can be found in Table 1-3. Positive LRs higher than 1 increase the odds of the disorder given a positive test, and negative LRs less than 1 decrease the odds of the disorder given a negative test.[22] However, it is the magnitude of the shifts in probability that determines the usefulness of a clinical test. Positive LRs higher than 10 and negative LRs close to zero often represent large and conclusive shifts in probability. An LR of 1 (either positive or negative) does not alter the probability that the patient does or does not have the particular disorder and is of little clinical value.[22] Once the LRs have been calculated, they can be applied to the nomogram (Fig. 1-4)[23] or a mathematical equation[24] can be used to determine more precisely the shifts in probability given a specific test result. Both methods are described in further detail later in the chapter.

Table 1-3 Interpretation of Likelihood Ratios

Positive Likelihood Ratio	Negative Likelihood Ratio	Interpretation
>10	<0.1	Generate large and often conclusive shifts in probability
5 to 10	0.1 to 0.2	Generate moderate shifts in probability
2 to 5	0.2 to 0.5	Generate small but sometimes important shifts in probability
1 to 2	0.5 to 1.0	Alter probability to a small and rarely important degree

Adapted from Jaeschke R, Guyatt GH, Sackett DL III. How to use an article about a diagnostic test. B. What are the results and will they help me in caring for my patients? *JAMA.* 1994;271:703-707.

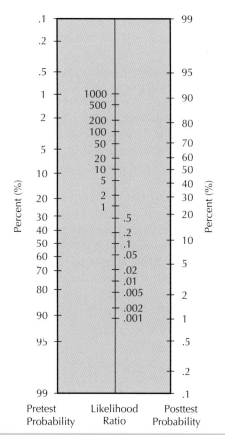

Figure 1-4

Fagan's nomogram. (Adapted with permission from Fagan TJ. Letter: nomogram for Bayes theorem. *N Engl J Med.* 1975;293:257. Copyright 2005, Massachusetts Medical Society. All rights reserved.)

If a diagnostic test exhibits a specificity of 1, the positive LR cannot be calculated because the equation will result in a zero for the denominator. In these circumstances, a suggestion has been made to modify the 2×2 contingency table by adding 0.5 to each cell in the table to allow for the calculation of LRs.[25]

Consider, for example, the diagnostic utility of the Crank test[5,26] in detecting labral tears in the shoulder compared with arthroscopic examination, the reference standard. This is revealed in a 2×2 contingency table (Table 1-4). The inability to calculate a positive LR becomes obvious in the following:

$$\text{Positive LR} = \text{Sensitivity} / (1 - \text{Specificity}) = 1/(1-1) = 1/0 \qquad (1-8)$$

The Reliability and Diagnostic Utility of the Orthopaedic Clinical Examination

Table 1-4 Results of the Crank Test in Detecting Labral Tears When Compared with the Reference Standard of Arthroscopic Examination

	Arthroscopic Examination Positive (n = 12)	Arthroscopic Examination Negative (n = 3)	
Crank Test Positive	10 a	0 b	PPV = 100 × 10 / 10 = 100 %
Crank Test Negative	c 2	d 3	NPV = 100 × 3 / 5 = 60 %
	Sensitivity = 100 % × 10 / 12 = 83 %	Specificity = 100 % × 3 / 3 = 100 %	

Because zero cannot be the denominator in a fraction, the 2×2 contingency table is modified by adding 0.5 to each cell.

Although the addition of 0.5 to each cell is the only reported method of modifying the contingency table to prevent zero in the denominator of an LR calculation, considering the changes that occur with the diagnostic properties of sensitivity, specificity, and predictive values, this technique has not been used in this text. In circumstances in which the specificity is zero and the positive LR cannot be calculated, it is documented as "undefined" (UD). In these cases, although we are not calculating the positive LR, the test is indicative of a large shift in probability.

Confidence Intervals

Calculations of sensitivity, specificity, and LRs are known as *point estimates*. That is, they are the single best estimates of the population values.[5] However, because point estimates are based on small subsets of people (samples), it is unlikely that they are a perfect representation of the larger population. It is more accurate, therefore, to include a range of values (*interval estimate*) in which the population value is likely to fall. A *confidence interval* (CI) is a range of scores around the point estimate that likely contains the population value.[27] Commonly, the 95% CI is calculated for studies investigating the diagnostic utility of the clinical examination. A 95% CI indicates the spread of scores in which we can be 95% confident that they contain the population value.[5] In this text, the 95% CI is reported for all studies that provided this information.

Pretest and Posttest Probability

Pretest probability is the likelihood that a patient exhibits a specific disorder before the clinical examination. Often prevalence rates are used as an indication of pretest probability, but when prevalence rates are unknown, the pretest probability is based on a combination of the patient's medical history, the results of previous tests, and the clinician's experience.[16] Determining the pretest probability is the first step in the decision-making process for clinicians. Pretest probability is an estimate by the clinician and can be expressed as a percentage (e.g., 75%, 80%) or as a qualitative measure (e.g., somewhat likely, very likely).[11,16] Once the pretest probability of a patient having a disorder is identified, tests and measures that have the potential to alter the probability should be selected for the physical examination. Posttest probability is the likelihood that a patient has a specific disorder after the clinical examination procedures have been performed.

Calculating Posttest Probability

As previously mentioned, LRs can assist with determining the shifts in probability that would occur following a given test result and depend on the respective LR ratios of that given test. The quickest method to determine the shifts in probability once an LR is known for a specific test is the nomogram (Fig. 1-5).[23] The nomogram is a diagram that illustrates the pretest probability on the left and the posttest probability on the right, with the LRs in the middle. To determine the shift in probability, a mark is placed on the nomogram representing the pretest probability. Then a mark is made on the nomogram at the level of the LR (either negative or positive). The two lines are

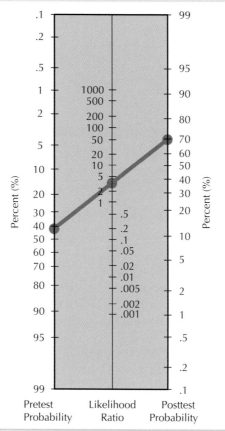

Figure 1-5

Nomogram representing the change in pretest probability from 42% if the test was positive (positive likelihood ratio = 4.2) to a posttest probability of 71%. (Adapted with permission from Fagan TJ. Letter: nomogram for Bayes theorem. *N Engl J Med*. 1975;293:257. Copyright 2005, Massachusetts Medical Society. All rights reserved.)

connected with a straight line and the line is carried through the right of the diagram. The point at which the line crosses the posttest probability scale indicates the shift in probability.

A more precise determination of the shift in probability can be calculated algebraically with the following formula[16]:

Step 1. Pretest odds = Pretest probability / 1 − Pretest probability   (1-9)

Step 2. Pretest odds × LR = Posttest odds   (1-10)

Step 3. Posttest odds / Posttest odds + 1 = Posttest probability   (1-11)

The clinician must make a determination of when the posttest probability is either low enough to rule out the presence of a certain disease or when the posttest probability is high enough that the clinician feels confident in having established the presence of a disorder. The level at which evaluation ceases and treatment begins is known as the *treatment threshold* (Fig. 1-6).[16]

Assessment of Study Quality

Once relevant articles are retrieved, the next step is critical analysis of their content for adequate methodologic rigor. It has been reported that the methodologic quality of studies investigating the diagnostic utility of the clinical examination is generally inferior to that of studies investigating the effectiveness of therapies.[28,29] Unfortunately, studies with significant methodologic flaws

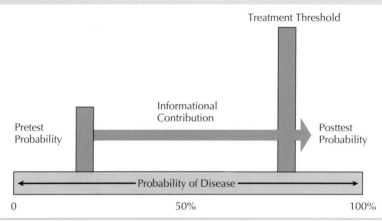

Figure 1-6
Treatment threshold. Clinicians must use the pretest probability and likelihood ratios to determine the treatment threshold as indicated in this illustration.

reporting the usefulness of specific tests and measures can lead to premature incorporation of ineffective tests. This can result in inaccurate diagnoses and poor patient management. Alternatively, identification and use of rigorously appraised clinical tests can improve patient care and outcomes.[29]

The Quality Appraisal for Reliability Studies (QAREL) was developed to assess the quality of diagnostic reliability studies.[30] The QAREL is an 11-item checklist developed in consultation with a reference group of experts in diagnostic research and quality appraisal that is used to assess a study's methodologic quality. Each item is scored as "yes," "no," "unclear," or "N/A." The QAREL has been found to be a reliable assessment tool when reviewers are given the opportunity to discuss the criteria by which to interpret each item.[31] Reliability of 9 of the 11 items was identified as good reliability, whereas reliability of only 2 of the 11 items was identified as fair reliability.[31] We have used the QAREL to evaluate each study related to reliability referenced in this text. For the purpose of this study we considered good quality to be ≥75% and fair quality to be between 74% and 50%. The percentages were calculated by dividing the number of "yes" responses by 11, minus the number of "N/A" responses. Green symbols indicate a high level of methodologic quality and imply that readers can be confident in study results. Yellow symbols indicate fair methodologic quality and imply that readers should interpret such study results with caution. Studies deemed to be of poor methodologic quality have not been included in the diagnostic utility tables throughout the chapters.

The Quality Assessment of Diagnostic Accuracy Studies (QUADAS) was developed to assess the quality of diagnostic accuracy studies.[32] A four-round Delphi panel identified 14 criteria that are used to assess a study's methodologic quality. Each item is scored as "yes," "no," or "unclear." The QUADAS is not intended to quantify a score for each study but rather provides a qualitative assessment of the study with the identification of weaknesses.[32] The QUADAS has demonstrated adequate agreement for the individual items in the checklist.[33] We have used the QUADAS to evaluate each study referenced in this text. For the purpose of this text we considered good quality to be ≥75% and fair quality to be between 74% and 50%. This was calculated by dividing the number of "yes" responses by 14 (the total number of criteria). Green symbols indicate a high level of methodologic quality and imply that readers can be confident in study results. Yellow symbols indicate fair methodologic quality and imply that readers should interpret such study results with caution. Studies deemed to be of poor methodologic quality have not been included in the diagnostic utility tables throughout the chapters.

Summary

It is important to consider the reliability and diagnostic utility of tests and measures before including them as components of the clinical examination. Tests and measures should demonstrate adequate reliability before they are used to guide clinical decision making. Throughout this text, the reliability of many tests and measures is reported. It is essential that clinicians consider these reported levels of reliability in the context of their own practice.

Before implementing tests and measures into the orthopaedic examination, it is first essential to consider each test's diagnostic utility. Table 1-5 summarizes the statistics related to diagnostic accuracy as well as the mathematical equations and operational definitions for each. The usefulness of a test or measure is most commonly considered in terms of the respective test's diagnostic properties. These can be described in terms of sensitivity, specificity, PPVs, and NPVs. However, perhaps the most useful diagnostic property is the LR, which can assist in altering the probability that a patient has a specific disorder.

No clinical test or measure provides absolute certainty as to the presence or absence of disease. However, clinicians can determine when enough data have been collected to alter the probability beyond the treatment threshold where the evaluation can cease, and therapeutic management can begin. Furthermore, careful methodologic assessment provides greater insight into the scientific rigor of each study and its performance, applicability, reliability, and reproducibility within a given clinical practice.

Table 1-5 2×2 Contingency Table and Statistics Used to Determine the Diagnostic Utility of a Test or Measure

	Reference Standard Positive	Reference Standard Negative
Diagnostic Test Positive	True-positive results a	False-positive results b
Diagnostic Test Negative	c False-negative results	d True-negative results

Statistic	Formula	Description
Overall accuracy	$(a+d)/(a+b+c+d)$	The percentage of individuals who are correctly diagnosed
Sensitivity	$a/(a+c)$	The proportion of patients with the condition who have a positive test result
Specificity	$d/(b+d)$	The proportion of patients without the condition who have a negative test result
Positive predictive value	$a/(a+b)$	The proportion of individuals with a positive test result who have the condition
Negative predictive value	$d/(c+d)$	The proportion of individuals with a negative test result who do not have the condition
Positive likelihood ratio	$\text{Sensitivity}/(1-\text{Specificity})$	If the test is positive, the increase in odds favoring the condition
Negative likelihood ratio	$(1-\text{Sensitivity})/\text{Specificity}$	If the test is positive, the decrease in odds favoring the condition

References

1. Sackett DL, Straws SE, Richardson WS, et al. *Evidence-Based Medicine: How to Practice and Teach EBM.* 2nd ed. London: Harcourt Publishers Limited; 2000.
2. Kassirer JP. Our stubborn quest for diagnostic certainty: a cause of excessive testing. *N Engl J Med.* 1989;320:1489–1491.
3. Lijmer JG, Mol BW, Heisterkamp S, et al. Empirical evidence of design-related bias in studies of diagnostic tests. *JAMA.* 1999;282:1061–1066.
4. Schwartz JS. Evaluating diagnostic tests: what is done–what needs to be done. *J G Intern Med.* 1986;1:266–267.
5. Portney LG, Watkins MP. *Foundations of Clinical Research: Applications to Practice.* 2nd ed. Upper Saddle River, NJ: Prentice Hall Health; 2000.
6. Rothstein JM, Echternach JL. *Primer on Measurement: An Introductory Guide to Measurement Issues.* Alexandria, VA: American Physical Therapy Association; 1999.
7. Domholdt E. *Physical Therapy Research.* 2nd ed. Philadelphia: WB Saunders; 2000.
8. Shrout PE. Measurement reliability and agreement in psychiatry. *Stat Methods Med Res.* 1998;7:301–317.
9. Van Genderen F, De Bie R, Helders P, Van Meeteren N. Reliability research: towards a more clinically relevant approach. *Phys Ther Rev.* 2003;8:169–176.
10. Bossuyt PMM, Reitsma JB, Bruns DE, et al. Towards complete and accurate reporting of studies of diagnostic accuracy: the STARD initiative. *Clin Chem.* 2003;49:1–6.
11. Fritz JM, Wainner RS. Examining diagnostic tests: an evidence-based perspective. *Phys Ther.* 2001;81:1546–1564.
12. Jaeschke R, Guyatt GH, Sackett III DL. How to use an article about a diagnostic test. A. Are the results of the study valid? *JAMA.* 1994;271:389–391.
13. Bossuyt PMM, Reitsma JB, Bruns DE, et al. The STARD statement for reporting studies of diagnostic accuracy: explanation and elaboration. *Clin Chem.* 2003;49:7–18.
14. McGinn T, Guyatt G, Wyer P, et al. Users' guides to the medical literature XXII: how to use articles about clinical decision rules. *JAMA.* 2000;284:79–84.
15. Greenhalgh T. Papers that report diagnostic or screening tests. *BMJ.* 1997;315:540–543.
16. Bernstein J. Decision analysis (current concepts review). *J Bone Joint Surg.* 1997;79:1404–1414.
17. Potter NA, Rothstein JM. Intertester reliability for selected clinical tests of the sacroiliac joint. *Phys Ther.* 1985;65:1671–1675.
18. Boyko EJ. Ruling out or ruling in disease with the most sensitive or specific diagnostic test: short cut or wrong turn? *Med Decis Making.* 1994;14:175–180.
19. Riddle DL, Stratford PW. Interpreting validity indexes for diagnostic tests: an illustration using the Berg balance test. *Phys Ther.* 1999;79:939–948.
20. Hayden SR, Brown MD. Likelihood ratio: a powerful tool for incorporating the results of a diagnostic test into clinical decision making. *Ann Emerg Med.* 1999;33:575–580.
21. Simel DL, Samsa GP, Matchar DB. Likelihood ratios with confidence: sample size estimation for diagnostic test studies. *J Clin Epidemiol.* 1991;44:763–770.
22. Jaeschke R, Guyatt GH, Sackett DL. How to use an article about a diagnostic test. B. What are the results and will they help me in caring for my patients? *JAMA.* 1994;271:703–707.
23. Fagan TJ. Letter: nomogram for Bayes theorem. *N Engl J Med.* 1975;293:257.
24. Sackett DL, Haynes RB, Guyatt GH, Tugwell P. *Clinical Epidemiology: A Basic Science for Clinical Medicine.* Boston: Little, Brown; 1991.
25. Wainner RS, Fritz JM, Irrgang JJ, et al. Reliability and diagnostic accuracy of the clinical examination and patient self-report measures for cervical radiculopathy. *Spine.* 2003;28:52–62.
26. Mimori K, Muneta T, Nakagawa T, Shinomiya K. A new pain provocation test for superior labral tears of the shoulder. *Am J Sports Med.* 1999;27:137–142.
27. Fidler F, Thomason N, Cumming G, et al. Editors can lead researchers to confidence intervals, but can't make them think. *Psychol Sci.* 2004;15:119–126.
28. Moons KGM, Biesheuvel CJ, Grobbee DE. Test research versus diagnostic research. *Clin Chem.* 2004;50:473–476.
29. Reid MC, Lachs MS, Feinstein AR. Use of methodological standards in diagnostic test research. *JAMA.* 1995;274:645–651.
30. Lucas NP, Macaskill P, Irwig L, Bogduk N. The development of a quality appraisal tool for studies of diagnostic reliability (QAREL). *J Clin Epidemiol.* 2010;63(8):854–861.
31. Lucas N, Macaskill P, Irwig L, et al. The reliability of a quality appraisal tool for studies of diagnostic reliability (QAREL). *BMC Med Res Methodol.* 2013;13:111.
32. Whiting P, Harbord R, Kleijnen J. No role for quality scores in systematic reviews of diagnostic accuracy studies. *BMC Med Res Methodol.* 2005;5:19.
33. Whiting PF, Weswood ME, Rutjes AW, et al. Evaluation of QUADAS, a tool for the quality assessment of diagnostic accuracy studies. *BMC Med Res Methodol.* 2006;6:9.

Temporomandibular Joint

Clinical Summary and Recommendations

Patient History	
Questions	• Screening instruments have been shown to be very good at identifying temporomandibular disorder (TMD) pain (+LR [likelihood ratio] of 33). • A subject complaint of "periodic restriction" (the inability to open the mouth as wide as was previously possible) has been found to be the best single history item to identify anterior disc displacement, both in patients with reducing discs and in those with nonreducing discs.

Physical Examination	
Palpation	• Reproducing pain during palpation of the temporomandibular joint (TMJ) and related muscles has been found to be moderately reliable and appears to demonstrate good diagnostic utility for identifying TMJ effusion confirmed by magnetic resonance imaging (MRI) and TMD when compared with a comprehensive physical examination. We recommend that palpation at least include the TMJ (+LR = 4.87 to 5.67), the temporalis muscle (+LR = 2.73 to 4.12), and the masseter muscle (+LR = 3.65 to 4.87). • If clinically feasible, pressure pain threshold (PPT) testing is helpful because it demonstrates superior diagnostic utility in identifying TMD when compared with a comprehensive physical examination.
Joint Sounds	• Detecting joint sounds (clicking and crepitus) during jaw motion is a generally unreliable sign demonstrating moderate diagnostic utility except in attempts to detect moderate to severe osteoarthritis (+LR = 4.79) and nonreducing anterior disc displacement (+LR = 2.6 to 15.2).
Range-of-Motion and Dynamic Movement Measurements	• Measuring mouth range of motion appears to be a highly reliable test, and when the range of motion is restricted or deviated from the midline, the measurement has moderate diagnostic utility in identifying nonreducing anterior disc displacement. • Detecting pain during motion is a less reliable sign, but it also demonstrates moderate to good diagnostic utility in identifying nonreducing anterior disc displacement and self-reported TMJ pain. • The combination of *motion restriction* and *pain during assisted opening* has been found to be the best combination for identifying nonreducing anterior disc displacement (+LR = 7.71). • Consistent with assessment of other body regions, assessment of "joint play" and "end feel" is highly unreliable and has unknown diagnostic utility.
Combination of Tests	• A combination of clinical examination findings has been shown to be beneficial in identifying disc displacement without reduction (5 positive tests +LR = 7.9)
Interventions	• Patients with TMD who report (1) *symptoms* ≥4/10 (*10* being severe pain) and (2) pain for 10 months' duration or less may benefit from nightly wearing of an occlusal stabilization splint, especially if they have (3) *nonreducing anterior disc displacement* and (4) show *improvement after 2 months* (+LR = 10.8 if all four factors are present).

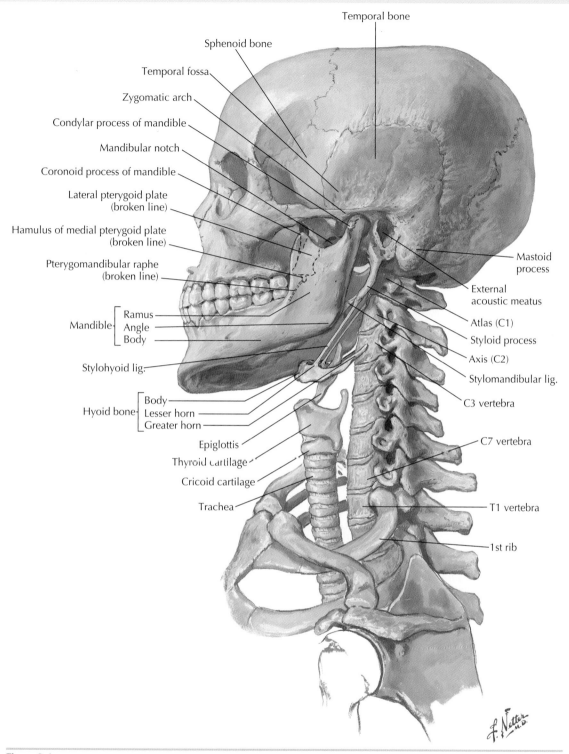

Temporal bone

Sphenoid bone

Temporal fossa

Zygomatic arch

Condylar process of mandible

Mandibular notch

Coronoid process of mandible

Lateral pterygoid plate
(broken line)

Hamulus of medial pterygoid plate
(broken line)

Pterygomandibular raphe
(broken line)

Mandible
- Ramus
- Angle
- Body

Stylohyoid lig.

Hyoid bone
- Body
- Lesser horn
- Greater horn

Epiglottis

Thyroid cartilage

Cricoid cartilage

Trachea

Mastoid
process

External
acoustic meatus

Atlas (C1)

Styloid process

Axis (C2)

Stylomandibular lig.

C3 vertebra

C7 vertebra

T1 vertebra

1st rib

Figure 2-1
Bony framework of head and neck.

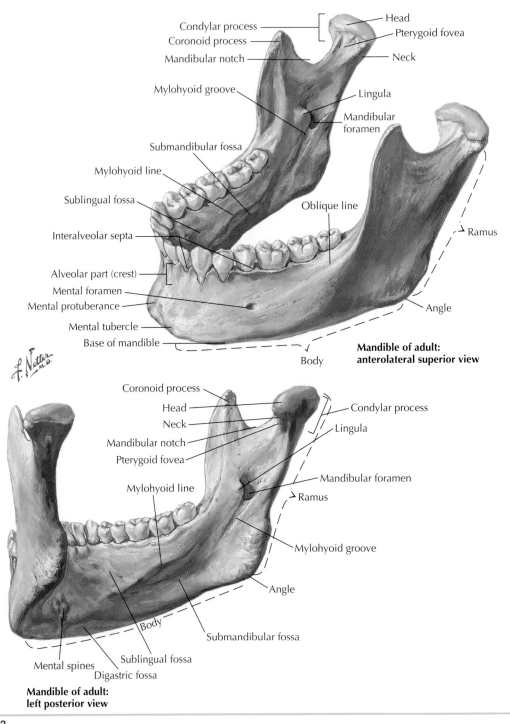

Condylar process
Coronoid process
Mandibular notch
Mylohyoid groove
Submandibular fossa
Mylohyoid line
Sublingual fossa
Interalveolar septa
Alveolar part (crest)
Mental foramen
Mental protuberance
Mental tubercle
Base of mandible

Head
Pterygoid fovea
Neck
Lingula
Mandibular foramen
Oblique line
Ramus
Angle
Body

**Mandible of adult:
anterolateral superior view**

Coronoid process
Head
Neck
Mandibular notch
Pterygoid fovea
Mylohyoid line
Condylar process
Lingula
Mandibular foramen
Ramus
Mylohyoid groove
Angle
Submandibular fossa
Body
Sublingual fossa
Mental spines
Digastric fossa

**Mandible of adult:
left posterior view**

Figure 2-2
Mandible.

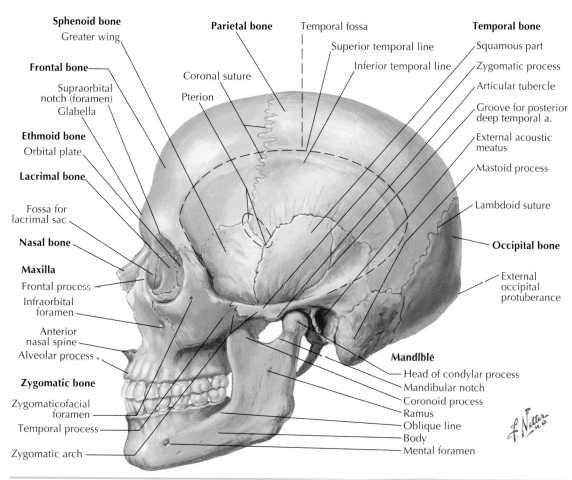

Sphenoid bone
Greater wing

Frontal bone

Supraorbital
notch (foramen)
Glabella

Ethmoid bone
Orbital plate

Lacrimal bone

Fossa for
lacrimal sac

Nasal bone

Maxilla
Frontal process
Infraorbital
foramen
Anterior
nasal spine
Alveolar process

Zygomatic bone
Zygomaticofacial
foramen
Temporal process
Zygomatic arch

Parietal bone

Coronal suture

Pterion

Temporal fossa

Superior temporal line

Inferior temporal line

Temporal bone
Squamous part
Zygomatic process
Articular tubercle
Groove for posterior
deep temporal a.
External acoustic
meatus
Mastoid process

Lambdoid suture

Occipital bone

External
occipital
protuberance

Mandible
Head of condylar process
Mandibular notch
Coronoid process
Ramus
Oblique line
Body
Mental foramen

Figure 2-3
Lateral skull.

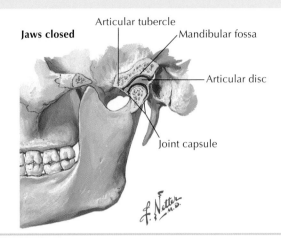

Jaws closed

Articular tubercle

Mandibular fossa

Articular disc

Joint capsule

Figure 2-4
Temporomandibular joint.

The temporomandibular joint (TMJ) is divided by an intraarticular biconcave disc that separates the joint cavity into two distinct functional components. The upper joint is a plane, or gliding, joint that permits translation of the mandibular condyles. The lower joint is a hinge joint that permits rotation of the condyles. The closed pack position of the TMJ is full occlusion. A unilateral restriction pattern primarily limits contralateral excursion but also affects mouth opening and protrusion.

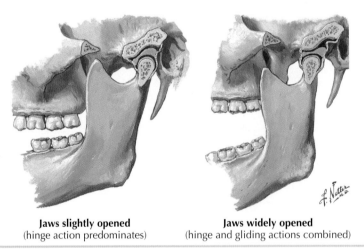

Jaws slightly opened
(hinge action predominates)

Jaws widely opened
(hinge and gliding actions combined)

Figure 2-5
Temporomandibular joint mechanics.

During mandibular depression from a closed mouth position, the initial movement occurs at the lower joint as the condyles pivot on the intraarticular disc. This motion continues to approximately 11 mm of depression. With further mandibular depression, motion begins to occur at the upper joint and causes anterior translation of the disc on the articular eminence. Normal mandibular depression is between 40 and 50 mm.

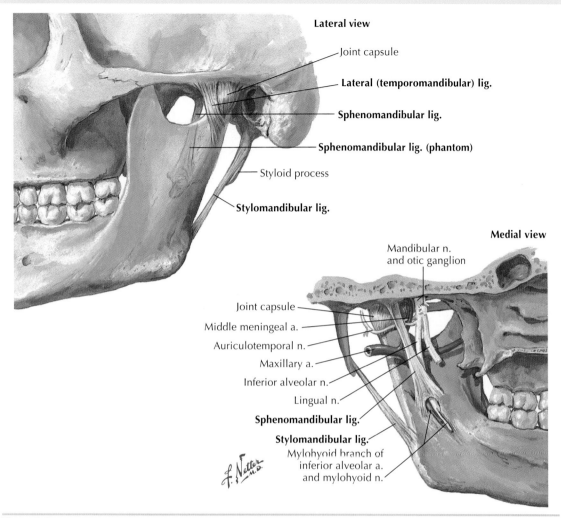

Lateral view
- Joint capsule
- **Lateral (temporomandibular) lig.**
- **Sphenomandibular lig.**
- **Sphenomandibular lig. (phantom)**
- Styloid process
- **Stylomandibular lig.**

Medial view
- Mandibular n. and otic ganglion
- Joint capsule
- Middle meningeal a.
- Auriculotemporal n.
- Maxillary a.
- Inferior alveolar n.
- Lingual n.
- **Sphenomandibular lig.**
- **Stylomandibular lig.**
- Mylohyoid branch of inferior alveolar a. and mylohyoid n.

Figure 2-6
Temporomandibular joint ligaments.

Ligaments	Attachments	Function
Temporomandibular	Thickening of anterior joint capsule extending from neck of mandible to zygomatic arch	Strengthen the TMJ laterally
Sphenomandibular	Sphenoid bone to mandible	Serve as a fulcrum for and reinforcer of TMJ motion
Stylomandibular	Styloid process to angle of mandible	Provide minimal support for joint

Muscles Involved in Mastication

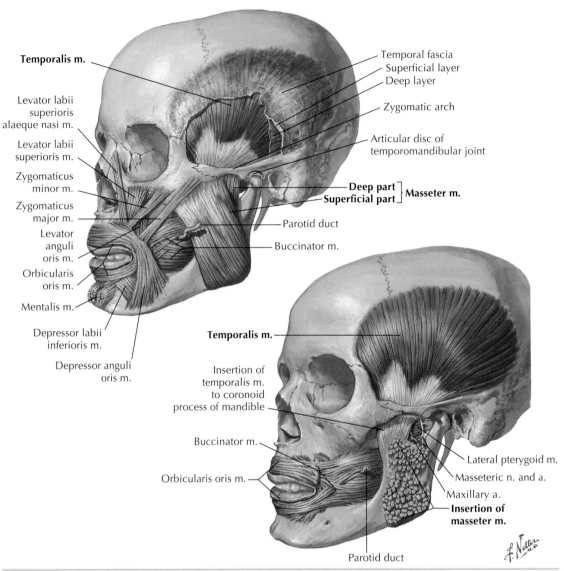

Figure 2-7
Muscles involved in mastication, lateral views.

Muscle	Proximal Attachment	Distal Attachment	Nerve and Segmental Level	Action
Temporalis	Temporal fossa	Coronoid process and anterior ramus of mandible	Deep temporal branches of mandibular nerve	Elevate mandible
Masseter	Inferior and medial aspects of zygomatic arch	Coronoid process and lateral ramus of mandible	Mandibular nerve via masseteric nerve	Elevate and protrude mandible

Muscles Involved in Mastication—cont'd

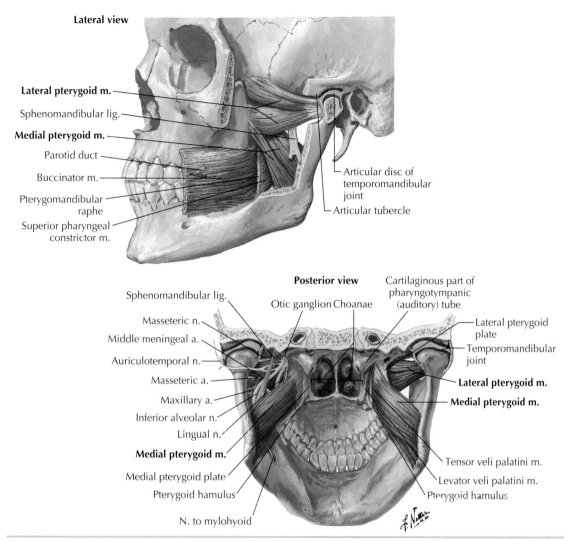

Lateral view

Lateral pterygoid m.

Sphenomandibular lig.

Medial pterygoid m.

Parotid duct

Buccinator m.

Pterygomandibular raphe

Superior pharyngeal constrictor m.

Articular disc of temporomandibular joint

Articular tubercle

Posterior view

Sphenomandibular lig.

Masseteric n.

Middle meningeal a.

Auriculotemporal n.

Masseteric a.

Maxillary a.

Inferior alveolar n.

Lingual n.

Medial pterygoid m.

Medial pterygoid plate

Pterygoid hamulus

N. to mylohyoid

Otic ganglion Choanae

Cartilaginous part of pharyngotympanic (auditory) tube

Lateral pterygoid plate

Temporomandibular joint

Lateral pterygoid m.

Medial pterygoid m.

Tensor veli palatini m.

Levator veli palatini m.

Pterygoid hamulus

Figure 2-8
Muscles involved in mastication, lateral and posterior views.

Muscle	Proximal Attachment	Distal Attachment	Nerve and Segmental Level	Action
Medial pterygoid	Medial surface of lateral pterygoid plate, pyramidal process of palatine bone, and tuberosity of maxilla	Medial aspect of mandibular ramus	Mandibular nerve via medial pterygoid nerve	Elevate and protrude mandible
Lateral pterygoid (superior head)	Lateral surface of greater wing of sphenoid bone	Neck of mandible, articular disc, and TMJ capsule	Mandibular nerve via lateral pterygoid nerve	Acting bilaterally: protrude and depress mandible
Lateral pterygoid (inferior head)	Lateral surface of lateral pterygoid plate			Acting unilaterally: laterally deviate mandible

Muscles of the Floor of the Mouth

Lateral, slightly inferior view

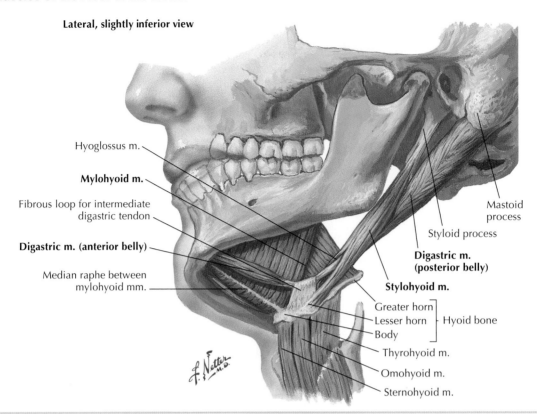

Figure 2-9
Floor of mouth, inferior view.

Muscle	Proximal Attachment	Distal Attachment	Nerve and Segmental Level	Action
Mylohyoid	Mylohyoid line of mandible	Hyoid bone	Mylohyoid nerve (branch of cranial nerve [CN] V_3)	Elevates hyoid bone
Stylohyoid	Styloid process of temporal bone	Hyoid bone	Cervical branch of facial nerve	Elevates and retracts hyoid bone
Geniohyoid	Inferior mental spine of mandible	Hyoid bone	C1 via hypoglossal nerve	Elevates hyoid bone anterosuperiorly
Digastric (anterior belly)	Digastric fossa of mandible	Intermediate tendon to hyoid bone	Mylohyoid nerve	Depresses mandible; raises and stabilizes hyoid bone
Digastric (posterior belly)	Mastoid notch of temporal bone		Facial nerve	

Muscles of the Floor of the Mouth—cont'd

Anteroinferior view

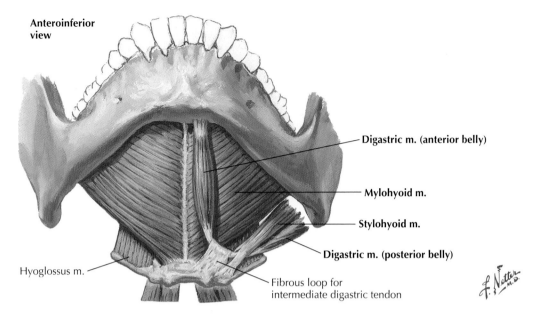

Digastric m. (anterior belly)

Mylohyoid m.

Stylohyoid m.

Digastric m. (posterior belly)

Hyoglossus m.

Fibrous loop for intermediate digastric tendon

Posterosuperior view

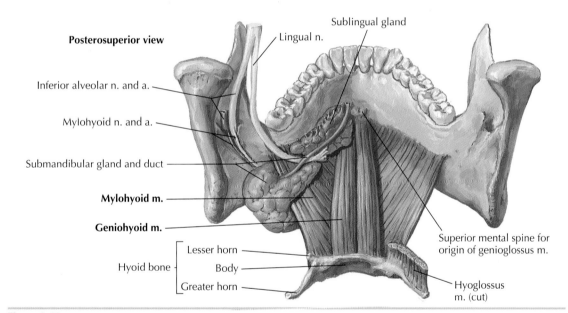

Sublingual gland

Lingual n.

Inferior alveolar n. and a.

Mylohyoid n. and a.

Submandibular gland and duct

Mylohyoid m.

Geniohyoid m.

Hyoid bone — Lesser horn, Body, Greater horn

Superior mental spine for origin of genioglossus m.

Hyoglossus m. (cut)

Figure 2-10
Floor of mouth, anteroinferior and posterosuperior views.

Mandibular Nerve

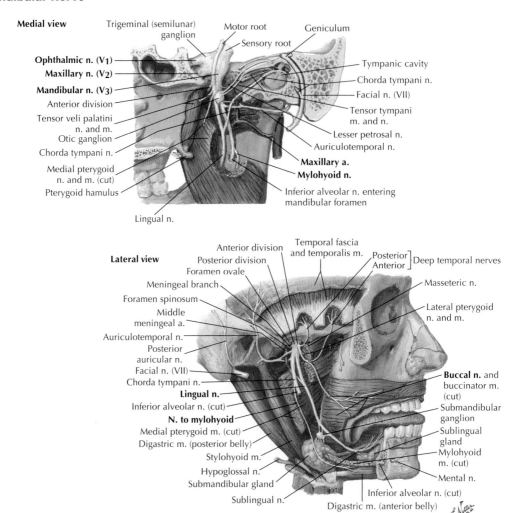

Figure 2-11
Mandibular nerve, medial and lateral views.

Nerves	Segmental Levels	Sensory	Motor
Mandibular	CN V$_3$	Skin of inferior third of face	Temporalis, masseter, lateral pterygoid, medial pterygoid, digastric, mylohyoid
Nerve to mylohyoid	CN V$_3$	No sensory	Mylohyoid
Buccal	CN V$_3$	Cheek lining and gingiva	No motor
Lingual	CN V$_3$	Anterior tongue and floor of mouth	No motor
Maxillary	CN V$_2$	Skin of middle third of face	No motor
Ophthalmic	CN V$_1$	Skin of superior third of face	No motor

CN V, trigeminal nerve.

Patient Reports	Initial Hypothesis
Patient reports jaw crepitus and pain during mouth opening and closing. Might also report limited opening with translation of the jaw to the affected side at the end range of opening	Possible osteoarthrosis Possible capsulitis Possible internal derangement consisting of an anterior disc displacement that does not reduce[1-3]
Patient reports jaw clicking and pain during opening and closing of the mouth	Possible internal derangement consisting of anterior disc displacement with reduction[1,4,5]
Patient reports limited motion to about 20 mm with no joint noise	Possible capsulitis Possible internal derangement consisting of an anterior disc displacement that does not reduce[1]

The Association of Oral Habits with Temporomandibular Disorders

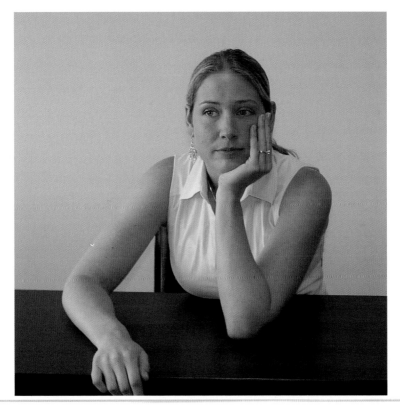

Figure 2-12
Frequent leaning of head on the palm.

Gavish and colleagues[6] investigated the association of oral habits with signs and symptoms of TMDs in 248 randomly selected female high school students. Although sensitivity and specificity were not reported, the results demonstrated that chewing gum, jaw play (nonfunctional jaw movements), chewing ice, and frequent leaning of the head on the palm were associated with the presence of TMJ disorders.

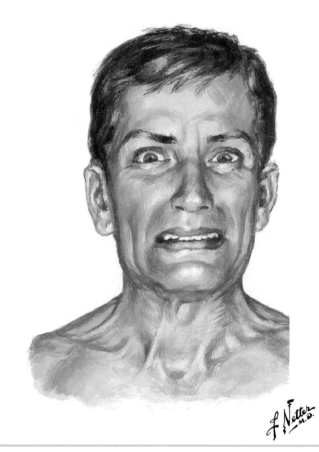

Figure 2-13
Temporomandibular joint pain.

Historical Finding and Study Quality	Description and Positive Findings	Population	Test-Retest Reliability
Visual analog scale (VAS)[7] ●	A 100-mm line, with ends defined as "no pain" and "worst pain imaginable"		$\kappa = .38$
Numerical scale[7] ●	An 11-point scale, with 0 indicating "no pain" and 10 representing "worst pain"	38 consecutive patients referred with TMD	$\kappa = .36$
Behavior rating scale[7] ●	A 6-point scale ranging from "minor discomfort" to "very strong discomfort"		$\kappa = .68$
Verbal scale[7] ●	A 5-point scale ranging from "no pain" to "very severe pain"		$\kappa = .44$

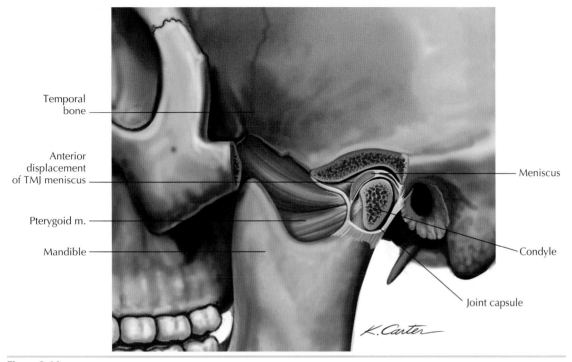

Figure 2-14
Anterior disc displacement.

Historical Finding and Study Quality	Description and Positive Findings	Population	Reference Standard	Sens	Spec	+LR	−LR
Clicking[8] ◖	Momentary snapping sound during opening or functioning			In presence of reducing disc			
				.82	.19	1.01	.95
				In presence of nonreducing disc			
				.86	.24	1.13	.58
Locking[8] ◖	Sudden onset of restricted movement during opening or closing	70 patients (90 TMJs) referred with complaints of craniomandibular pain	Anterior disc displacement via MRI	In presence of reducing disc			
				.53	.22	.68	2.14
				In presence of nonreducing disc			
				.86	.52	1.79	.27
Restriction after clicking[8] ◖	Inability to open as wide as was previously possible after clicking			In presence of reducing disc			
				.26	.40	.43	1.85
				In presence of nonreducing disc			
				.66	.74	2.54	.46

Continued

Historical Finding and Study Quality	Description and Positive Findings	Population	Reference Standard	Sens	Spec	+LR	−LR
Periodic restriction[8] ●	Periodic inability to open as wide as was previously possible			In presence of reducing disc			
				.60	.90	6.0	.44
				In presence of nonreducing disc			
				.12	.95	2.4	.93
Continuous restriction[8] ●	Continuous inability to open as wide as was previously possible			In presence of reducing disc			
				.35	.26	.47	2.5
				In presence of nonreducing disc			
				.78	.62	2.05	.35
Function related to joint pain[8] ●				In presence of reducing disc			
				.82	.10	.91	1.8
				In presence of nonreducing disc			
				.96	.24	1.26	.17
Complaint of clicking[8] ●				In presence of reducing disc			
				.28	.24	.37	3.00
				In presence of nonreducing disc			
				.82	.69	2.65	.26
Complaint of movement-related pain[8] ●	Not reported			In presence of reducing disc			
				.71	.31	1.03	.94
				In presence of nonreducing disc			
				.74	.36	1.16	.72
Complaint of severe restriction[8] ●				In presence of reducing disc			
				.60	.65	1.71	.62
				In presence of nonreducing disc			
				.38	.93	5.43	.67

Reliability of Self-Reported Temporomandibular Pain

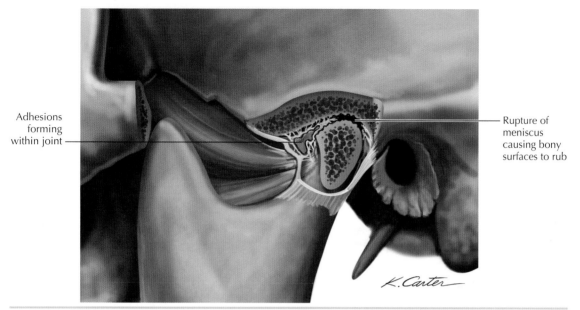

Adhesions forming within joint

Rupture of meniscus causing bony surfaces to rub

Figure 2-15
Temporomandibular arthrosis.

Historical Finding and Study Quality	Description and Positive Findings	Population	Reliability
TMD pain screening questionnaire[10] ●	See diagnostic table on following page. Participants were asked same questions 2 to 7 days apart	549 participants: 212 with pain-related TMD, 116 with TMD, 80 with odontalgia, 45 with headache without TMD pain, and 96 healthy controls	ICC − .83
Self-report of TMJ pain[9] ●	See diagnostic table on following page. Participants were asked same questions 2 weeks apart	120 adolescents: 60 with self-reported TMJ pain and 60 age- and sex-matched controls	Test-retest κ = .83 (.74, .93)

Diagnostic Utility of Self-Reported Temporomandibular Pain

Historical Finding and Study Quality	Description and Positive Findings	Population	Reference Standard	Sens	Spec	+LR	−LR

TMD pain screening questionnaire[10] ◆	Participants were asked:
	(1) "In the last 30 days, on average, how long did any pain in your jaw or temple area on either side last?"
	  (a) There was no pain
	  (b) Pain lasted from a very brief time to more than a week, but it did stop
	  (c) Pain was continuous
	(2) "In the last 30 days, have you had pain or stiffness in your jaw on awakening?"
	  (a) No
	  (b) Yes
	(3) "In the last 30 days, did […] chewing hard or tough food […] change any pain (i.e., make it better or make it worse) in your jaw or temple area on either side?"
	  (a) No
	  (b) Yes
	An (a) response received 0 points, a (b) response received 1 point, and a (c) response received 2 points.
	The test was positive for scores of 2 or higher
		549 participants: 212 with pain-related TMD, 116 with TMJ disorder, 80 with odontalgia, 45 with headache without TMD pain, and 96 healthy controls	RDC/TMD assessment protocol	.99	.97	33.0	.01

Self-report of TMJ pain[9] ●	Participants were asked: (1) "Do you have pain in your temple, face, TMJ, or jaw once a week or more?" (2) "Do you have pain when you open your mouth wide or chew once a week or more?" If answer was "yes" to either question, test was positive	120 adolescents: 60 with self-reported TMJ pain and 60 age- and sex-matched controls	RDC/TMD diagnosis of myofascial pain or arthralgia, arthritis, and arthrosis	.98	.90	9.8 (4.8, 20.0)	.02 (.00, .16)

RDC/TMD, Research Diagnostic Criteria for Temporomandibular Disorders
diagnostic accuracy statistics reported for participants with pain-related TMD versus healthy controls.

The Diagnostic Criteria for Temporomandibular Disorders (DC/TMD) provides evidence-based criteria for assessing patients with TMD. It superseded the Research Diagnostic Criteria for Temporomandibular Disorders (RDC/TMD) as of 2014 and is intended for immediate implementation in both clinical and research settings.[11] All tools required for clinical implementation are available at the International RDC-TMD Consortium website (www.rdc-tmdinternational.org/, accessed February 2015). A summary of the DC/TMD is presented here along with the associated reliability and diagnostic utility statistics. However, because the sources of the statistical estimates were not always clear, we were unable to assess the quality of the studies that provided the reliability and diagnostic utility values. The previous version of RDC/TMD showed fair to moderate agreement for most diagnoses and no to slight agreement for some diagnoses.

Diagnosis	History	Examination	Interexaminer Reliability	Sens	Spec	+LR	−LR
Myalgia	Positive for both: 1. Pain in jaw, temple, ear, front of ear 2. Pain modified with jaw movement, function, or parafunction	Positive for both: 1. Confirmation of pain in temporalis or masseter muscle 2. Report of familiar pain with one or more of following: (a) Palpation of temporalis muscle; (b) Palpation of masseter muscle; (c) Maximum unassisted or assisted opening movement	κ = .94 (.83, 1.00)	.90	.99	90.0	.10
Local myalgia	Positive for both: 1. Pain in jaw, temple, ear, or front of ear 2. Pain modified with jaw movement, function, or parafunction	Positive for all: 1. Confirmation of pain in temporalis or masseter muscle 2. Report of familiar pain with palpation of temporalis or masseter muscle 3. Report of pain localized to site of palpation	Not reported	Not established	Not established	Not established	Not established
Myofascial pain	Positive for both: 1. Pain in jaw, temple, ear, or front of ear 2. Pain modified with jaw movement, function, or parafunction	Positive for all: 1. Confirmation of pain in temporalis or masseter muscle 2. Report of familiar pain with palpation of temporalis or masseter muscle 3. Report of pain spreading beyond site of palpation but within boundary of muscle	Not reported	Not established	Not established	Not established	Not established

Continued

Diagnosis	History	Examination	Interexaminer Reliability	Sens	Spec	+LR	−LR
Myofascial pain with referral	Positive for both: 1. Pain in jaw, temple, ear, or front of ear 2. Pain modified with jaw movement, function, or parafunction	Positive for all: 1. Confirmation of pain in temporalis or masseter muscle 2. Report of familiar pain with palpation of temporalis or masseter muscle 3. Report of pain at site beyond boundary of muscle palpated	$\kappa = .85$ (.55, 1.00)	.86	.98	43.0	.14
Arthralgia	Positive for both: 1. Pain in jaw, temple, ear, or front of ear 2. Pain modified with jaw movement, function, or parafunction	Positive for both: 1. Confirmation of pain in area of TMJ 2. Report of familiar pain in TMJ with at least one of the following provocation tests: (a) Palpation of lateral pole or around lateral pole (b) Maximum unassisted or assisted opening, right or left lateral, or protrusive movement	$\kappa = .86$ (.75, .97)	.89	.98	44.5	.11
Headache attributed to TMD	Positive for both: 1. Headache of any type in temple 2. Headache modified with jaw movement, function, or parafunction	Positive for both: 1. Confirmation of headache in area of temporalis muscle 2. Report of familiar headache in temple with at least one of the following provocation tests: (a) Palpation of temporalis muscle (b) Maximum unassisted or assisted opening, right or left lateral, or protrusive movement	Not reported	.89	.87	6.85	.13

Note: Reliability and validity are derived from the datasets of the Validation Project and TMJ Impact Project Finalization of DC/TMD.[11]

Diagnosis	History	Examination	Interexaminer Reliability	Sens	Spec	+LR	−LR
Disc displacement with reduction	Positive for at least one: 1. In last 30 days, any TMJ noise present with jaw movement or function 2. Patient reports any noise present during examination	Positive for at least one: 1. Clicking, popping, and/or snapping noise during both opening and closing movements, detected with palpation during at least one of three repetitions of jaw opening and closing movements 2. Clicking, popping, and/or snapping noise detected with palpation during at least one of three repetitions of opening or closing movements AND right or left lateral or protrusive movement(s)	κ = .58 (.33, .84)	.34	.92	4.25	.72
Disc displacement with reduction with intermittent locking	Positive for both: 1. In last 30 days, any TMJ noise with jaw movement or function or patient reports any noise present during examination 2. In last 30 days, jaw locks with limited mouth opening and then unlocks	Positive for at least one: 1. Clicking, popping, and/or snapping noise during both opening and closing movements, detected with palpation during at least one of three repetitions of jaw opening and closing movements 2. Clicking, popping, and/or snapping noise detected with palpation during at least one of three repetitions of opening or closing movements AND right or left lateral or protrusive movement	Not reported	.38	.98	19.0	.63

Continued

Temporomandibular Joint

2

Diagnosis	History	Examination	Interexaminer Reliability	Sens	Spec	+LR	−LR
Disc displacement without reduction with limited opening	Positive for both: 1. Jaw locked so that mouth would not open all the way 2. Limitation in jaw opening severe enough to limit jaw opening and interfere with ability to eat	Positive for the following: 1. Maximum assisted opening (passive stretch) movement, including vertical incisal overlap less than 40 mm	Not reported	.80	.97	26.7	.21
Disc displacement without reduction without limited opening	Positive for both of the following in the past: 1. Jaw locked so that mouth would not open all the way 2. Limitation in jaw opening severe enough to limit jaw opening and interfere with ability to eat	Positive for the following: 1. Maximum assisted opening (passive stretch) movement, including vertical incisal overlap of 40 mm or more	$\kappa = .84$ (.38, 1.00)	.54	.79	2.57	.58
Degenerative joint disease	Positive for at least one: 1. In last 30 days, any TMJ noise present with jaw movement or function 2. Patient reports any noise present during examination	Positive for the following: 1. Crepitus detected with palpation during at least one of the following: opening, closing, right or left lateral movement, or protrusive movement	$\kappa = .33$ (.01, .65)	.55	.61	1.41	.74
Subluxation	Positive for both: 1. In last 30 days, jaw locking or catching in a wide-open mouth position so could not close from wide-open position 2. Inability to close mouth from wide-open position without a self-maneuver	No examination findings required	Not reported	.98	1.00	Undefined	.02

Note: Reliability and validity are derived from the datasets of the Validation Project and TMJ Impact Project Finalization of DC/TMD.[11]

Reliability in Determining the Presence of Pain during Muscle Palpation

Finding and Study Quality	Description and Positive Findings	Population	Interexaminer Reliability
Masseter[12] ◆	Examiner palpates the origin, body, and insertion of the masseter muscle	27 TMD patients	κ (Right) = .78 (Left) = .56
Temporalis[12] ◆	Examiner palpates the origin, body, and insertion of the temporalis muscle		κ (Right) = .87 (Left) = .91
Tendon of temporalis[12] ◆	Examiner palpates the tendon of the temporalis muscle		κ (Right) = .53 (Left) = .48
Extraoral[13] ◉	Examiner palpates the temporalis, masseter, posterior cervical, and sternocleidomastoid muscles	64 healthy volunteers	κ = .91
Intraoral[13] ◉	Examiner palpates tendon of the temporalis, lateral pterygoid, and masseter muscles and body of the tongue		κ = .90
Masseter[14] ◉	Examiner palpates the midbelly of the masseter muscle	79 randomly selected patients referred to craniomandibular disorder department	κ = .33
Temporalis[14] ◉	Examiner palpates the midbelly of the temporalis muscle		κ = .42
Medial pterygoid[14] ◉	Examiner palpates the insertion of the medial pterygoid muscle		κ = .23
Masseter[15] ◉	Examiner palpates the superficial and deep portions of the masseter muscle	79 patients referred to TMD and orofacial pain department	κ = .33
Temporalis[15] ◉	Examiner palpates the anterior and posterior aspects of the temporalis muscle		κ = .42
Medial pterygoid[15] attachment ◉	Examiner palpates the medial pterygoid muscles extraorally		κ = .23

Reliability in Determining the Presence of Pain during Temporomandibular Joint Regional Palpation

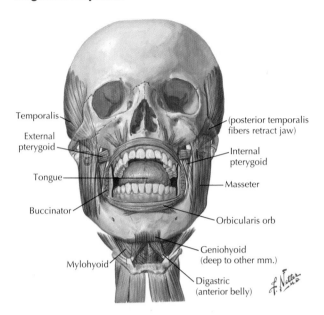

Temporalis
External pterygoid
Tongue
Buccinator
Mylohyoid
(posterior temporalis fibers retract jaw)
Internal pterygoid
Masseter
Orbicularis orb
Geniohyoid (deep to other mm.)
Digastric (anterior belly)

Figure 2-16
Musculature of the temporomandibular joint.

Finding and Study Quality	Description and Positive Findings	Population	Reliability
Retromandibular region[12] ◆			Interexaminer κ (Right) = .56 (Left) = .50
Submandibular region[12] ◆	Examiner palpation consistent with RDC/TMD guidelines	27 TMD patients	Interexaminer κ (Right) = .73 (Left) = .68
Lateral pterygoid area[12] ◆			Interexaminer κ (Right) = .50 (Left) = .37
Lateral pole and posterior attachment of TMJ[12] ◆			Interexaminer κ (Right) = .43 (Left) = .46
Lateral palpation[16] ●	Examiner palpates anterior to the ear over the TMJ	61 patients with TMJ pain	Intraexaminer κ = .53
Posterior palpation[14] ●	Examiner palpates TMJ through external meatus	61 patients with TMJ pain	Intraexaminer κ = .48
Palpation of TMJ[14] ●	Examiner palpates the lateral and dorsal aspects of the condyle	79 randomly selected patients referred to craniomandibular disorder department	Interexaminer κ = .33
Masseter[15] ●	Examiner palpates the superficial and deep portions of the masseter muscle		Interexaminer κ = .33
Palpation of TMJ[15] ●	Examiner palpates the lateral pole of the condyle in open and closed mouth positions. The dorsal pole is palpated posteriorly through the external auditory meatus	79 patients referred to TMD and orofacial pain department	Interexaminer κ = .33

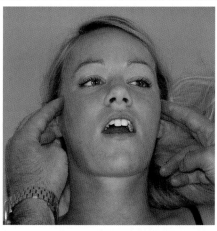

Lateral palpation of the temporomandibular joint

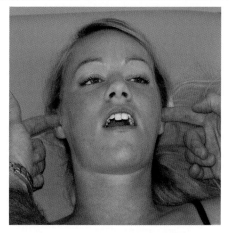

Posterior palpation of the temporomandibular joint through external auditory meatus

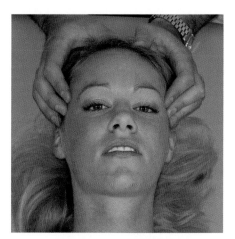

Palpation of the temporalis

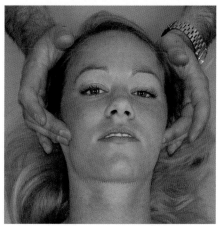

Palpation of the masseter

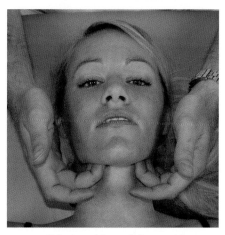

Palpation of the medial pterygoid

Figure 2-17
Palpation tests.

Diagnostic Utility of Palpation in Identifying Temporomandibular Conditions

Test and Study Quality	Description and Positive Findings	Population	Reference Standard	Sens	Spec	+LR	−LR
Lateral palpation[16] ◆	Examiner palpates the lateral pole of the condyle with the index finger. Positive if pain is present	61 patients with TMJ pain	Presence of TMJ effusion via MRI	.83	.69	2.68	.25
Posterior palpation[16] ◆	Examiner palpates the posterior portion of the condyle with the little finger in the patient's ear. Positive if pain is present			.85	.62	2.24	.24
Palpation[17] ◐	Palpation of lateral and posterior aspects of the TMJ and assessment of pain response with active movements. Positive if patient reports pain	84 patients with symptoms of TMJ pain	TMJ synovitis via arthroscopic investigation	.92	.21	1.16	.38
Palpation[18] ◐	Examiner palpates lateral and posterior aspects of the TMJ with one finger and determines the presence of tenderness	200 consecutive patients with TMJ disease	TMJ synovitis via arthroscopic investigation	.88	.36	1.38	.33
Tender joint on palpation[8] ◐	Examiner palpates the lateral and posterior aspects of the joint. Positive if pain is present	70 patients (90 TMJs) referred with complaints of craniomandibular pain	Detecting anterior disc displacement via MRI	In presence of reducing disc			
				.38	.41	.64	1.51
				In presence of nonreducing disc			
				.66	.67	2.0	.51
Palpation[19] ◐	Examiner palpates the TMJ laterally and posteriorly, the temporalis muscle, and the masseter muscle. Pain recorded via VAS using a cutoff value to maximize sensitivity and specificity	147 patients referred for craniomandibular complaints and 103 asymptomatic individuals	Patient report of tenderness in masticatory muscles, pre-auricular area, or TMJ in past month	.75	.67	2.27	.37
Palpation of temporalis muscle[20] ◐				Right side*			
				.60	.78	2.73	.51
				Left side*			
	Performed with index and middle fingers for 2 to 4 seconds with approximately 3 pounds of pressure on the muscle and 2 pounds of pressure on the joint. Pain recorded via VAS with cutoff values at 1 standard deviation from the mean*	40 patients diagnosed with TMD and 40 asymptomatic patients	TMD diagnosis from RCD/TMD evaluation	.70	.83	4.12	.36
Palpation of TMJ[20] ◐				Right side*			
				.68	.88	5.67	.36
				Left side*			
				.73	.85	4.87	.32
Palpation of masseter muscle[20] ◐				Right side*			
				.73	.85	4.87	.32
				Left side*			
				.73	.80	3.65	.34

*Gomes and colleagues[20] also calculated sensitivity and specificity for cutoff values of 1.5 and 2 standard deviations. Values showed almost perfect specificity but poor sensitivity.

Diagnostic Utility of Pressure Pain Thresholds in Identifying Temporomandibular Disorder

Test and Study Quality	Description and Positive Findings	Population	Reference Standard	Sens	Spec	+LR	−LR
PPT of temporalis muscle[20]	Used pressure algometer fitted with a rubber tip. PPT defined as lightest pressure to cause pain. Cutoff values represent 1 standard deviation from the mean*	40 patients diagnosed with TMD and 40 asymptomatic patients	TMD diagnosis from RCD/TMD evaluation	Right side			
				.68	.88	5.67	.36
				Left side			
				.63	.90	6.30	.41
PPT of TMJ[20]				Right side			
				.56	.95	11.20	.46
				Left side			
				.75	.95	15.00	.26
PPT of masseter muscle[20]				Right side			
				.75	.90	7.50	.28
				Left side			
				.78	.90	7.80	.24
PPT of anterior temporalis muscle[21]	Used pressure algometer pressed into relaxed muscle belly. PPT defined as lightest pressure to cause pain. Cutoff values chosen from receiver operator curve when specificity was .91	99 women with dental or intraarticular TMJ pain		.77	.91	8.37	.25
PPT of middle temporalis muscle[21]				.73	.91	7.93	.30
PPT of posterior temporalis muscle[21]				.67	.91	7.28	.36
PPT of masseter muscle[21]				.55	.91	5.98	.50

PPT, pressure pain threshold.

*Gomes and colleagues[20] also calculated sensitivity and specificity for cutoff values of 1.5 and 2 standard deviations. Values showed almost perfect specificity but poor sensitivity.

Temporomandibular Joint

2

Reliability of Detecting Joint Sounds during Active Motion

Test and Study Quality	Description and Positive Findings	Population	Reliability
TMJ sounds[12] ◆	Presence of joint noises is recorded by examiner during mouth opening	27 TMD patients	Interexaminer κ (Right) = .52 (Left) = .25
Click sounds during mouth opening[16] ◉	During mouth opening, examiner records the presence of a click sound	61 patients with TMJ pain	Intraexaminer κ = .12
Clicking during active maximal mouth opening[14] ◉	Intensity of clicking and crepitation is graded on a scale of 0 to 2 from "none" to "clearly audible"	79 randomly selected patients referred to craniomandibular disorder department	Interexaminer κ = .70
Joint noise[14] ◉	Presence of joint noises is recorded by examiner		Interexaminer κ = .24
Opening[15] ◉	Examiner records the presence of joint sounds during mandibular opening, lateral excursion to right and left, and protrusion	79 patients referred to TMD and orofacial pain department	Interexaminer κ = .59
Lateral excursion, right[15] ◉			Interexaminer κ = .57
Lateral excursion, left[15] ◉			Interexaminer κ = .50
Protrusion[15] ◉			Interexaminer κ = .47
Joint sounds during opening of the mouth[22] ◉	Identification of click or crepitus with palpation or auscultation during described motion	40 individuals with TMJ pain	Interexaminer κ Click (right): .94 Crepitus (right): .95 Click (left): .95 Crepitus (left): .83
Joint sounds during closing of the mouth[22] ◉			Interexaminer κ Click (right): .87 Crepitus (right): .93 Click (left): .88 Crepitus (left): .93
Joint sounds during protrusion of the mouth[22] ◉			Interexaminer κ Click (right): .66 Crepitus (right): .66 Click (left): .81 Crepitus (left): .78
Joint sounds during laterotrusion right[22] ◉			Interexaminer κ Click (right): .87 Crepitus (right): .59 Click (left): .92 Crepitus (left): 1.0
Joint sounds during laterotrusion left[22] ◉			Interexaminer κ Click (right): .47 Crepitus (right): .77 Click (left): .80 Crepitus (left): .88

Reliability of Detecting Joint Sounds during Joint Play

Test and Study Quality	Description and Positive Findings	Population	Reliability
Joint noise during joint play[14] ◐	Examiner records presence of joint noise during traction and translation	79 randomly selected patients referred to craniomandibular disorder department	Interexaminer $\kappa = -.01$
Traction, right[15] ◐	Examiner moves the mandibular condyle in an inferior direction for traction and in a mediolateral direction for translation. Examiner records presence of joint sound during translation and traction	79 patients referred to TMD and orofacial pain department	Interexaminer $\kappa = -.02$
Traction, left[15] ◐			Interexaminer $\kappa = .66$
Translation, right[15] ◐			Interexaminer $\kappa = .07$
Translation, left[15] ◐			Interexaminer $\kappa = -.02$

Temporomandibular Joint

Diagnostic Utility of Clicking in Identifying Temporomandibular Conditions

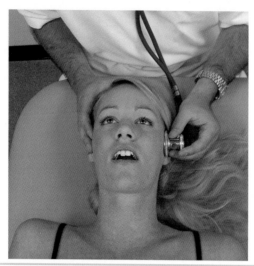

Figure 2-18
Auscultation performed with a stethoscope.

Test and Study Quality	Description and Positive Findings	Population	Reference Standard	Sens	Spec	+LR	−LR
Clicking[23] ◆	Examiner palpated and auscultated TMJs. Positive defined as reciprocal click occurring during opening and closing movements and elimination for TMJ clicking on protrusive opening and closing movements	53 patients referred to an oral clinic (105 TMJs)	Anterior disc displacement *with* reduction via MRI	.38	.81	2.0	.76
Clicking[3] ◆	Examiner palpates the lateral aspect of the TMJ during opening and closing. Examiner records audible, palpable clicking	146 patients attending TMJ and craniofacial pain clinic	Anterior disc displacement *with* reduction via MRI	.51	.83	3.0	.59
Clicking[16] ◆	Examiner auscultates for sounds during joint movement. Presence of a click sound is considered positive	61 patients with TMJ pain	Presence of TMJ effusion via MRI	.69	.51	1.41	.61
Reproducible clicking[8] ●	Auscultation with a stethoscope. Considered positive if observed at least four times during five repetitions of mouth opening	70 patients (90 TMJs) referred with complaints of craniomandibular pain	Detecting anterior disc displacement via MRI	In presence of reducing disc			
				.10	.40	.17	2.25
				In presence of nonreducing disc			
				.71	.90	7.10	.32
Reciprocal clicking[8] ● (see Video 2-1)	Auscultation with a stethoscope. Considered positive if a click on opening is followed by a click on closing			In presence of reducing disc			
				.40	.52	.83	1.15
				In presence of nonreducing disc			
				.76	.95	15.2	.25

Diagnostic Utility of Crepitus in Identifying Temporomandibular Conditions

Test and Study Quality	Description and Positive Findings	Population	Reference Standard	Sens	Spec	+LR	−LR
Presence of crepitus[16] ◆	Examiner auscultates for sounds during joint movement. Presence of grating or grinding noise is considered positive	61 patients with TMJ pain	Presence of TMJ effusion via MRI	.85	.30	1.21	.50
Presence of crepitus[17] ◐	Osteoarthritis based on presence of crepitus during auscultation. Presence of crepitus is considered positive	84 patients with symptoms of TMJ pain	TMJ osteoarthritis via arthroscopic investigation	.70	.43	1.23	.70
Presence of crepitus[18] ◐	Auscultation performed with stethoscope. Presence of crepitus is considered positive	200 consecutive patients with TMJ disease	TMJ osteoarthritis via arthroscopic investigation	Minor osteoarthritis[#]			
				.45	.84	2.81	.65
				Severe osteoarthritis[#]			
				.67	.86	4.79	.38
Joint sound test right[22] ◐	Crepitus sound while opening the mouth	35 patients with 53 painful TMJs	Disc dislocation without reduction confirmed via MRI	.71	.77	2.97	.38*
Joint sound test left[22] ◐				.63	.76	2.63	.49*

[#]Minor osteoarthritis is defined as the presence of smooth, glossy white surfaces of the disc and fibrocartilage. Severe osteoarthritis is defined as the presence of one or more of the following features: (1) pronounced fibrillation of the articular cartilage and disc; (2) exposure of subchondral bone; and (3) disc perforation.
*Values were calculated by the authors of this text.

Temporomandibular Joint

2

Reliability of Range-of-Motion Measurements of the Temporomandibular Joint during Mouth Opening

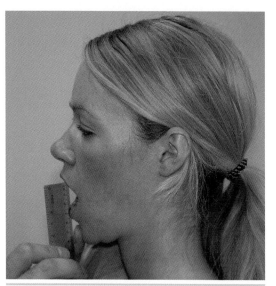

Figure 2-19
Measurement of mouth opening active range of motion.

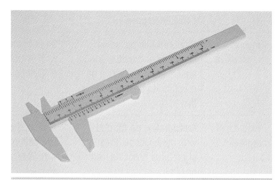

Figure 2-20
Plastic vernier caliper used to measure mandibular position.

Test and Study Quality		Description and Positive Findings	Population	Reliability
Opening[25] ◆	Without TMJ disorder	Patient is instructed to open mouth as much as possible without causing pain. Interincisal distance is measured to the nearest millimeter with a plastic ruler	15 subjects with TMJ disorder and 15 subjects without this disorder	Interexaminer ICC = .98 Intraexaminer ICC = .77 to .89
	With TMJ disorder			Interexaminer ICC = .99 Intraexaminer ICC = .94
Unassisted opening without pain[12] ◆			27 TMD patients	Interexaminer ICC = .83
Maximum unassisted opening[12] ◆				Interexaminer ICC = .89
Maximum assisted opening[12] ◆				Interexaminer ICC = .93
Unassisted opening without pain[26] ●	In older adults	Measured in millimeters with ruler consistent with RMC/TMD guidelines	43 asymptomatic older adults (age 68 to 96 years) and 44 asymptomatic young adults (age 18 to 45 years)	Interexaminer ICC = .88 (.78, .94)
	In young adults			Interexaminer ICC = .91 (.83, .95)
Maximum unassisted opening[26] ●	In older adults			Interexaminer ICC = .95 (.91, .97)
	In young adults			Interexaminer ICC = .98 (.96, .99)
Maximum assisted opening[26] ●	In older adults			Interexaminer ICC = .96 (.92, .98)
	In young adults			Interexaminer ICC = .98 (.96, .99)

Reliability of Range-of-Motion Measurements of the Temporomandibular Joint

Test and Study Quality		Description and Positive Findings	Population	Reliability
Overbite[25] ◆	Without TMJ disorder	A horizontal line is made on the lower incisor at the level of the upper incisor with the TMJ closed. The vertical distance between the line, and the superior aspect of the lower incisor is measured		Interexaminer ICC = .98 Intraexaminer ICC = .90 to .96
	With TMJ disorder			Interexaminer ICC = .95 Intraexaminer ICC = .90 to .97
Excursion, left[25] ◆	Without TMJ disorder			Interexaminer ICC = .95 Intraexaminer ICC = .91 to .92
	With TMJ disorder	Vertical marks are made in the median plane on the anterior surface of the lower central incisors in relationship to the upper central incisors. Patient is instructed to move the jaw as far lateral as possible, and the measurement is recorded		Interexaminer ICC = .94 Intraexaminer ICC = .85 to .92
Excursion, right[25] ◆	Without TMJ disorder		15 subjects with TMJ disorder and 15 subjects without TMJ disorder	Interexaminer ICC = .90 Intraexaminer ICC = .70 to .87
	With TMJ disorder			Interexaminer ICC = .96 Intraexaminer ICC = .75 to .82
Protrusion[25] ◆	Without TMJ disorder	Two vertical lines are made on the first upper and lower canine incisors. Subject is instructed to move the jaw as far forward as possible, and a measurement is made between the two marks		Interexaminer ICC = .95 Intraexaminer ICC = .85 to .93
	With TMJ disorder			Interexaminer ICC = .98 Intraexaminer ICC = .89 to .93
Overjet[25] ◆	Without TMJ disorder	The horizontal distance between the upper and lower incisors is measured when the mouth is closed		Interexaminer ICC = 1.0 Intraexaminer ICC = .98
	With TMJ disorder			Interexaminer ICC = .99 Intraexaminer ICC = .98 to .99
Lateral excursion, right[12] ◆				Interexaminer ICC = .41
Lateral excursion, left[12] ◆			27 TMD patients	Interexaminer ICC = .40
Horizontal overbite[12] ◆				Interexaminer ICC = .79
Vertical overlap[12] ◆				Interexaminer ICC = .70
Maximum laterotrusion[26] ◉	In older adults	Measured in millimeters with ruler consistent with RMC/TMD guidelines	43 older as-ymptomatic adults (age 68 to 96 years) and 44 young asymptomatic adults (age 18 to 45 years)	Interexaminer ICC = .71 (.45, .84)
	In young adults			Interexaminer ICC = .77 (.57, .88)
Maximum protrusion[26] ◉	In older adults			Interexaminer ICC = .78 (.59, .88)
	In young adults			Interexaminer ICC = .90 (.81, .95)

Temporomandibular Joint

2

Reliability of Range-of-Motion Measurements of the Temporomandibular Joint—cont'd

Test and Study Quality	Description and Positive Findings	Population	Reliability
Opening[27]	A plastic vernier caliper was used to measure mandibular position	30 healthy subjects	Interexaminer ICC = .95 Intraexaminer ICC = .97
Protrusion[27]			Interexaminer ICC = .77 Intraexaminer ICC = .95
Laterotrusion right[27]			Interexaminer ICC = .50 Intraexaminer ICC = .90
Laterotrusion left[27]			Interexaminer ICC = .42 Intraexaminer ICC = .92
Overbite[27]			Interexaminer ICC = .70 Intraexaminer ICC = .93
Overjet[27]			Interexaminer ICC = .70 Intraexaminer ICC = .96
Joint mobility[22]	The examiner palpates mandibular condyles during active motion. Reduction in mobility of one condyle during mandibular depression is considered positive	40 individuals with TMJ pain	Interexaminer κ Right: .54 Left: .55

Reliability of Joint Play and End-Feel Assessment of the Temporomandibular Joint

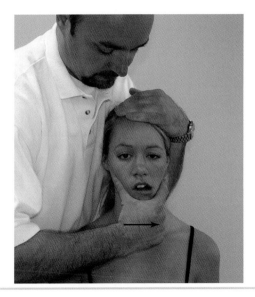

Figure 2-21
Translation of mandible, left.

Test and Study Quality		Description and Positive Findings	Population	Reliability
Traction and translation[14]	Restriction of movement	Examinor records the presence of restriction of movement at end feel during traction and translation of the TMJ	79 randomly selected patients referred to craniomandibular disorder department	Interexaminer κ = .08
	End feel			Interexaminer κ = .07
Traction, right[15]	Joint play			Interexaminer κ = −.03
	End feel			Interexaminer κ = −.05
Traction, left[15]	Joint play	Examiner moves the mandibular condyle in an inferior direction for traction and a mediolateral direction for translation. The extent of joint play and end feel is graded as "normal" or "abnormal"	79 patients referred to TMD and orofacial pain department	Interexaminer κ = .08
	End feel			Interexaminer κ = .20
Translation, right[15]	Joint play			Interexaminer κ = −.05
	End feel			Interexaminer κ = −.05
Translation, left[15]	Joint play			Interexaminer κ = −.10
	End feel			Interexaminer κ = −.13

Diagnostic Utility of Limited Range of Motion in Identifying Anterior Disc Displacement

Test and Study Quality	Description and Positive Findings	Population	Reference Standard	Sens	Spec	+LR	−LR
Restriction of condylar trans-lation[3] ◆	Examiner asks patient to maximally open mouth while palpating condylar movement. Examiner records any limitation of condylar translation	146 patients attending TMJ and craniofacial pain clinic	Anterior disc displacement *without* reduction via MRI	.69	.81	3.63	.38
Restriction of range of functional opening[3] ◆	Examiner asks patient to maximally open mouth and measures the distance in millimeters. Less than 40 mm is considered a restriction			.32	.83	1.88	.82
Restriction of range of functional opening[8] ◉	Measurement is taken at the end range of active mouth opening. Definition of positive not reported	70 patients (90 TMJs) referred with complaints of cranio-mandibular pain	Anterior disc displacement via MRI	In presence of reducing disc			
				.38	.21	.48	2.95
				In presence of nonreducing disc			
				.86	.62	2.26	.23
Restriction of range of pas-sive opening[8] ◉	Measurement is taken at the end range of passive mouth opening after 15 seconds. Definition of positive not reported			In presence of reducing disc			
				.29	.29	.41	2.45
				In presence of nonreducing disc			
				.76	.69	2.45	.35
Restricted translation[8] ◉	Not reported			In presence of reducing disc			
				.15	.38	.24	2.24
				In presence of nonreducing disc			
				.66	.81	3.47	.42
Restricted protrusion[8] ◉	Measurement is taken at the end range of active mandibular protrusion. Definition of positive not reported			In presence of reducing disc			
				.29	.38	.47	1.87
				In presence of nonreducing disc			
				.62	.64	1.72	.59
Restricted contralateral movement[8] ◉	Measurement is taken at the end of contralateral movement from the midline. Definition of positive not reported			In presence of reducing disc			
				.15	.34	.23	2.50
				In presence of nonreducing disc			
				.66	.76	2.75	.45
Laterotrusion test right[24] ◉	Reduced range of motion to the opposite side	35 patients with 53 painful TMJs	Diagnosis of disc dislocation that does not reduce via MRI	.71	.59	1.73	.43*
Laterotrusion test left[24] ◉				.38	.52	.79	1.2*

*Values were calculated by the authors of this text.

Diagnostic Utility of Deviations in Movement in Identifying Anterior Disc Displacement

Test and Study Quality	Description and Positive Findings	Population	Reference Standard	Sens	Spec	+LR	−LR
Deviation of mandible[3] ◆	Patient is asked to maximally open the mouth. If the midline of the upper and lower incisors does not line up, then the test is considered positive	146 patients attending TMJ and craniofacial pain clinic	Anterior disc displacement *without* reduction via MRI	.32	.87	2.46	.78
Deviation test right[24] ◐	The jaw moves ipsilateral while moving mouth	35 patients with 53 painful TMJs	Diagnosis of disc dislocation that does not reduce via MRI	.57	.77	2.48	.56*
Deviation test left[24] ◐				.63	.71	2.17	.52*
Deviation of mandible with correction[8] ◐	Examiner observes active mouth opening. Test is considered positive if a deviation occurs and the mandible returns to midline	70 patients (90 TMJs) referred with complaints of craniomandibular pain	Anterior disc displacement via MRI	In presence of reducing disc			
				.14	.57	.33	1.51
				In presence of nonreducing disc			
				.44	.83	2.59	.67
Deviation of mandible without correction[8] ◐	Examiner observes active mouth opening. Test is considered positive if the mandible does not return to midline after deviation			In presence of reducing disc			
				.18	.41	.31	2.0
				In presence of nonreducing disc			
				.66	.83	3.88	.41

*Values were calculated by the authors of this text.

Temporomandibular Joint

2

Reliability of Determining the Presence of Pain during Dynamic Movements

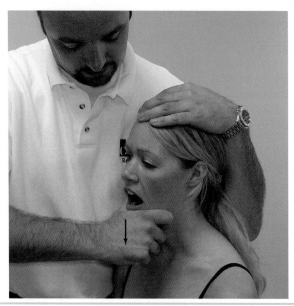

Figure 2-22
Assessment of pain during passive opening.

Test and Study Quality	Description and Positive Findings	Population	Reliability
Mandibular movements[16]	Patient is asked if pain is felt during opening, closing, lateral excursion, protrusion, and retrusion	61 patients with TMJ pain	Intraexaminer κ = .43
Maximum assisted opening[16]	Examiner applies overpressure to the end range of mandibular depression		Intraexaminer κ = −.05
Pain on opening[15]	Patient is asked to maximally open mouth	79 patients referred to TMD and orofacial pain department	Interexaminer κ = .28
Pain on lateral excursion, right[15]	Patient is asked to move the mandible in a lateral direction as far as possible		Interexaminer κ = .28
Pain on lateral excursion, left[15]			Interexaminer κ = .28
Pain on protrusion[15]	Patient is asked to actively protrude the jaw		Interexaminer κ = .36
Passive opening[14]	At the end of active opening the examiner applies a passive stretch to increase mouth opening	79 randomly selected patients referred to cranio-mandibular disorder department	Interexaminer κ = .34
Active opening[14]	Patient is asked to open mouth as wide as possible		Interexaminer κ = .32
Pain on mouth opening[22]	Pain with movement	40 patients with TMJ pain	Interexaminer κ Right: .79 Left: .89
Pain on protrusion[22]			Interexaminer κ Right: .44 Left: .57
Pain on right laterotrusion[22]			Interexaminer κ Right: .75 Left: .60
Pain on left laterotrusion[22]			Interexaminer κ Right: .64 Left: .71

Reliability of Detecting Pain during Resistance Tests

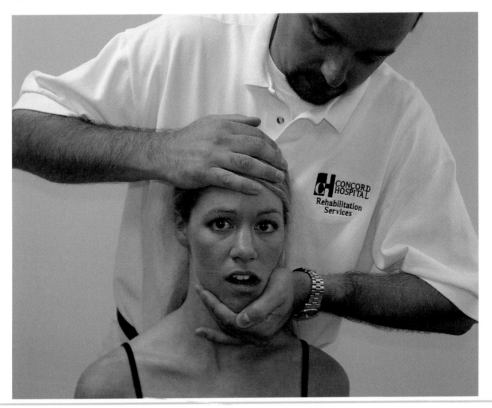

Figure 2-23
Manual resistance applied during lateral deviation.

Test and Study Quality	Description and Positive Findings	Population	Reliability
Dynamic tests[16] ◐	Patient performs opening, closing, lateral excursion, protrusion, and retrusion movements while examiner applies resistance	61 patients with TMJ pain	Intraexaminer $\kappa = .20$
Opening[15] ◐	Examiner applies isometric resistance during opening, closing, and lateral excursions to the right and left of the TMJ. The presence of pain is recorded	79 patients referred to TMD and orofacial pain department	Interexaminer $\kappa = .24$
Closing[15] ◐			Interexaminer $\kappa = .30$
Lateral excursion, right[15] ◐			Interexaminer $\kappa = .28$
Lateral excursion, left[15] ◐			Interexaminer $\kappa = .26$
Static pain test[14] ◐	The examiner applies resistance against the patient's mandible in upward, downward, and lateral directions	79 randomly selected patients referred to craniomandibular disorder department	Interexaminer $\kappa = .15$
Isometric test[22] ◐	Isometric resistance contra-lateral results in ipsilateral pain	40 patients with TMJ pain	Interexaminer κ Right = .78 Left = .75

Reliability of Determining the Presence of Pain during Joint Play

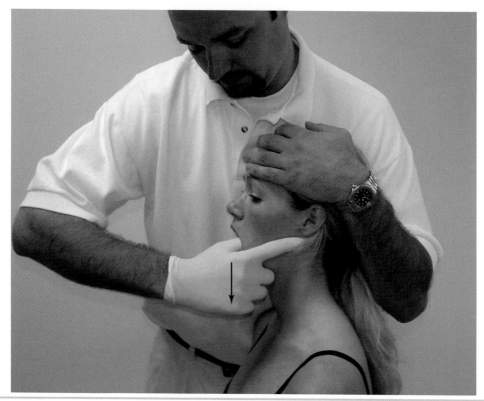

Figure 2-24
Temporomandibular traction.

Test and Study Quality	Description and Positive Findings	Population	Reliability
Traction, right[12] ◆	Examiner moves the mandibular condyle in an inferior direction for traction and a mediolateral direction for translation. The presence of pain is recorded	79 patients referred to TMD and orofacial pain department	Interexaminer ICC = −.08
Traction, left[12] ◆			Interexaminer ICC = .25
Translation, right ◆			Interexaminer ICC = .50
Translation, left[12] ◆			Interexaminer ICC = .28
Joint play test[13] ●	Examiner performs passive traction and translation movements	61 patients with TMJ pain	Intraexaminer ICC = .20
Joint play test[15] ●	Examiner applies a traction and a translation (mediolateral) force through the TMJ	79 randomly selected patients referred to craniomandibular disorder department	Interexaminer ICC = .46

Diagnostic Utility of Pain in Identifying Temporomandibular Conditions

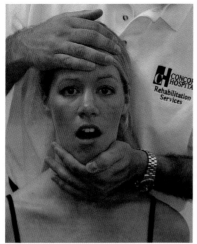 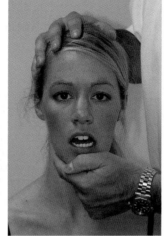

Mouth opening   Mouth closing

Figure 2-25
Manual resistance applied during mouth opening and closing.

Test and Study Quality	Description and Positive Findings	Population	Reference Standard	Sens	Spec	+LR	−LR
Pain during mandibular movements[16] ◆	Patient is asked to open, close, protrude, retrude, and perform lateral excursion of the mandible. Positive if pain present			.82	.61	2.10	.30
Pain during maximum opening and overpressure[16] ◆	Patient is asked to perform the movements above while examiner applies resistance. Positive if pain present	61 patients with TMJ pain	Presence of TMJ effusion via MRI	.93	.16	.95	4.38
Pain during dynamic tests[16] ◆	Patient is instructed to open the mouth as wide as possible, and examiner applies overpressure. Positive if pain present			.74	.44	1.32	.59
Pain during joint play[16] ◆	Examiner passively performs translation and traction of the TMJ. Positive if pain present			.80	.39	1.31	.51
TMJ pain during assisted opening[3] ◆ (see Video 2-2)	At the end of maximal mouth opening, examiner applies 2 to 3 pounds of overpressure. The presence or absence of pain is recorded	146 patients attending TMJ and craniofacial pain clinic	Anterior disc displacement *without* reduction via MRI	.55	.91	6.11	.49

Diagnostic Utility of Pain in Identifying Temporomandibular Conditions—cont'd

Test and Study Quality	Description and Positive Findings	Population	Reference Standard	Sens	Spec	+LR	−LR
Joint pain on opening[8] ◐	Patient is asked to open mouth as wide as possible. Positive if pain present	70 patients (90 TMJs) referred with complaints of cranio-mandibular pain	Anterior disc displacement via MRI	In presence of reducing disc			
				.44	.31	.64	1.81
				In presence of nonreducing disc			
				.74	.57	1.72	.46
Pain with contralateral motion[8] ◐	Patient is asked to perform lateral excursion contralateral to the side of joint involvement. Positive if pain present			In presence of reducing disc			
				.60	.69	1.94	.58
				In presence of nonreducing disc			
				.34	.93	4.86	.71
Dynamic/static[19] ◐	Manual resistance was applied during mouth opening, closing, protrusion, and lateral deviation. Pain was recorded via VAS using a cutoff value to maximize sensitivity and specificity	147 patients referred for cranio-mandibular complaints and 103 asymptomatic individuals	Patient report of tenderness in masticatory muscles, preauricular area, or temporomandibular area in past month	.63	.93	.90	.40
Active movements[19] ◐	Patient was asked to maximally depress mandible, protrude it, and deviate it right and left. Pain was recorded via VAS using a cutoff value to maximize sensitivity and specificity			.87	.67	2.64	.19
Passive movements[19] ◐	At the end of maximal mouth opening, examiner gently applied overpressure. Pain was recorded via VAS using a cutoff value to maximize sensitivity and specificity			.80	.64	2.22	.31
Isometric test right[24] ◐	Isometric resistance contralateral produces ipsilateral pain	35 patients with 53 painful TMJs	Diagnosis of disc dislocation that does not reduce via MRI	.57	.68	1.78	.63*
Isometric test left[24] ◐				.38	.62	1.0	1.0*
Joint provocation test right[24] ◐	Pain evoked by palpation of retrodiscal tissue			1.0	.27	1.36	0*
Joint provocation test left[24] ◐				1.0	.19	1.23	0*

*Values were calculated by the authors of this text.

Reliability of the Compression Test

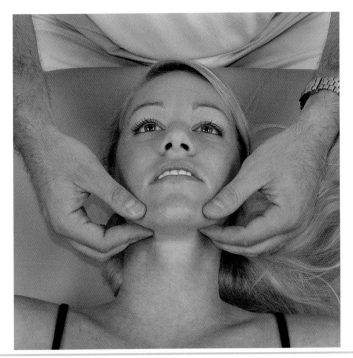

Figure 2-26
Bilateral temporomandibular compression.

Test and Study Quality		Description and Positive Findings	Population	Reliability
Compression, right[15]	Pain	The examiner loads the intraarticular structures by moving the mandible in a dorsocranial direction. The presence of pain and joint sounds are recorded	79 patients referred to TMD and orofacial pain department	Interexaminer κ = .19
	Sounds			Not reported
Compression, left[15]	Pain			Interexaminer κ = .47
	Sounds			Interexaminer κ = 1.0
Compression[13]	Pain		79 randomly selected patients referred to craniomandibular disorder department	Interexaminer κ = .40
	Joint noises			Interexaminer κ = .66

Temporomandibular Joint

2

Diagnostic Utility of Combined Tests for Detecting Anterior Disc Displacement with Reduction

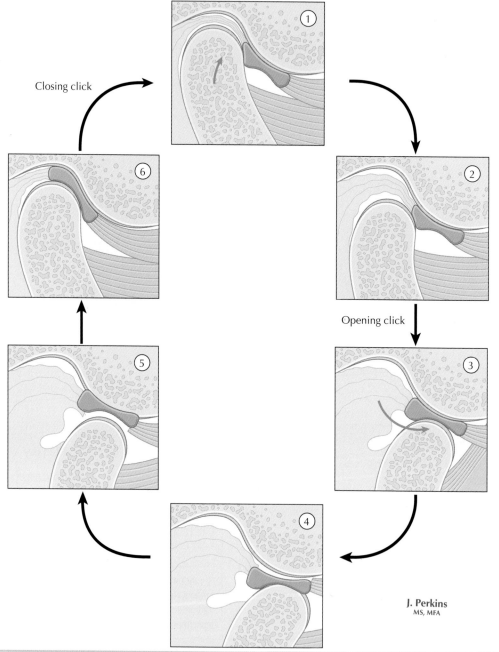

Figure 2-27
Anterior disc displacement with reduction.

Diagnostic Utility of Combined Tests for Detecting Anterior Disc Displacement with Reduction—cont'd

Test and Study Quality	Description and Positive Findings	Population	Reference Standard	Sens	Spec	+LR	−LR
No deviation of mandible; no pain during assisted opening[3] ◆				.76	.30	1.09	.80
No deviation of mandible; no limitation of opening[3] ◆				.76	.27	1.04	.89
No deviation of mandible; no restriction of condylar translation[3] ◆				.75	.37	1.19	.68
No deviation of mandible; clicking[3] ◆				.51	.85	3.40	.58
No deviation of mandible; no pain during opening; no limitation of opening[3] ◆	See previous descriptions under single test items	146 patients attending TMJ and craniofacial pain clinic	Anterior disc displacement with reduction via MRI	.71	.35	1.09	.83
No deviation of mandible; no pain during opening; no limitation of opening; no restriction of condylar translation[3] ◆				.68	.37	1.00	.86
No deviation of mandible; no pain during opening; no limitation of opening; no restriction of condylar translation; clicking[3] ◆				.44	.86	3.14	.65

Diagnostic Utility of Combined Tests for Detecting Anterior Disc Displacement without Reduction

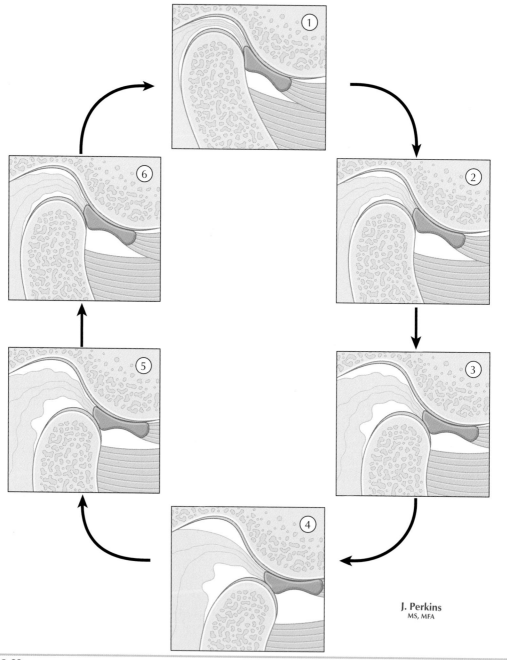

J. Perkins
MS, MFA

Figure 2-28
Anterior disc displacement without reduction.

Diagnostic Utility of Combined Tests for Detecting Anterior Disc Displacement without Reduction—cont'd

Test and Study Quality	Description and Positive Findings	Population	Reference Standard	Sens	Spec	+LR	−LR
Motion restriction; no clicking[3] ◆	See previous descriptions under single test items	146 patients attending TMJ and craniofacial pain clinic	Anterior disc displacement *without* reduction via MRI	.61	.82	3.39	.48
Motion restriction; pain during assisted opening[3] ◆				.54	.93	7.71	.49
Motion restriction; limitation of maximal mouth opening[3] ◆				.31	.87	2.38	.79
Motion restriction; deviation of mandible[3] ◆				.30	.90	3.0	.78
Motion restriction; no clicking, TMJ pain with assistive opening[3] ◆				.46	.94	7.67	.59
Motion restriction; no clicking; TMJ pain with assistive opening; limitation of maximum mouth opening[3] ◆				.22	.96	5.50	.81
Motion restriction; no clicking; TMJ pain with assistive opening; limitation of maximum mouth opening; deviation of mandible[3] ◆				.11	.98	5.5	.91
Clinical diagnosis using history and combined tests[28] ◆	Examination using Clinical Diagnostic Criteria for Temporomandibular Disorders (CDC/TMD)	69 patients referred with TMD	Anterior disc displacement *without* reduction via MRI	.75	.83	4.41	.3
Dental stick test right[24] ⊚ Dental stick test left[24] ⊚ Isometric test right[24] ⊚ Isometric test left[24] ⊚ Joint provocation test right[24] ⊚ Joint provocation test left[24] ⊚ Joint sound test right[24] ⊚ Joint sound test left[24] ⊚ Deviation test right[24] ⊚ Deviation test left[24] ⊚ Laterotrusion test right[24] ⊚ Laterotrusion test left[24] ⊚ Joint mobility right[24] ⊚ Joint mobility left[24] ⊚	See previous descriptions under single test items	35 patients with 53 painful TMJs	Anterior disc displacement without reduction via MRI	1 or more positive test	1.0	.09	1.1
				2 or more positive test	1.0	.27	1.37
				3 or more positive test	1.0	.55	2.22
				4 or more positive test	.71	.82	3.94
				5 or more positive test	.71	.91	7.89
				6 or more positive test	.43	.91	4.78
				7 or more positive test	.29	.95	5.8

2 Temporomandibular Joint

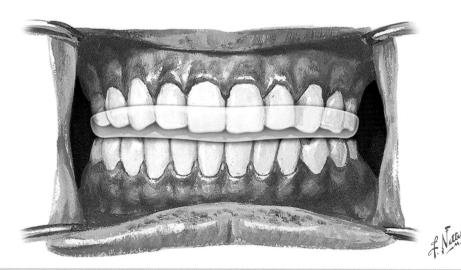

Figure 2-29
Occlusal stabilization splint.

Predicting Treatment Success with Nightly Wear of Occlusal Stabilization Splint

Test and Study Quality	Description and Positive Findings	Population	Reference Standard	Sens	Spec	+LR	−LR*
Time since pain[29] ◆	42 weeks or less			.62 (.49, .73)	.69 (.54, .80)	2.0 (1.3, 3.0)	.55
Baseline pain level[29] ◆	40 mm or more on VAS			.48 (.35, .60)	.72 (.57, .83)	1.7 (1.0, 2.7)	.72
Change in VAS level at 2 months[29] ◆	15 mm or more on VAS			.72 (.75, .93)	.91, (.64, .88)	3.9 (2.3, 6.5)	.31
Disc displacement without reduction[29] ◆	As observed on MRI	119 consecutive patients referred to TMD clinic diagnosed with unilateral TMJ arthralgia	Treatment success (more than 70% reduction in VAS) after 6 months with nightly wear of occlusal stabilization splint	.25 (.15, .37)	.91 (.79, .97)	2.7 (1.0, 6.8)	.82
Four positive tests[29] ◆	Four of the four findings listed above			.10 (.04, .20)	.99 (.90, 1.00)	10.8 (.62, 188.1)	.91
Three or more positive tests[29] ◆	Three or four of the four findings listed above			.23, (.14, .36)	.91 (.79, .97)	2.5 (.97, 6.4)	.85
Two or more positive tests[29] ◆	Two to four of the four findings listed above			.49 (.37, .62)	.85 (.72, .93)	3.3 (1.7, 6.6)	.60

VAS, visual analog scale.
*−LRs were not reported in the study and, therefore, were calculated by the authors of this book.

Predicting Treatment Failure with Nightly Wear of Occlusal Stabilization Splint

Test and Study Quality	Description and Positive Findings	Population	Reference Standard	Sens	Spec	+LR	−LR*
Time since pain[29] ◆	More than 43 weeks	119 consecutive patients referred to TMD clinic diagnosed with unilateral TMJ arthralgia	Treatment failure after 6 months with nightly wear of occlusal stabilization splint	.56 (.45, .67)	.65 (.47, .79)	1.68	.68 (.52, .89)
Baseline pain level[29] ◆	Less than 40 mm on VAS			.76 (.65, .84)	.68 (.50, .82)	2.38	.36 (.24, .54)
Change in VAS level at 2 months[29] ◆	9 mm or less on VAS			.82 (.71, .89)	.97 (.84, .99)	27.33	.19 (.12, .30)
Disc displacement with reduction[29] ◆	As observed on MRI			.10 (.05, .19)	.57 (.40, .73)	.23	1.59 (1.42, 1.78)
Four positive tests[29] ◆	Four of the four findings listed above			.96 (.67, 1.0)	.76 (.67, .84)	4.00	.05 (.00, .77)
Three or more positive tests[29] ◆	Three or four of the four findings listed above			.19 (.09, .36)	.96 (.89, .99)	4.75	.84 (.72, .98)
Two or more positive tests[29] ◆	Two to four of the four findings listed above			.38 (.23, .55)	.78 (.67, .86)	1.73	.80 (.62, 1.0)

VAS, visual analog scale.

*−LRs were not reported in the study and, therefore, were calculated by the authors of this book.

Outcome Measure	Scoring and Interpretation	Test-Retest Reliability	MCID
Mandibular Function Impairment Questionnaire (MFIQ)	Users rate perceived level of difficulty on a Likert scale ranging from 0 (no difficulty) to 4 (very great difficulty or impossible without help) on a series of 17 questions about jaw function. The sum item score for function impairment ranges from 0 to 68, with higher scores representing more disability	Spearman's r = .69 to .96[30,31]	14[30]
Numeric Pain Rating Scale (NPRS)	Users rate their level of pain on an 11-point scale ranging from 0 to 10, with high scores representing more pain. Often asked as current pain or least, worst, and average pain in the past 24 hours	ICC = .72[32]	2[33,34]

MCID, minimum clinically important difference.

1. Barclay P, Hollender LG, Maravilla KR, Truelove EL. Comparison of clinical and magnetic resonance imaging diagnosis in patients with disc displacement in the temporomandibular joint. *Oral Surg Oral Med Oral Pathol Oral Radiol Endod.* 1999;88:37–43.

2. Cholitgul W, Nishiyama H, Sasai T, et al. Clinical and magnetic resonance imaging findings in temporomandibular joint disc displacement. *Dentomaxillofac Radiol.* 1997;26:183–188.

3. Orsini MG, Kuboki T, Terada S, et al. Clinical predictability of temporomandibular joint disc displacement. *J Dent Res.* 1999;78:650–660.

4. Gross AR, Haines T, Thomson MA, et al. Diagnostic tests for temporomandibular disorders: an assessment of the methodologic quality of research reviews. *Man Ther.* 1996;1:250–257.

5. Haley DP, Schiffman EL, Lindgren BR, et al. The relationship between clinical and MRI findings in patients with unilateral temporomandibular joint pain. *J Am Dent Assoc.* 2001;132:476–481.

6. Gavish A, Halachmi M, Winocur E, Gazit E. Oral habits and their association with signs and symptoms of temporomandibular disorders in adolescent girls. *J Oral Rehabil.* 2000;27:22–32.

7. Magnusson T, List T, Helkimo M. Self-assessment of pain and discomfort in patients with temporomandibular disorders: a comparison of five different scales with respect to their precision and sensitivity as well as their capacity to register memory of pain and discomfort. *J Oral Rehabil.* 1995;22:549–556.

8. Stegenga B, de Bont LG, van der Kuijl B, Boering G. Classification of temporomandibular joint osteoarthrosis and internal derangement. 1. Diagnostic significance of clinical and radiographic symptoms and signs. *Cranio.* 1992;10:96–106. discussion 116-117.

9. Nilsson IM, List T, Drangsholt M. The reliability and validity of self-reported temporomandibular disorder pain in adolescents. *J Orofac Pain.* 2006;20:138–144.

10. Gonzalez YM, Schiffman E, Gordon SM, et al. Development of a brief and effective temporomandibular disorder pain screening questionnaire: reliability and validity. *J Am Dent Assoc.* 2011;142(10):1183–1191.

11. Schiffman E, Ohrbach R, Truelove E, et al. Diagnostic Criteria for Temporomandibular Disorders (DC/TMD) for clinical and research applications: recommendations of the International RDC/TMD Consortium Network and Orofacial Pain Special Interest Group. *J Oral Facial Pain Headache.* 2014;28(1):6–27.

12. Leher A, Graf K, PhoDuc JM, Rammelsberg P. Is there a difference in the reliable measurement of temporomandibular disorder signs between experienced and inexperienced examiners? *J Orofac Pain.* 2005;19:58–64.

13. Dworkin SF, LeResche L, DeRouen T, et al. Assessing clinical signs of temporomandibular disorders: reliability of clinical examiners. *J Prosthet Dent.* 1990;63:574–579.

14. Lobbezoo-Scholte AM, de Wijer A, Steenks MH, Bosman F. Interexaminer reliability of six orthopaedic tests in diagnostic subgroups of craniomandibular disorders. *J Oral Rehabil.* 1994;21:273–285.

15. de Wijer A, Lobbezoo-Scholte AM, Steenks MH, Bosman F. Reliability of clinical findings in temporomandibular disorders. *J Orofac Pain.* 1995;9:181–191.

16. Manfredini D, Tognini F, Zampa V, Bosco M. Predictive value of clinical findings for temporomandibular joint effusion. *Oral Surg Oral Med Oral Pathol Oral Radiol Endod.* 2003;96:521–526.

17. Israel HA, Diamond B, Saed-Nejad F, Ratcliffe A. Osteoarthritis and synovitis as major pathoses of the temporomandibular joint: comparison of clinical diagnosis with arthroscopic morphology. *J Oral Maxillofac Surg.* 1998;56:1023–1027. discussion 1028.

18. Holmlund AB, Axelsson S. Temporomandibular arthropathy: correlation between clinical signs and symptoms and arthroscopic findings. *Int J Oral Maxillofac Surg.* 1996;25:178–181.

19. Visscher CM, Lobbezoo F, de Boer W, et al. Clinical tests in distinguishing between persons with or without craniomandibular or cervical spinal pain complaints. *Eur J Oral Sci.* 2000;108:475–483.

20. Gomes MB, Guimaraes JP, Guimaraes FC, Neves AC. Palpation and pressure pain threshold: reliability and validity in patients with temporomandibular disorders. *Cranio.* 2008;26:202–210.

21. Silva RS, Conti PC, Lauris JR, et al. Pressure pain threshold in the detection of masticatory myofascial pain: an algometer-based study. *J Orofac Pain.* 2005;19:318–324.

22. Julsvoll EH, Vollestad NK, Opseth G, Robinson HS. Inter-tester reliability of selected clinical tests for long-standing temporomandibular disorders. *J Man Manip Ther.* 2017;25(4):182–189.

23. Marpaung CM, Kalaykova SI, Lobbezoo F, Naeije M. Validity of functional diagnostic examination for temporomandibular joint displacement with reduction. *J Oral Rehabil.* 2014;41:243–249.

24. Julsvoll EH, Vollestanbd NK, Robinson HS. Validation of clinical tests for patients with long standing painful temporomandibular disorders with anterior disc displacement without reduction. *Man Ther.* 2016;21:109–119.

25. Walker N, Bohannon RW, Cameron D. Discriminant validity of temporomandibular joint range of motion measurements obtained with a ruler. *J Orthop Sports Phys Ther.* 2000;30:484–492.

26. Hassel AJ, Rammelsberg P, Schmitter M. Interexaminer reliability in the clinical examination of temporomandibular disorders: influence of age. *Community Dent Oral Epidemiol.* 2006;34:41–46.

27. Best N, Best S, Loudovici-Krug D, Smolenski UC. Measurement of mandible movements using a vernier caliper: an evaluation of the intrasession, intersession and interobserver reliability. *Cranio.* 2013;31(3):176–180.

2

Temporomandibular Joint

28. Emshoff R, Innerhofer K, Rudisch A, Bertram S. Clinical versus magnetic resonance imaging findings with internal derangement of the temporomandibular joint: an evaluation of anterior disc displacement without reduction. *J Oral Maxillofac Surg.* 2002;60(1):36–41.

29. Emshoff R, Rudisch A. Likelihood ratio methodology to identify predictors of treatment outcome in temporomandibular joint arthralgia patients. *Oral Surg Oral Med Oral Pathol Oral Radiol Endod.* 2008;106:525–533.

30. Kropmans TJ, Dijkstra PU, van Veen A, et al. The smallest detectable difference of mandibular function impairment in patients with a painfully restricted temporomandibular joint. *J Dent Res.* 1999;78:1445–1449.

31. Undt G, Murakami K, Clark GT, et al. Cross-cultural adaptation of the JPF-Questionnaire for German-speaking patients with functional temporomandibular joint disorders. *J Craniomaxillofac Surg.* 2006;34:226–233.

32. Li L, Liu X, Herr K. Postoperative pain intensity assessment: a comparison of four scales in Chinese adults. *Pain Med.* 2007;8:223–234.

33. Farrar JT, Berlin JA, Strom BL. Clinically important changes in acute pain outcome measures: a validation study. *J Pain Symptom Manage.* 2003;25:406–411.

34. Farrar JT, Portenoy RK, Berlin JA, et al. Defining the clinically important difference in pain outcome measures. *Pain.* 2000;88:287–294.

Cervical Spine | 3

Clinical Summary and Recommendations

Patient History	
Complaints	• The utility of the patient history has been studied only in the context of identifying cervical radiculopathy. Subjective reports of symptoms were generally not helpful, with diagnoses including complaints of "weakness," "numbness," "tingling," "burning," or "arm pain." • The patient complaints most useful in diagnosing cervical radiculopathy were *(1) a report of symptoms most bothersome in the scapular area* (+LR [likelihood ratio] = 2.30) and *(2) a report that symptoms improve with moving the neck* (+LR = 2.23).
Physical Examination	
Screening	• Traditional neurologic screening (sensation, reflex, and manual muscle testing [MMT]) is of moderate utility in identifying cervical radiculopathy. Sensation testing (pinprick at any location) and MMT of the muscles in the lower arm and hand are unhelpful. Muscle stretch reflex (MSR) and MMT of the muscles in the upper arm (especially the biceps brachii muscle) exhibit good diagnostic utility and are recommended. • A 2012 systematic review[1] evaluating the accuracy of the Canadian C-Spine Rule (CCR) and the NEXUS Low-Risk Criteria in screening for clinically important cervical spine injury in patients following blunt trauma concluded that the CCR appears to have better diagnostic accuracy than the NEXUS Criteria at ruling out clinically important cervical spine injuries that require diagnostic imaging. We recommend use of the CCR because it has been consistently shown to have perfect sensitivity (−LR = .00).
Range-of-Motion and Manual Assessment	• Measuring the cervical range of motion is consistently reliable but is of unknown diagnostic utility. • The results of studies assessing the reliability of passive intervertebral motion are highly variable, but generally, the results show that this maneuver has poor reliability as an assessment for limitations of movement and moderate reliability as an assessment for pain. • Assessing for both pain and limited movement during manual assessment is highly sensitive for zygapophyseal joint pain and is recommended to rule out zygapophyseal involvement (−LR = .00 to .23).
Special Tests	• Although of questionable reliability, multiple studies demonstrate the high diagnostic utility of Spurling's test in identifying cervical radiculopathy, cervical disc prolapse, and neck pain (+LR = 1.9 to 18.6). • Using a combination of *Spurling's A test, the upper limb tension test A, a distraction test,* and assessment for *cervical rotation* of less than 60 degrees to the ipsilateral side is very good for identifying cervical radiculopathy and is recommended (+LR = 30.3 if all four factors are present). • Using a combination of *gait deviation, the Hoffmann test, the inverted supinator sign, the Babinski test,* and *age more than 45 years* is very good at identifying cervical myelopathy and is recommended (+LR = 30.9 if three of five factors are present).
Interventions	• Factors associated with improvement from cervical thrust manipulation in patients with neck pain include symptom duration of less than 38 days, a positive expectation that manipulation will help, a side-to-side difference in cervical rotation range of motion of 10 degrees or greater, and pain with posteroanterior spring testing of the middle cervical spine (+LR 13.5 if three or more of the four factors are present).

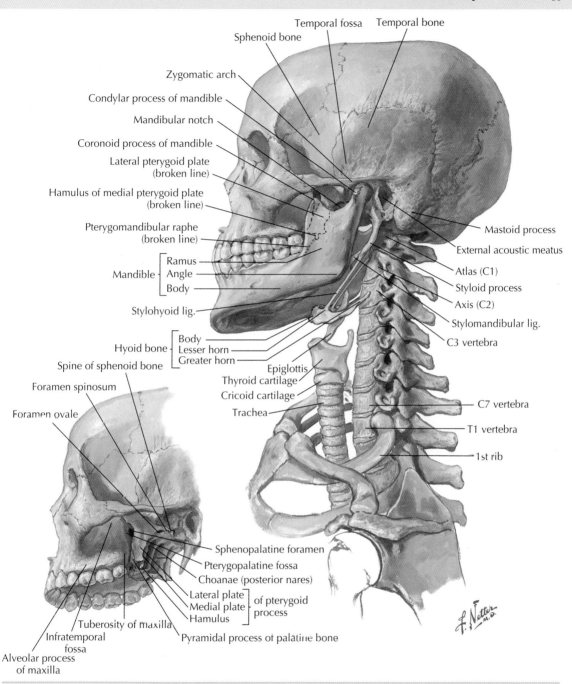

Figure 3-1
Bony framework of the head and neck.

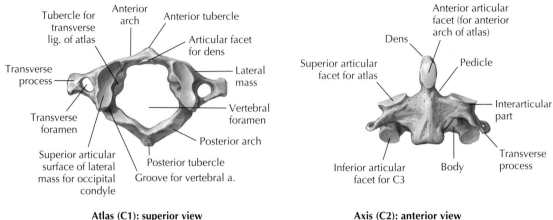

Atlas (C1): superior view

Axis (C2): anterior view

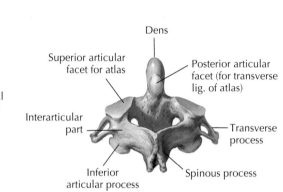

Atlas (C1): inferior view

Axis (C2): posterosuperior view

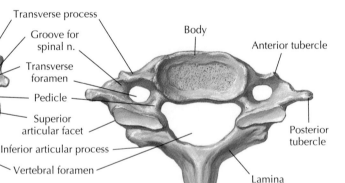

4th cervical vertebra: superior view

7th cervical vertebra: superior view

Figure 3-2
Cervical vertebrae.

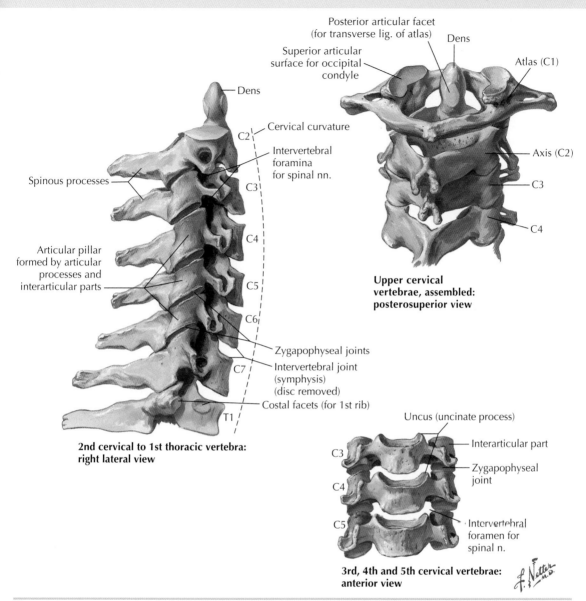

Figure 3-3
Joints of the cervical spine.

Joint	Type and Classification	Closed Packed Position	Capsular Pattern
Atlantooccipital	Synovial: plane	Not reported	Not reported
Atlantoodontoid/dens	Synovial: trochoid	Extension	Not reported
Atlantoaxial apophyseal joints	Synovial: plane	Extension	Not reported
C3-C7 Apophyseal joints	Synovial: plane	Full extension	Limitation in side-bending = rotation = extension
C3-C7 Intervertebral joints	Amphiarthrodial	Not applicable	Not applicable

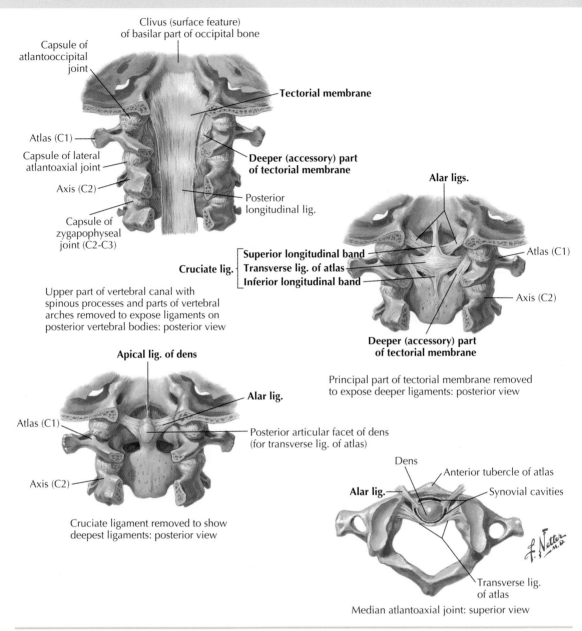

Figure 3-4
Ligaments of the atlantooccipital joint.

Ligaments	Attachments	Function
Alar	Sides of dens to lateral aspects of foramen magnum	Limits ipsilateral head rotation and contralateral side-bending
Ligaments	Attachments	Function
Apical	Dens to posterior aspect of foramen magnum	Limits separation of dens from occiput
Tectorial membrane	Body of C2 to occiput	Limits forward flexion
Cruciform ligament (superior longitudinal)	Transverse ligament to occiput	Maintains contact between dens and anterior arch of atlas
Cruciform ligament (transverse)	Extends between lateral tubercles of C1	
Cruciform ligament (inferior)	Transverse ligament to body of C2	

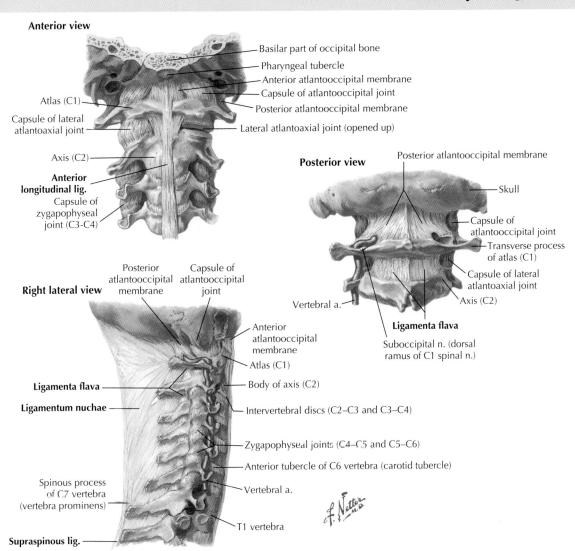

Figure 3-5
Spinal ligaments.

Ligaments	Attachments	Function
Anterior longitudinal	Extends from anterior sacrum to anterior tubercle of C1. Connects anterolateral vertebral bodies and discs	Maintains stability of vertebral body joints and prevents hyperextension of vertebral column
Posterior longitudinal	Extends from sacrum to C2. Runs within vertebral canal attaching posterior vertebral bodies	Prevents hyperflexion of vertebral column and posterior disc protrusion
Ligamentum nuchae	An extension of supraspinous ligament (occipital protuberance to C7)	Prevents cervical hyperflexion
Ligamenta flava	Attaches lamina above each vertebra to lamina below	Prevents separation of vertebral lamina
Supraspinous	Connects apices of spinous processes C7-S1	Limits separation of spinous processes
Interspinous	Connects adjoining spinous processes C1-S1	Limits separation of spinous processes
Intertransverse	Connects adjacent transverse processes of vertebrae	Limits separation of transverse processes

Anterior Muscles of the Neck

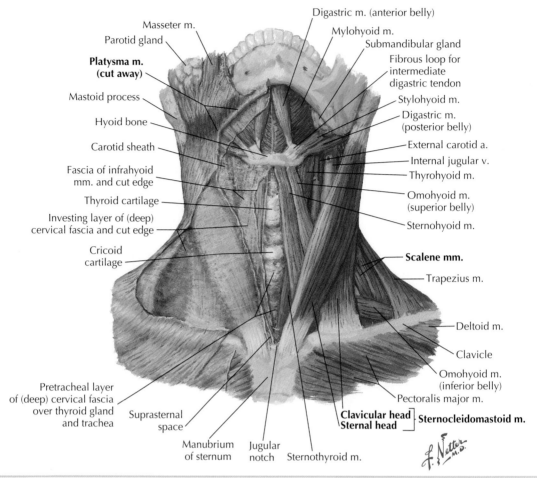

Figure 3-6
Anterior muscles of the neck.

Muscle	Proximal Attachment	Distal Attachment	Nerve and Segmental Level	Action
Sternocleidomas-toid	Lateral aspect of mastoid process and lateral superior nuchal line	Sternal head: anterior aspect of manubrium Clavicular head: su-peromedial aspect of clavicle	Spinal root of acces-sory nerve	Neck flexion, ipsilateral side-bending, and contralateral rotation
Scalene (anterior)	Transverse processes of vertebrae C4-C6	First rib	C4, C5, C6	Elevates first rib, ipsilateral side-bending, and contralateral rotation
Scalene (middle)	Transverse processes of vertebrae C1-C4	Superior aspect of first rib	Ventral rami of cervi-cal spinal nerves	Elevates first rib, ipsilateral side-bending, contralateral rotation
Scalene (posterior)		External aspect of second rib	Ventral rami of cervical spinal nerves C3, C4	Elevates second rib, ipsilateral side-bending, contralateral rotation
Platysma	Inferior mandible	Fascia of pectoralis major and deltoid	Cervical branch of facial nerve	Draws skin of neck superiorly with clenched jaw, draws corners of mouth inferiorly

Suprahyoid and Infrahyoid Muscles

Muscle	Proximal Attachment	Distal Attachment	Nerve and Segmental Level	Action
Suprahyoids				
Mylohyoid	Mandibular mylohyoid line	Hyoid bone	Mylohyoid nerve	Elevates hyoid bone, floor of mouth, and tongue
Geniohyoid	Mental spine of mandible	Body of hyoid bone	Hypoglossal nerve	Elevates hyoid bone anterosuperiorly, widens pharynx
Stylohyoid	Styloid process of temporal bone	Body of hyoid bone	Cervical branch of facial nerve	Elevates and retracts hyoid bone
Digastric	Anterior belly: digastric fossa of mandible Posterior belly: mastoid notch of temporal bone	Greater horn of hyoid bone	Anterior belly: mylohyoid nerve Posterior belly: facial nerve	Depresses mandible and raises hyoid
Infrahyoids				
Sternohyoid	Manubrium and medial clavicle	Body of hyoid bone	Branch of ansa cervicalis (C1, C2, C3)	Depresses hyoid bone after it has been elevated
Omohyoid	Superior border of scapula	Inferior aspect of hyoid bone	Branch of ansa cervicalis (C1, C2, C3)	Depresses and retracts hyoid bone
Sternothyroid	Posterior aspect of manubrium	Thyroid cartilage	Branch of ansa cervicalis (C2, C3)	Depresses hyoid bone and larynx
Thyrohyoid	Thyroid cartilage	Body and greater horn of hyoid bone	Hypoglossal nerve (C1)	Depresses hyoid bone, elevates larynx

Cervical Spine

3

Suprahyoid and Infrahyoid Muscles—cont'd

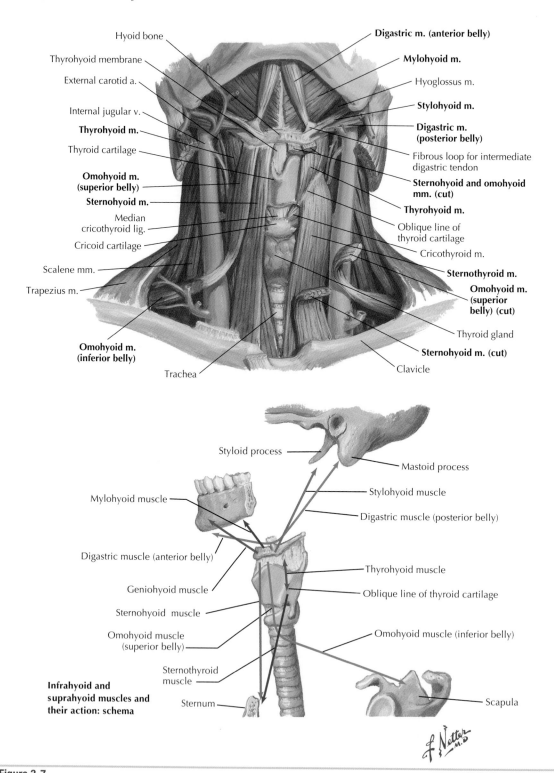

Figure 3-7
Suprahyoid and infrahyoid muscles.

Scalene and Prevertebral Muscles

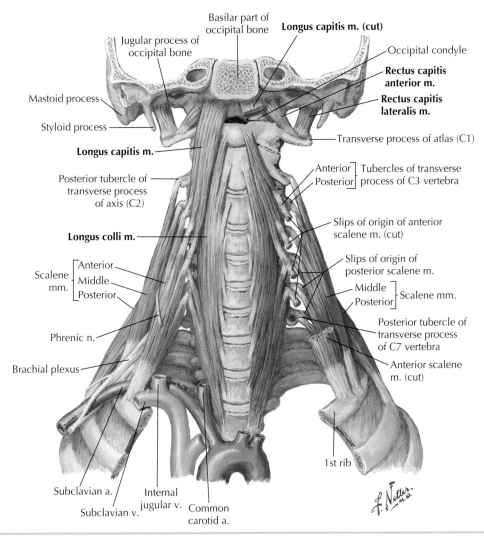

Basilar part of
occipital bone

Longus capitis m. (cut)

Jugular process of
occipital bone

Occipital condyle

**Rectus capitis
anterior m.**

**Rectus capitis
lateralis m.**

Mastoid process

Styloid process

Transverse process of atlas (C1)

Longus capitis m.

Posterior tubercle of
transverse process
of axis (C2)

Anterior ⎤ Tubercles of transverse
Posterior ⎦ process of C3 vertebra

Slips of origin of anterior
scalene m. (cut)

Longus colli m.

Slips of origin of
posterior scalene m.

Anterior
Scalene   Middle
mm.   Posterior

Middle ⎤ Scalene mm.
Posterior ⎦

Posterior tubercle of
transverse process
of C7 vertebra

Phrenic n.

Anterior scalene
m. (cut)

Brachial plexus

1st rib

Subclavian a.

Internal
jugular v.   Common
Subclavian v.   carotid a.

Figure 3-8
Scalene and prevertebral muscles.

Muscle	Proximal Attachment	Distal Attachment	Nerve and Segmental Level	Action
Longus capitis	Basilar aspect of occipital bone	Anterior tubercles of transverse processes C3-C6	Ventral rami of C1-C3 spinal nerves	Flexes head on neck
Longus colli	Anterior tubercle of C1, bodies of C1-C3, and transverse processes of C3-C6	Bodies of C3-T3 and transverse processes of C3-C5	Ventral rami of C2-C6 spinal nerves	Neck flexion, ipsilateral side-bending, and rotation
Rectus capitis anterior	Base of skull anterior to occipital condyle	Anterior aspect of lateral mass of C1	Branches from loop between C1 and C2 spinal nerves	Flexes head on neck
Rectus capitis lateralis	Jugular process of occipital bone	Transverse process of C1		Flexes head and assists in stabilizing head on neck

Posterior Muscles of the Neck

Muscle	Proximal Attachment	Distal Attachment	Nerve and Segmental Level	Action
Upper trapezius	Superior nuchal line, occipital protuberance, nuchal ligament, spinous processes of C7-T12	Lateral clavicle, acromion, and spine of scapula	Spinal root of accessory nerve	Elevates scapula
Levator scapulae	Transverse processes of C1-C4	Superomedial border of scapula	Dorsal scapular nerve (C3, C4, C5)	Elevates scapula and inferiorly rotates glenoid fossa
Semispinalis capitis and cervicis	Cervical and thoracic spinous processes	Superior spinous processes and occipital bone	Dorsal rami of spinal nerves	Bilaterally: extends neck Unilaterally: ipsilateral side-bending
Splenius capitis and cervicis	Spinous processes of T1-T6 and ligamentum nuchae	Mastoid process and lateral superior nuchal line	Dorsal rami of middle cervical spinal nerves	Bilaterally: head and neck extension Unilaterally: ipsilateral rotation
Longissimus capitis and cervicis	Superior thoracic transverse processes and cervical transverse processes	Mastoid process of temporal bone and cervical transverse processes	Dorsal rami of cervical spinal nerves	Head extension, ipsilateral side-bending, and rotation of head and neck
Spinalis cervicis	Lower cervical spinous processes of vertebrae	Upper cervical spinous processes of vertebrae	Dorsal rami of spinal nerves	Bilaterally: extends neck Unilaterally: ipsilateral side-bending of neck
Suboccipital Muscles				
Rectus capitis posterior major	Spinous process of C2	Lateral inferior nuchal line of occipital bone	Suboccipital nerve (C1)	Head extension and ipsilateral rotation
Rectus capitis posterior minor	Posterior arch of C1	Medial inferior nuchal line	Suboccipital nerve (C1)	Head extension and ipsilateral rotation
Obliquus capitis superior	Transverse process of C1	Occipital bone	Suboccipital nerve (C1)	Head extension and side-bending
Obliquus capitis inferior	Spinous process of C2	Transverse process of C1	Suboccipital nerve (C1)	Ipsilateral neck rotation

Posterior Muscles of the Neck—cont'd

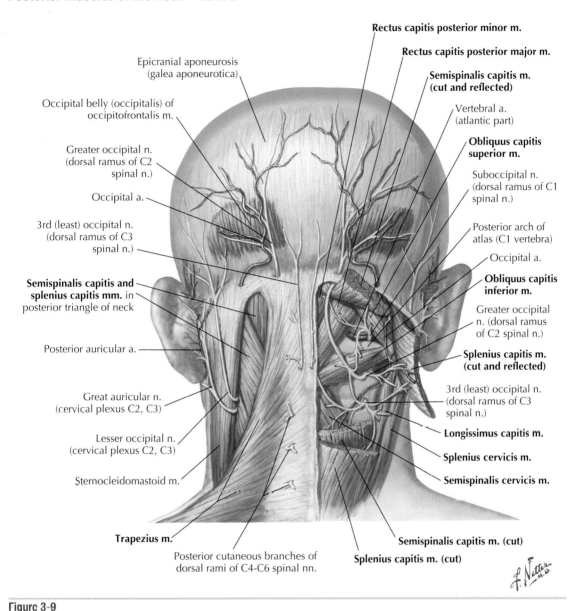

Rectus capitis posterior minor m.

Rectus capitis posterior major m.

Semispinalis capitis m. (cut and reflected)

Vertebral a. (atlantic part)

Obliquus capitis superior m.

Suboccipital n. (dorsal ramus of C1 spinal n.)

Posterior arch of atlas (C1 vertebra)

Occipital a.

Obliquus capitis inferior m.

Greater occipital n. (dorsal ramus of C2 spinal n.)

Splenius capitis m. (cut and reflected)

3rd (least) occipital n. (dorsal ramus of C3 spinal n.)

Longissimus capitis m.

Splenius cervicis m.

Semispinalis cervicis m.

Epicranial aponeurosis (galea aponeurotica)

Occipital belly (occipitalis) of occipitofrontalis m.

Greater occipital n. (dorsal ramus of C2 spinal n.)

Occipital a.

3rd (least) occipital n. (dorsal ramus of C3 spinal n.)

Semispinalis capitis and splenius capitis mm. in posterior triangle of neck

Posterior auricular a.

Great auricular n. (cervical plexus C2, C3)

Lesser occipital n. (cervical plexus C2, C3)

Sternocleidomastoid m.

Trapezius m.

Posterior cutaneous branches of dorsal rami of C4-C6 spinal nn.

Semispinalis capitis m. (cut)

Splenius capitis m. (cut)

Figure 3-9
Posterior muscles of the neck.

Cervical Spine

Nerves	Segmental Levels	Sensory	Motor
Dorsal scapular	C4, C5	No sensory	Rhomboids, levator scapulae
Suprascapular	C4, C5, C6	No sensory	Supraspinatus, infraspinatus
Nerve to subclavius	C5, C6	No sensory	Subclavius
Lateral pectoral	C5, C6, C7	No sensory	Pectoralis major
Medial pectoral	C8, T1	No sensory	Pectoralis major Pectoralis minor
Long thoracic	C5, C6, C7	No sensory	Serratus anterior
Medial cutaneous of arm	C8, T1	Medial aspect of arm	No motor
Medial cutaneous of forearm	C8, T1	Medial aspect of forearm	No motor
Upper subscapular	C5, C6	No sensory	Subscapularis
Lower subscapular	C5, C6, C7	No sensory	Subscapularis, teres major
Thoracodorsal	C6, C7, C8	No sensory	Latissimus dorsi
Axillary	C5, C6	Lateral shoulder	Deltoid, teres minor
Radial	C5, C6, C7, C8, T1	Dorsal lateral aspect of hand, including the thumb and up to the base of digits 2 and 3	Triceps brachii, brachioradialis, anconeus, extensor carpi radialis longus, extensor carpi radialis brevis
Median	C5, C6, C7, C8, T1	Palmar aspect of lateral hand, including lateral half of digit 4, dorsal distal half of digits 1-3, and lateral border of digit 4	Pronator teres, flexor carpi radialis, palmaris longus, flexor digitorum superficialis, flexor pollicis longus, flexor digitorum profundus (lateral half), pronator quadratus, lumbricals to digits 2 and 3, thenar muscles
Ulnar	C8, T1	Medial border of both palmar and dorsal hand, including medial half of digit 4	Flexor carpi ulnaris, flexor digitorum profundus (medial half), palmar interossei, adductor pollicis, palmaris brevis, dorsal interossei, lumbricals to digits 4 and 5, hypothenar muscles
Musculocutaneous	C5, C6, C7	Lateral forearm	Coracobrachialis, biceps brachii, brachialis

Cervical Spine

3

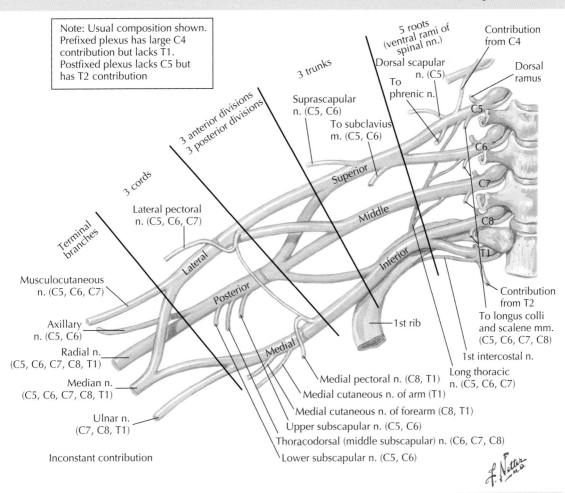

Note: Usual composition shown.
Prefixed plexus has large C4
contribution but lacks T1.
Postfixed plexus lacks C5 but
has T2 contribution

5 roots
(ventral rami of
spinal nn.)

Contribution
from C4

3 trunks

Dorsal scapular
n. (C5)

Dorsal
ramus

Suprascapular
n. (C5, C6)

To
phrenic n.

3 anterior divisions
3 posterior divisions

To subclavius
m. (C5, C6)

C5

C6

3 cords

Superior

C7

Lateral pectoral
n. (C5, C6, C7)

Middle

C8

Terminal
branches

Lateral

T1

Inferior

Musculocutaneous
n. (C5, C6, C7)

Posterior

Contribution
from T2

Axillary
n. (C5, C6)

1st rib

To longus colli
and scalene mm.
(C5, C6, C7, C8)

Radial n.
(C5, C6, C7, C8, T1)

Medial

1st intercostal n.

Median n.
(C5, C6, C7, C8, T1)

Medial pectoral n. (C8, T1)

Long thoracic
n. (C5, C6, C7)

Medial cutaneous n. of arm (T1)

Ulnar n.
(C7, C8, T1)

Medial cutaneous n. of forearm (C8, T1)

Upper subscapular n. (C5, C6)

Inconstant contribution

Thoracodorsal (middle subscapular) n. (C6, C7, C8)

Lower subscapular n. (C5, C6)

Figure 3-10
Nerves of the neck.

History	Initial Hypotheses
Patient reports diffuse nonspecific neck pain that is exacerbated by neck movements	Mechanical neck pain[2] Cervical facet syndrome[3] Cervical muscle strain or sprain
Patient reports pain in certain postures that is alleviated by positional changes	Upper crossed postural syndrome
Traumatic mechanism of injury with complaint of nonspecific cervical symptoms that are exacerbated in the vertical positions and relieved with the head supported in the supine position	Cervical instability, especially if patient reports dysesthesias of the face occurring with neck movement
Reports of nonspecific neck pain with numbness and tingling into one upper extremity	Cervical radiculopathy
Reports of neck pain with bilateral upper extremity symptoms with occasional reports of loss of balance or lack of coordination of the lower extremities	Cervical myelopathy

Cervical Zygapophyseal Pain Syndromes

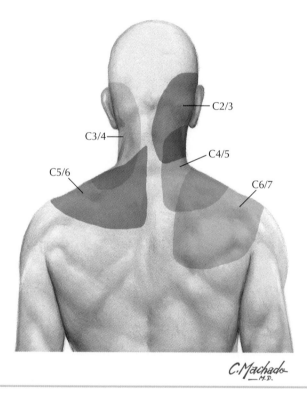

Figure 3-11

Pain referral patterns. Distribution of zygapophyseal pain referral patterns as described by Dwyer and colleagues.[4] (Dwyer A, Aprill C, Bogduk N. Cervical zygapophyseal joint pain patterns. I: A study in normal volunteers. *Spine.* 1990;15:453-457.)

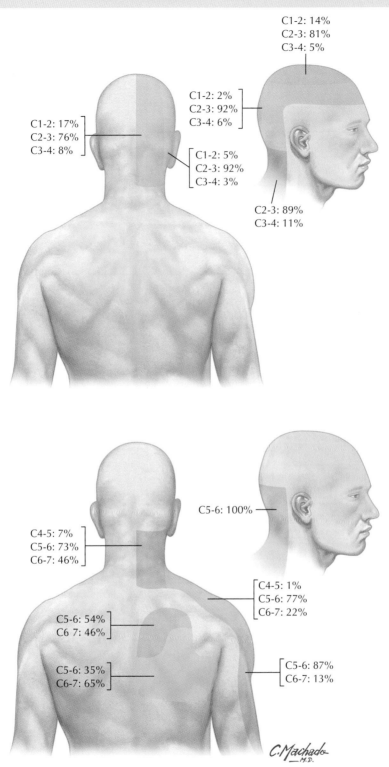

C1-2: 14%
C2-3: 81%
C3-4: 5%

C1-2: 2%
C2-3: 92%
C3-4: 6%

C1-2: 17%
C2-3: 76%
C3-4: 8%

C1-2: 5%
C2-3: 92%
C3-4: 3%

C2-3: 89%
C3-4: 11%

C5-6: 100%

C4-5: 7%
C5-6: 73%
C6-7: 46%

C4-5: 1%
C5-6: 77%
C6-7: 22%

C5-6: 54%
C6 7: 46%

C5-6: 35%
C6-7: 65%

C5-6: 87%
C6-7: 13%

Figure 3-12
Pain referral patterns. Probability of zygapophyseal joints at the segments indicated being the source of pain, as described by Cooper and colleagues.[5] (Cooper G, Bailey B, Bogduk N. Cervical zygapophysial joint pain maps. *Pain Med.* 2007;8:344-353.)

Historical Question and Study Quality	Possible Responses	Population	Interexaminer Reliability
Mode of onset[6] ◆	Gradual, sudden, or traumatic	22 patients with mechanical neck pain	$\kappa = .72$ (.47, .96)
Nature of neck symptoms[6] ◆	Constant or intermittent		$\kappa = .81$ (.56, 1.0)
Prior episode of neck pain[6] ◆	Yes or No		$\kappa = .90$ (.70, 1.0)
Turning the head aggravates symptoms[6] ◆	Yes or No		(Right) $\kappa = -.04$ (2.11, .02)* (Left) $\kappa = 1.0$ (1.0, 1.0)
Looking up and down aggravates symptoms[6] ◆	Yes or No		(Down) $\kappa = .79$ (.51, 1.0) (Up) $\kappa = .80$ (.55, 1.0)
Driving aggravates symptoms[6] ◆	Yes or No		$\kappa = -.06$ (−.39, .26)*
Sleeping aggravates symptoms[6] ◆	Yes or No		$\kappa = .90$ (.72, 1.0)
Which of the following symptoms are most bothersome for you?[7] ◆	• Pain • Numbness and tingling • Loss of feeling	50 patients with suspected cervical radiculopathy or carpal tunnel syndrome	$\kappa = .74$ (.55, .93)
Where are your symptoms most bothersome?[7] ◆	• Neck • Shoulder or shoulder blade • Arm above elbow • Arm below elbow • Hands and/or fingers		$\kappa = .83$ (.68, .96)
Which of the following best describes the behavior of your symptoms?[7] ◆	• Constant • Intermittent • Variable		$\kappa = .57$ (.35, .79)
Does your entire affected limb and/or hand feel numb?[7] ◆	Yes or No		$\kappa = .53$ (.26, .81)
Do your symptoms keep you from falling asleep?[7] ◆	Yes or No		$\kappa = .70$ (.48, .92)
Do your symptoms improve with moving your neck?[7] ◆	Yes or No		$\kappa = .67$ (.44, .90)

*Question had a high percentage of agreement but a low κ because 95% of participants answered "yes."

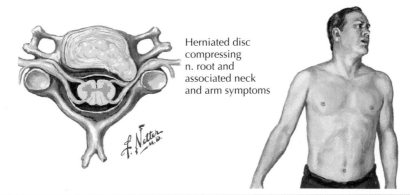

Herniated disc
compressing
n. root and
associated neck
and arm symptoms

Figure 3-13
Cervical radiculopathy.

Complaint and Study Quality	Description and Positive Findings	Population	Reference Standard	Sens	Spec	+LR	−LR
Weakness[8] ◆	Not specifically described	183 patients referred to electrodiagnostic laboratories	Cervical radiculopathy via electrodiagnostics	.65	.39	1.07	.90
Numbness[8] ◆				.79	.25	1.05	.84
Arm pain[8] ◆				.65	.26	.88	1.35
Neck pain[8] ◆				.62	.35	.95	1.09
Tingling[8] ◆				.72	.25	.96	1.92
Burning[8] ◆				.33	.63	.89	1.06

Complaint and Study Quality	Description and Positive Findings	Population	Reference Standard	Sens	Spec	+LR	−LR*
Which of the following symptoms are most bothersome for you?[7] ◆	Pain	82 consecutive patients referred to electrophysiologic laboratory with suspected diagnosis of cervical radiculopathy or carpal tunnel syndrome	Cervical radiculopathy via needle electromyography and nerve conduction studies	.47 (.23, .71)	.52 (.41, .65)	.99 (.56, 1.7)	1.02
	Numbness and tingling			.47 (.23, .71)	.56 (.42, .68)	1.1 (.6, 1.9)	.95
	Loss of feeling			.06 (.00, .17)	.92 (.85, .99)	.74 (.09, 5.9)	1.02
Where are your symptoms most bothersome?[7] ◆	Neck			.19 (.00, .35)	.90 (.83, .98)	1.9 (.54, 6.9)	.90
	Shoulder or scapula			.38 (.19, .73)	.84 (.75, .93)	2.3 (1.0, 5.4)	.74
	Arm above elbow			.03 (.14, .61)	.93 (.86, .99)	.41 (.02, 7.3)	1.04
	Arm below elbow			.06 (.00, .11)	.84 (.75, .93)	.39 (.05, 2.8)	1.12
	Hands and/or fingers			.38 (.14, .48)	.48 (.36, .61)	.73 (.37, 1.4)	1.29
Which of the following best describes the behavior of your symptoms?[7] ◆	Constant			.12 (.00, .27)	.84 (.75, .93)	.74 (.18, 3.1)	1.05
	Intermittent			.35 (.13, .58)	.62 (.50, .74)	.93 (.45, 1.9)	1.05
	Variable			.53 (.29, .77)	.54 (.42, .66)	1.2 (.68, 1.9)	.87
Does your entire affected limb and/or hand feel numb?[7] ◆	Yes or No			.24 (.03, .44)	.73 (.62, .84)	.87 (.34, 2.3)	1.04
Do your symptoms keep you from falling asleep?[7] ◆				.47 (.23, .71)	.60 (.48, .72)	1.19 (.66, 2.1)	.88
Do your symptoms improve with moving your neck?[7] ◆				.65 (.42, .87)	.71 (.60, .82)	2.23 (1.3, 3.8)	.49

*—LR in this table has been calculated by the authors.

Reliability of Sensation Testing

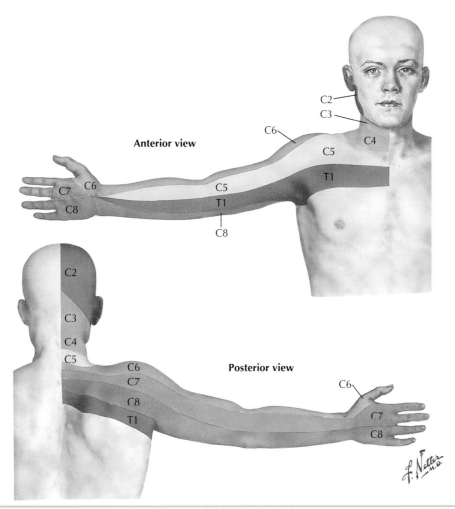

Figure 3-14
Dermatomes of the upper limb.

Cervical Spine 3

Test and Study Quality	Description and Positive Findings	Population	Reliability
Identifying sensory deficits in extremities[9] ◆	No details given	8924 adult patients who presented to emergency department after blunt trauma to head/neck and had Glasgow Coma Score of 15	Interexaminer κ = .60

Diagnostic Utility of Pinprick Sensation Testing for Cervical Radiculopathy

Test and Study Quality	Description and Positive Findings	Population	Reference Standard	Sens	Spec	+LR	−LR
C5 Dermatome[7] ◆		82 consecutive patients referred to electrophysiologic laboratory with suspected diagnosis of cervical radiculopathy or carpal tunnel syndrome	Cervical radiculopathy via needle electromyography and nerve conduction studies	.29 (.08, .51)	.86 (.77, .94)	2.1 (.79, 5.3)	.82 (.60, 1.1)
C6 Dermatome[7] ◆	Pinprick sensation testing. Graded as "normal" or "abnormal"			.24 (.03, .44)	.66 (.54, .78)	.69 (.28, 1.8)	1.16 (.84, 1.6)
C7 Dermatome[7] ◆				.18 (.00, .36)	.77 (.66, .87)	.76 (.25, 2.3)	1.07 (.83, 1.4)
C8 Dermatome[7] ◆				.12 (.00, .27)	.81 (.71, .90)	.61 (.15, 2.5)	1.09 (.88, 1.4)
T1 Dermatome[7] ◆				.18 (.00, .36)	.79 (.68, .89)	.83 (.27, 2.6)	1.05 (.81, 1.4)
Decreased sensation to pinprick[8] ◆	Not specifically described	183 patients referred to electrodiagnostic laboratories	Cervical radiculopathy via electrodiagnostics	.49	.64	1.36	.80

Reliability of Manual Muscle Testing

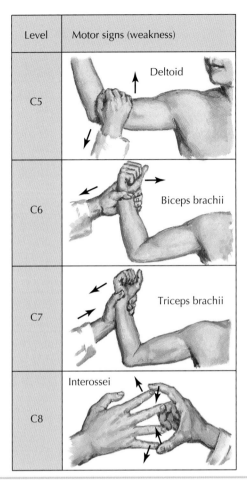

Level	Motor signs (weakness)
C5	Deltoid
C6	Biceps brachii
C7	Triceps brachii
C8	Interossei

Figure 3-15
Manual muscle testing of the upper limb.

Test and Study Quality	Description and Positive Findings	Population	Reliability
Identifying motor deficits in the extremities[9] ◆	No details given	8924 adult patients who presented to emergency department after blunt trauma to head/neck and had Glasgow Coma Score of 15	Interexaminer κ = .93

Diagnostic Utility of Manual Muscle Testing for Cervical Radiculopathy

Test and Study Quality	Description and Positive Findings	Population	Reference Standard	Sens	Spec	+LR	−LR
MMT deltoid[7] ◆	Standard strength testing using methods of Kendall and McCreary. Graded as "normal" or "abnormal"	82 consecutive patients referred to electrophysiologic laboratory with suspected diagnosis of cervical radiculopathy or carpal tunnel syndrome	Cervical radiculopathy via needle electromyography and nerve conduction studies	.24 (.03, .44)	.89 (.81, .97)	2.1 (.70, 6.4)	.86 (.65, 1.1)
MMT biceps brachii[7] ◆				.24 (.03, .44)	.94 (.88, 1.0)	3.7 (1.0, 13.3)	.82 (.62, 1.1)
MMT extensor carpi radialis longus/brevis[7] ◆				.12 (.00, .27)	.90 (.83, .98)	1.2 (.27, 5.6)	.98 (.81, 1.2)
MMT triceps brachii[7] ◆				.12 (.00, .27)	.94 (.88, 1.0)	1.9 (.37, 9.3)	.94 (.78, 1.1)
MMT flexor carpi radialis[7] ◆				.06 (.00, .17)	.89 (.82, .97)	.55 (.07, 4.2)	1.05 (.91, 1.2)
MMT abductor pollicis brevis[7] ◆				.06 (.00, .17)	.84 (.75, .93)	.37 (.05, 2.7)	1.12 (.95, 1.3)
MMT first dorsal interosseus[7] ◆				.03 (.00, .10)	.93 (.87, .99)	.40 (.02, 7.0)	1.05 (.94, 1.2)

Diagnostic Utility of Muscle Stretch Reflex Testing for Cervical Radiculopathy

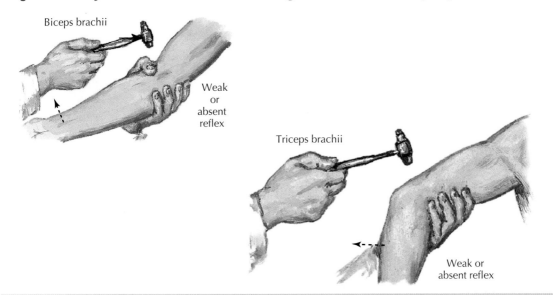

Figure 3-16
Reflex testing.

Test and Study Quality	Description and Positive Findings	Population	Reference Standard	Sens	Spec	+LR	−LR
Biceps brachii MSR[7] ◆	Tested bilaterally using standard reflex hammer. Graded as "normal" or "abnormal"	82 consecutive patients referred to electrophysiologic laboratory with suspected diagnosis of cervical radiculopathy or carpal tunnel syndrome	Cervical radiculopathy via needle electromyography and nerve conduction studies	.24 (.3, .44)	.95 (.90, 1.0)	4.9 (1.2, 20.0)	.80 (.61, 1.1)
Brachioradialis MSR[7] ◆				.06 (.00, .17)	.95 (.90, 1.9)	1.2 (.14, 11.1)	.99 (.87, 1.1)
Triceps MSR[7] ◆				.03 (.00, .10)	.93 (.87, .99)	.40 (.02, 7.0)	1.05 (.94, 1.2)
Biceps[8] ◆	Not specifically described	183 patients referred to electrodiagnostic laboratories	Cervical radiculopathy via electrodiagnostics	.10	.99	10.0	.91
Triceps[8] ◆				.10	.95	2.0	.95
Brachioradialis[8] ◆				.08	.99	8.0	.93

Cervical Spine

3

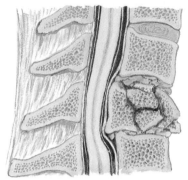

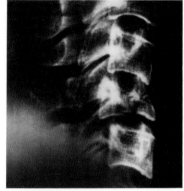

X-ray film: Type III fracture of C5

Type III. Fracture through entire vertebral body with fragmentation of its anterior portion. Posterior cortex intact but projects into spinal canal causing damage to cord and/or nerve roots

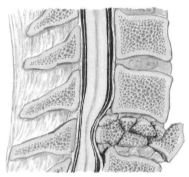

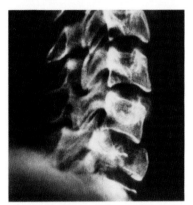

X-ray film: Type IV fracture of C6

Type IV. "Burst" fracture. Entire vertebral body crushed, with intraspinal bone fragments

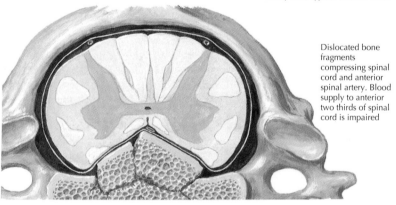

Dislocated bone fragments compressing spinal cord and anterior spinal artery. Blood supply to anterior two thirds of spinal cord is impaired

Figure 3-17
Compression fracture of the cervical spine.

NEXUS Low-Risk Criteria[10]

Cervical spine radiography is indicated for patients with trauma unless they meet all of the following criteria:	1. No posterior midline cervical spine tenderness
	2. No evidence of intoxication
	3. Normal level of alertness
	4. No focal neurologic deficit
	5. No painful distracting injuries

Diagnostic Utility of the Clinical Examination for Identifying Cervical Spine Injury

Test and Study Quality	Description and Positive Findings	Population	Reference Standard	Sens	Spec	+LR	−LR
NEXUS Low-Risk Criteria[11] ◆	See Figure 3-18	34,069 patients who presented to emergency department after blunt trauma and had cervical spine radiography	Clinically important cervical spine injury demonstrated by radiography, computed tomography (CT), or magnetic resonance imaging (MRI)	.99 (.98, 1.0)	.13 (.13, .13)	1.14	.08
NEXUS Low-Risk Criteria[12] ◆		320 elderly patients (65 years or older) who presented to emergency department after blunt trauma	Clinically important cervical spine injury demonstrated by CT	.66	.60	1.65	.57
NEXUS Low-Risk Criteria[13] ◆	See Figure 3-18	8924 alert adult patients who presented to emergency department after blunt trauma to head/neck	Clinically important cervical spine injury defined as any fracture, dislocation, or ligamentous instability demonstrated by radiography, CT, and/or a telephone follow-up	.93 (.87, .96)	.38 (.37, .39)	1.50	.18
NEXUS Low-Risk Criteria[10] ◆		7430 alert adult patients who presented to emergency department after blunt trauma to head/neck		.91 (.85, .94)	.37 (.36, .38)	1.44	.24
Canadian C-Spine Rule[10] ◆				.99 (.96, 1.0)	.45 (.44, .46)	1.80	.02
Canadian C-Spine Rule[9] ◆	See Figure 3-18	8924 alert adult patients who presented to emergency department after blunt trauma to head/neck		1.0 (.98, 1.0)	.43 (.40, .44)	1.75	.00
Canadian C-Spine Rule[14] ◖				1.0 (.94, 1.0)	.44 (.43, .45)	1.79	.00
Physician judgment[14] ◖	Physicians were asked to estimate the probability that the patient would have a clinically important cervical spine injury by circling one of the following: 0%, 1%, 2%, 3%, 4%, 5%, 10%, 20%, 30%, 40%, 50%, 75%, or 100%	6265 alert adult patients who presented to emergency department after trauma to head/neck	Clinically important cervical spine injury demonstrated by radiography, CT, and/or a telephone follow-up	.92 (.82, .96)	.54 (.53, .55)	2.00	.15

Continued

Cervical Spine

3

Diagnostic Utility of the Clinical Examination for Identifying Cervical Spine Injury—cont'd

Test and Study Quality	Description and Positive Findings	Population	Reference Standard	Sens	Spec	+LR	−LR
Clinical examination[15]	Patient history, including mechanism of injury and subjective complaints of neck pain and/or neurologic deficits, followed by physical examination of tenderness to palpation, abnormalities to palpation, and neurologic deficits	534 patients consulting a level I trauma center after blunt trauma to head/neck	Cervical fracture via CT	.77	.55	1.70	.42
	Among subset of patients with a Glasgow Coma Score of 15 (i.e., alert), who were not intoxicated, and who did not have a distracting injury			.67	.62	1.76	.54

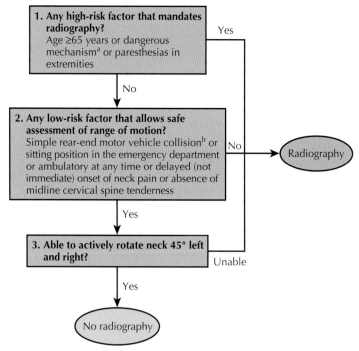

1. Any high-risk factor that mandates radiography?
Age ≥65 years or dangerous mechanism[a] or paresthesias in extremities

→ Yes

2. Any low-risk factor that allows safe assessment of range of motion?
Simple rear-end motor vehicle collision[b] or sitting position in the emergency department or ambulatory at any time or delayed (not immediate) onset of neck pain or absence of midline cervical spine tenderness

No →

Radiography

3. Able to actively rotate neck 45° left and right?

Unable

Yes

No radiography

[a] A dangerous mechanism is considered to be a fall from an elevation of 3 feet or greater or three to five stairs; an axial load to the head (e.g., diving); a motor vehicle collision at high speed (>100 km/hr) or with rollover or ejection.

[b] A simple rear-end motor vehicle collision excludes being pushed into oncoming traffic, being hit by a bus or a large truck, a rollover, or being hit by a high-speed vehicle.

Figure 3-18
Canadian C-Spine Rule. (See Stiell IG, Clement CM, McKnight RD, et al. The Canadian C-spine rule versus the NEXUS low-risk criteria in patients with trauma. *N Engl J Med.* 2003;349:2510-2518.)

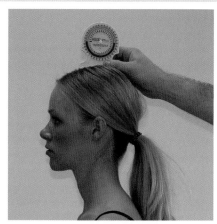

Positioning of inclinometer to measure
flexion and extension

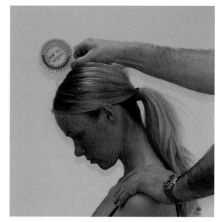

Measurement of flexion

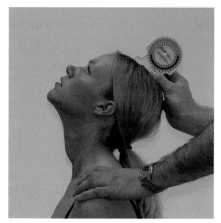

Measurement of extension

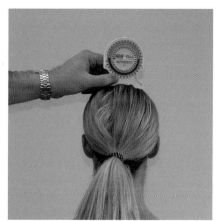

Positioning of inclinometer
to measure side bending

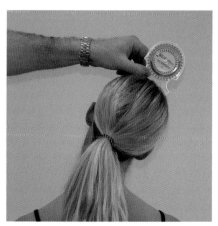

Measurement of side-
bending to the right

Figure 3-19
Range of motion.

Reliability of Measuring Range of Motion

Test and Study Quality	Instrumentation	Population	Interexaminer Reliability
Extension[16] ◆	Inclinometer	30 patients with neck pain	ICC = .86 (.73, .93)
Flexion[16] ◆			ICC = .78 (.59, .89)
Rotation in flexion[16] ◆			(Right) ICC = .78 (.60, .89) (Left) ICC = .89 (.78, .95)
Lateral bending[16] ◆			(Right) ICC = .87 (.75, .94) (Left) ICC = .85 (.70, .92)
Rotation[16] ◆			(Right) ICC = .86 (.74, .93) (Left) ICC = .91 (.82, .96)
Flexion[6] ◆	Inclinometer	22 patients with mechanical neck pain	ICC = .75 (.50, .89)
Extension[6] ◆			ICC = .74 (.48, .88)
Side-bending[6] ◆			(Right) ICC = .66 (.33, .84) (Left) ICC = .69 (.40, .86)
Rotation[6] ◆	Goniometer		(Right) ICC = .78 (.55, .90) (Left) ICC = .77 (.52, .90)
Flexion[7] ◆	Inclinometer	50 patients with suspected cervical radiculopathy or carpal tunnel syndrome	ICC = .79 (.65, .88)
Extension[7] ◆			ICC = .84 (.70, .95)
Left rotation[7] ◆	Goniometer		ICC = .75 (.59, .85)
Right rotation[7] ◆			ICC = .63 (.22, .82)
Left side-bending[7] ◆	Inclinometer		ICC = .63 (.40, .78)
Right side-bending[7] ◆			ICC = .68 (.62, .87)
Flexion[17] ◉	Cervical range-of-motion (CROM) instrument	60 patients with neck pain	ICC = .58
Extension[17] ◉			ICC = .97
Right side-bending[17] ◉			ICC = .96
Left side-bending[17] ◉			ICC = .94
Right rotation[17] ◉			ICC = .96
Left rotation[17] ◉			ICC = .98
Protraction[17] ◉			ICC = .49
Retraction[17] ◉			ICC = .35

ICC, intraclass correlation coefficient.

Reliability of Measuring Range of Motion—cont'd

Test and Study Quality	Instrumentation	Population	Interexaminer Reliability
Flexion-extension[18]	Inclinometer and CROM	30 asymptomatic subjects	Inclinometer ICC = .84 CROM ICC = .88
Side-bending[18]			Inclinometer ICC = .82 CROM ICC = .84
Rotation[18]			Inclinometer ICC = .81 CROM ICC = .92
Flexion[19]	CROM, universal goniometer, and visual estimation	60 patients in whom the assessment of CROM testing would be appropriate during the physical therapy evaluation	CROM ICC = .86 Goniometer ICC = .57 Visual estimation ICC = .42
Extension[19]			CROM ICC = .86 Goniometer ICC = .79 Visual estimation ICC = .42
Left side-bending[19]			CROM ICC = .73 Goniometer ICC = .79 Visual estimation ICC = .63
Right side-bending[19]			CROM ICC = .73 Goniometer ICC = .79 Visual estimation ICC = .63
Left rotation[19]			CROM ICC = .82 Goniometer ICC = .54 Visual estimation ICC = .70
Right rotation[19]			CROM ICC − .92 Goniometer ICC = .62 Visual estimation ICC = .82
Cervical flexion[20]	Inclinometer	22 individuals with neck pain	ICC = .41 (−.16, .71)
Cervical extension[20]			ICC = .59 (.24, .81)
Cervical side-bending[20]			ICC = .75 (.59, .86)
Cervical rotation[20]	Goniometer		ICC = .31 (−.03, .55)
Cervical flexion[21]	Inclinometer	21 individuals with shoulder pain	ICC = .82 (.62, .92)
Cervical extension[21]			ICC = .87 (.70, .95)
Cervical side-bending[21]			Right: ICC = .52 (.14, .77) Left: ICC = .42 (.01, .71)
Cervical rotation[21]	Goniometer		Right: ICC = .25 (−.15, .59) Left: ICC = .26 (−.17, .61)
Cervical flexion[22]	Goniometer	19 healthy subjects	Tested on 2 sessions: ICC = .79 and .92
Cervical extension[22]			Tested on 2 sessions: ICC = .92 and .79
Cervical side-bending[22]			Tested on 2 sessions: Right: ICC = .89 and .87 Left: ICC = .89 and .87
Cervical rotation[22]			Tested on 2 sessions: Right: ICC = .90 and .88 Left: ICC = .83 and .90

3

Cervical Spine

Diagnostic Utility of Pain Responses during Active Physiologic Range of Motion

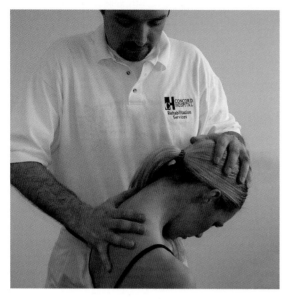

Testing flexion with overpressure

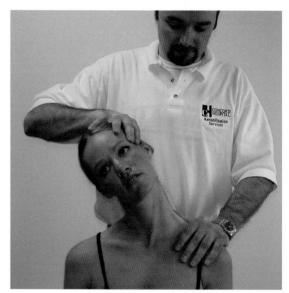

Testing side-bending with overpressure

Figure 3-20
Overpressure testing.

Test and Measure Quality	Test Procedure and Determination of Positive Findings	Population	Reference Standard	Sens	Spec	+LR	−LR
Active flexion and extension of the neck[23] ●	Active flexion and extension performed to the extremes of the range. Positive if subject reported pain with procedure	75 males (22 with neck pain)	Patient reports of neck pain	.27	.90	2.70	.81

Reliability of Cervical Strength and Endurance Testing

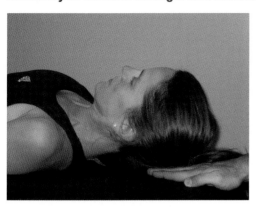

Figure 3-21
Cervical flexor endurance.

Test and Study Quality	Description and Positive Findings	Population	Reliability
Neck flexor muscle endurance test[24] ◆	With patient supine with knees flexed, examiner's hand is placed behind occiput and the subject gently flexes the upper neck and lifts the head off the examiner's hand while retaining the upper neck flexion. The test was timed and terminated when the subject was unable to maintain the position of the head off the examiner's hand	21 patients with postural neck pain	Interexaminer ICC = .93 (.86, .97)
Chin tuck neck flexion test[6] ◆	With patient supine, subject tucks the chin and lifts the head approximately 1 inch. The test was timed with a stopwatch and terminated when the patient's position deviated	22 patients with mechanical neck pain	Interexaminer ICC = .57 (.14, .81)
Cervical flexor endurance[25] ●	With patient supine, knees flexed, and chin maximally retracted, subject lifts the head slightly. The test was timed with a stopwatch and terminated when the subject lost maximal retraction, flexed the neck, or could not continue	27 asymptomatic subjects	Intraexaminer ICC = 0.74 (.50, .87) Interexaminer Test #1 ICC = .54 (.31, .73) Test #2 ICC = .66 (.46, .81)
Cervical flexor endurance[26] ●	With patient supine with knees flexed and chin maximally retracted, subject lifts the head approximately 1 inch. The test was timed with a stopwatch and terminated when the subject lost maximal retraction	20 asymptomatic subjects	Intraexaminer ICC = .82–.91 Interexaminer ICC = .67–.78
		20 patients with neck pain	Interexaminer ICC = .67
Craniocervical flexion test[27] ●	With patient supine with a pressure biofeedback unit placed suboccipitally, subject performs a gentle head-nodding action of craniocervical flexion for five 10-second incremental stages of increasing range (22, 24, 26, 28, and 30 mm Hg). Performance was measured by the highest level of pressure the individual could hold for 10 seconds	10 asymptomatic subjects	Intraexaminer κ = .72
Cervical flexor endurance[28] ●	With patient supine with knees flexed, subject holds the tongue on the roof of the mouth and breathes normally. Subject then lifts his or her head off the table and holds it as long as possible with the neck in a neutral position. The test was timed with a stopwatch and terminated when the head moved more than 5 degrees either forward or backward	30 patients with grade II whiplash-associated disorders	Interexaminer ICC = .96

Reliability of Cervical Strength and Endurance Testing—cont'd

Test and Study Quality	Description and Positive Findings	Population	Reliability
Neck flexor endurance test[20] ◐	With patient supine with knees flexed and chin maximally retracted, subject lifts the head approximately 1 inch. The test was timed with a stopwatch and terminated when the subject lost maximal retraction	22 individuals with neck pain	Interexaminer ICC = .70 (.40, .87)
Neck flexor endurance test[29] ◐	With patient supine with knees flexed and chin maximally retracted, subject lifts the head approximately 1 inch. The test was timed with a stopwatch and terminated when the subject lost maximal retraction	22 individuals with neck pain	Interexaminer ICC = .73 (.45, .88)

Reliability of Cervical Movement Control Tests

Test and Study Quality	Description and Positive Findings	Population	Interexaminer Reliability
Active cervical extension in sitting[30] ◆	Patient is asked to "look toward the ceiling back with the eyes as far as possible." Positive if: Dominant upper cervical extension with minimal movement of the head posteriorly		κ = .73 (.29, .91)
Return to neutral from the cervical extension position in sitting[30] ◆	Patient asked to "return to neutral from the cervical extension position." Positive if: Initiates movement with sternocleidomastoid or anterior scalene muscles resulting in lower cervical flexion but not upper cranio-cervical flexion	15 patients with chronic neck pain	κ = .69 (.44, .90)
Active cervical rotation in sitting[30] ◐	Patient is asked to "rotate your head and neck as far as you can to each side while maintaining the plane of your face vertical and your eyes horizontal." Positive if: Rotation to either side occurs with concurrent/simultaneous lateral flexion, extension or flexion, and/or forward translation of the head and neck		κ = .81 (.58, 1.0)

Reliability of Assessing Limited Passive Intervertebral Motion

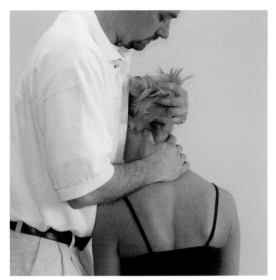

Testing rotation of C1-C2

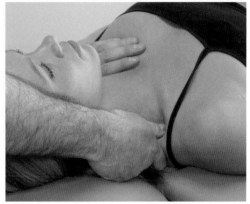

Testing of stiffness of 1st rib

Figure 3-22
Assessing limited passive intervertebral motion.

Test and Study Quality	Description and Positive Findings	Population	Interexaminer Reliability
Rotation of C1-C2[31] ◆	With patient seated, C2 is stabilized while C1 is rotated on C2 until the end of passive range of motion. Positive if decreased rotation is seen on one side compared with the contralateral side		κ = .28
Lateral flexion of C2-C3[31] ◆	With patient supine, examiner's left hand stabilizes the patient's head while the right hand performs side-bending flexion of C2-C3 until the end of passive range of motion. This is repeated in the contralateral direction. Positive if lateral flexion on one side is reduced compared with contralateral side	61 patients with nonspecific neck problems	κ = .43
Flexion and extension[31] ◆	With patient side-lying, examiner stabilizes the patient's neck with one hand while palpating the movement at C7-T1 with the other. Positive if flexion and extension are "stiff" compared with the vertebrae superior and inferior		κ = .36
First rib[31]◆	With patient supine, the cervical spine is rotated toward the side being tested. The first rib is pressed in a ventral and caudal direction. Positive if the rib is more "stiff" than the contralateral side		κ = .35

Reliability of Assessing Limited Passive Intervertebral Motion—cont'd

Test and Study Quality	Description and Positive Findings	Population	Interexaminer Reliability
Identification of hypomobile segment[32] ◆	With subject sitting, examiner palpates passive physiologic intervertebral motion at each cervical vertebra in rotation and lateral flexion and determines the most hypomobile segment	Three asymptomatic patients with single-level congenital fusions in the cervical spine (two at C2-C3 and one at C5-C6)	$\kappa = .68$
C0-C1[20] ◐	The therapist maximally flexes the lower cervical spine in supine and rotates the head to both directions. The rotation should be approximately 45 degrees and the therapist makes a determination if the range is normal hypomobile or hypermobile		$\kappa = .15\ (-.06, .49)$
C1-C2[20] ◐	Patient is supine and cervical spine is rotated approximately 30 degrees. An anterior to posterior glide through the occiput is performed and determined to be normal, hypomobile, or hypermobile	22 individuals with neck pain	$\kappa = .31\ (.04, .58)$
C2-C3[20] ◐			$\kappa = .30\ (.01, .56)$
C3-C4[20] ◐	Performed with the patient in supine. The therapist applies a lateral force through the articular pillar or the target segment. The therapist determines if the mobility is normal, hypomobile, or hypermobile		$\kappa = .22\ (-.07, .48)$
C4-C5[20] ◐			$\kappa = .43\ (.16, .67)$
C5-C6[20] ◐			$\kappa = .30\ (.01, .57)$
C6-C7[20] ◐			$\kappa = .23\ (-.07, .49)$

Reliability of Assessing Limited and Painful Passive Intervertebral Motion

Test and Study Quality	Description and Positive Findings	Population	Interexaminer Reliability			
			Limited Movements		Pain	
			Right	Left	Right	Left
C0-C1[6] ◆	With patient supine, examiner cradles the occiput with both hands and rotates the head 30 degrees toward the side to be tested; an anterior-to-posterior glide is performed to assess the amount of available motion compared with the contralateral side	22 patients with mechanical neck pain	$\kappa = -.26$ (−.57, .07)	$\kappa = .46$ (.06, .86)	$\kappa = -.52$ (−.09, −.14)	$\kappa = .08$ (−.37, .54)
C1-C2[6] ◆	With patient supine, examiner passively and maximally flexes the neck and then performs passive cervical rotation to one side and then to the other. The amount of motion to each side is compared, and if one side is determined to have less motion, it is considered to be "hypomobile"		$\kappa = .72$ (.43, .91)	$\kappa = .74$ (.40, 1.0)	$\kappa = .15$ (−.05, .36)	$\kappa = -.16$ (−.56, .22)
C0-C1[33] ◆	With patient supine, passive flexion is performed. Motion is classified as "limited" or "not limited" and patient pain response is assessed on 11-point numeric pain rating (NPR) scale		$\kappa = .29$	Not reported	ICC = .73	Not reported
C1-C2[33] ◆	With patient supine, rotation is performed and classified as "limited" or "not limited." Patient pain response is assessed on 11-point NPR scale	32 patients with neck pain	$\kappa = .20$	$\kappa = .37$	ICC = .56	ICC = .35
C2-C3[33] ◆			$\kappa = .34$	$\kappa = .63$	ICC = .50	ICC = .78
C3-C4[33] ◆			$\kappa = .20$	$\kappa = .26$	ICC = .62	ICC = .75
C4-C5[33] ◆	With patient supine, fixation of lower segment with side-bending to the right and left. Motion classified as "limited" or "not limited" and patient pain response assessed on 11-point NPR scale		$\kappa = .16$	$\kappa = -.09$	ICC = .62	ICC = .55
C5-C6[33] ◆			$\kappa = .17$	$\kappa = .09$	ICC = .66	ICC = .65
C6-C7[33] ◆			$\kappa = .34$	$\kappa = .03$	ICC = .59	ICC = .22
C7-T1[33] ◆			$\kappa = .08$	$\kappa = .14$	ICC = .45	ICC = .34
T1-T2[33] ◆			$\kappa = .33$	$\kappa = .46$	ICC = .80	ICC = .54

3

Cervical Spine

Reliability of Assessing Limited and Painful Passive Intervertebral Motion—cont'd

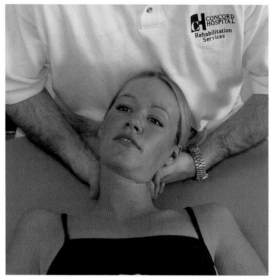

Testing side-bending of C5-C6

Figure 3-23
Assessing limited and painful passive intervertebral motion.

Test and Study Quality	Description and Positive Findings	Population	Interexaminer Reliability	
			Limited Movements	**Pain**
C2[6] ◆			κ = .01 (−.35, .38)	κ = .13 (−.04, .31)
C3[6] ◆	Posterior-to-anterior spring testing centrally over the spinous process of the vertebrae. Mobility judged as "normal," "hypomobile," or "hypermobile" and as "painful" or "not painful"	22 patients with mechanical neck pain	κ = .10 (−.25, .44)	κ = .13 (−.21, .47)
C4[6] ◆			κ = .10 (−.22, .40)	κ = .27 (−.12, .67)
C5[6] ◆			κ = .10 (−.15, .35)	κ = .12 (−.09, .42)
C6[6] ◆			κ = .01 (−.21, .24)	κ = .55 (.22, .88)
C7[6] ◆			κ = .54 (0.2, .88)	κ = .90 (.72, 1.0)
C0-C1 lateral glide[16] ◆			κ = .81 (.72, .91)	κ =32 (.15, .49)
C0-C1 lateral bend[16] ◆			κ = .35 (.08, .62)	κ = .35 (.15, .55)
C1-C2 rotation in full flexion[16] ◆			κ = .21 (.08, .34)	κ = .36 (.24, .49)
C1-C2 full lateral flexion[16] ◆	Mobility was recorded as "normal" or "hypomobile" when compared with the contralateral side. Pain reproduction recorded as "pain" or "no pain"	30 patients with neck pain	κ = .30 (.17, .43)	κ = .61 (.50, .72)
C2 lateral glide[16] ◆			κ = .46 (.33, .59)	κ = .42 (.28, .56)
C3 lateral glide[16] ◆			κ = .25 (.12, .38)	κ = .29 (.16, .43)
C4 lateral glide[16] ◆			κ = .27 (.13, .40)	κ = .65 (.54, .76)
C5 lateral glide[16] ◆			κ = .18 (.03, .33)	κ = .55 (.43, .67)
C6 lateral glide[16] ◆			κ = −.07 (−.34, .20)	κ = .76 (.64, .87)

Reliability of Assessing Passive Mobility in the Upper Cervical Spine for Detecting Ligament and Membrane Injuries

Test and Study Quality	Description and Positive Findings	Population	Reliability
Alar ligament, right[34] ◐	Passive stretching of the ligament or membrane by the examiner with the patient sitting in a chair is compared with MRI findings. Positive for examination if subjectively rated to have moderate or extensively increased motion by examiner. Positive for MRI when more than one third of structure showed increased signal intensity	92 subjects with chronic whiplash-associated disorder and 30 healthy individuals	Interexaminer $\kappa = .71$ (.58, .83)
Alar ligament, left[34] ◐			$\kappa = .69$ (.57, .82)
Transverse ligament[34] ◐			$\kappa = .69$ (.55, .83)
Tectorial membrane[34] ◐			$\kappa = .93$ (.83, 1.03)
Atlantooccipital membrane[34] ◐			$\kappa = .97$ (.92, 1.03)

Diagnostic Utility of Assessing Passive Mobility in the Upper Cervical Spine for Detecting Ligament and Membrane Injuries

Test and Study Quality	Description and Positive Findings	Population	Reference Standard	Sens	Spec	+LR	−LR
Alar ligament, right[34] ◆	Passive stretching of the ligament or membrane by examiner with the patient sitting in a chair is compared with MRI findings. Positive for examination if subjectively rated to have moderate or extensively increased motion by examiner. Positive for MRI when more than one third of structure showed increased signal intensity	92 subjects with chronic whiplash-associated disorder and 30 healthy individuals	MRI	.69 (.56, .81)	1.00 (1.00, 1.00)	Undefined	.31
Alar ligament, left[34] ◆				.72 (.60, .84)	.96 (.91, 1.00)	18	.29
Transverse ligament[34] ◆				.65 (.51, .79)	.99 (.96, 1.01)	65	.35
Tectorial membrane[34] ◆				.94 (.82, 1.06)	.99 (.97, 1.01)	94	.06
Atlantooccipital membrane[34] ◆				.96 (.87, 1.04)	1.00 (1.00, 1.00)	Undefined	.04

Cervical Spine

3

Diagnostic Utility of the Sharp-Purser Test for Cervical Instability

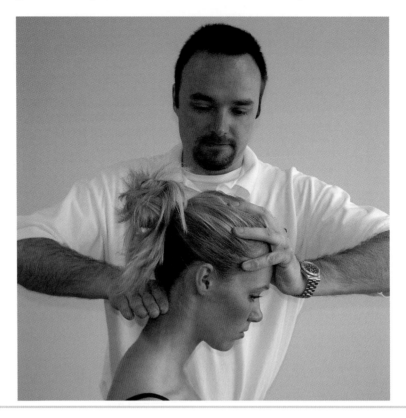

Figure 3-24
Sharp-Purser test.

Test and Study Quality	Description and Positive Findings	Population	Reference Standard	Sens	Spec	+LR	−LR
Sharp-Purser test[35] ● (see Video 3-1)	Patient sits with neck in a semiflexed position. Examiner places palm of one hand on patient's forehead and index finger of the other hand on the spinous process of axis. When posterior pressure is applied through the forehead, a sliding motion of the head posteriorly in relation to axis indicates a positive test for atlantoaxial instability	123 consecutive outpatients with rheumatoid arthritis	Full flexion and extension lateral radiographs. Atlantodens interval greater than 3 mm was considered abnormal	.69	.96	17.25	.32

Diagnostic Utility of Assessing Limited and Painful Passive Intervertebral Motion

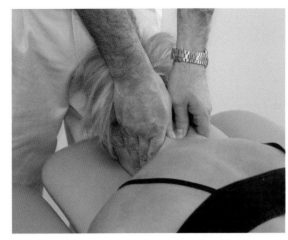

Posteroanterior central glides to the mid cervical spine

Figure 3-25
Assessing limited and painful passive intervertebral motion.

Test and Study Quality	Description and Positive Findings	Population	Reference Standard	Sens	Spec	+LR	−LR
Manual examination[36] ◆	Subjective examination, followed by central posterior-to-anterior glides, followed by passive physiologic intervertebral movements of flexion, extension, side-bending, and rotation. Joint dysfunction is diagnosed if the examiner concludes that the joint demonstrates an abnormal end feel and abnormal quality of resistance to motion and there is reproduction of pain	173 patients with cervical pain	Level of zygapophyseal pain via radiologically controlled diagnostic nerve block	.89 (.82, .96)	.47 (.37, .57)	1.7 (1.2, 2.5)	.23
Manual examination[37] ◆		20 patients with cervical pain		1.0 (.81, 1.0)*	1.0 (.51, 1.0)*	Unde-fined	.00
Identification of hypomobile segment[32] ◉	With subject sitting, examiner palpates passive physiologic intervertebral motion at each cervical vertebra in rotation and lateral flexion and determines the most hypomobile segment	Three asymptomatic patients with single-level congenital fusions in cervical spine (two at C2-C3 and one at C5-C6)	Level of congenital cervical fusion	.98	.74	3.77	.03

*Confidence intervals were not originally reported by Jull and colleagues[37] but were later calculated and presented by King and colleagues.[36]

Reliability of Assessing Pain with Palpation

Test and Study Quality		Description and Positive Findings	Population	Interexaminer Reliability
Midline neck tenderness[9] ◆		No details given	8924 adult patients who presented to emergency department after blunt trauma to head/neck and had Glasgow Coma Score of 15	κ = .78
Posterolateral neck tenderness[9] ◆				κ = .32
Maximal tenderness at midline[9] ◆				κ = .72
Upper cervical spinous process[38] ◉		Patient supine. Graded as "no tenderness," "moderate tenderness," or "marked tenderness"	52 patients referred for cervical myelography	κ = .47
Lower cervical spinous process[38] ◉				κ = .52
Right side of neck[38] ◉				κ = .24
Suprascapular area[38] ◉				(Right) κ = .42 (Left) κ = .44
Scapular area[38] ◉				(Right) κ = .34 (Left) κ = .56
Zygapophyseal joint pressure[39] ◉	High cervical	Method of classification for high, middle, and low not described		κ = .14 (−.12, .39)
	Middle cervical			κ = .37 (.12, .85)
	Low cervical			κ = .31 (.28, .90)
Occiput[39] ◉		No details	24 patients with headaches	(Right) κ = .00 (−1.00, .77) (Left) κ = .16 (−.31, .61)
Mastoid process[39] ◉				κ = .77 (.34, 1.00)
Sternocleidomastoid muscle[39] ◉	Insertion	Sternocleidomastoid insertion on occiput (minor occipital nerve)		(Right) κ = .68 (.29, 1.00) (Left) κ = .35 (−.17, .86)
	Anterior	Just anterior to sternocleidomastoid muscle border		(Right) κ = .35 (−.17, .86) (Left) κ = .55 (.10, .99)
	Middle	At sternocleidomastoid muscle border		(Right) κ = .52 (.12, .92) (Left) κ = .42 (.01, .82)
	Posterior	Just posterior to sternocleidomastoid muscle border		(Right) κ = .60 (.19, 1.00) (Left) κ = .87 (.62, 1.00)

Reliability of Assessing Pain with Palpation with and without a Patient History

Test and Study Quality	Description and Positive Findings	Population	Interexaminer Reliability	
			Without Knowledge of History	With Knowledge of History
Spinous processes C2-C3[40] ◆	No details given	100 patients with neck and/or shoulder problems with or without radiating pain	$\kappa = .60$	$\kappa = .49$
Spinous processes C4-C7[40] ◆			$\kappa = .42$	$\kappa = .50$
Spinous processes T1-T3[40] ◆			$\kappa = .55$	$\kappa = .79$
Paraspinal joints C1-C3[40] ◆			$\kappa = .32$	$\kappa = .22$
Paraspinal joints C4-C7[40] ◆			$\kappa = .34$	$\kappa = .55$
Paraspinal joints T1-T3[40] ◆			$\kappa = .41$	$\kappa = .51$
Neck muscles[40] ◆			$\kappa = .32$	$\kappa = .46$
Brachial plexus[40] ◆			$\kappa = .27$	$\kappa = .22$
Paraspinal muscles[40] ◆			$\kappa = -.04$	$\kappa = .46$

Reliability of Assessing Pain with Palpation in Patients with Cervicogenic Headache

Test and Study Quality	Description and Positive Findings	Population	Interexaminer Reliability
Articular pillars C0-C1[41] ◆	Patient prone with neck in neutral position. Examiner applies progressive unilateral posteroanterior pressure over articular pillars. Positive if patient's headache symptoms are reproduced	60 patients with cervicogenic headache based on criteria developed by International Headache Society	$\kappa = .64 \,(.40, .88)$
Articular pillars C1-C2[41] ◆			$\kappa = .71 \,(.51, .91)$
Articular pillars C2-C3[41] ◆			$\kappa = .70 \,(.52, .88)$
Articular pillars C3-C4[41] ◆			$\kappa = .61 \,(.37, .85)$

Diagnostic Utility of Assessing Pain with Palpation

Test and Measure Quality	Test Procedure and Determination of Positive Findings	Population	Reference Standard	Sens	Spec	+LR	−LR
Palpation over the facet joints in the cervical spine[23] ◑	Articulations were palpated 2 cm lateral to the spinous process. Positive if patient reported pain with procedure	75 males (22 with neck pain)	Patient reports of neck pain	.82	.79	3.90	.23

Reliability of Postural Assessment

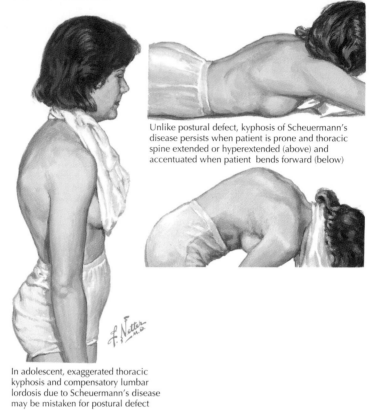

Unlike postural defect, kyphosis of Scheuermann's disease persists when patient is prone and thoracic spine extended or hyperextended (above) and accentuated when patient bends forward (below)

In adolescent, exaggerated thoracic kyphosis and compensatory lumbar lordosis due to Scheuermann's disease may be mistaken for postural defect

Figure 3-26
Thoracic kyphosis.

Reliability of Muscle Length Assessment

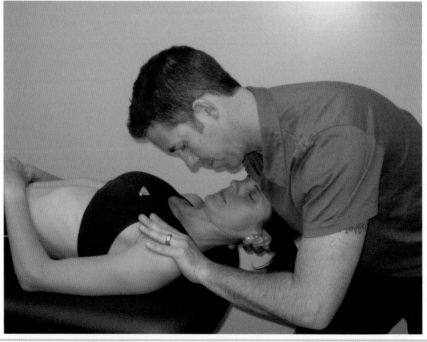

Figure 3-27
Muscle length assessment.

Reliability of Spurling's and Neck Compression Tests

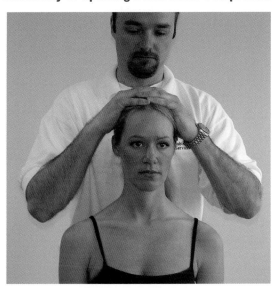

Figure 3-28
Cervical compression test.

Cervical Spine   3

Test and Study Quality		Description and Positive Findings	Population	Interexaminer Reliability
Straight compression[40] ◆		Patient seated with examiner standing behind patient. Examiner exerts pressure on head. Positive if pain is provoked	100 patients with neck and/or shoulder problems with or without radiating pain	$\kappa = .34$ without knowledge of patient history $\kappa = .44$ with knowledge of patient history
Spurling's A[7] ◆		Patient seated with neck side-bent toward ipsilateral side; 7 kg of overpressure is applied	50 patients with suspected cervical radiculopathy or carpal tunnel syndrome	$\kappa = .60$ (.32, .87)
Spurling's B[7] ◆		Patient seated with extension and side-bending/rotation to ipsilateral side; 7 kg of overpressure is applied		$\kappa = .62$ (.25, .99)
Spurling's to the right[40] ◆		Cervical compression performed with patient seated. Examiner passively rotates and side-bends head to right or left and applies compression force of 7 kg. Presence and location of pain, paresthesias, or numbness are recorded	100 patients with neck and/or shoulder problems with or without radiating pain	$\kappa = .37$ without knowledge of patient history $\kappa = .28$ with knowledge of patient history
Spurling's to the left[40] ◆				$\kappa = .37$ without knowledge of patient history $\kappa = .46$ with knowledge of patient history
Neck compression with[38]: ●	Right shoulder/arm pain	Cervical compression performed with patient sitting. Examiner passively rotates and side-bends the head to the right and/or left. A compression force of 7 kg is applied. Presence and location of pain, paresthesias, or numbness are recorded	52 patients referred for cervical myelography	(Right) $\kappa = .61$ (Left) Not available
	Left shoulder/arm pain			(Right) Not available (Left) $\kappa = .40$
	Right forearm/hand pain			(Right) $\kappa = .77$ (Left) $\kappa = .54$
	Left forearm/hand pain			(Right) Not available (Left) $\kappa = .62$
Spurling's test[20] ●		Patient seated with neck side-bent toward ipsilateral side; 7 kg of overpressure is applied	22 individuals with neck pain	$\kappa = .13$ (−.19, .45)

Diagnostic Utility of Spurling's Test

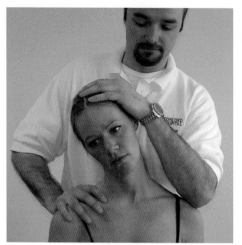

Spurling's A test

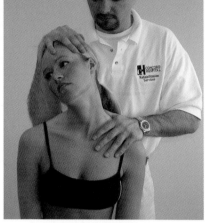

Spurling's B test

Figure 3-29
Spurling's test.

Test and Study Quality	Description and Positive Findings	Population	Reference Standard	Sens	Spec	+LR	−LR
Spurling's A[7] ◆	Patient is seated, the neck is side-bent toward the ipsilateral side, and 7 kg of overpressure is applied (see Fig. 3-29). Positive if symptoms are reproduced	82 consecutive patients referred to electrophysiologic laboratory with suspected diagnosis of cervical radiculopathy or carpal tunnel syndrome	Cervical radiculopathy via needle electromyography and nerve conduction studies	.50 (.27, .73)	.86 (.77, .94)	3.5 (1.6, 7.5)	.58 (.36, .94)
Spurling's B[7] ◆	Patient seated. Extension and side-bending/rotation to the ipsilateral side and then 7 kg of overpressure is applied (see Fig. 3-29). Positive if symptoms are reproduced			.50 (.27, .73)	.74 (.63, .85)	1.9 (1.0, 3.6)	.67 (.42, 1.1)

Diagnostic Utility of Spurling's Test—cont'd

Test and Study Quality	Description and Positive Findings	Population	Reference Standard	Sens	Spec	+LR	−LR
Spurling's test[42] ◆ (see Video 3-2)	The patient's neck is extended and rotated for the suspected involved side prior to axial compression. Positive with radicular pain that radiates into the upper extremity	257 patients who had symptoms of unilateral cervical radiculopathy lasting for at least 4 weeks	Cervical radiculopathy via CT scanning	.95	.94	15.8	.05
Spurling's test[43] ◆	The patient's neck is extended and laterally flexed toward the involved side, and downward axial pressure is applied on the head. Positive if radicular pain or tingling in the upper limb is reproduced or aggravated	50 patients presenting to neurosurgery with neck and arm pain suggestive of radicular pain	Soft lateral cervical disc prolapse via MRI	.93 (.84, 1.0)	.95 (.86, 1.0)	18.6	.07
Spurling's test[44] ◉	Patient side-bends and extends the neck, and examiner applies compression. Positive if pain or tingling that starts in the shoulder radiates distally to the elbow	255 consecutive patients referred to physiatrist for upper extremity nerve disorders	Cervical radiculopathy via electrodiagnostic testing	.30	.93	4.29	.75
Spurling's test[23] ◉	Extension of the neck with rotation and side-bending to the same side. Positive if subject reports pain with procedure	75 males (22 with neck pain)	Patient reports of neck pain	.77	.92	9.63	.25
Spurling's test[45] ◉	Patient was seated, and the examiner pushed patient's head downward while the head was laterally flexed to the affected side. Reproduction of pain was considered a positive finding	97 patients who referred to an electrodiagnostic center with neck and arm pain	Electrodiagnostic studies	Acute: .47 Chronic: .147	Acute: .85 Chronic: .85	Acute: 3.1* Chronic: .98*	Acute: .62 Chronic: 1.0

*Values were calculated by the authors of this text.

Reliability of Neck Distraction and Traction Tests

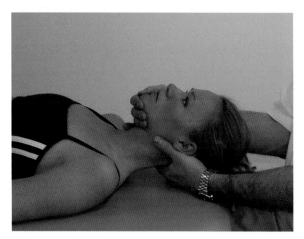

Neck distraction test

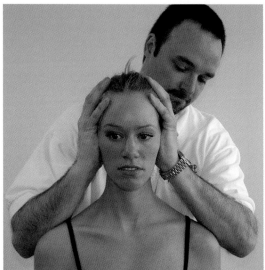

Traction test

Figure 3-30
Neck distraction and traction tests.

Test and Study Quality	Description and Positive Findings	Population	Interexaminer Reliability
Neck distraction test[7] ◆	With patient supine, examiner grasps patient under chin and occiput while slightly flexing patient's neck while applying distraction force of 14 pounds. Positive if symptoms are reduced	50 patients with suspected cervical radiculopathy or carpal tunnel syndrome	κ = .88 (.64, 1.0)
Traction[40] ◆	With patient seated, examiner stands behind patient with hands underneath each maxilla and thumbs on the back of the head. Positive if symptoms are reduced during traction	100 patients with neck and/or shoulder problems with or without radiating pain	κ = .56 without knowledge of history κ = .41 with knowledge of history
Axial manual traction[38] ◉	With patient supine, examiner applies axial distraction force of 10-15 kg. Positive if radicular symptoms decrease	52 patients referred for cervical myelography	κ = .50
Distraction test[20] ◉	With patient supine, examiner grasps patient under chin and occiput while slightly flexing patient's neck while applying distraction force of 14 pounds. Positive if symptoms are reduced	22 individuals with neck pain	κ = .35 (.07, .63)

Reliability of Cervical Flexion-Rotation Test

Test and Study Quality	Description and Positive Findings	Population	Interexaminer Reliability
Cervical flexion-rotation test[46]	With patient supine and the cervical spine passively maximally flexed, the examiner passively rotates head left and right. Positive if subject reports onset of pain or if examiner encounters firm resistance at an estimated range of motion that is reduced by more than 10 degrees from normal of 44 degrees	15 subjects with cervicogenic headache evaluated on headache-free days and 10 asymptomatic subjects	$\kappa = .50$

Cervical Spine

3

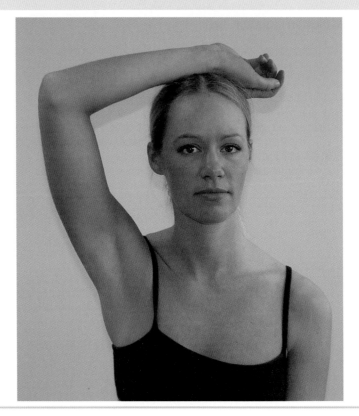

Figure 3-31
Shoulder abduction test.

Reliability of Shoulder Abduction Test

Test and Study Quality	Description and Positive Findings	Population	Interexaminer Reliability
Shoulder abduction test[7] ◆	Patient is seated and asked to place the symptomatic extremity on head. Positive if symptoms are reduced	50 patients with suspected cervical radiculopathy or carpal tunnel syndrome	$\kappa = .20$ (.00, .59)
Shoulder abduction test[38] ●	Patient is seated and asked to raise the symptomatic extremity above the head. Positive if symptoms are reduced	52 patients referred for cervical myelography	(Right) $\kappa = .21$ (Left) $\kappa = .40$

Diagnostic Utility of Shoulder Abduction Test

Test and Study Quality	Description and Positive Findings	Population	Reference Standard	Sens	Spec	+LR	−LR
Shoulder abduction test[45] ●	The patient was seated and actively placed the palm of the affected extremity on top of the head. Positive signs were noted if this position relieved radicular pain	97 patients who referred to an electrodiagnostic center with neck and arm pain	Electrodiagnostic studies	Acute: .558 Chronic: .21	Acute: .85 Chronic: .85	Acute: 3.7* Chronic: 1.4*	Acute: .52* Chronic: .93*

*Values were calculated by the authors of this text.

Reliability of Neural Tension Tests

Test and Study Quality	Description and Positive Findings	Population	Interexaminer Reliability
Upper limb tension test A[7] ◆	With patient supine, examiner performs the following movements: 1. Scapular depression 2. Shoulder abduction 3. Forearm supination 4. Wrist and finger extension 5. Shoulder lateral rotation 6. Elbow extension 7. Contralateral/ipsilateral cervical side-bending Positive response defined by any of the following: 1. Patient symptoms reproduced 2. Side-to-side differences in elbow extension of more than 10 degrees 3. Contralateral cervical side-bending increases symptoms or ipsilateral side-bending decreases symptoms	50 patients with suspected cervical radiculopathy or carpal tunnel syndrome	$\kappa = .76\ (.51, 1.0)$
Upper limb tension test B[7] ◆	With patient supine and shoulder abducted 30 degrees, examiner performs the following movements: 1. Scapular depression 2. Shoulder medial rotation 3. Full elbow extension 4. Wrist and finger flexion 5. Contralateral/ipsilateral cervical side-bending Positive response defined by any of the following: 1. Patient symptoms reproduced 2. Side-to-side differences in wrist flexion of more than 10 degrees 3. Contralateral cervical side-bending increases symptoms or ipsilateral side-bending decreases symptoms		$\kappa = .83\ (.65, 1.0)$
Brachial plexus test[38] ●	With patient supine, examiner abducts the humerus to the limit of pain-free motion and then adds lateral rotation of the arm and elbow flexion. If no limitation of motion is noted, the humerus is abducted to 90 degrees. The appearance of symptoms is recorded	52 patients referred for cervical myelography	(Right) $\kappa = .35$ Left was not calculated because prevalence of positive findings was less than 10%
Upper limb tension test[20] ●	With patient supine, examiner performs the following movements: 1. Scapular depression 2. Shoulder abduction 3. Forearm supination 4. Wrist and finger extension 5. Shoulder lateral rotation 6. Elbow extension 7. Contralateral/ipsilateral cervical side-bending Positive response defined by any of the following: 1. Patient symptoms reproduced side-to-side differences in elbow extension of more than 10 degrees 2. Contralateral cervical side-bending increases symptoms or ipsilateral side-bending decreases symptoms	22 individuals with neck pain	$\kappa = .36\ (.04, .68)$

Cervical Spine

3

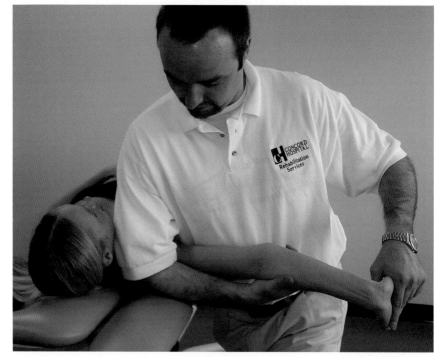

Test A

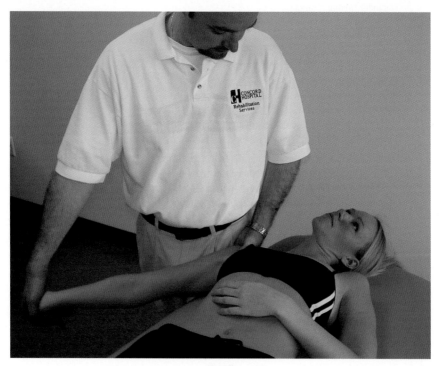

Test B

Figure 3-32
Upper limb tension tests.

Diagnostic Utility of Neural Tension Tests for Cervical Radiculopathy

Test and Study Quality	Description and Positive Findings	Population	Reference Standard	Sens	Spec	+LR	−LR
Upper limb tension test A[7] ●	With patient supine, examiner performs the following movements: 1. Scapular depression 2. Shoulder abduction 3. Forearm supination 4. Wrist and finger extension 5. Shoulder lateral rotation 6. Elbow extension 7. Contralateral and ipsilateral cervical side-bending Positive response defined by any of the following: 1. Patient symptoms reproduced 2. Side-to-side differences in elbow extension of more than 10 degrees 3. Contralateral cervical side-bending increases symptoms or ipsilateral side-bending decreases symptoms	82 consecutive patients referred to electrophysiologic laboratory with suspected diagnosis of cervical radiculopathy or carpal tunnel syndrome	Cervical radiculopathy via needle electromyography and nerve conduction studies	.97 (.90, 1.0)	.22 (.12, .33)	1.3 (1.1, 1.5)	.12 (.01, 1.9)
Upper limb tension test B[7] ●	With patient supine and patient's shoulder abducted 30 degrees, examiner performs the following movements: 1. Scapular depression 2. Shoulder medial rotation 3. Full elbow extension 4. Wrist and finger flexion 5. Contralateral and ipsilateral cervical side-bending Positive response defined by any of the following: 1. Patient symptoms reproduced 2. Side-to-side differences in wrist flexion of more than 10 degrees 3. Contralateral cervical side-bending increases symptoms or ipsilateral side-bending decreases symptoms			.72 (.52, .93)	.33 (.21, .45)	1.1 (.77, 1.5)	.85, (.37, 1.9)

Continued

Cervical Spine

3

Diagnostic Utility of Neural Tension Tests for Cervical Radiculopathy—cont'd

Test and Study Quality	Description and Positive Findings	Population	Reference Standard	Sens	Spec	+LR	−LR
Upper limb tension test[23] ●	With patient seated and arm in extension, abduction and external rotation of the glenohumeral joint, extension of the elbow, the forearm in supination, and the wrist and fingers in extension. Contralateral flexion of the neck is added. Positive if patient reported pain with procedure	75 males (22 with neck pain)	Patient reports of neck pain	.77	.94	12.83	.25
Upper limb tension test[45] ●	The patient was supine while the affected arm was placed on his/her body. In the first step, the arm was abducted passively by the examiner with the patient's forearm in pronation and elbow in flexion. Then the forearm was supinated, and the elbow extended. Finally, the patient's wrist was extended. Reproduction of the pain in any step was considered as a positive sign	97 patients who referred to an electrodiagnostic center with neck and arm pain	Electrodiagnostic studies	Acute: .605 Chronic: .353	Acute: .40 Chronic: .40	Acute: 1.0* Chronic: .59*	Acute: .99* Chronic: 1.6*

*Values were calculated by the authors of this text.

Reliability of the Arm Squeeze Test in Distinguishing Cervical Nerve Root Compression from Shoulder Pain

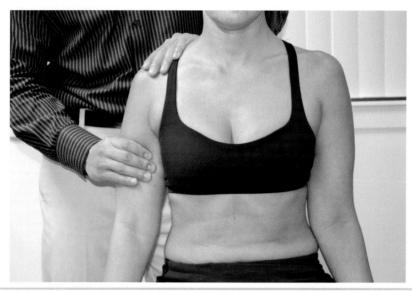

Figure 3-33
Arm squeeze test.

Test and Study Quality	Description and Positive Findings	Population	Reliability
Arm squeeze test[47] ● (see Video 3-3)	Examiner squeezes the middle third of the patient's upper arm with thumb on patient's triceps and fingers on patient's biceps with moderate compression (5.9 to 8.1 kg). Positive if patient reports 3 points or higher on visual analog scale (VAS) with pressure on middle third of upper arm compared with acromioclavicular joint and subacromial area	305 patients with cervical nerve root compression, 903 patients with rotator cuff tear, and 350 healthy volunteers	Intraexaminer $\kappa = .87$ (.85, .89) Interexaminer $\kappa = .81$ (.79, .82)

Diagnostic Utility of the Arm Squeeze Test in Distinguishing Cervical Nerve Root Compression from Shoulder Pain

Test and Study Quality	Description and Positive Findings	Population	Reference Standard	Sens	Spec	+LR	−LR
Arm squeeze test[47] ◆	Examiner squeezes the middle third of the patient's upper arm with thumb on patient's triceps and fingers on patient's biceps with moderate compression (5.9 to 8.1 kg). Positive if patient reports 3 points or higher on VAS with pressure on middle third of upper arm compared with acromioclavicular joint and subacromial area	305 patients with cervical nerve root compression, 903 patients with rotator cuff tear, and 350 healthy volunteers	Diagnosis of cervical nerve root compression (C5-T1) based on clinical examination, electromyography, x-rays, and MRI	.96 (.85, .99)	.96 (.86, .98)	24	.04

Cervical Spine 3

Diagnostic Utility of Brachial Plexus Compression for Cervical Cord Compression

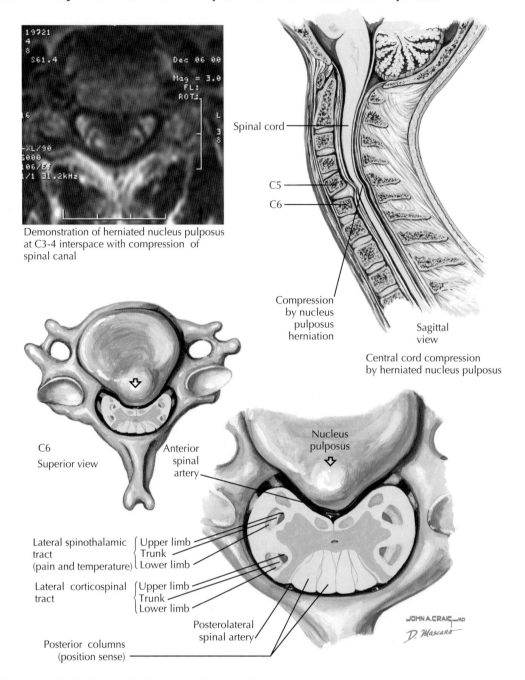

Demonstration of herniated nucleus pulposus at C3-4 interspace with compression of spinal canal

Spinal cord

C5

C6

Compression by nucleus pulposus herniation

Sagittal view

Central cord compression by herniated nucleus pulposus

C6
Superior view

Anterior spinal artery

Nucleus pulposus

Lateral spinothalamic tract (pain and temperature) { Upper limb / Trunk / Lower limb

Lateral corticospinal tract { Upper limb / Trunk / Lower limb

Posterolateral spinal artery

Posterior columns (position sense)

JOHN A. CRAIG—AD
D. Mascaro

Figure 3-34
Cervical disc herniation causing cord compression.

Test and Study Quality	Description and Positive Findings	Population	Reference Standard	Sens	Spec	+LR	−LR
Compression of brachial plexus[48] ●	Firm compression and squeezing of the brachial plexus with the thumb. Positive only when pain radiates to the shoulder or upper extremity	65 patients who had undergone MRI of cervical spine as result of radiating pain	Cervical cord compression via MRI	.69	.83	4.06	.37

Reliability of Tests for Cervical Myelopathy

Test and Study Quality	Description and Positive Findings	Population	Interexaminer Reliability
Hoffmann sign[49] ◆	With the patient standing or sitting, the clinician stabilizes the proximal interphalangeal joint of the middle finger and applies a stimulus to the middle finger by "flicking" the fingernail between his thumb and index finger into a flexed position. Positive with adduction of the thumb and flexion of the fingers		$\kappa = .76$ (.56, .96)
Deep tendon reflex test[49] ◆	In biceps tendon testing, the patient assumes a sitting position while the clinician places the patient's slightly supinated forearm on the clinician's own forearm, ensuring relaxation. The clinician's thumb is placed on the patient's biceps tendon, and the clinician strikes his own thumb with quick strikes of a reflex hammer. In triceps tendon testing, the sitting patient's elbow is flexed passively via shoulder elevation to approximately 90 degrees. The clinician then places his thumb over the distal aspect of the triceps tendon and applies a series of quick strikes of the reflex hammer to his own thumb. Positive with hyperreflexia	51 patients with cervical pain as primary complaint	$\kappa = .73$ (.50, .95)
Inverted supinator sign[49] ◆	With the patient in a seated position, the clinician places the patient's slightly pronated forearm on his forearm to ensure relaxation. The clinician applies a series of quick strikes near the styloid process of the radius at the attachment of the brachioradialis tendon. The test is performed in the same manner as a brachioradialis tendon reflex test. Positive with finger flexion or slight elbow extension		$\kappa = .52$ (.26, .78)
Suprapatellar quadriceps test[49] ◆	With the patient sitting with his or her feet off the ground, the clinician applies quick strikes of the reflex hammer to the suprapatellar tendon. Positive with hyperreflexive knee extension		$\kappa = .68$ (.46, .89)
Hand withdrawal reflex[49] ◆	With the patient sitting or standing, the clinician grasps the patient's palm and strikes the dorsum of the patient's hand with a reflex hammer. Positive with abnormal flexor response		$\kappa = .55$ (.34, .82)
Babinski sign[49] ◆	With the patient supine, the clinician supports the patient's foot in neutral and applies stimulation to the plantar aspect of the foot (typically from lateral to medial from heel to metatarsal) with the blunt end of a reflex hammer. Positive with great toe extension and fanning of the second through fifth toes		$\kappa = .56$ (.24, .89)
Clonus[49] ◆	With the patient sitting with his or her feet off the ground, the clinician applies a quick stretch to the Achilles tendon via rapid passive dorsiflexion of the ankle. Positive when ankle "beats" in and out of dorsiflexion for at least three beats		$\kappa = .66$ (.03, .99)

Cervical Spine 3

Diagnostic Utility of Tests for Cervical Myelopathy

Test and Study Quality	Description and Positive Findings	Popula-tion	Reference Standard	Sens	Spec	+LR	−LR
Hoffmann sign[49] ◆	With the patient standing or sitting, the clinician stabilizes the proximal interphalangeal joint of the middle finger and applies a stimulus to the middle finger by "flicking" the fingernail between his thumb and index finger into a flexed position. Positive with adduction of the thumb and flexion of the fingers			.44 (.28, .58)	.75 (.63, .86)	1.8 (.80, 4.1)	.70 (.50, 1.1)
Deep tendon reflex test[49] ◆	In biceps tendon testing, clinician places the patient's slightly supinated forearm on his own forearm, ensuring relaxation. The clinician's thumb is placed on the patient's biceps tendon, and the clinician strikes his own thumb with quick strikes of a reflex hammer. In triceps tendon testing, the patient's elbow is flexed passively via shoulder elevation to approximately 90 degrees. The clinician then places his thumb over the distal aspect of the triceps tendon and applies a series of quick strikes of the reflex hammer to his own thumb. Positive with hyperreflexia	51 patients with cervical pain as primary complaint	Cervical myelopathy via MRI	.44 (.28, .59)	.71 (.59, .82)	1.5 (.70, 3.4)	.80 (.50, 1.2)
Inverted supinator sign[49] ◆	With the patient in a seated position, the clinician places the patient's slightly pronated forearm on his forearm to ensure relaxation. The clinician applies a series of quick strikes near the styloid process of the radius at the attachment of the brachioradialis tendon. The test is performed in the same manner as a brachioradialis tendon reflex test. Positive with finger flexion or slight elbow extension			.61 (.44, .74)	.78 (.65, .88)	2.8 (1.2, 6.4)	.50 (.30, .90)
Supra-patellar quadriceps test[49] ◆	With the patient sitting with his or her feet off the ground, the clinician applies quick strikes of the reflex hammer to the suprapatellar tendon. Positive with hyperreflexive knee extension			.56 (.39, .72)	.33 (.22, .46)	.80 (.50, 1.3)	1.3 (.60, 2.8)

Diagnostic Utility of Tests for Cervical Myelopathy—cont'd

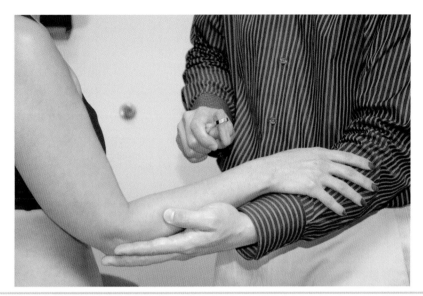

Figure 3-35
Inverted supinator sign.

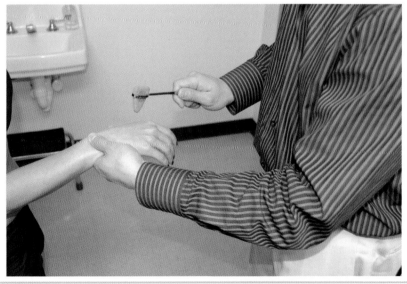

Figure 3-36
Hand withdrawal reflex.

Diagnostic Utility of Tests for Cervical Myelopathy—cont'd

Test and Study Quality	Description and Positive Findings	Popula-tion	Reference Standard	Sens	Spec	+LR	−LR
Hand withdrawal reflex[49] ◆	With the patient sitting or standing, the clinician grasps the patient's palm and strikes the dorsum of the patient's hand with a reflex hammer. Positive with abnormal flexor response	82 con-secutively referred patients with suspected cervical ra-diculopathy or CTS	Electro-physiologic examina-tion	.41 (.25, .58)	.63 (.51, .75)	1.1 (.50, 2.3)	.90 (.60, 1.5)
Babinski sign[49] ◆	With the patient supine, the clinician supports the patient's foot in neutral and applies stimulation to the plantar aspect of the foot (typically from lateral to medial from heel to metatarsal) with the blunt end of a reflex hammer. Positive with great toe extension and fanning of the second through fifth toes			.33 (.19, .41)	.92 (.81, .98)	4.0 (1.1, 16.6)	.70 (.60, .90)
Clonus[49] ◆	With the patient sitting with his or her feet off the ground, the clinician applies a quick stretch to the Achilles tendon via rapid passive dorsiflexion of the ankle. Positive when ankle "beats" in and out of dorsiflexion for at least three beats			.11 (.30, .16)	.96 (.90, .99)	2.7 (.40, 20.1)	.90 (.80, 1.1)
Hoffman sign[50] ◉	Examiner uses their thumb to press on the patient's middle fingernail. The exam-iner then slid the thumb of the patient's distal end of the fingernail causing the distal phalanx to flick back into extension. A positive response is noted if the patient flexed the distal phalanx of both the thumb and index finger	85 indi-viduals with cervical-spondylosis related problems	Magnetic resonance imaging	.76	.93	10.9*	.26*
Tromner sign[50] ◉	The examiner flicks the volar surface of the distal phalanx of the patient's middle finger. A positive response is noted if the patient flexed the distal phalanx of both the thumb and index finger			.94	.82	5.2*	.07*
Inverted radial reflex[50] ◉	The examiner supports the patient's arm in a neutral position between supination and pronation with the wrist in ulnar deviation. The radial aspect of the forearm was tapped 6 cm from the radial styloid process. A positive response was noted if there was an involuntary flexion of the ipsilateral fingers			.76	.86	5.4*	.28*
Babinski[50] ◉	The examiner rubbed the lateral border of the patient's foot with the blunt end of a reflex hammer in a proximal to distal direction then medially across the ball of the foot. A positive sign was noted if extension of the great toe and fanning of the lesser toes occurred			.36	1.0	Infin-ity*	.64*

*Values were calculated by the authors of this text.

Diagnostic Utility of Clusters of Tests for Cervical Myelopathy

Cook and colleagues[51] identified a test item cluster, or an optimal combination of clinical examination tests, that may be useful in identifying patients with cervical myelopathy. The five clinical findings listed below demonstrated the capacity to rule out cervical myelopathy when clustered into one of five positive findings and rule in cervical myelopathy when clustered into three of five positive findings.

Test and Study Quality	Description and Positive Findings	Population	Reference Standard	Sens	Spec	+LR	−LR
Gait deviation + Positive Hoffmann test + Inverted supinator sign + Positive Babinski test + Age over 45 years[51] ●	One of five positive tests	249 consecutive patients with primary complaint of cervical pain or dysfunction seen at university spine surgery center	Diagnosis of cervical myelopathy was confirmed or ruled out using MRI	.94 (.89, .97)	.31 (.27, .32)	1.4 (1.2, 1.4)	.18 (.12, .42)
	Three of five positive tests			.19 (.15, .20)	.99 (.97, .99)	30.9 (5.5, 181.8)	.81 (.79, .87)

Cervical Spine

3

Diagnostic Utility of Clusters of Tests for Cervical Radiculopathy

Wainner and colleagues[7] identified a test item cluster, or an optimal combination of clinical examination tests, that can determine the likelihood that a patient is presenting with cervical radiculopathy. The four predictor variables most likely to identify patients presenting with cervical radiculopathy are the upper limb tension test A, the Spurling's A test, the distraction test, and cervical rotation of less than 60 degrees to the ipsilateral side.

Test and Study Quality	Description and Positive Findings	Population	Reference Standard	Sens	Spec	+LR	−LR
Upper limb tension test A + Spurling's A test + Distraction test + Cervical rotation of less than 60 degrees to the ipsilateral side[7] ◆	All four tests positive	82 consecutive patients referred to electrophysiologic laboratory with suspected diagnosis of cervical radiculopathy or carpal tunnel syndrome	Cervical radiculopathy via needle electromyography and nerve conduction studies	.24 (.05, .43)	.99 (.97, 1.0)	30.3 (1.7, 38.2)	Not reported
	Any three tests positive			.39 (.16, .61)	.94 (.88, 1.0)	6.1 (2.0, 18.6)	
	Any two tests positive			.39 (.16, .61)	.56 (.43, .68)	.88 (1.5, 2.5)	

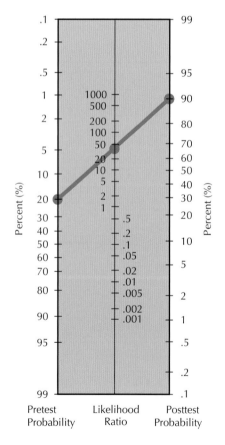

Figure 3-37

Fagan's nomogram. Considering the 20% prevalence or pretest probability of cervical radiculopathy in the study by Wainner and colleagues, the nomogram demonstrates the major shifts in probability that occur when all four tests from the cluster are positive (see Wainner RS, Fritz JM, Irrgang JJ, et al. Reliability and diagnostic accuracy of the clinical examination and patient self-report measures for cervical radiculopathy. *Spine.* 2003;28:52-62). (Reprinted with permission from Fagan TJ. Letter: Nomogram for Bayes theorem. *N Engl J Med.* 1975;293:257. Copyright 2005, Massachusetts Medical Society. All rights reserved.)

Clinical Prediction Rule to Identify Patients with Neck Pain Who Are Likely to Benefit from Cervical Thrust Manipulation

Puentedura and colleagues[52] developed a clinical prediction rule for identifying patients with neck pain who are likely to benefit from cervical thrust manipulation. The result of their study demonstrated that if three or more of the four attributes (symptom duration less than 38 days, positive expectation that manipulation will help, side-to-side difference in cervical rotation range of motion of 10 degrees or more, and pain with posteroanterior spring testing of the middle cervical spine) were present, the +LR was 13.5 (95% CI 1.0, 328.3) and the probability of experiencing a successful outcome improved from 39% to 90%.

Diagnostic Utility of Single Factors and Combinations of Factors for Identifying a Positive Short-Term Clinical Outcome for Cervical Radiculopathy

We used the baseline examination and physical therapy interventions received to investigate predictors for short-term improvement in patients with cervical radiculopathy.[53] Patients were treated at the discretion of their physical therapist for a mean of 6.4 visits over an average of 28 days. In addition to identifying the single factors most strongly associated with improvement, we used logistic regression to identify the combination of factors most predictive of short-term improvement.

Test and Study Quality	Description and Positive Findings	Population	Reference Standard	Sens	Spec	+LR	−LR
Age less than 54 years[53] ◆	Self-report			.76 (.64, .89)	.52 (.38, .67)	1.5 (1.2, 2.1)	
Dominant arm is not affected[53] ◆	Self-report			.74 (.62, .86)	.52 (.38, .67)	1.5 (1.1, 2.2)	
Looking down does not worsen symptoms[53] ◆	Self-report	96 patients referred to physical therapy with cervical radiculopathy as defined by being positive on all four items in Wainner's diagnostic test item cluster[7] (see previous section on Diagnostic Utility of Clusters of Tests for Cervical Radiculopathy)	Improvement at physical therapy discharge as defined by surpassing the minimal detectable change in all outcome measures	.68 (.55, .81)	.48 (.34, .62)	1.3 (.93, 1.8)	
More than 30 degrees of cervical flexion[53] ◆	Patient sitting. Used an inclinometer after two warm-up repetitions			.56 (.42, .70)	.59 (.44, .73)	1.4 (.89, 2.1)	Not reported
Age less than 54 years + Dominant arm is not affected + Looking down does not worsen symptoms + Provided with multimodal treatment, including manual therapy, cervical traction, and deep neck flexor muscle strengthening for 50% or more of visits[53] ◆	All four tests positive			.18 (.07, .29)	.98 (.94, 1.0)	8.3 (1.9, 63.9)	
	Any three tests positive			.68 (.55, .81)	.87 (.77, .97)	5.2 (2.4, 11.3)	
	Any two tests positive			.94 (.87, 1.0)	.37 (.23, .51)	1.5 (1.2, 1.9)	
	Any one test positive			1.0 (1.0, 1.0)	.08 (.01, .20)	1.1 (1.0, 2.0)	

Cervical Spine

3

Diagnostic Utility of Historical and Physical Examination Findings for Immediate Improvement with Cervical Manipulation

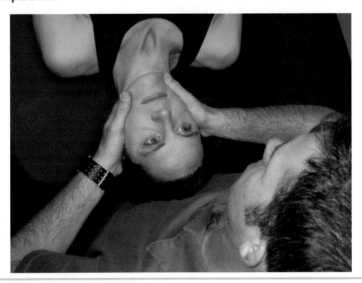

Figure 3-38
Cervical manipulation. Delivered by Tseng and colleagues at the discretion of the therapist to the most hypomobile segments. "Once a hypomobile segment was localized, the manipulator carefully flexed and sidebent the patient's neck to lock the facet joints of other spinal segments until the barrier was reached. A specific cervical manipulation with a high-velocity, low-amplitude thrust force was then exerted on the specific, manipulable lesion to gap the facet." (See Tseng YL, Wang WT, Chen WY, et al. Predictors for the immediate responders to cervical manipulation in patients with neck pain. *Man Ther.* 2006;11:306-315.)

Test and Study Quality	Description and Positive Findings	Population	Reference Standard	Sens	Spec	+LR	−LR
Initial Neck Disability Index score over 11.5 + Bilateral involvement pattern + Not performing sedentary work for longer than 5 hours/day + Feeling better while moving the neck + Without feeling worse while extending the neck + Diagnosis of spondylosis without radiculopathy[54] ◆	Five or six tests positive	100 patients referred to physical therapy for neck pain	Immediate improvement after cervical manipulation as determined by any of the following: 1. Decrease of 50% or more in score on NPRS 2. Score of 4 or higher (much improved) on Global Rating of Change (GROC) scale 3. Patient satisfaction rating of "very satisfied" after manipulation	.07 (.00, .13)	1.00 (1.00, 1.00)	Undefined	Not reported
	Any four tests positive			.40 (.28, .52)	.93 (.84, 1.00)	5.33 (1.72, 16.54)	
	Any three tests positive			.43 (.31, .56)	.78 (.65, .90)	1.93 (1.01, 3.67)	
	Any two tests positive			.08 (.01, .15)	.57 (.42, .73)	.20 (.08, .49)	
	Any one test positive			.02 (−.02, .05)	.75 (.62, .88)	.07 (.01, .50)	

Diagnostic Utility of a Cluster of Historical and Physical Examination Findings for Immediate Improvement with Thoracic Manipulation

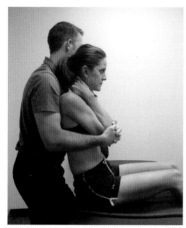
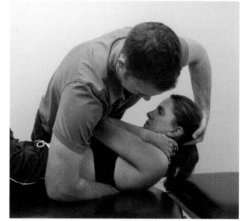

All patients received a standardized series of 3 thrust manipulations directed at the thoracic spine. In the first technique (A), with the patient sitting, the therapist uses his or her sternum as a fulcrum on the patient's middle thoracic spine and applies a high-velocity distraction thrust in an upward direction. The second and third techniques (B) are delivered supine. The therapist uses his or her body to push down through the patient's arms to perform a high-velocity, low-amplitude thrust directed toward either T1 through T4 or T5 through T8.[46]

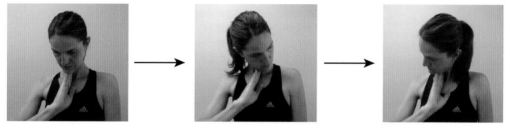

After the manipulations, patients were instructed in a cervical range-of-motion exercise to perform 3-4 times/day.[46]

Figure 3-39
Thoracic spine manipulation and active range of motion.

Diagnostic Utility of Historical and Physical Examination Findings for Improvement with Three Weeks of Mechanical Cervical Traction

Test and Study Quality	Description and Positive Findings	Population	Reference Standard	Sens	Spec	+LR	−LR
Neck distraction test[55] ◆	Patient lies supine and the neck is comfortably positioned. Examiner securely grasps the patient's head under the occiput and chin and gradually applies an axial traction force of up to approximately 30 pounds. Positive response defined by reduction of symptoms	68 patients referred to physical therapy with neck pain with or without upper extremity symptoms	Improvement after six treatments over 3 weeks of mechanical cervical traction and postural/deep neck flexor strengthening exercise as determined by a score of +7 or higher ("a very great deal better") on GROC scale	.83 (.66, .93)	.50 (.35, .65)	1.67 (1.18, 2.45)	.33 (.14, .73)
Shoulder abduction test[55] ◆	While sitting, the patient is instructed to place the hand of the affected extremity on the head in order to support the extremity in the scapular plane. Positive response defined by alleviation of symptoms			.33 (.19, .51)	.87 (.73, .94)	2.53 (1.01, 6.50)	.77 (.55, 1.00)
Positive ULTT A[55] ◆	With patient supine, examiner performs the following movements: 1. Scapular depression 2. Shoulder abduction 3. Forearm supination 4. Wrist and finger extension 5. Shoulder lateral rotation 6. Elbow extension 7. Contralateral and ipsilateral cervical side-bending Positive response defined by reproduction of symptoms			.80 (.63, .90)	.37 (.23, .53)	1.27 (.93, 1.75)	.54 (.23, 1.18)

ULTT, upper limb tension test.

Diagnostic Utility of Historical and Physical Examination Findings for Improvement with Three Weeks of Mechanical Cervical Traction—cont'd

Test and Study Quality	Description and Positive Findings	Population	Reference Standard	Sens	Spec	+LR	−LR
Pain with manual muscle testing[55] ◆	No details given	68 patients referred to physical therapy with neck pain with or without upper extremity symptoms	Improvement after six treatments over 3 weeks of mechanical cervical traction and postural/deep neck flexor strengthening exercise as determined by a score of +7 or higher ("a very great deal better") on the GROC scale	.63 (.46, .78)	.71 (.55, .83)	2.19 (1.27, 3.92)	.52 (.30, .82)
Body mass index score of 28.4 or higher[55] ◆				.67 (.49, .81)	.68 (.53, .81)	2.11 (1.26, 3.66)	.49 (.27, .81)
Frequency of past episodes[55] ◆				.70 (.48, .85)	.67 (.47, .82)	2.10 (1.15, 4.08)	.45 (.21, .87)
Symptoms distal to the shoulder[35] ◆				.67 (.49, .81)	.58 (.42, .72)	1.58 (1.01, 2.53)	.58 (.32, .99)
Headaches[55] ◆				.43 (.27, .61)	.55 (.40, .70)	.97 (.56, 1.65)	1.02 (.65, 1.57)
Diminished strength[55] ◆				.43 (.27, .61)	.76 (.61, .87)	1.83 (.92, 3.69)	.74 (.50, 1.04)
Peripheralization with central posteroanterior motion testing at lower cervical C4-C7 spine[55] ◆				.37 (.22, .54)	.82 (.67, .91)	1.99 (.90, 4.47)	.78 (.54, 1.04)
Ipsilateral rotation of less than 60 degrees[55] ◆				.43 (.27, .61)	.66 (.50, .79)	1.27 (.69, 2.31)	.86 (.57, 1.26)
Patient-reported neck stiffness[55] ◆				.43 (.27, .61)	.34 (.21, .50)	.66 (.40, 1.02)	1.65 (.97, 2.88)
Flexion active range of motion of less than 55 degrees[55] ◆				.60 (.42, .75)	.55 (.40, .70)	1.34 (.84, 2.14)	.72 (.42, 1.19)
Age of 55 years or older[55] ◆				.47 (.30, .64)	.89 (.76, .96)	4.43 (1.74, 11.89)	.60 (.40, .81)
Ipsilateral side-bending of less than 40 degrees[55] ◆				.73 (.56, .86)	.45 (.30, .60)	1.33 (.92, 1.93)	.60 (.29, 1.14)

GROC scale, Global Rating of Change scale.

Diagnostic Utility of a Cluster of Historical and Physical Examination Findings for Improvement with Three Weeks of Mechanical Cervical Traction

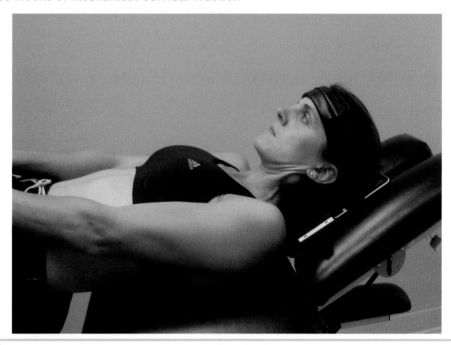

Figure 3-40
Cervical traction. The cervical traction in this study was performed with the patient supine and the legs supported on a stool. The neck was flexed to 24 degrees for patients with full cervical range of motion and to 15 degrees otherwise. The traction force was set at 10 to 12 pounds initially and adjusted upward during the first treatment session to optimally relieve symptoms. Each traction session lasted approximately 15 minutes and alternated between 60 seconds of pull and 20 seconds of release at 50% force. (See Raney NH, Petersen EJ, Smith TA, et al. Development of a clinical prediction rule to identify patients with neck pain likely to benefit from cervical traction and exercise. *Eur Spine J.* 2009;18(3):382-391.)

Test and Study Quality	Description and Positive Findings	Population	Reference Standard	Sens	Spec	+LR	−LR
Age 55 years or older + Positive shoulder abduction test + Positive ULTT A + Symptom peripheralization with central posteroanterior motion testing at lower cervical (C4-C7) spine + Positive neck distraction test[55] ◆	At least four tests positive	68 patients referred to physical therapy with neck pain with or without upper extremity symptoms	Improvement after six treatments over 3 weeks of mechanical cervical traction and postural/ deep neck flexor strengthening exercise as determined by a score of +7 or higher ("a very great deal better") on the GROC scale	.30 (.17, .48)	1.0 (.91, 1.0)	23.1 (2.50, 227.9)	.71 (.53, .85)
	At least three tests positive			.63 (.46, .78)	.87 (.73, .94)	4.81 (2.17, 11.4)	.42 (.25, .65)
	At least two tests positive			.30 (.17, .48)	.97 (.87, 1.00)	1.44 (1.05, 2.03)	.40 (.16, .90)
	At least one test positive			.07 (.02, .21)	.97 (.87, 1.00)	1.15 (.97, 1.4)	.21 (.03, 1.23)

GROC scale, Global Rating of Change scale; ULTT, upper limb tension test.

Outcome Measure	Scoring and Interpretation	Test-Retest Reliability	MCID
Neck Disability Index (NDI)	Users are asked to rate the difficulty of performing 10 functional tasks on a scale of 0 to 5 with different descriptors for each task. A total score out of 100 is calculated by summing each score and doubling the total. The answers provide a score between 0 and 100, with higher scores representing more disability	ICC = .64[56] ◆	10.2[56]
Fear-Avoidance Beliefs Questionnaire (FABQ)	Users are asked to rate their level of agreement with statements concerning beliefs about the relationship between physical activity, work, and their back pain ("neck" can be substituted for "back"). Level of agreement is answered on a Likert-type scale ranging from 0 (completely disagree) to 7 (completely agree). The FABQ is composed of two parts: a seven-item work subscale (FABQW) and a four-item physical activity subscale (FABQPA). Each scale is scored separately, with higher scores representing higher levels of fear avoidance	FABQW: ICC = .82 FABQPA: ICC = .66[57] ●	Not available
Numeric Pain Rating Scale (NPRS)	Users rate their level of pain on an 11-point scale ranging from 0 to 10, with high scores representing more pain. Often asked as "current pain" and "least," "worst," and "average pain" in the past 24 hours	ICC = .76[58] ●	1.3[58]

MCID, minimum clinically important difference.

Cervical Spine

3

References

1. Michaleff ZA, Maher CG, Verhagen AP, et al. Accuracy of the Canadian C-spine rule and NEXUS to screen for clinically important cervical spine injury in patients following blunt trauma: a systematic review. *CMAJ*. 2012;184(16):E867–E876.
2. Bogduk N. Neck pain. *Aust Fam Physician*. 1984;13:26–30.
3. Lord SM, Barnsley L, Wallis BJ, Bogduk N. Chronic cervical zygapophysial joint pain after whiplash. A placebo-controlled prevalence study. *Spine*. 1996;21:1737–1744. discussion 1744-1745.
4. Dwyer A, Aprill C, Bogduk N. Cervical zygapophyseal joint pain patterns. I: a study in normal volunteers. *Spine*. 1990;15:453–457.
5. Cooper G, Bailey B, Bogduk N. Cervical zygapophysial joint pain maps. *Pain Med*. 2007;8:344–353.
6. Cleland JA, Childs JD, Fritz JM, Whitman JM. Interrater reliability of the history and physical examination in patients with mechanical neck pain. *Arch Phys Med Rehabil*. 2006;87:1388–1395.
7. Wainner RS, Fritz JM, Irrgang JJ, et al. Reliability and diagnostic accuracy of the clinical examination and patient self-report measures for cervical radiculopathy. *Spine*. 2003;28:52–62.
8. Lauder TD, Dillingham TR, Andary M, et al. Predicting electrodiagnostic outcome in patients with upper limb symptoms: are the history and physical examination helpful? *Arch Phys Med Rehabil*. 2000;81:436–441.
9. Stiell IG, Wells GA, Vandemheen KL, et al. The Canadian C-spine rule for radiography in alert and stable trauma patients. *JAMA*. 2001;286:1841–1848.
10. Stiell IG, Clement CM, McKnight RD, et al. The Canadian C-spine rule versus the NEXUS low-risk criteria in patients with trauma. *N Engl J Med*. 2003;349:2510–2518.
11. Hoffman JR, Mower WR, Wolfson AB, et al. Validity of a set of clinical criteria to rule out injury to the cervical spine in patients with blunt trauma. National Emergency X-Radiography Utilization Study Group. *N Engl J Med*. 2000;343:94–99.
12. Goode T, Young A, Wilson SP, et al. Evaluation of cervical spine fracture in the elderly: can we trust our physical examination? *Am Surg*. 2014;80(2):182–184.
13. Dickinson G, Stiell IG, Schull M, et al. Retrospective application of the NEXUS low-risk criteria for cervical spine radiography in Canadian emergency departments. *Ann Emerg Med*. 2004;43:507–514.
14. Bandiera G, Stiell IG, Wells GA, et al. The Canadian C-spine rule performs better than unstructured physician judgment. *Ann Emerg Med*. 2003;42:395–402.
15. Duane TM, Dechert T, Wolfe LG, et al. Clinical examination and its reliability in identifying cervical spine fractures. *J Trauma*. 2007;62:1405–1410.
16. Piva SR, Erhard RE, Childs JD, Browder DA. Intertester reliability of passive intervertebral and active movements of the cervical spine. *Man Ther*. 2006;11:321–330.
17. Olson SL, O'Connor DP, Birmingham G, et al. Tender point sensitivity, range of motion, and perceived disability in subjects with neck pain. *J Orthop Sports Phys Ther*. 2000;30:13–20.
18. Hole DE, Cook JM, Bolton JE. Reliability and concurrent validity of two instruments for measuring cervical range of motion: effects of age and gender. *Man Ther*. 1995;1:36–42.
19. Youdas JW, Carey JR, Garrett TR. Reliability of measurements of cervical spine range of motion: comparison of three methods. *Phys Ther*. 1991;71:98–104. discussion 105-106.
20. Hanney WJ, George SZ, Young I, et al. Inter-rater reliability of the physical examination in patients with neck pain. *Physiother Theory Pract*. 2014;30:345–352.
21. Burns SA, Cleland JA, Carpenter K, Mintken P. Interrater reliability of the cervicothoracic and shoulder physical examination in patients with primary complaint of shoulder pain. *Phys Ther Sport*. 2015;18:46–55.
22. Nazim Farooq M, Mohseni Bandpei MA, Ali M, Ali Khan G. Reliability of the universal goniometer for assessing active cervical range of motion in asymptomatic healthy persons. *Pak J Med Sci*. 2016;32(2):457–461.
23. Sandmark H, Nisell R. Validity of five common manual neck pain provoking tests. *Scand J Rehabil Med*. 1995;27:131–136.
24. Edmondston SJ, Wallumrod ME, Macleid F, et al. Reliability of isometric muscle endurance tests in subjects with postural neck pain. *J Manipulative Physiol Ther*. 2008;31:348–354.
25. Olson LE, Millar AL, Dunker J, et al. Reliability of a clinical test for deep cervical flexor endurance. *J Manipulative Physiol Ther*. 2006;29:134–138.
26. Harris KD, Heer DM, Roy TC, et al. Reliability of a measurement of neck flexor muscle endurance. *Phys Ther*. 2005;85:1349–1355.
27. Chiu TT, Law EY, Chiu TH. Performance of the craniocervical flexion test in subjects with and without chronic neck pain. *J Orthop Sports Phys Ther*. 2005;35:567–571.
28. Kumbhare DA, Balsor B, Parkinson WL, et al. Measurement of cervical flexor endurance following whiplash. *Disabil Rehabil*. 2005;27:801–807.
29. Lourenco AS, Lameiras C, Silva AG. Neck flexor and extensor muscle endurance in subclinical neck pain: Intrarater reliability, standard error of measurement, minimal detectable change, and comparison with asymptomatic participants in a university student population. *J Manipulative Physiol Ther*. 2016;39:427–433.
30. Segarra V, Duenas L, Torres R, et al. Inter- and intra-tester reliability of a battery of cervical movement control dysfunction tests. *Man Ther*. 2015;20:570–579.
31. Smedmark V, Wallin M, Arvidsson I. Inter-examiner reliability in assessing passive intervertebral motion of the cervical spine. *Man Ther*. 2000;5:97–101.

32. Humphreys BK, Delahaye M, Peterson CK. An investigation into the validity of cervical spine motion palpation using subjects with congenital block vertebrae as a "gold standard. *BMC Musculoskelet Disord.* 2004;5:19.

33. Pool JJ, Hoving JL, de Vet HC, et al. The interexaminer reproducibility of physical examination of the cervical spine. *J Manipulative Physiol Ther.* 2004;27:84–90.

34. Kaale BR, Krakenes J, Albrektsen G, Wester K. Clinical assessment techniques for detecting ligament and membrane injuries in the upper cervical spine region: a comparison with MRI results. *Man Ther.* 2008;13(5):397–403.

35. Uitvlugt G, Indenbaum S. Clinical assessment of atlantoaxial instability using the Sharp-Purser test. *Arthritis Rheum.* 1988;31:918–922.

36. King W, Lau P, Lees R, Bogduk N. The validity of manual examination in assessing patients with neck pain. *Spine J.* 2007;7:22–26.

37. Jull G, Bogduk N, Marsland A. The accuracy of manual diagnosis for cervical zygapophysial joint pain syndromes. *Med J Aust.* 1988;148:233–236.

38. Viikari-Juntura E. Interexaminer reliability of observations in physical examinations of the neck. *Phys Ther.* 1987;67:1526–1532.

39. Van Suijlekom HA, De Vet HC, Van Den Berg SG, Weber WE. Interobserver reliability in physical examination of the cervical spine in patients with headache. *Headache.* 2000;40:581–586.

40. Bertilson BC, Grunnesjo M, Strender LE. Reliability of clinical tests in the assessment of patients with neck/shoulder problems: impact of history. *Spine.* 2003;28:2222–2231.

41. Hall T, Briffa K, Hopper D, Robinson K. Reliability of manual examination and frequency of symptomatic cervical motion segment dysfunction in cervicogenic headache. *Man Ther.* 2010;15(6):542–546.

42. Shabat S, Leitner Y, David R, Folman Y. The correlation between Spurling test and imaging studies in detecting cervical radiculopathy. *J Neuroimaging.* 2012;22(4):375–378.

43. Shah KC, Rajshekhar V. Reliability of diagnosis of soft cervical disc prolapse using Spurling's test. *Br J Neurosurg.* 2004;18:480–483.

44. Tong HC, Haig AJ, Yamakawa K. The Spurling test and cervical radiculopathy. *Spine.* 2002;27:156–159.

45. Ghasemi M, Golabchi K, Mousavi SA, et al. The value of provocative tests in diagnosis of cervical radiculopathy. *J Res Med Sci.* 2013;18(Suppl 1):S35–S38.

46. Hall T, Briffa K, Hopper D, Robinson K. Long-term stability and minimal detectable change of the cervical flexion-rotation test. *J Orthop Sports Phys Ther.* 2010;40(4):225–229.

47. Gumina S, Carbone S, Albino P, et al. Arm squeeze test: a new clinical test to distinguish neck from shoulder pain. *Eur Spine J.* 2013;22(7):1558–1563.

48. Uchihara T, Furukawa T, Tsukagoshi H. Compression of brachial plexus as a diagnostic test of cervical cord lesion. *Spine.* 1994;19:2170–2173.

49. Cook C, Roman M, Stewart KM, et al. Reliability and diagnostic accuracy of clinical special tests for myelopathy in patients seen for cervical dysfunction. *J Orthop Sports Phys Ther.* 2009;39(3):172–178.

50. Chaiyamongkol W, Laohawiriyakamol T, Tangtrakulwanich B, et al. The significance of the Tromner sign in cervical spondylitic patient. *Clin Spin Surg.* 2017;30:E1315–E1320.

51. Cook C, Brown C, Isaacs R, et al. Clustered clinical findings for diagnosis of cervical spine myelopathy. *J Man Manip Ther.* 2010;18(4):175–180.

52. Puentedura EJ, Cleland JA, Landers MR, et al. Development of a clinical prediction rule to identify patients with neck pain likely to benefit from thrust joint manipulation to the cervical spine. *J Orthop Sports Phys Ther.* 2012;42(7):577–592.

53. Cleland JA, Fritz JM, Whitman JM, Heath R. Predictors of short-term outcome in people with a clinical diagnosis of cervical radiculopathy. *Phys Ther.* 2007;87:1619–1632.

54. Tseng YL, Wang WT, Chen WY, et al. Predictors for the immediate responders to cervical manipulation in patients with neck pain. *Man Ther.* 2006;11:306–315.

55. Raney NH, Petersen EJ, Smith TA, et al. Development of a clinical prediction rule to identify patients with neck pain likely to benefit from cervical traction and exercise. *Eur Spine J.* 2009;18(3):382–391.

56. Young BA, Walker MJ, Strunce JB, et al. Responsiveness of the Neck Disability Index in patients with mechanical neck disorders. *Spine J.* 2009;9(10):802–808.

57. Grotle M, Brox JI, Vollestad NK. Reliability, validity and responsiveness of the fear-avoidance beliefs questionnaire: methodological aspects of the Norwegian version. *J Rehabil Med.* 2006;38:346–353.

58. Cleland JA, Childs JD, Whitman JM. Psychometric properties of the Neck Disability Index and Numeric Pain Rating Scale in patients with mechanical neck pain. *Arch Phys Med Rehabil.* 2008;89:69–74.

3

Cervical Spine

Thoracolumbar Spine | 4

Clinical Summary and Recommendations

Patient History

Complaints	• A few subjective complaints appear to be useful in identifying specific spinal pathologic conditions. A report of "no pain when seated" is the answer to the single question with the best diagnostic utility for lumbar spinal stenosis (+LR [likelihood ratio] = 6.6). "Pain not relieved by lying down," "back pain at night," and "morning stiffness for longer than 1/2 hour" are all somewhat helpful in identifying ankylosing spondylitis (+LR = 1.51 to 1.57). Subjective complaints of weakness, numbness, tingling, and/or burning do not appear to be especially helpful, at least in identifying lumbar radiculopathy.

Physical Examination

Neurologic Screening	• Traditional neurologic screening (sensation, reflex, and manual muscle testing) is reasonably useful in identifying lumbar radiculopathy. When tested in isolation, weakness with manual muscle testing and, even more so, reduced reflexes are suggestive of lumbar radiculopathy, especially at the L3-L4 spinal levels. Sensation testing (vibration and pinprick) alone does not seem to be especially useful. However, when changes in reflexes, muscular strength, and sensation are found in conjunction with a positive straight-leg raise test, lumbar radiculopathy is highly likely (+LR = 6.0). • In addition, a finding of decreased sensation (vibration and pinprick), muscle weakness, or reflex changes is modestly helpful in identifying lumbar spinal stenosis (+LR = 2.1 to 2.8).
Range-of-Motion, Strength, and Manual Assessment	• Measuring both thoracolumbar range of motion and motor control, as well as trunk strength, has consistently been shown to be reliable, but the findings are of unknown diagnostic utility. • The results of studies assessing the reliability of passive intervertebral motion (PIVM) are highly variable, but generally, the reports are of poor reliability when assessing for limited or excessive movement and of moderate reliability when assessing for pain. • Diagnostic studies assessing PIVM suggest that abnormal segmental motion is moderately useful both in identifying radiographic hypomobility/hypermobility and in predicting the responses to certain conservative treatments. However, restricted PIVM may have little or no association with low back pain.
Special Tests	• The centralization phenomenon (movement of symptoms from distal/lateral regions to more central regions) has been shown to be both highly reliable and decidedly useful in identifying painful lumbar discs (+LR = 6.9). • The straight-leg raise test, crossed straight-leg raise test, and slump test have all been shown to be moderately useful in identifying nerve root impingement and disc pathologic conditions, including bulges, herniations, and extrusions. • Palpation of gluteal trigger points appears to be helpful in both identifying and ruling out radicular low back pain (+LR = 8.6, −LR = .28). • A 2011 systematic review[1] identified the passive lumbar extension test as a useful clinical test in identifying lumbar segmental instability (+LR = 8.8). • Both the Romberg test and a two-stage treadmill test have been found to be moderately useful in identifying lumbar spinal stenosis.
Interventions	• Patients with low back pain of less than 16 days' duration and no symptoms distal to the knees and/or patients who meet at least four out of the five criteria proposed by Flynn and colleagues[2] should be treated with lumbosacral manipulation. • Patients with low back pain who meet at least three out of the five criteria proposed by Hicks[3] should be treated with lumbar stabilization exercises.

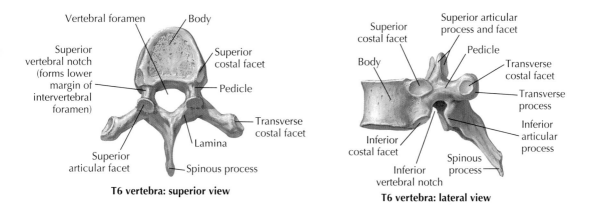

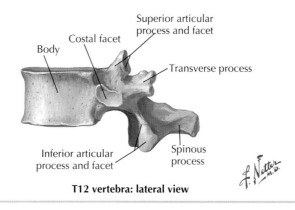

Figure 4-1
Thoracic vertebrae.

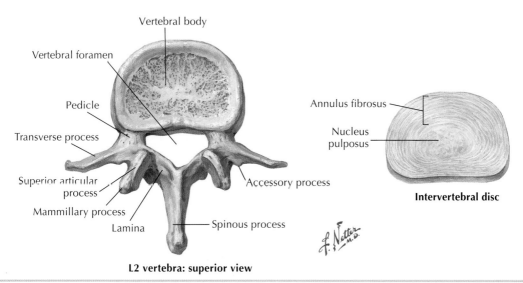

Figure 4-2
Lumbar vertebrae.

Thoracolumbar Spine

4

Joints of the Thoracic Spine

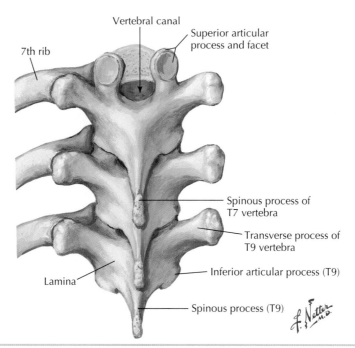

Figure 4-3
T7, T8, and T9 vertebrae, posterior view.

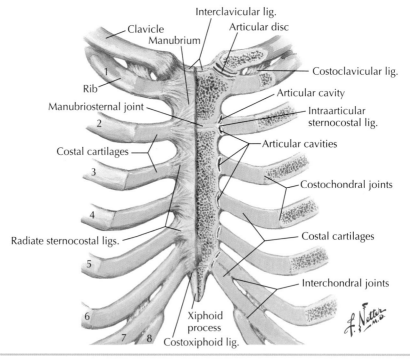

Figure 4-4
Sternocostal articulations, anterior view.

Joints of the Thoracic Spine—cont'd

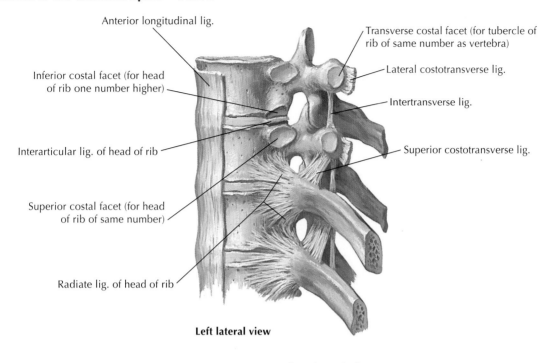

Anterior longitudinal lig.

Transverse costal facet (for tubercle of
rib of same number as vertebra)

Inferior costal facet (for head
of rib one number higher)

Lateral costotransverse lig.

Intertransverse lig.

Interarticular lig. of head of rib

Superior costotransverse lig.

Superior costal facet (for head
of rib of same number)

Radiate lig. of head of rib

Left lateral view

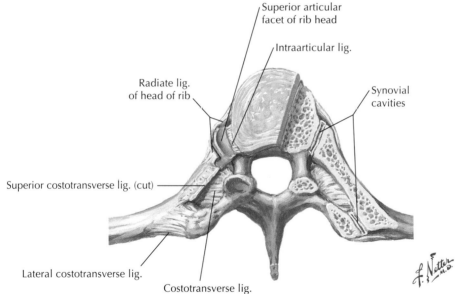

Superior articular
facet of rib head

Intraarticular lig.

Radiate lig.
of head of rib

Synovial
cavities

Superior costotransverse lig. (cut)

Lateral costotransverse lig.

Costotransverse lig.

Transverse section: superior view

Figure 4-5
Costovertebral joints.

Thoracolumbar Spine

4

Joints of the Thoracic Spine—cont'd

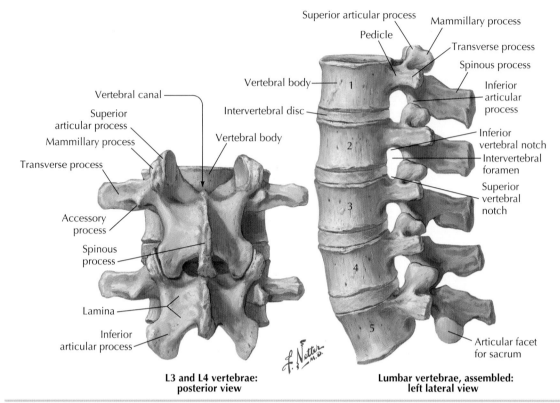

Figure 4-6
Lumbar spine.

Thoracolumbar Joints	Type and Classification	Closed Packed Position	Capsular Pattern
Zygapophyseal joints	Synovial: plane	Extension	Lumbar: significant limitation of side-bending bilaterally and limitations of flexion and extension Thoracic: limitation of extension, side-bending, and rotation; less limitation of flexion
Intervertebral joints	Amphiarthrodial	Not applicable	Not applicable

Thoracic Spine	Type and Classification	Closed Packed Position	Capsular Pattern
Costotransverse	Synovial	Not reported	Not reported
Costovertebral	Synovial	Not reported	Not reported
Costochondral	Synchondroses	Not reported	Not reported
Interchondral	Synovial	Not reported	Not reported
Sternocostal (first joint)	Amphiarthrodial	Not applicable	Not applicable
Sternocostal (second to seventh joints)	Synovial	Not reported	Not reported

Costovertebral Ligaments

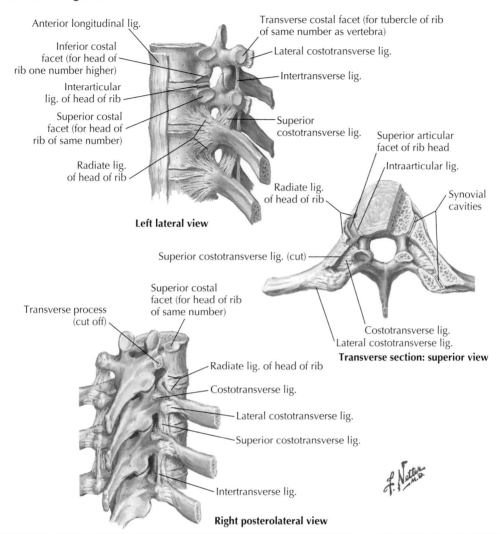

Left lateral view

Anterior longitudinal lig.

Inferior costal facet (for head of rib one number higher)

Interarticular lig. of head of rib

Superior costal facet (for head of rib of same number)

Radiate lig. of head of rib

Transverse costal facet (for tubercle of rib of same number as vertebra)

Lateral costotransverse lig.

Intertransverse lig.

Superior costotransverse lig.

Superior articular facet of rib head

Intraarticular lig.

Synovial cavities

Radiate lig. of head of rib

Superior costotransverse lig. (cut)

Superior costal facet (for head of rib of same number)

Transverse process (cut off)

Radiate lig. of head of rib

Costotransverse lig.

Lateral costotransverse lig.

Superior costotransverse lig.

Intertransverse lig.

Costotransverse lig.
Lateral costotransverse lig.

Transverse section: superior view

Right posterolateral view

Figure 4-7
Costovertebral ligaments.

Ligaments	Attachments	Function
Radiate sternocostal	Costal cartilage to the anterior and posterior aspects of the sternum	Reinforces joint capsule
Interchondral	Connect adjacent borders of articulations between costal cartilages 6 and 7, 7 and 8, and 8 and 9	Reinforces joint capsule
Radiate ligament of head of rib	Lateral vertebral body to head of rib	Prevents separation of rib head from vertebra
Costotransverse	Posterior aspect of rib to anterior aspect of transverse process of vertebra	Prevents separation of rib from transverse process
Intraarticular	Crest of the rib head to intervertebral disc	Divides joint into two cavities

Thoracolumbar Spine

4

Thoracolumbar Ligaments

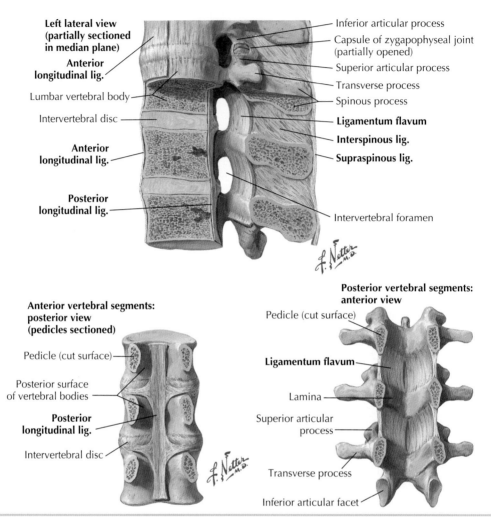

Figure 4-8
Thoracolumbar ligaments.

Ligaments	Attachments	Function
Anterior longitudinal	Extends from anterior sacrum to anterior tubercle of C1. Connects anterolateral vertebral bodies and discs	Maintains stability and prevents excessive extension of spinal column
Posterior longitudinal	Extends from the sacrum to C2. Runs within the vertebral canal attaching the posterior vertebral bodies	Prevents excessive flexion of spinal column and posterior disc protrusion
Ligamenta flava	Binds the lamina above each vertebra to the lamina below	Prevents separation of the vertebral laminae
Supraspinous	Connect spinous processes of C7-S1	Limits separation of spinous processes
Interspinous	Connect spinous processes of C1-S1	Limits separation of spinous processes
Intertransverse	Connect adjacent transverse processes of vertebrae	Limits separation of transverse processes
Iliolumbar	Transverse processes of L5 to posterior aspect of iliac crest	Stabilizes L5 and prevents anterior shear

Thoracolumbar Muscles: Superficial Layers

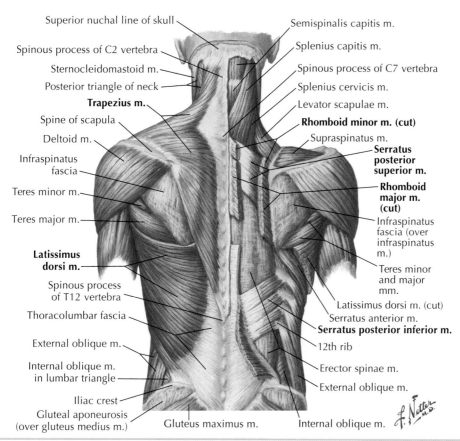

Superior nuchal line of skull

Spinous process of C2 vertebra

Sternocleidomastoid m.

Posterior triangle of neck

Trapezius m.

Spine of scapula

Deltoid m.

Infraspinatus fascia

Teres minor m.

Teres major m.

Latissimus dorsi m.

Spinous process of T12 vertebra

Thoracolumbar fascia

External oblique m.

Internal oblique m. in lumbar triangle

Iliac crest

Gluteal aponeurosis (over gluteus medius m.)

Gluteus maximus m.

Semispinalis capitis m.

Splenius capitis m.

Spinous process of C7 vertebra

Splenius cervicis m.

Levator scapulae m.

Rhomboid minor m. (cut)

Supraspinatus m.

Serratus posterior superior m.

Rhomboid major m. (cut)

Infraspinatus fascia (over infraspinatus m.)

Teres minor and major mm.

Latissimus dorsi m. (cut)

Serratus anterior m.

Serratus posterior inferior m.

12th rib

Erector spinae m.

External oblique m.

Internal oblique m.

Thoracolumbar Spine

4

Figure 4-9
Muscles of the back, superficial layers.

Muscles	Proximal Attachment	Distal Attachment	Nerve and Segmental Level	Action
Latissimus dorsi	Spinous processes of T6-T12, thoracolumbar fascia, iliac crest, inferior four ribs	Intertubercular groove of humerus	Thoracodorsal nerve (C6, C7, C8)	Humerus extension, adduction, and internal rotation
Trapezius (middle)	Superior nuchal line, occipital protuberance, nuchal ligament, spinous processes of T1-T12	Lateral clavicle, acromion, and spine of scapula	Accessory nerve (CN XI)	Retracts scapula
Trapezius (lower)				Depresses scapula
Rhomboid major	Spinous processes of T2-T5	Inferior medial border of scapula	Dorsal scapular nerve (C4, C5)	Retracts scapula, inferiorly rotates glenoid fossa, stabilizes scapula to thoracic wall
Rhomboid minor	Spinous processes of C7-T1 and nuchal ligament	Superior medial border of scapula		
Serratus posterior superior	Spinous processes of C7-T3, ligamentum nuchae	Superior surface of ribs 2-4	Intercostal nerves 2-5	Elevates ribs
Serratus posterior inferior	Spinous processes of T11-L2	Inferior surface of ribs 8-12	Ventral rami of thoracic spinal nerves 9-12	Depresses ribs

CN, Cranial nerve.

Thoracolumbar Muscles: Intermediate Layer

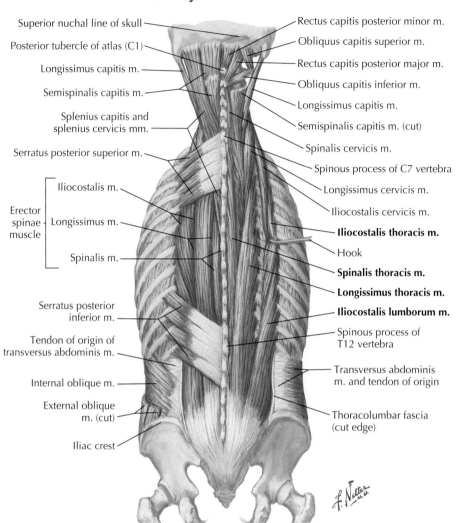

Superior nuchal line of skull
Posterior tubercle of atlas (C1)
Longissimus capitis m.
Semispinalis capitis m.
Splenius capitis and splenius cervicis mm.
Serratus posterior superior m.
Iliocostalis m.
Erector spinae muscle
Longissimus m.
Spinalis m.
Serratus posterior inferior m.
Tendon of origin of transversus abdominis m.
Internal oblique m.
External oblique m. (cut)
Iliac crest

Rectus capitis posterior minor m.
Obliquus capitis superior m.
Rectus capitis posterior major m.
Obliquus capitis inferior m.
Longissimus capitis m.
Semispinalis capitis m. (cut)
Spinalis cervicis m.
Spinous process of C7 vertebra
Longissimus cervicis m.
Iliocostalis cervicis m.
Iliocostalis thoracis m.
Hook
Spinalis thoracis m.
Longissimus thoracis m.
Iliocostalis lumborum m.
Spinous process of T12 vertebra
Transversus abdominis m. and tendon of origin
Thoracolumbar fascia (cut edge)

Figure 4-10
Muscles of the back, intermediate layer.

Muscles	Proximal Attachment	Distal Attachment	Nerve and Segmental Level	Action
Iliocostalis thoracis	Iliac crest, posterior sacrum, spinous processes of sacrum and inferior lumbar vertebrae, supraspinous ligament	Cervical transverse processes and superior angles of lower ribs	Dorsal rami of spinal nerves	Bilaterally: extend spinal column Unilaterally: side-bend spinal column
Iliocostalis lumborum		Inferior surface of ribs 4-12		
Longissimus thoracis		Thoracic transverse processes and superior surface of ribs		
Longissimus lumborum		Transverse process of lumbar vertebrae		
Spinalis thoracis		Upper thoracic spinous processes		

Thoracolumbar Muscles: Deep Layer

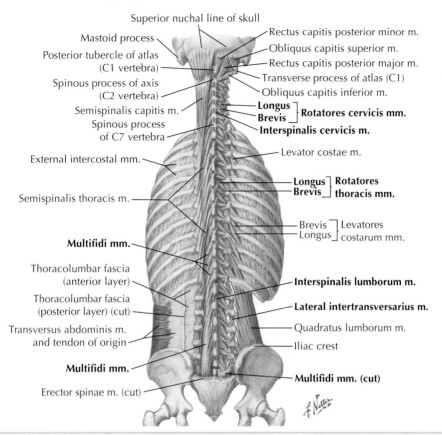

Figure 4-11
Muscles of the back, deep layer.

Muscles	Proximal Attachment	Distal Attachment	Nerve and Segmental Level	Action
Rotatores	Transverse processes of vertebrae	Spinous process of vertebra one to two segments above origin	Dorsal rami of spinal nerves	Vertebral stabilization, assists with rotation and extension
Interspinalis	Superior aspect of cervical and lumbar spinous processes	Inferior aspect of spinous process superior to vertebrae of origin	Dorsal rami of spinal nerves	Extension and rotation of vertebral column
Intertransversarius	Cervical and lumbar transverse processes	Transverse process of adjacent vertebrae	Dorsal and ventral rami of spinal nerves	Bilaterally stabilizes vertebral column. Ipsilaterally side-bends vertebral column
Multifidi	Sacrum, ilium, transverse processes of T1-T3, articular processes of C4-C7	Spinous process of vertebra two to four segments above origin	Dorsal rami of spinal nerves	Stabilizes vertebrae

Anterior Abdominal Wall

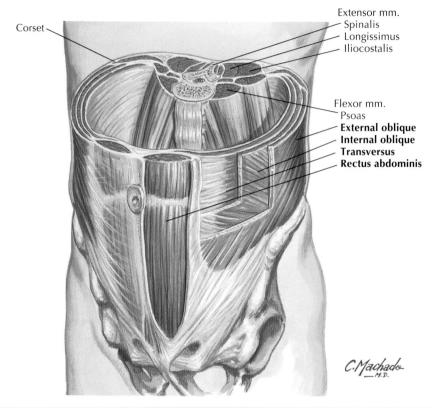

Figure 4-12
Dynamic "corset" concept of lumbar stability.

Muscles	Proximal Attachment	Distal Attachment	Nerve and Segmental Level	Action
Rectus abdominis	Pubic symphysis and pubic crest	Costal cartilages 5-7 and xiphoid process	Ventral rami of T6-T12	Flexes trunk
Internal oblique	Thoracolumbar fascia, anterior iliac crest, and lateral inguinal ligament	Inferior border of ribs 10-12, linea alba, and pecten pubis	Ventral rami of T6-L1	Flexes and rotates trunk
External oblique	External aspects of ribs 5-12	Anterior iliac crest, linea alba, and pubic tubercle	Ventral rami of T6-T12 and subcostal nerve	Flexes and rotates trunk
Transversus abdominis	Internal aspects of costal cartilages 7-12, thoracolumbar fascia, iliac crest, and lateral inguinal ligament	Linea alba, pecten pubis, and pubic crest	Ventral rami of T6-L1	Supports abdominal viscera and increases intraabdominal pressure

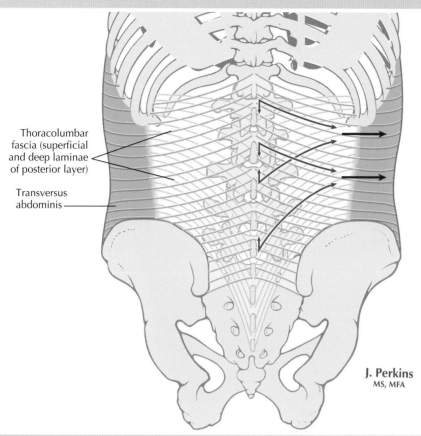

Thoracolumbar fascia (superficial and deep laminae of posterior layer)

Transversus abdominis

J. Perkins
MS, MFA

Figure 4-13
Transverse abdominis. The transverse abdominis exerts a force through the thoracolumbar fascia, creating a stabilizing force through the lumbar spine. (From Kay AG. An extensive literature review of the lumbar multifidus: biomechanics. *J Man Manip Ther.* 2001;9:17-39.)

The thoracolumbar fascia is a dense layer of connective tissue running from the thoracic region to the sacrum.[4] It is composed of three separate and distinct layers: anterior, middle, and posterior. The middle and posterior layers blend together to form a dense fascia referred to as the *lateral raphe*.[5] The posterior layer consists of two distinctly separate laminae. The superficial lamina fibers are angled downward and the deep lamina fibers are angled upward. Bergmark[6] has reported that the thoracolumbar fascia serves three purposes: (1) to transfer forces from muscles to the spine, (2) to transfer forces between spinal segments, and (3) to transfer forces from the thoracolumbar spine to the retinaculum of the erector spinae muscles. The transverse abdominis attaches to the middle layer of the thoracolumbar fascia and exerts a force through the lateral raphe, resulting in a cephalad tension through the deep layer and a caudal tension through the superficial layer of the posterior lamina.[4,5,7] The result is a stabilizing force exerted through the lumbar spine, which has been reported to provide stability and assist with controlling intersegmental motion of the lumbar spine.[8-10]

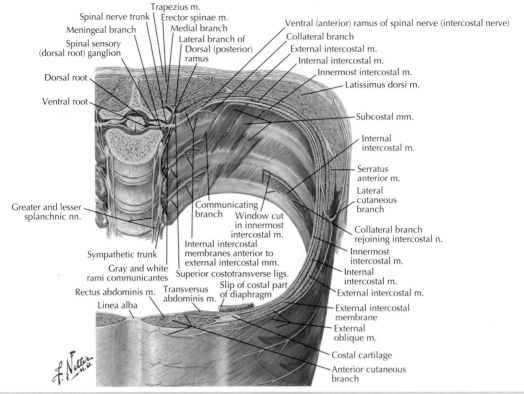

Figure 4-14
Nerves of the thoracic spine.

Nerve Ventral Rami	Segmental Level	Sensory	Motor
Intercostals	T1-T11	Anterior and lateral aspect of the thorax and abdomen	Intercostals, serratus posterior, levator costarum, transversus thoracis
Subcostals	T12		Part of external oblique
Dorsal rami	T1-T12	Posterior thorax and back	Splenius, iliocostalis, longissimus, spinalis, interspinales, intertransversarii, multifidi, semispinalis, rotatores
Subcostal nerve	T12	Lateral hip	External oblique
Iliohypogastric nerve	T12, L1	Posterolateral gluteal region	Internal oblique, transverse abdominis
Ilioinguinal	L1	Superior medial thigh	Internal oblique, transverse abdominis
Genitofemoral	L1, L2	Superior anterior thigh	No motor
Lateral cutaneous	L2, L3	Lateral thigh	No motor
Branch to iliacus	L2, L3, L4	No sensory	Iliacus
Femoral nerve	L2, L3, L4	Thigh via cutaneous nerves	Iliacus, sartorius, quadriceps femoris, articularis genu, pectineus
Obturator nerve	L2, L3, L4	Medial thigh	Adductor longus, adductor brevis, adductor magnus (adductor part), gracilis, obturator externus
Sciatic	L4, L5, S1, S2, S3	Hip joint	Knee flexors and all muscles of the lower leg and foot

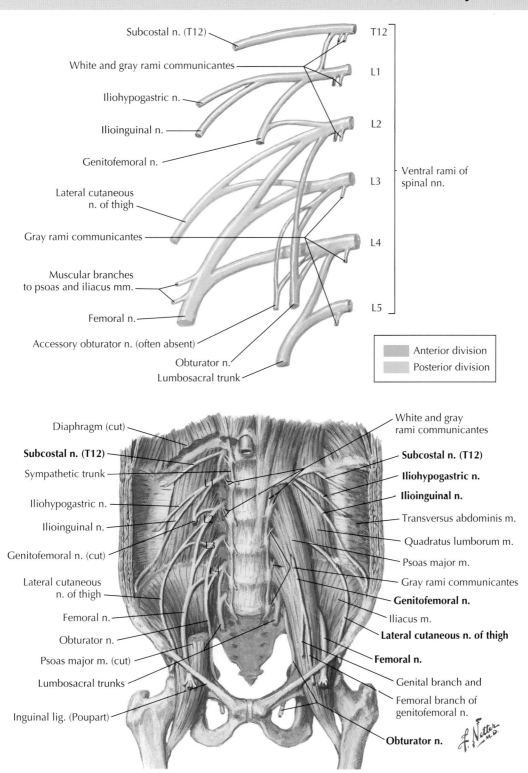

Subcostal n. (T12)

White and gray rami communicantes

Iliohypogastric n.

Ilioinguinal n.

Genitofemoral n.

Lateral cutaneous n. of thigh

Gray rami communicantes

Muscular branches to psoas and iliacus mm.

Femoral n.

Accessory obturator n. (often absent)

Obturator n.

Lumbosacral trunk

T12

L1

L2

L3

L4

L5

Ventral rami of spinal nn.

Anterior division

Posterior division

Diaphragm (cut)

Subcostal n. (T12)

Sympathetic trunk

Iliohypogastric n.

Ilioinguinal n.

Genitofemoral n. (cut)

Lateral cutaneous n. of thigh

Femoral n.

Obturator n.

Psoas major m. (cut)

Lumbosacral trunks

Inguinal lig. (Poupart)

White and gray rami communicantes

Subcostal n. (T12)

Iliohypogastric n.

Ilioinguinal n.

Transversus abdominis m.

Quadratus lumborum m.

Psoas major m.

Gray rami communicantes

Genitofemoral n.

Iliacus m.

Lateral cutaneous n. of thigh

Femoral n.

Genital branch and

Femoral branch of genitofemoral n.

Obturator n.

Figure 4-15
Nerves of the lumbar spine.

Thoracolumbar Spine

4

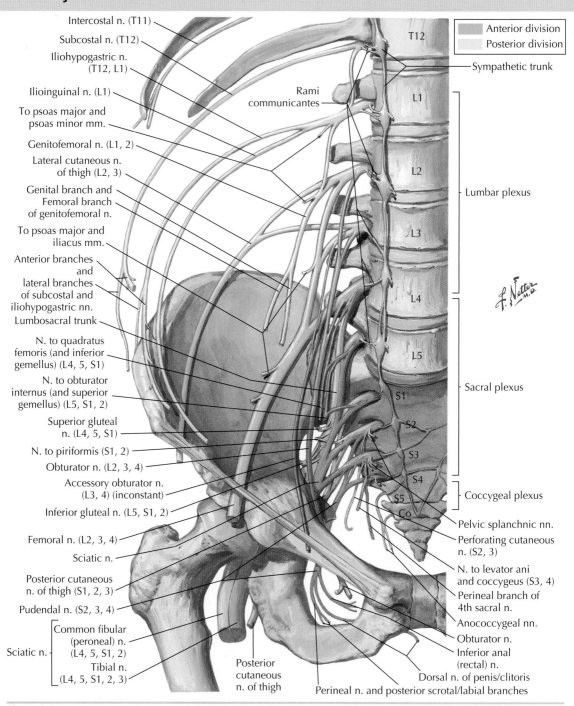

Intercostal n. (T11)
Subcostal n. (T12)
Iliohypogastric n. (T12, L1)
Ilioinguinal n. (L1)
To psoas major and psoas minor mm.
Genitofemoral n. (L1, 2)
Lateral cutaneous n. of thigh (L2, 3)
Genital branch and Femoral branch of genitofemoral n.
To psoas major and iliacus mm.
Anterior branches and lateral branches of subcostal and iliohypogastric nn.
Lumbosacral trunk
N. to quadratus femoris (and inferior gemellus) (L4, 5, S1)
N. to obturator internus (and superior gemellus) (L5, S1, 2)
Superior gluteal n. (L4, 5, S1)
N. to piriformis (S1, 2)
Obturator n. (L2, 3, 4)
Accessory obturator n. (L3, 4) (inconstant)
Inferior gluteal n. (L5, S1, 2)
Femoral n. (L2, 3, 4)
Sciatic n.
Posterior cutaneous n. of thigh (S1, 2, 3)
Pudendal n. (S2, 3, 4)

Sciatic n.
Common fibular (peroneal) n. (L4, 5, S1, 2)
Tibial n. (L4, 5, S1, 2, 3)

Rami communicantes

T12
L1
L2
L3
L4
L5
S1
S2
S3
S4
S5
Co

Anterior division
Posterior division
Sympathetic trunk

Lumbar plexus

Sacral plexus

Coccygeal plexus

Pelvic splanchnic nn.
Perforating cutaneous n. (S2, 3)
N. to levator ani and coccygeus (S3, 4)
Perineal branch of 4th sacral n.
Anococcygeal nn.
Obturator n.
Inferior anal (rectal) n.
Dorsal n. of penis/clitoris

Posterior cutaneous n. of thigh
Perineal n. and posterior scrotal/labial branches

Figure 4-16
Nerves of the lumbar spine.

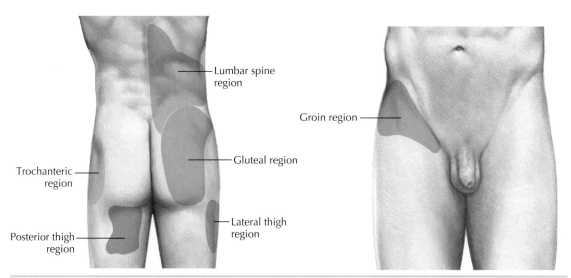

Figure 4-17
Lumbar zygapophyseal joint pain referral patterns. Zygapophyseal pain patterns of the lumbar spine as described by Fukui and colleagues. Lumbar zygapophyseal joints L1-L2, L2-L3, and L4-L5 always referred pain to the lumbar spine region. Primary referral to the gluteal region was from L5-S1 (68% of the time). Levels L2-L3, L3-L4, L4-L5, and L5-S1 occasionally referred pain to the trochanteric region (10% to 16% of the time). Primary referral to the lateral thigh, posterior thigh, and groin regions was most often from L3-L4, L4-L5, and L5-S1 (5% to 30% of the time). (From Fukui S, Ohseto K, Shiotani M, et al. Distribution of referred pain from the lumbar zygapophyseal joints and dorsal rami. *Clin J Pain.* 1997;13:303-307.)

Area of Pain Referral	Percentage of Patients Presenting with Pain (n = 176 Patients with Low Back Pain)*
Left groin	15%
Right groin	3%
Left buttock	42%
Right buttock	15%
Left thigh	38%
Right thigh	38%
Left calf	27%
Right calf	15%
Left foot	31%
Right foot	8%

*Prevalence of pain referral patterns in patients with zygapophyseal joint pain syndromes as confirmed by diagnostic blocks.[11] In a subsequent study,[12] it was determined that in a cohort of 63 patients with chronic low back pain, the prevalence of zygapophyseal joint pain was 40%.

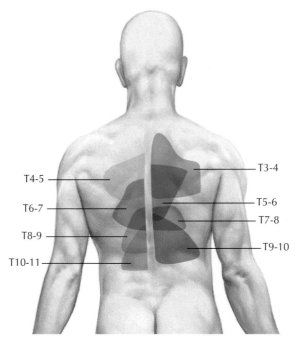

T4-5

T6-7

T8-9

T10-11

T3-4

T5-6

T7-8

T9-10

As described by Dreyfuss et al.[12a]

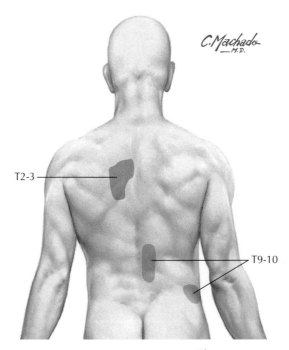

T2-3

T9-10

As described by Fukui et al.[12b]

Figure 4-18
Zygapophyseal pain patterns of the thoracic spine.

Historical Question and Study Quality		Population	Reliability
Increased pain with[15] ◆	Sitting	A random selection of 91 patients with low back pain	Interexaminer κ = .49
	Standing		Interexaminer κ = 1.0
	Walking		Interexaminer κ = .56
	Lying down		Interexaminer κ = .41
Pain with sitting[16] ◆		95 patients with low back pain	Interexaminer κ = .99 to 1.0
Pain with bending[16] ◆			Interexaminer κ = .98 to .99
Increased pain with coughing/sneezing[15] ◆		A random selection of 91 patients with low back pain	Interexaminer κ = .64
Patient report of[13] ◉	Foot pain	Two separate groups of patients with low back pain (n₁ = 50, n₂ = 33)	Interexaminer κ = .12 to .73
	Leg pain		Interexaminer κ = .53 to .96
	Thigh pain		Interexaminer κ = .39 to .78
	Buttock pain		Interexaminer κ = .33 to .44
	Back pain		Interexaminer κ = −.19 to .16
Increased pain with[14] ◉	Sitting	53 subjects with a primary complaint of low back pain	Test-retest κ = .46
	Standing		Test-retest κ = .70
	Walking		Test-retest κ = .67
Pain with bending[14] ◉		53 subjects with a primary complaint of low back pain	Test-retest κ = .65
Pain with bending[13] ◉		Two separate groups of patients with low back pain (n₁ = 50, n₂ = 33)	Interexaminer κ = .51 to .56
Increased pain with coughing[14] ◉		53 subjects with a primary complaint of low back pain	Test-retest κ = .75
Pain with pushing/lifting/carrying[14] ◉			Test-retest κ = .77 to .89

Thoracolumbar Spine

4

Historical Question and Study Quality	Patient Population	Reference Standard	Sens	Spec	+LR	−LR
Age ≥ 75[17] ◐	669 patients >55 years of age seen in primary care for 1st episode of low back pain with or without leg pain	Radiologic diagnosis of vertebral fracture	.45 (.28, .62)	.85 (.82, .88)	3.1 (2.0, 4.7)	.60 (.50, .90)
Trauma[17] ◐			.21 (.07, .35)	.97 (.95, .98)	6.2 (2.8, 13.5)	.80 (.50, 1.3)
Osteoporosis[17] ◐			.38 (.21, .54)	.88 (.86, .91)	3.2 (1.9, 5.2)	.70, (.50, .90)
Back pain intensity score ≥7/10[17] ◐			.67 (.51, .83)	.63 (.59, .67)	1.8 (1.4, 2.3)	.50 (.30, .90)
Thoracic back pain[17] ◐			.42 (.26, .59)	.78 (.75, .81)	1.9 (1.3, 3.0)	.70 (.50, 1.0)
≥1/5 of above features[17] ◐			.88 (.77, .99)	.42 (.38, .46)	1.5 (1.3, 1.8)	.30 (.10, .70)
≥2/5 of above features[17] ◐			.70 (.54, .85)	.81 (.78, .84)	3.6 (2.8, 4.8)	.40 (.20, .60)
≥3/5 of above features[17] ◐			.30 (.15, .46)	.95 (.93, .97)	5.8 (3.2, 10.8)	.70 (.60, .90)
Any of the following 4 factors: 1. Anticoagulant use 2. Decreased sensation of physical exam 3. Pain that is worse at night 4. Pain that persists despite appropriate treatment[18] ◐	329 adult patients presenting to emergency department with nontraumatic low back pain	Serious outcome as the identification of any one of the following underlying pathologies within 30 days of the initial visit: compression fracture, osteomyelitis, spinal abscess, malignancy, cauda equina syndrome, severe disc prolapse requiring surgery, any condition requiring immediate intervention (i.e., abdominal aortic aneurysm, retroperitoneal tumor, bleeding or infection that required treatment, spinal stenosis requiring surgery, or death)	.91 (.71, .99)	.55 (.49, .61)	2.0 (1.7, 2.4)	.17 (.04, .62)

Historical Question and Study Quality	Patient Population	Reference Standard	Sens	Spec	+LR	−LR
Age over 65 years[19] ◆	93 patients with low back pain 40 years old or older	Lumbar spinal stenosis per attending physician's impression; 88% also supported by computed tomography (CT) or magnetic resonance imaging (MRI)	.77 (.64, .90)	.69 (.53, .85)	2.5	.33
Pain below knees?[19] ◆			.56 (.41, .71)	.63 (.46, .80)	1.5	.70
Pain below buttocks?[19] ◆			.88 (.78, .98)	.34 (.18, .50)	1.3	.35
No pain when seated?[19] ◆			.46 (.30, .62)	.93 (.84, 1.0)	6.6	.58
Severe lower extremity pain?[19] ◆			.65 (.51, .79)	.67 (.51, .83)	2.0	.52
Symptoms improved while seated?[19] ◆			.52 (.37, .67)	.83 (.70, .96)	3.1	.58
Worse when walking?[19] ◆			.71 (.57, .85)	.30 (.14, .46)	1.0	.97
Numbness[19] ◆			.63 (.49, .74)	.59 (.42, .76)	1.5	.63
Poor balance[19] ◆			.70 (.56, .84)	.53 (.36, .70)	1.5	.57
Do you get pain in your legs with walking that is relieved by sitting?[20] ⬤	45 patients with low back and leg pain and self-reported limitations in walking tolerance	Lumbar spinal stenosis per MRI or CT imaging	.81 (.66, .96)	.16 (.00, .32)	.82 (.63, 1.1)	1.27
Are you able to walk better when holding onto a shopping cart?[20] ⬤			.63 (.42, .85)	.67 (.40, .93)	1.9 (.80, 4.5)	.55
Sitting reported as best posture with regard to symptoms[20] ⬤			.89 (.76, 1.0)	.39 (.16, .61)	1.5 (.90, 2.4)	.28
Walking/standing reported as worst posture with regard to symptoms[20] ⬤			.89 (.76, 1.0)	.33 (.12, .55)	1.3 (.80, 2.2)	.33

4

Thoracolumbar Spine

Historical Question and Study Quality	Patient Population	Reference Standard	Sens	Spec	+LR	−LR
Patient reports of:						
Weakness[21] ◆	170 patients with low back and leg symptoms	Lumbosacral radiculopathy per electrodiagnostics	.70	.41	1.19	.73
Numbness[21] ◆			.68	.34	1.03	.94
Tingling[21] ◆			.67	.31	.97	1.06
Burning[21] ◆			.40	.60	1.0	1.0

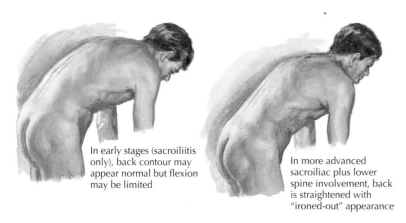

In early stages (sacroiliitis only), back contour may appear normal but flexion may be limited

In more advanced sacroiliac plus lower spine involvement, back is straightened with "ironed-out" appearance

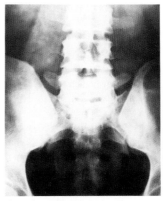

Bilateral sacroiliitis is early radiographic sign. Thinning of cartilage and bone condensation on both sides of sacroiliac joints

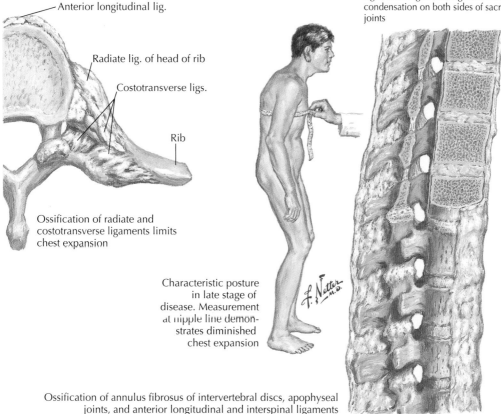

Anterior longitudinal lig.

Radiate lig. of head of rib

Costotransverse ligs.

Rib

Ossification of radiate and costotransverse ligaments limits chest expansion

Characteristic posture in late stage of disease. Measurement at nipple line demonstrates diminished chest expansion

Ossification of annulus fibrosus of intervertebral discs, apophyseal joints, and anterior longitudinal and interspinal ligaments

Figure 4-19
Ankylosing spondylitis.

Clinical Symptom and Study Quality	Patient Population	Reference Standard	Sens	Spec	+LR	−LR
Pain not relieved by lying down[22] ◆	449 randomly selected patients with low back pain	The New York criteria and radiographic confirmation of ankylosing spondylitis	.80	.49	1.57	.41
Back pain at night[23] ◆			.71	.53	1.51	.55
Morning stiffness for longer than ½ hour[22] ◆			.64	.59	1.56	.68
Pain or stiffness relieved by exercise[22] ◆			.74	.43	1.30	.60
Age of onset 40 years or less[22] ◆			1.0	.07	1.07	.00

Thoracolumbar Spine

4

Diagnostic Utility of Sensation Testing, Manual Muscle Testing, and Reflex Testing for Lumbosacral Radiculopathy

Test and Study Quality		Description and Positive Findings	Population	Reference Standard	Sens	Spec	+LR	−LR
Sensation (vibration and pinprick)[21] ◆		Considered abnormal when either vibration or pinprick was reduced on the side of the lesion	170 patients with low back and lower extremity symptoms	Electrodiagnostic testing. Radiculopathy defined as the presence of positive sharp waves; fibrillation potentials; complex repetitive discharges; high-amplitude, long-duration motor unit potentials; reduced recruitment; or increased polyphasic motor unit potentials (of more than 30%) in two or more muscles innervated by the same nerve root level but different peripheral nerves	.50	.62	1.32	.81
Weakness[21] ◆	Gastrocnemius and soleus	Weakness was defined as any grade of less than 5/5			S1 = .47	S1 = .76	1.96	.70
	Extensor hallucis longus				L5 = .61	L5 = .55	1.36	.71
	Hip flexors				L3-L4 = .70	L3-L4 = .84	4.38	.36
	Quadriceps				L3-L4 = .40	L3-L4 = .89	3.64	.67
Reflexes[21] ◆	Achilles	Considered abnormal when the reflex on the side of the lesion was reduced compared with the opposite side			S1 = .47	S1 = .9	4.70	.59
	Patellar				L3-L4 = .50	L3-L4 = .93	7.14	.54
Reflexes[24] ◆	Achilles	Test is positive if reflex is absent	100 patients with lumbar disc herniation diagnosed by MRI	Lumbar disc herniation diagnosed by MRI with level of herniation intraoperatively confirmed	S1 = .83	S1 = .57	1.93	.30
	Medial hamstring				L5 = .76	L5 = .85	5.07	.28
	Patellar				L3-L4 = .88	L3-L4 = .86	6.29	.14
Reflexes + Weakness + Sensory[21] ◆		All three abnormal		Electrodiagnostic testing. Radiculopathy defined as the presence of positive sharp waves; fibrillation potentials; complex repetitive discharges; high-amplitude, long-duration motor unit potentials; reduced recruitment; or increased polyphasic motor unit potentials (of more than 30%) in two or more muscles innervated by the same nerve root level but different peripheral nerves	.12	.97	4.00	.91
Reflexes + Weakness + Sensory + Straight-leg raise test[21] ◆		All four abnormal	170 patients with low back and lower extremity symptoms		.06	.99	6.00	.95
		Any of four abnormal			.87	.35	1.34	.37

Level of Herniation	Pain	Numbness	Weakness	Atrophy	Reflexes
L3-4 disc; 4th lumbar nerve root	Lower back, hip, posterolateral thigh, anterior leg	Antero-medial thigh and knee	Quadriceps	Quadriceps	Knee jerk diminished
L4-5 disc; 5th lumbar nerve root	Over sacro-iliac joint, hip, lateral thigh, and leg	Lateral leg, web of great toe	Dorsiflexion of great toe and foot; difficulty walking on heels; foot drop may occur	Minor	Changes uncommon (absent or diminished posterior tibial reflex)
L5-S1 disc; 1st sacral nerve root	Over sacro-iliac joint, hip, postero-lateral thigh, and leg to heel	Back of calf; lateral heel, foot and toe	Plantar flexion of foot and great toe may be affected; difficulty walking on toes	Gastrocne-mius and soleus	Ankle jerk diminished or absent
Massive midline protrusion	Lower back, thighs, legs, and/or perineum depending on level of lesion; may be bilateral	Thighs, legs, feet, and/or perineum; variable; may be bilateral	Variable paralysis or paresis of legs and/or bowel and bladder inconti-nence	May be extensive	Ankle jerk diminished or absent

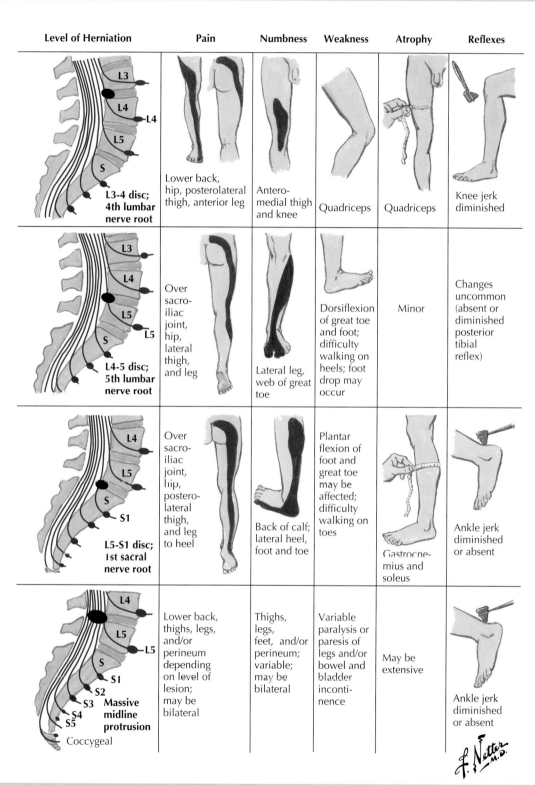

Figure 4-20
Clinical features of herniated lumbar nucleus pulposus.

Thoracolumbar Spine

4

Diagnostic Utility of Sensation Testing, Manual Muscle Testing, and Reflex Testing for Lumbar Spinal Stenosis

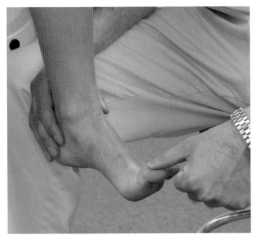

Strength testing of extensor
hallucis longus muscle

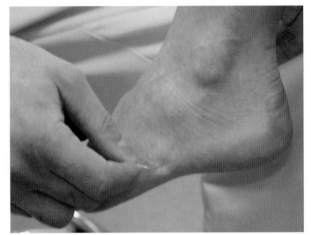

Pinprick test

Figure 4-21
Lumbar spinal stenosis testing.

Test and Study Quality	Description and Positive Findings	Population	Reference Standard	Sens	Spec	+LR	−LR
Vibration deficit[19] ◆	Assessed at the first metatarsal head with a 128-Hz tuning fork. Considered abnormal if patient did not perceive any vibration			.53 (.38, .68)	.81 (.67, .95)	2.8	.58
Pinprick deficit[19] ◆	Sensation tested at the dorsomedial foot, dorsolateral foot, and medial and lateral calf. Graded as "decreased" or "normal"	93 patients with back pain with or without radiation to the lower extremities	Diagnosis of spinal stenosis by retrospective chart review and confirmed by MRI or CT	.47 (.32, .62)	.81 (.67, .95)	2.5	.65
Weakness[19] ◆	Strength of knee flexors, knee extensors, and hallucis longus muscles was tested. Graded from 0 (no movement) to 5 (normal)			.47 (.32, .62)	.78 (.64, .92)	2.1	.68
Absent Achilles reflex[19] ◆	Reflex testing of the Achilles tendon. Graded from 0 (no response) to 4 (clonus)			.46 (.31, .61)	.78 (.64, .92)	2.1	.69

Reliability of Range-of-Motion Measurements

Measurement and Study Quality	Instrumentation	Population	Reliability	
			Intraexaminer*	Interexaminer
Active rotation in standing[28] ◆	Patients stood with a horizontal bar resting on their shoulders. A plumb weight hung from the end of the bar to the floor	24 asymptomatic golfers	ICC (right) = .86 (.70, .94) ICC (left) = .80 (.58, .92)	ICC (right) = .74 (.49, .88) ICC (left) = .78 (.56, .90)
Thoracolumbar flexion[29] ◆	iPhone inclinometer application	30 asymptomatic adult participants	ICC = .97 (.93, .98)	ICC = .98 (.95, .99)
Thoracolumbar extension[29] ◆			ICC = .80 (.58, .90)	ICC = .81 (.60, .91)
Thoracolumbar lateral flexion[29] ◆			ICC (right) = .82 (.61, .91) ICC (left) = .84 (.67, .92)	ICC (right) = .93 (.86, .97) ICC (left) = .90 (.77, .96)
Lumbar flexion[30] ◆	Single inclinometer	49 patients with low back pain referred for flexion-extension radiographs	Interexaminer ICC = .60 (.33, .79)	
Lumbar extension[30] ◆			Interexaminer ICC = .61 (.37, .78)	
Lumbar flexion[31] ◆		123 patients with low back pain of less than 90 days' duration	Interexaminer ICC = .74 (.60, .84)	
Lumbar extension[31] ◆			Interexaminer ICC = .61 (.42, .75)	

Continued

Thoracolumbar Spine

4

Reliability of Range-of-Motion Measurements—cont'd

Measurement and Study Quality	Instrumentation	Population	Reliability	
			Intraexaminer*	Interexaminer
Forward bending[25] ◆	Measured distance from fingertips to floor	Heterogeneous group (n = 98) including participants with low back pain and/or pelvic girdle pain and participants with no pain	Not tested	ICC = .93 (.90, .95)
Forward bending[26] ◉		30 patients with back pain and 20 asymptomatic subjects (only asymptomatic subjects were used for intraexaminer comparisons)	Intraclass correlation coefficient (ICC) = .95 (.89, .99)	ICC = .99 (.98, .10)
Lateral bending[26] ◉	Measured distance that fingertip slid down lateral thigh		ICC (right) = .99 (.95, 1.0) ICC (left) = .94 (.82, .98)	ICC (right) = .93 (.89, .96) ICC (left) = .95 (.91, .97)
Trunk rotation[26] ◉	Patients sat with horizontal bar on sternum. Plumb weight hung down to floor, and angle was measured with a protractor		ICC (right) = .92 (.76, .97) ICC (left) = .96 (.87, .99)	ICC (right) = .82 (.70, .89) ICC (left) = .85 (.75, .91)
Modified Schober test[26] ◉	Distances between lumbosacral junction, 5 cm below, and 10 cm above, were measured with patient in erect standing position and while maximally bending forward		ICC = .87 (.68, .96)	ICC = .79 (.67, .88)
Modified Schober test[25] ◆		Heterogeneous group (n = 98) including participants with low back pain and/or pelvic girdle pain and participants with no pain	Not tested	ICC = .77 (.67, .84)
Flexion Extension Left rotation Right rotation Left side-bending Right side-bending[27] ◉	Back range-of-motion instrument	47 asymptomatic students	ICC = .91 ICC = .63 ICC = .56 ICC = .57 ICC = .92 ICC = .89	ICC = .77 ICC = .35 ICC = .37 ICC = .35 ICC = .81 ICC = .89

*In the case of multiple examiners, intraexaminer estimates are presented for the first examiner only.

Reliability of Range-of-Motion Measurements—cont'd

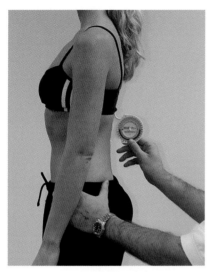

Inclinometer placement at the spinous process of the 12th thoracic vertebra

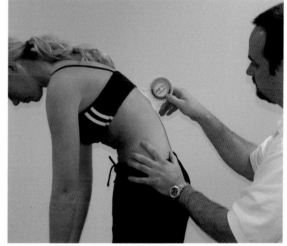

Measurement of thoracolumbar flexion

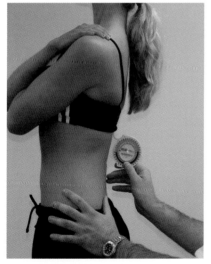

Measurement of thoracolumbar extension

Figure 4-22
Range-of-motion measurement.

Thoracolumbar Spine

4

Reliability of Pain Provocation during Range-of-Motion Measurements

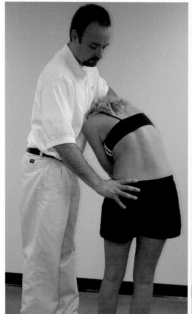 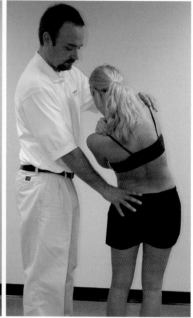

| Flexion, side-bending, and rotation | Extension, side-bending, and rotation |

Figure 4-23
Pain provocation during active movements.

Test and Study Quality	Description and Positive Findings	Population	Reliability
Side-bending[23] ◆	Patient stands with arms at sides. Patient slides hand down the outside of the thigh	35 patients with low back pain	$\kappa = .60$ (.40, .79)
Rotation[23] ◆	Patient stands with arms at sides. Patient rotates the trunk		$\kappa = .17$ (−.08, .42)
Side-bend rotation[23] ◆	Patient stands with arms at sides. Patient moves the pelvis to one side, creating a side-bend rotation to the opposite side		$\kappa = .29$ (.06, .51)
Flexion, side-bending, and rotation[23] ◆	Patient stands and the therapist guides the patient into lumbar flexion, then side-bending, then rotation		$\kappa = .39$ (.18, .61)
Extension, side-bending, and rotation[23] ◆	Patient stands and the therapist guides the patient into lumbar extension, then side-bending, then rotation		$\kappa = .29$ (.06, .52)
Thoracic rotation, right[32] ◆	Patient places hands on the opposite shoulders and rotates the trunk as far as possible in each direction. Examiner then determines the effect of each movement on the patient's symptoms as "no effect," "increases symptoms," or "decreases symptoms"	22 patients with mechanical neck pain	$\kappa = -.03$ (−.11, .04)
Thoracic rotation, left[32] ◆			$\kappa = 0.7$ (.40, 1.0)

Reliability of Assessing Thoracolumbar Strength and Endurance

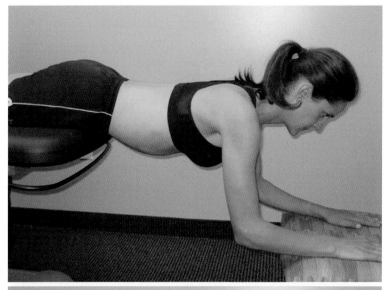

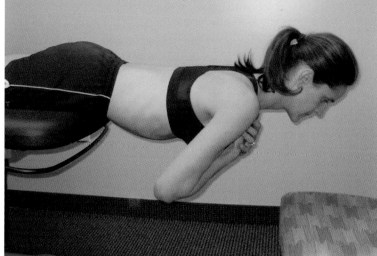

Figure 4-24
Modified Biering-Sorensen test.

Thoracolumbar Spine

4

Reliability of Assessing Thoracolumbar Strength and Endurance—cont'd

Measurement and Study Quality	Description and Positive Findings	Population	Reliability
30-second chair stand test[33] ◆	With arms crossed on chest, patients were directed to stand up and sit down from a chair as many times as possible within 30 seconds	38 patients with low back pain	Test-retest ICC = .94 (.89, .97)
Abdominal muscle endurance[34] ●	Supine participants were asked to elevate their legs off the table with hips and knees at 90° and maintain the position for as long as possible. Hold time was recorded in seconds	31 office workers with subacute low back pain	Test-retest ICCs = [men] .97 (.96, .99) [women] .96 (.92, .99)
Lumbar muscle endurance[34] ●	Prone participants were asked to lift their chest and maintain the position for as long as possible. Hold time was recorded in seconds		Test-retest ICCs = [men] .97 (.94, .98) [women] .96 (.94, .98)
Abdominal muscle endurance[26] ●	From a supine hook-lying position, the patient curls up to touch fingertips to the superior patellae and holds the position for as long as possible. Time in seconds is measured with a stopwatch	30 patients with back pain and 20 asymptomatic subjects (only asymptomatic subjects were used for intraexaminer comparisons)	Intraexaminer ICC = .90 (.75, .97) Interexaminer ICC = .92 (.87, .96)
Modified Biering-Sorensen test[26] ●	Patient starts prone with pelvis and legs supported on couch and trunk hanging off the edge supported by a chair. The patient then extends the trunk and holds a neutral position for as long as possible. Time in seconds is measured with a stopwatch		Intraexaminer ICC = .92 (.75, .97) Interexaminer ICC = .91 (.85, .95)

Reliability of Postural Assessment

Test and Study Quality	Description and Positive Findings	Population	Interexaminer Reliability
Forward head[32] ◆	"Yes" if the patient's external auditory meatus was anteriorly deviated (anterior to the lumbar spine)		$\kappa = -.10 \ (-.20, .00)$
Excessive shoulder protraction[32] ◆	"Yes" if the patient's acromions were anteriorly deviated (anterior to the lumbar spine)		$\kappa = .83 \ (.51, 1.0)$
C7-T2 excessive kyphosis[32] ◆	Recorded as "normal" (no deviation), "excessive kyphosis," or "diminished kyphosis." *Excessive kyphosis* was defined as an increase in the convexity, and *diminished kyphosis* was defined as a flattening of the convexity of the thoracic spine (at each segmental group)	22 patients with mechanical neck pain	$\kappa = .79 \ (.51, 1.0)$
T3-T5 excessive kyphosis[32] ◆			$\kappa = .69 \ (.30, 1.0)$
T3-T5 decreased kyphosis[32] ◆			$\kappa = .58 \ (.22, .95)$
T6-T10 excessive kyphosis[32] ◆			$\kappa = .90 \ (.74, 1.0)$
T6-T10 decreased kyphosis[32] ◆			$\kappa = .90 \ (.73, 1.0)$
Kyphosis[35] ◉	With patient standing, examiner inspects posture from the side. Graded as "present" or "absent"	111 adults age 60 years of age or older with chronic low back pain and 20 asymptomatic patients	$\kappa = .21$
Scoliosis[35] ◉	With patient standing, examiner runs finger along spinous processes. Patient bends over and examiner assesses height of paraspinal musculature. Graded as "present" or "absent"		$\kappa = .33$
Functional leg length discrepancy[35] ◉	Compared height of bilateral iliac crests with patient standing. Graded as "symmetric" or "asymmetric"		$\kappa = .00$
Scoliosis[36] ◉	Adam's forward bend test: one side of ribs is higher than other side during standing forward bending. Graded as "present" or "absent"	111 asymptomatic adolescents aged 12-14 years	$\kappa = .32 \ (.04, .60)$
Shoulder height asymmetry[36] ◉	Graded as "present" or "absent"		$\kappa = .20 \ (.10, .28)$

Thoracolumbar Spine

4

Reliability of Assessment for Generalized Hypermobility

Test and Study Quality	Description and Positive Findings	Population	Interexaminer Reliability
Knee extension[36]	Graded as "present" or "absent"	111 asymptomatic adolescents aged 12-14 years	(Right) $\kappa = .12$ (−.15, .38) (Left) $\kappa = .32$ (−.17, .81)
Elbow extension[36]			(Right) $\kappa = .60$ (.40, .79) (Left) $\kappa = .50$ (.31, .69)
Thumb abduction/opposition with wrist flexion[36]			(Right) $\kappa = .70$ (.47, .93) (Left) $\kappa = .70$ (.48, .92)
5th finger extension[36]			(Right) $\kappa = .49$ (−.11, 1.0) (Left) $\kappa = .39$ (−.15, .93)
Trunk/hip flexion[36]			$\kappa = 1.0$ (1.0, 1.0)
Beighton Score ≥ 4[36]	Number of positive tests above (shoulder height asymmetry, knee extension, elbow extension, thumb abduction/opposition with wrist flexion, trunk/hip flexion) out of 9. Each side (right vs. left) counted as one point		$\kappa = .65$ (.33, .97)
Beighton Score ≥ 5[36]			$\kappa = .56$ (.11, 1.0)

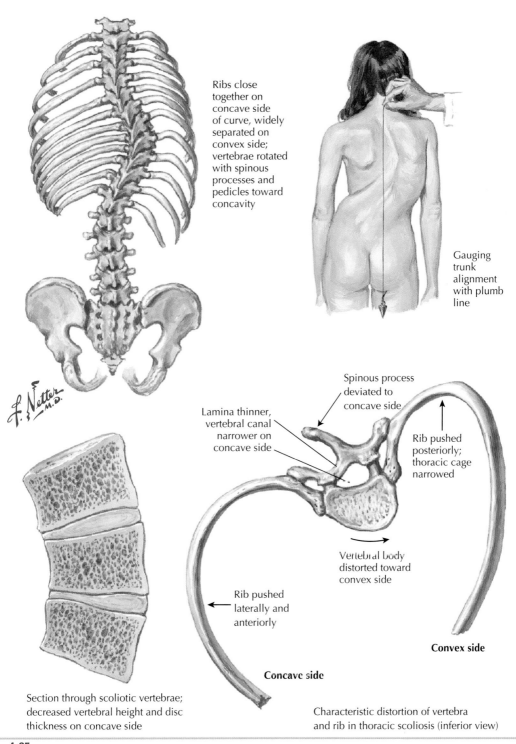

Ribs close together on concave side of curve, widely separated on convex side; vertebrae rotated with spinous processes and pedicles toward concavity

Gauging trunk alignment with plumb line

Spinous process deviated to concave side

Lamina thinner, vertebral canal narrower on concave side

Rib pushed posteriorly; thoracic cage narrowed

Vertebral body distorted toward convex side

Rib pushed laterally and anteriorly

Convex side

Concave side

Section through scoliotic vertebrae; decreased vertebral height and disc thickness on concave side

Characteristic distortion of vertebra and rib in thoracic scoliosis (inferior view)

Thoracolumbar Spine

4

Figure 4-25
Pathologic anatomy of scoliosis.

Reliability of Tests for Lumbar Motor Control

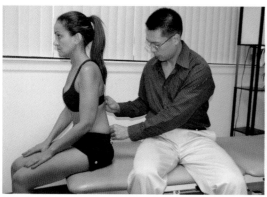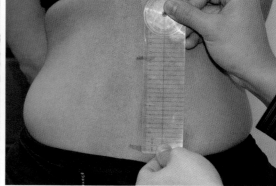

Figure 4-26
Sitting forward lean.

Test and Study Quality	Description and Positive Findings	Population	Interexaminer Reliability
Repositioning[37] ◆	Subject seated with feet supported and with low back in neutral. A 5-cm tape measure is taped at S1 (0 cm) and marked by a laser pointer. The subject is instructed to actively move the pelvis twice from maximum anterior tilt to maximum posterior tilt. Subject then repositions the pelvis back to neutral, and the distance is measured between S1 (0 cm) and the laser pointer		ICC = .90 (.81, .94)
Sitting forward lean[37] ◆	Subject seated with feet supported and low back in neutral. S1 and a point 10 cm above S1 are marked. Subject instructed to maintain distance between the two points while performing 5 repetitions of hip flexion to a maximum of 120 degrees. The distance between marks (0 cm and 10 cm) is measured		ICC = .96 (.92, .98)
Sitting knee extension[37] ◆	Same setup as for the repositioning test but with feet unsupported. The low back is in neutral with a 5-cm tape measure taped at S1 (0 cm) and marked by a laser pointer. Five repetitions of active knee extension to −10 degrees are performed while maintaining the pelvis in neutral. The distance is measured between S1 (0 cm) and the laser pointer	25 subjects with non-specific low back pain and 15 subjects without it	ICC = .95 (.90, .97)
Bent knee fall-out[37] ◆	Subject supine with one knee flexed 120 degrees and pelvis in neutral. A 5-cm tape measure is placed between the right and left anterior superior iliac spines, with a 0-cm mark and laser pointer placed lateral to the anterior superior iliac spine opposite the bent leg (with the laser pointing medially to the 0-cm mark). Five repetitions of abduction/external hip rotation of the bent leg to 45 degrees are performed. Movement of the pelvis is measured between 0 cm on the tape measure and the laser pointer		ICC = .94 (.88, .97)
Leg lowering[37] ◆	Subject supine with hips at 90 degrees of flexion, knees in maximum relaxed flexion, and low back in neutral. A pressure biofeedback unit is placed under the low back and inflated to 40 mm Hg. The subject is asked to actively push the low back downward, increasing the pressure to 45 mm Hg. Then the subject is instructed to lower the feet to just above the surface of the plinth. Five repetitions are performed while attempting to maintain 45 mm Hg. Pressure is recorded when the feet are as close as possible to the plinth		ICC = .98 (.96, .99)

Reliability of Tests for Lumbar Motor Control—cont'd

Test and Study Quality	Description and Positive Findings	Population	Interexaminer Reliability
Knee lift[38] ◆	"Stand with your feet together and your arms lifted to shoulder height away from your body. Lift one knee to hip-height. Bring your foot back down again." Score is composite of 7 possible incorrect test components	21 patients with low back pain and 17 healthy participants	ICC = .68 (.47, .82)
Static lunge[38] ◆	"Stand with one foot in front of the other. Keep feet hips-width apart. Lift the back heel from the floor, hold out your arms sideways, keep your back straight and kneel down toward the floor." Score is composite of 5 possible incorrect test components		ICC = .79 (.65, .88)
Dynamic lunge[38] ◆	"Stand up straight with your feet together and arms lifted above your head. Step forward into a lunge and maintain your trunk in an upright position. Step back to the starting position." Score is composite of 6 possible incorrect test components		ICC = .80 (.68, .89)
Single-leg squat[39] ◆	Subjects were asked to put their hands on their hips and balance on their leg of choice. If able to balance for 5 seconds, then they were asked to slowly squat down to about 45 degrees of knee bend and slowly return to standing. Graded on a scale from 0-3 points	23 healthy participants	ICC = .14 (.00, .44)
Supine bridge[39] ◆	Subjects were asked to lie down on their backs on the exam table and bend their hips and knees. They were then asked to raise their pelvis up until their back was straight and hold for 5 seconds. If able to hold for 5 seconds, they were asked to lift 1 leg and extend the knee. If able to hold for 5 more seconds, then they were asked to alternate legs and hold for 5 more seconds. Graded on a scale from 0-3 points		ICC = .40 (.16, .64)
Side bridge[39] ◆	From side-lying with knees bent, subjects were asked to raise their pelvis to make their back straight (supported on knee and forearm). If they could hold this posture for 5 seconds, then they returned to the starting position and were asked to extend their legs out straight and again lift their pelvis from the table and try to make their back straight (supported on ankle and forearm). If they could hold this for 5 seconds, they were asked to raise their upper leg about 30 degrees for 5 more seconds. Graded on a scale from 0-3 points		ICC = .69 (.50, .83)
Prone bridge[39] ◆	Subjects were asked to roll onto their stomachs and prop themselves up on their forearms and toes until their back was straight. If they could hold this posture for 5 seconds, then they were asked to raise 1 leg off the table for 5 seconds, then alternate legs for another 5 seconds. Graded on a scale from 0-3 points		ICC = .46 (.22, .68)
Core score[39] ◆	The individual scores from the 4 above tests were combined to create a composite score out of 12 points		ICC = .68 (.49, .83)

4

Thoracolumbar Spine

Reliability of Assessing Limited or Excessive Passive Intervertebral Motion

Test and Study Quality	Description and Positive Findings	Population	Reliability
Posterior-to-anterior stiffness[40] ◆	Each level of the lumbar spine was evaluated for segmental dysfunction. With patient prone, examiner assessed posterior-to-anterior stiffness and multifidus hypertonicity. With patient side-lying, side flexion and ventral flexion were assessed by moving the patient's legs. After performing all four examination procedures, examiners identified the level of maximal dysfunction	60 patients with low back pain	Intraexaminer κ = .54 Intraexaminer (±1 level) κ = .64 Interexaminer κ = .23 Interexaminer (±1 level) κ = .52
Segmental side flexion[41] ◆			Intraexaminer κ = .57 Intraexaminer (±1 level) κ = .69 Interexaminer κ = .22 Interexaminer (±1 level) κ = .45
Segmental ventral flexion[41] ◆			Intraexaminer κ = .31 Intraexaminer (±1 level) κ = .45 Interexaminer κ = .22 Interexaminer (±1 level) κ = .44
Multifidus hypertonicity[41] ◆			Intraexaminer κ = .51 Intraexaminer (±1 level) κ = .60 Interexaminer κ = .12 Interexaminer (±1 level) κ = .57
Maximal level of segmental dysfunction[41] ◆			Intraexaminer κ = .60 Intraexaminer (±1 level) κ = .70 Interexaminer κ = .21 Interexaminer (±1 level) κ = .57
Segmental mobility testing[46] ◆	With patient side-lying with hips and knees flexed, examiner assesses mobility while passively moving the patient. Examiner determines whether mobility of the segment is "decreased," "normal," or "increased"	71 patients with low back pain	Interexaminer κ = .54
Hypermobility at any level[30] ◆	With patient prone, examiner applies a posteroanterior force to the spinous process of each lumbar vertebra. Mobility of each segment is judged as "normal," "hypermobile," or "hypomobile"	49 patients with low back pain referred for flexion-extension radiographs	Interexaminer κ = .48 (.35, .61)
Hypomobility at any level[30] ◆			Interexaminer κ = .38 (.22, .54)
Identification of a mis-aligned vertebra[45] ◆	Static palpation is used to determine the relationship of one vertebra to the vertebra below	21 symptomatic and 25 asymptomatic subjects	Interexaminer κ ranged from −.04 to .03, with a mean of .00
Passive motion palpation[45] ◆	Passive motion palpation is performed, and the segment is considered fixated if a hard end feel is noted during the assessment	21 symptomatic and 25 asymptomatic subjects	Interexaminer κ = ranged from −.03 to .23, with a mean of .07
Determination of segmental fixations[44] ◐		60 asymptomatic volunteers	Intraexaminer κ ranged from −.09 to .39 Interexaminer κ ranged from −.06 to .17

Reliability of Assessing Limited or Excessive Passive Intervertebral Motion—cont'd

Test and Study Quality	Description and Positive Findings	Population	Reliability
Upper lumbar segmental mobility[43] ◐	With patient prone, examiner applies a posteroanterior force to the spinous process and lumbar facets of each lumbar vertebra. Mobility of each segment is judged as "normal" or "restricted"	39 patients with low back pain	(Spinous) Interexaminer κ =.02 (−.27, .32) (Left facet) Interexaminer κ =.17 (−.14, .48) (Right facet) Interexaminer κ = −.01 (−.33, .30)
Lower lumbar segmental mobility[43] ◐			(Spinous) Interexaminer κ = −.05 (−.36, .27) (Left facet) Interexaminer κ = −.17 (−.41, .06) (Right facet) Interexaminer κ = −.12 (−.41, .18)
Identifying the least mobile segment[40] ◐	With patient prone, examiner applies a posteroanterior force to the spinous process of each lumbar vertebra	29 patients with central low back pain	Interexaminer κ = .71 (.48, .94)
Identifying the most mobile segment[40] ◐			Interexaminer κ = .29 (−.13, .71)
Segmental mobility[42] ◐	With patient side-lying, examiner palpates adjacent spinous processes while moving the patient's legs to produce passive flexion and extension of the lumbar spine. Segmental mobility was graded on a 5-point scale	20 patients with low back pain	Interexaminer κ ranged from −.25 to .53 depending on examiners and vertebral level
Determination of posteroanterior spinal stiffness[47] ◐	Five raters tested lumbar spinal levels for posteroanterior mobility and graded each on an 11-point scale ranging from "markedly reduced stiffness" to "markedly increased stiffness"	40 asymptomatic individuals	Interexaminer ICC in the first study = .55 (.32, .79) Interexaminer ICC in the second study = .77 (.57, .89)
Posteroanterior mobility testing[48] ◐	With the patient prone, examiner evaluates posteroanterior motion mobility. Mobility is scored on a 9-point scale ranging from "severe excess motion" to "no motion," and the presence of pain is recorded	18 patients with low back pain	Interexaminer ICC = .25 (.00, .39)
Segmental mobility testing[49] ◐	With patient prone, examiner applies an anteriorly directed force over the spinous process of the segment to be tested. Examiner grades the mobility as "hypermobile," "normal," or "hypomobile"	63 patients with current low back pain	Interexaminer κ ranged from −.20 to .26 depending on level tested
Detection of a segmental lesion at T11-L5/S1[50] ◐	Two clinicians used visual postural analysis, pain descriptions, leg length discrepancy, neurologic examination, motion palpation, static palpation, and any special orthopaedic tests to determine the level of segmental lesion	19 patients with chronic mechanical low back pain	Intraexaminer κ = −.08 to .43 Interexaminer κ = −.16 to .25

4

Thoracolumbar Spine

Reliability of Assessing Painful Passive Intervertebral Motion

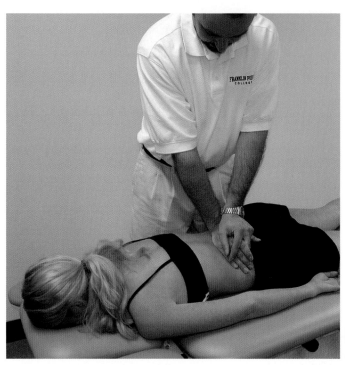

Figure 4-27
Assessment of posteroanterior segmental mobility.

Test and Study Quality	Description and Positive Findings	Population	Reliability	
			Intraexaminer	**Interexaminer**
Pain with lumbar mobility testing[52] ◆	With patient prone, examiner applies a posteroanterior (PA) or lateral force to the spinous processes and lumbar facets of each lumbar vertebra. Response at each segment is judged as "painful" or "not painful." Process was repeated in flexion and extension and reliability estimates are average of all spinal levels and all positions	18 patients with subacute nonspecific low back pain	(PA spinous) Interexaminer κ = .43 (.31, .54) (PA left facet) Interexaminer κ = .43 (.36, .50) (PA right facet) Interexaminer κ = .42 (.34, .49) (Left lateral spinous) Interexaminer κ = .52 (.36, .68) (Right lateral spinous) Interexaminer κ = .43 (.33, .52)	
Pain during mobility testing[30] ◆	With patient prone, examiner applies an anteriorly directed force over the spinous processes of the segment to be tested. Considered positive if pain is reproduced	49 patients with low back pain referred for flexion-extension radiographs	Interexaminer κ = .57 (.43, .71)	
Pain provocation[49] ◗		63 patients with current low back pain	Interexaminer κ ranged from .25 to .55 depending on the segmental level tested	

Reliability of Assessing Painful Passive Intervertebral Motion—cont'd

Test and Study Quality	Description and Positive Findings	Population	Reliability	
			Intraexaminer	Interexaminer
Spring test T10-T7[51] ◐	With patients in the prone position the therapist applies a postero-anterior force to the spinous processes of T7-L5. The pressure of each force is held for 20 seconds. Considered positive if the force produces pain	84 subjects, of whom 53% reported experiencing low back symptoms within the last 12 months	κ = .73 (.39 to 1.0)	κ =.12 (−.18 to .41)
Spring test L2-T11[51] ◐			κ = .78 (.49 to 1.0)	κ = .36 (.07 to .66)
Spring test L5-L3[51] ◐			κ = .56 (.18 to .94)	κ = .41 (.12 to .70)
Pain with upper lumbar mobility testing[43] ◐	With patient prone, examiner applies a posteroanterior force to the spinous processes and lumbar facets of each lumbar vertebra. Response at each segment is judged as "painful" or "not painful"	39 patients with low back pain	(Spinous) Interexaminer κ =.21 (−.10, .53) (Left facet) Interexaminer κ = .46 (.17, .75) (Right facet) Interexaminer κ = .38 (.06, .69)	
Pain with lower lumbar mobility testing[43] ◐			(Spinous) Interexaminer κ = .57 (.32, .83) (Left facet) Interexaminer κ = .73 (.51, .95) (Right facet) Interexaminer κ = .52 (.25, .79)	

Thoracolumbar Spine **4**

Diagnostic Utility of Assessing Limited and Painful Passive Intervertebral Motion

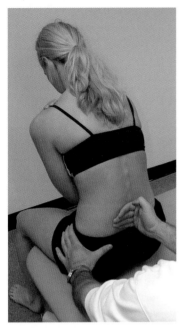

Motion palpation, seated

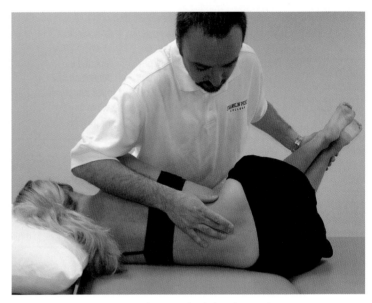

Motion palpation of side-bending, right

Figure 4-28
Segmental mobility examination.

Test and Study Quality	Description and Positive Findings	Popula-tion	Reference Standard	Sens	Spec	+LR	−LR
Active range of motion[53] ◆	Quantity of forward-bending active range of motion. Rated as "hypomobile," "normal," or "hypermobile"		Flexion and extension lateral radiographs. Segments were considered hypomobile if motion was more than 2 standard deviations from the mean of a normal population	.75 (.36, .94)	.60 (.27, .86)	1.88 (.57, 6.80)	.42 (.07, 1.90)
Abnormality of segmental motion (Abn-ROM)[53] ◆	Examiner judged presence of abnormal segmental motion during active range of motion. Rated as "hypomobile," "normal," or "hypermobile"			.43 (.19, .71)	.88 (.70, .96)	3.60 (.84, 15.38)	.65 (.28, 1.06)
Passive accessory intervertebral motion (PAIVM)[53] ◆	Examiner applies central posteroanterior pressure. Passive accessory intervertebral motion was rated as "hypomobile," "normal," or "hypermobile"	9 patients with low back pain		.75 (.36, .94)	.35 (.20, .55)	1.16 (.44, 3.03)	.71 (.12, 2.75)
Passive physiologic intervertebral motion (PPIVM)[53] ◆	With patient side-lying, examiner palpates amount of PPIVM during forward bending. Rated as "hypomobile," "normal," or "hypermobile"			.42 (.19, .71)	.89 (.71, .96)	3.86 (.89, 16.31)	.64 (.28, 1.04)
Motion palpation[54] ◐	Palpation of a motion segment during either passive or active motion. Examiners evaluated for limited motion (i.e., "fixation"). Patient's pain reaction was noted after motion palpation of each segment	184 twins	Self-reported low back pain	.42	.57	.98	1.02

Diagnostic Utility of Assessing Excessive Passive Intervertebral Motion

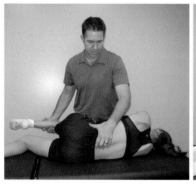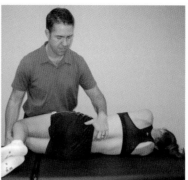

Lumbar flexion   Lumbar extension

Figure 4-29
Assessing lumbar passive physiologic intervertebral motion (PPIVM).

Test and Study Quality	Description and Positive Findings	Population	Reference Standard	Sens	Spec	+LR	−LR
Passive accessory intervertebral motion (PAIVM)[55] ◆	Examiner applies central posteroanterior pressure. PAIVM was rated as "hypomobile," "normal," or "hypermobile"			**Rotational Lumbar Segmental Instability**			
				.33 (.12, .65)	.88 (.83, .92)	2.74 (1.01, 7.42)	.76 (.48, 1.21)
				Translational Lumbar Segmental Instability			
			Flexion and extension lateral radiographs. Segments were considered hypermobile if motion was more than 2 standard deviations from the mean of a normal population	.29 (.14, .50)	.89 (.83, .93)	2.52 (1.15, 5.53)	.81 (.61, 1.06)
Flexion passive physiologic intervertebral motion (PPIVM)[55] ◆	With patient side-lying, examiner palpates amount of PPIVM during forward bending. Rated as "hypomobile," "normal," or "hypermobile"	Patients with a new episode of recurrent or chronic low back pain		**Rotational Lumbar Segmental Instability**			
				.05 (.01, .36)	.99 (.96, 1.00)	.12 (.21, 80.3)	.96 (.83, 1.11)
				Translational Lumbar Segmental Instability			
				.05 (.01, .22)	.99 (.97, 1.00)	8.73 (.57, 134.7)	.96 (.88, 1.05)
Extension PPIVM[55] ◆	With patient side-lying, examiner palpates amount of PPIVM during backward bending. Rated as "hypomobile," "normal," or "hypermobile"			**Rotational Lumbar Segmental Instability**			
				.22 (.06, .55)	.97 (.94, .99)	8.40 (1.88, 37.55)	.80 (.56, 1.13)
				Translational Lumbar Segmental Instability			
				.16 (.06, .38)	.98 (.94, .99)	7.07 (1.71, 29.2)	.86 (.71, 1.05)

Thoracolumbar Spine   4

Reliability of Identifying Segmental Levels

Procedure Performed and Quality	Description of Procedure	Patient Population	Interexaminer Reliability
Detection of segmental levels in the lumbar spine[56] ◆	With patient prone, examiner identifies nominated levels of the lumbar spine. Examiner marks the specific level with a pen containing ink that can only be seen under ultraviolet light	20 patients with low back pain	$\kappa = .69$
Identification of lumbar spinous process using multiple bony landmarks[57] ◆	With the patient prone, each examiner used all of the following landmarks to determine the location of the spinous processes for L1-L4: 1. Identification of T12 by the smaller size of its spinous process compared with that of L1 to determine the location of L1. 2. Identification of 12th ribs and their attachment site at T12 to determine the location of T12 and its spinous process and, subsequently, the location of L1. 3. Identification of iliac crests to approximately determine the location of the vertebral body of L4. 4. Identification of sacral base to determine the location of L5. 5. Identification of L5 spinous process by the smaller size of its spinous process to determine the location of L4. Accuracy of the skin marker placement over the corresponding spinous process determined by radiograph	60 subjects age 20 to 60 years	$\kappa = .81$ (.79, .83)
Examiner judgment of marked segmental level[48] ◐	With the patient prone, one spinous process is arbitrarily marked on each patient. Examiners identify the level of the marked segment	18 patients with low back pain	ICC = .69 (.53, .82)

Reliability of Identifying Tenderness to Palpation

Procedure Performed and Quality	Description of Procedure	Patient Population	Interexaminer Reliability
Osseous pain of each joint T11/L1-L5/S1[45] ◆	With the subject prone, examiner applies pressure over the bony structures of each joint	21 symptomatic and 25 asymptomatic subjects	Mean κ for all levels = .48
Intersegmental tenderness[46] ◆	With patient prone, examiner palpates the area between the spinous processes. Increased tenderness is considered positive	71 patients with low back pain	κ = .55
Lumbar paravertebral myofascial pain[35] ●	Reports of pain with deep thumb pressure (4 kg)		κ = .34
Piriformis myofascial pain[35] ●			κ = .66
Tensor fasciae latae myofascial pain[35] ●			κ = .75
Fibromyalgia tender points[35] ●	Reports of pain with enough pressure to blanch thumbnail at: 1. Occiput at suboccipital muscle insertions 2. Low cervical region at the anterior aspects of the intertransverse spaces at C5-C7 3. Trapezius, midpoint of upper border 4. Supraspinatus at origin 5. Rib 2 at the second costochondral junction 6. 2 cm distal to the epicondyle 7. Medial fat pad of the knee 8. Greater trochanter 9. Gluteal at upper outer quadrant of buttocks	111 adults age 60 years with chronic low back pain and 20 asymptomatic subjects	κ = .87

4

Thoracolumbar Spine

Diagnostic Utility of Gluteal Trigger Points in Differentiating Radicular and Nonradicular Low Back Pain

Test and Study Quality	Description and Positive Findings	Population	Reference Standard	Sens	Spec	+LR	−LR
Presence of gluteal muscle trigger points[58] ◆	Palpated using "flat palpation." Considered present when taut band, tenderness, and pain recognition	325 patients with low back pain	Combination of clinical exam and MRI findings. Radicular low back pain defined as pain below the knee and/or neuro-logic symptoms	.74 (.67, .80)	.91 (.86, .95)	8.6 (5.0, 15.0)	.28 (.22, .36)

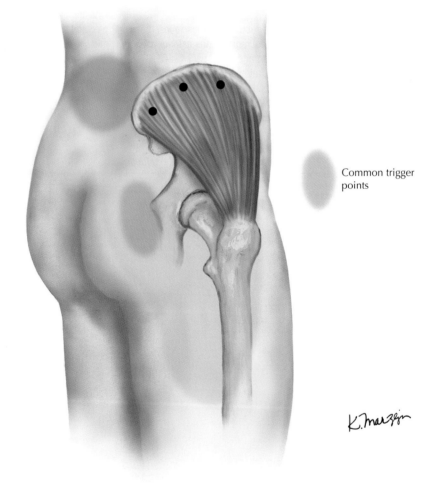

Common trigger points

Figure 4-30
Common trigger points and associated referred pain in the gluteus medius muscle. *Black dots* are "common trigger points." *Blue areas* are "referred pain."

Reliability of Assessing Lumbopelvic Muscle Function via Palpation

Procedure Performed and Quality	Description of Procedure	Patient Population	Interexaminer Reliability
Abdominal drawing-in maneuver (ADIM)[59] ◆	In supine "hook-lying" (hips and knees flexed), patients were instructed to gently draw the naval towards the spine. The transversus abdominus (TrA) muscles were palpated just medially to the anterior superior iliac crest (ASIS). The ADIM was considered successful when a slow preferential TrA muscle contraction could be palpated for 10 seconds	38 patients with low back pain and 15 healthy volunteers	$\kappa = .71$ (.41, 1.0)
Multifidus lift test L4-L5[60] ◆	Participant prone with arms flexed to approximately 120 degrees and elbows flexed to approximately 90 degrees, the patient is instructed to raise contralateral arm toward the ceiling approximately 5 cm. Test is positive when little or no palpable contraction of the muscle is identified during the arm lift	32 adults with current low back pain	$\kappa = .75$ (.52, .97)
Multifidus lift test L5-S1[60] ◆			$\kappa = .81$ (.62, 1.00)

In addition to testing reliability, Kaping and colleagues (Kaping et al., 2015) also tested the association of manual and ultrasonic assessment of transverse abdominis (TrA) function during the abdominal drawing-in maneuver (ADIM) and its ability to discriminate patients with low back pain from the healthy volunteers. Although manual assessment was poorly correlated to ultrasonic measures ($r = .13–.40$), it was moderately good at identifying patients with low back pain (sensitivity = .30, specificity = .73).

Thoracolumbar Spine

4

Reliability of Identifying the Centralization Phenomenon

Test and Study Quality	Description and Positive Findings	Population	Interexaminer Reliability
Centralization and directional preference[61] ◆	Two examiners with more than 5 years of training in the McKenzie method evaluated all patients and determined whether centralization occurred during repeated movements. If centralization occurred, the clinician recorded the directional preference	39 patients with low back pain	κ if centralization occurred = .70
			κ related to centralization and directional preference = .90
Judgments of centralization[62] ◆	Therapists (without formal training in McKenzie methods) and students viewed videotapes of patients undergoing a thorough examination by one therapist. All therapists and students watching the videos were asked to make an assessment regarding the change in symptoms based on movement status	12 patients receiving physical therapy for low back pain	Between physical therapists κ = .82 (.81, .84) Between physical therapy students κ = .76 (.76, .77)
Status change with flexion in sitting[31] ◆			κ = .55 (.28, .81)
Status change with repeated flexion in sitting[31] ◆	10 different examiners assessed symptom change (centralization, peripheralization, or no change) with single or repeated movements	123 patients with low back pain of less than 90 days' duration	κ = .46 (.23, .69)
Status change with extension[31] ◆			κ = .51 (.29, .72)
Status change with repeated extension[31] ◆			κ =.15 (.06, .36)
Status change with sustained prone extension[31] ◆			κ = .28 (.10, .47)

Diagnostic Utility of the Centralization Phenomenon

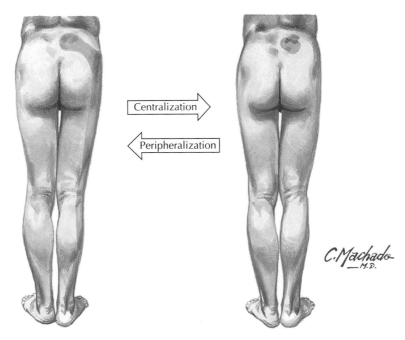

During specific movements, range of motion and movement of pain noted. Movement of pain from peripheral to central location (centralization) predicts outcome and appropriateness of therapy.

Figure 4-31
Centralization of pain.

Test and Study Quality	Description and Positive Findings	Population	Reference Standard	Sens	Spec	+LR	−LR
Centralization[63] ◆	Centralization present if pain in the furthermost region from midline was abolished or reduced with a McKenzie-styled repeated motion examination	69 patients with persistent low back pain with or without referred leg pain	At least one painful disc adjacent to a nonpainful disc with discography	.40 (.28, .54)	.94 (.73, .99)	6.9 (1.0, 47.3)	.63 (.49, .82)

Thoracolumbar Spine 4

Reliability of the Straight-Leg Raise Test

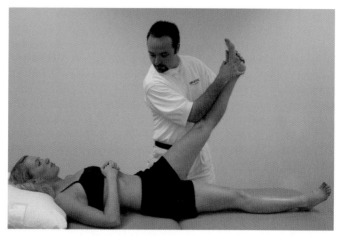

Straight-leg raise

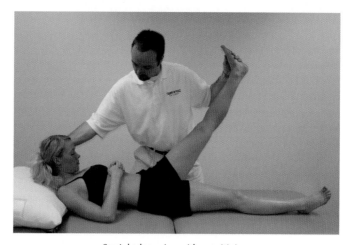

Straight-leg raise with sensitizing
maneuver of cervical flexion

Figure 4-32
Straight-leg raise test.

Test and Study Quality	Description and Positive Findings	Population	Interexaminer Reliability
Passive straight-leg raise test[15] ◆	With patient supine, examiner passively flexes the hip and extends the knee. Examiner measures the angle of straight-leg raising and determines if symptoms occurred in a dermatomal fashion	91 patients with low back pain randomly selected	For typical dermatomal pain, $\kappa = .68$ For any pain in the leg, $\kappa = .36$ For straight-leg raising of less than 45 degrees, $\kappa = .43$
Passive straight-leg raise test[64] ⬤	With patient supine, examiner maintains the knee in extension while passively flexing the hip. The hip is flexed until examiner feels resistance. A range-of-motion measurement is recorded	18 physiotherapy students	ICC Right = .86, Left = .83
Passive straight-leg raise test[65] ⬤	Passive elevation of the leg with knee extended. Considered positive if pain in the low back or buttock is experienced	27 patients with low back pain	$\kappa = .32$

Diagnostic Utility of the Straight-Leg Raise Test for Detecting Disc Bulge or Herniation

Deville and colleagues[66] compiled the results of 15 studies investigating the accuracy of the straight-leg raise test for detecting disc herniation. Ten of the studies included information about both the sensitivity and specificity of the straight-leg raise test and were used for statistical pooling of estimates. However, numerous variations of the straight-leg raise maneuver have been reported, and no consistency was noted among the studies selected for the Deville and colleagues review. Similarly, a 2010 Cochrane Review[67] investigating the accuracy of the straight-leg raise test for detecting disc herniation used nine studies for statistical pooling of estimates; all nine were the same as those used by the Deville and colleagues study, reported above. The results of each study, as well as the pooled estimates, are listed here.

Straight-Leg Raise Study and Quality	Description and Positive Findings	Reference Standard	Sens	Spec	+LR	−LR
Straight-leg raise test **2000 Meta-analysis**[66] ◆	With the patient supine, the knee fully extended, and the ankle in neutral dorsiflexion, examiner then passively flexes the hip while maintaining the knee in extension. Positive test defined by reproduction of sciatic pain between 30 degrees and 60 to 75 degrees	Herniated lumbar disc observed during surgery. Herniation was defined as an extruded, protruded, and bulging disc or a sequestrated disc in most studies	.91 (.82, .94)	.26 (.16, .38)	1.23	.35
Straight-leg raise test **2011 Meta-analysis**[67] ◆			.92 (.87, .95)	.28 (.18, .40)	1.3	.29
Straight-leg raise test[69] ◆	With patient supine, examiner slowly lifts the symptomatic straight leg until maximal hip flexion is reached or the patient asks to stop. The angle between the leg and the table is measured. Positive if reproduction of familiar radicular pain occurs	MRI findings of disc extrusions in 99 patients with lumbar radicular symptoms referred for epidural steroid injection	.59 (.41, .75)	.53 (.41, .64)	1.3 (.84, 1.9)	.77 (.47, 1.3)
		MRI findings of high-grade sub-articular nerve root compression in 99 patients with lumbar radicular symptoms referred for epidural steroid injection	.93 (.66, 1.0)	.57 (.45, .67)	2.1 (1.6, 2.8)	.13 (.02, .84)
Straight-leg raise test[70] ◆	As above. Positive test defined by reproduction of pain distal to the knee between 30° and 70° of hip flexion	Electrodiagnostic evidence of S1 nerve root compression in 506 patients with unilateral radicular low back pain referred for electrodiagnosis of the lower extremity	.63 (.58, .69)	.46 (.39, .53)	1.2 (1.0, 1.4)	.80 (.64, .98)
Modified Brag-gard test[70] ◆	Same as the straight-leg raise test with the addition of passive ankle dorsiflexion when patients could achieve 70° of hip flexion without leg symptoms		.69 (.60, .77)	.76 (.57, .77)	2.1 (1.5, 2.9)*	.46 (.33, .62)
Straight-leg raise test[68] ◉	With patient supine, examiner slowly lifts the symptomatic straight leg until maximal hip flexion is reached or the patient asks to stop. The angle between the leg and the table is measured. Positive if reproduction of familiar radicular pain occurs	MRI findings of disc bulges, herniations, and/or extrusions in 75 patients with complaints of acute or recurrent low back and/or leg pain of 12 weeks' duration or less	.52 (.42, .58)	.89 (.79, .95)	4.73	.54

*+LR was found to be 4.2 (2.8, 5.7) in acute (pain less than 3 weeks) patients.

Diagnostic Utility of the Crossed Straight-Leg Raise Test for Detecting Disc Bulging or Herniation

Deville and colleagues[66] also compiled the results of eight studies investigating the accuracy of the crossed straight-leg raise test for detecting disc herniation. Five of the studies included information about both the sensitivity and specificity of the crossed straight-leg raise test and were used for statistical pooling of estimates. Similarly, a 2010 Cochrane Review[67] investigating the accuracy of the crossed straight-leg raise test for detecting disc herniation used five studies for statistical pooling of estimates. Four of the five studies used for the pooled estimate were the same as those used by the Deville and colleagues[66] study, reported above. The results of each study, as well as the pooled estimates, are listed here.

Crossed Straight-Leg Raise Study and Quality	Description and Positive Findings	Reference Standard	Sens	Spec	+LR	−LR
Crossed straight-leg raise test **2000 Metaanalysis**[66] ◆	Performed identically to the straight-leg raise test except the uninvolved lower extremity is lifted. A positive test is defined as reproducing pain in the involved lower extremity	Herniated lumbar disc observed during surgery. Herniation was defined as extruded, protruded, and bulging disc or sequestrated disc in most studies	.29 (.24, .34)	.88 (.86, .90)	2.42	.81
Crossed straight-leg raise test **2011 Metaanalysis**[67] ◆			.28 (.22, .35)	.90 (.85, .94)	2.8	.80

Reliability of the Slump Test

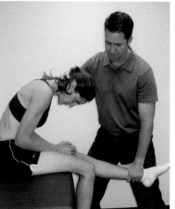
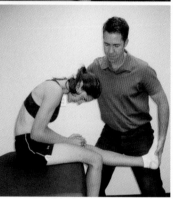
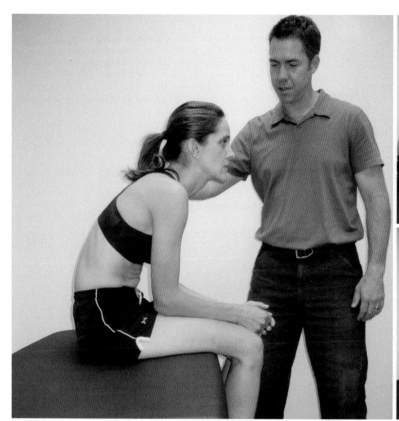

Thoracolumbar Spine 4

Figure 4-33
Slump test.

Test and Study Quality	Description and Positive Findings	Population	Intraexaminer Reliability
Knee extension range of motion during the slump test[71] ●	Subject sitting maximally slumped with one thigh flexed 25 degrees to the horizontal plane. Starting with the knee at 90 degrees and maximal ankle dorsiflexion, the knee was slowly extended to maximal discomfort and measured with an electrogoniometer	20 asymptomatic subjects	With cervical flexion: ICC = .95 With cervical extension: ICC = .95

Diagnostic Utility of the Slump Test for Detecting Disc Extrusions, Bulging or Herniation, and Nerve Root Compression

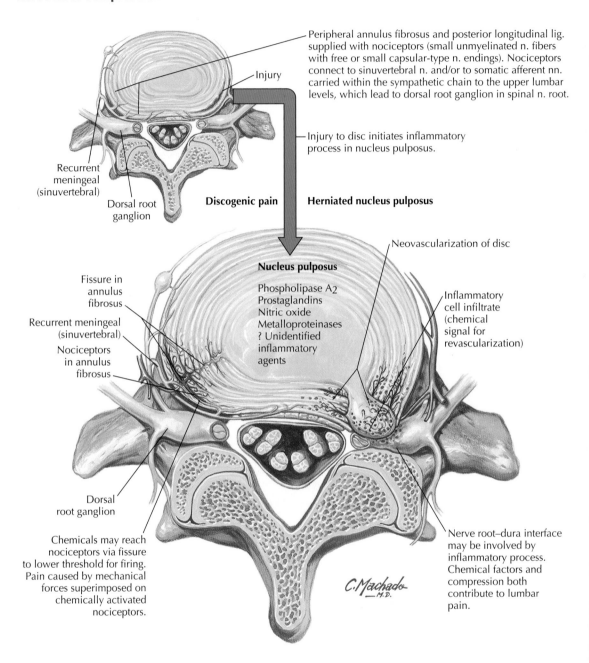

Injury

Peripheral annulus fibrosus and posterior longitudinal lig. supplied with nociceptors (small unmyelinated n. fibers with free or small capsular-type n. endings). Nociceptors connect to sinuvertebral n. and/or to somatic afferent nn. carried within the sympathetic chain to the upper lumbar levels, which lead to dorsal root ganglion in spinal n. root.

Recurrent
meningeal
(sinuvertebral)

Dorsal root
ganglion

Injury to disc initiates inflammatory process in nucleus pulposus.

Discogenic pain   **Herniated nucleus pulposus**

Neovascularization of disc

Nucleus pulposus

Phospholipase A2
Prostaglandins
Nitric oxide
Metalloproteinases
? Unidentified
inflammatory
agents

Fissure in
annulus
fibrosus

Recurrent meningeal
(sinuvertebral)

Nociceptors
in annulus
fibrosus

Inflammatory
cell infiltrate
(chemical
signal for
revascularization)

Dorsal
root ganglion

Chemicals may reach
nociceptors via fissure
to lower threshold for firing.
Pain caused by mechanical
forces superimposed on
chemically activated
nociceptors.

Nerve root–dura interface
may be involved by
inflammatory process.
Chemical factors and
compression both
contribute to lumbar
pain.

C. Machado
—M.D.

Figure 4-34
Role of inflammation in lumbar pain.

Diagnostic Utility of the Slump Test for Detecting Disc Extrusions, Bulging or Herniation, and Nerve Root Compression—cont'd

Test and Study Quality	Description and Positive Findings	Population	Reference Standard	Sens	Spec	+LR	−LR
Slump test[69] ◆	Sitting with the back straight, the patient is encouraged to slump into lumbar and thoracic flexion while looking straight ahead. Then the patient fully flexes the neck and extends one knee. Last, the patient dorsiflexes the ipsilateral foot. Positive if reproduction of familiar radicular pain occurs	99 patients with lumbar radicular symptoms referred for epidural steroid injection	MRI findings of disc extrusions	.78 (.59, .89)	.36 (.26, .48)	1.2 (.93, 1.6)	.61 (.29, 1.3)
			MRI findings of high-grade subarticular nerve root compression	1.0 (.77, 1.0)	.38 (.27, .49)	1.6 (1.4, 1.9)	0.0
Slump test[68] ◆		75 patients with complaints of acute or recurrent low back pain and/or leg pain of 12 weeks' duration or less	MRI findings of disc bulges, herniations, and/or extrusions	.84 (.74, .90)	.83 (.73, .90)	4.94	.19
Slump test[72] ◆		21 individuals with low back pain with or without radiating leg pain	Neuropathic pain as determined by a standard neurosensory examination including a straight-leg raise (but not slump) test	.91 (.62, .98)	.70 (.40, .89)	3.0 (1.2, 8.0)	.13 (.02, .88)
Slump test + location of symptoms[72] ◆	As above, but positive test only in the case of symptoms below the knee			.55 (.28, .79)	1.0 (.72, 1.0)	11.9 (.76, 187.8)	.48 (.26, .90)

Thoracolumbar Spine 4

Reliability of the Slump Knee Bend Test

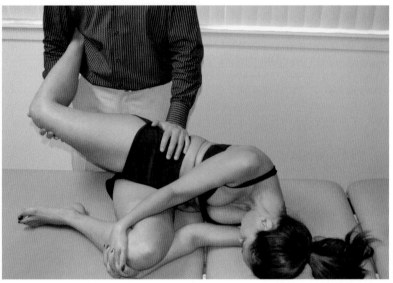

Figure 4-35
Slump knee bend test.

Test and Study Quality	Description and Positive Findings	Population	Intraexaminer Reliability
Slump knee bend test[73] ◆ (see Video 4-1)	Subject side-lying with no pillow, slightly "cuddling" underside leg with cervical and thoracic spines flexed. Clinician stands behind subject supporting upper leg in neutral (no adduction/abduction). With the subject's upper knee flexed, clinician extends the hip until symptom is evoked. The subject is asked to extend the neck. Positive if symptom diminishes with neck extension	Sixteen patients with radicular leg pain	$\kappa = .71$ (.33, 1.00)

Diagnostic Utility of the Slump Knee Bend Test in Detecting Disc Extrusions and Nerve Root Compression

Test and Study Quality	Description and Positive Findings	Population	Reference Standard	Sens	Spec	+LR	−LR
Slump knee bend test[69] ◆	Patient side-lying on the nonaffected side, assesses the presence/absence of neural mechanosensitivity (L2-4) using a combination of thoracolumbar, cervical, and knee flexion, and hip extension. Positive if one of the maneuvers reproduced symptoms and the symptoms were different from the contralateral side	99 patients with lumbar radicular symptoms referred for epidural steroid injection	MRI findings of disc extrusions	.43 (.16, .75)	.64 (.35, .85)	1.2 (.37, 3.8)	.90 (.41, 2.0)
			MRI findings of high-grade subarticular nerve root compression	1.0 (.21, 1.0)	.65 (.41, .83)	2.8 (1.5, 5.4)	0.0
Slump knee bend test[73] ◆	Patient side-lying on the nonaffected side, assesses the presence/absence of neural mechanosensitivity (L2-4) using a combination of thoracolumbar, cervical, and knee flexion, and hip extension. Positive if one of the maneuvers reproduced symptoms and the symptoms were different from the contralateral side	16 patients with radicular leg pain	MRI findings of nerve root compression	1.00 (.40, 1.00)	.83 (.52, .98)	6.00 (1.58, 19.4)	0.0 (0.0, .60)

Thoracolumbar Spine 4

Reliability of Tests for Lumbar Segmental Instability

Test and Study Quality	Description and Positive Findings	Population	Interexaminer Reliability
Passive lumbar extension test (PLET)[74] ◆	With the patient prone, both legs are passively raised about 30 cm from bed level and then pulled gently. Positive if the patient experiences severe low back pain, or reports the low back feels heavy or about to "come off"	40 adults with recurrent or chronic low back pain	κ = .46 (.20, .72)
Lumbar flexion ROM > 53° [74] ◆	Measured standing to full forward bending with a bubble inclinometer read at T12-L1 and S2. Lumbar flexion ROM is the difference between 2 readings		κ = .48 (.16, .80)
Lack of hypomobility[74] ◆	Measured prone by placing posterior to anterior (PA) pressure on each lumbar spinous process. Positive when no lumbar segments are judged to be hypomobile (stiff)		κ = −.02 (−.22, .18)
Average passive straight-leg raise > 90°[74] ◆	Measured supine with a bubble inclinometer on the tibial crest. The leg is passively raised to the maximum tolerable level		κ = .77 (.47, 1.1)
Hip extension test[75] ◆	Prone patient extends one hip at a time. Positive if lateral shift, rotation, or hyperextension of the lumbar spine occurs	42 patients with chronic low back pain	κ = .72 (left) κ = .76 (right)
Altered lumbopelvic rhythm[76] ◆	Hip motion greater than lumbar spine motion during the first third of forward bending and/or lumbar spine motion greater than hip motion during the last third of forward bending	102 subjects with current low back pain, history of low back pain, or no low back pain	κ = .83 (.73, .93)
Sagittal plane deviation from midline[76] ◆	Movement away from the primary sagittal plane (flexion/extension), including rotations and/or lateral flexion		κ = .60 (.50, .69)
Instability catch[76] ◆	Patient experiences a sudden acclimation of deceleration of trunk movements outside the primary plane of movement		κ = .46 (.31, .61)
Any of the above 3 aberrant[76] movements ◆	As above		κ = .53 (.43, .64)
Any of the 5 aberrant[76] movements ◆	As above plus painful arc in flexion and/or return from flexion		κ = .68 (.747, .89)
Painful arc in flexion[49] ◉	Patient reports symptoms at a particular point in the movement but the symptoms are not present before or after the movement	63 patients with current low back pain	κ = .69 (.54, .84)
Painful arc on return from flexion[49] ◉	Patient experiences symptoms when returning from the flexed position		κ = .61 (.44, .78)
Instability catch[49] ◉	Patient experiences a sudden acclimation of deceleration of trunk movements outside the primary plane of movement		κ = .25 (−.10, .60)
Gower sign[49] ◉	Patient pushes up from thighs with the hands when returning to upright from a flexed position		κ = .00 (−1.09, 1.09)
Reversal of lumbopelvic rhythm[49] ◉	On attempting to return from the flexed position, the patient bends the knees and shifts the pelvis anteriorly		κ = .16 (−.15, .46)
Aberrant movement pattern[49] ◉			κ = .60 (.47, .73)
Aberrant movement pattern[31] ◆	If the patient demonstrates any of the above five possible movement patterns, the patient is considered to be positive for an aberrant movement pattern	123 patients with low back pain of less than 90 days' duration	κ = .18 (−.07, .43)
Aberrant movement pattern[77] ◉		30 patients with low back pain	κ = .64 (.32, .90)
Aberrant motion[74] ◆		40 adults with recurrent or chronic low back pain	κ = .79 (.39, 1.2)

Reliability of Tests for Lumbar Segmental Instability—cont'd

Test and Study Quality	Description and Positive Findings	Population	Interexaminer Reliability
Trendelenburg[78] ◆	While standing, the patient flexes one hip to 30 degrees and lifts the ipsilateral pelvis above the transiliac line. The test is positive if the patient cannot hold the position for 30 seconds or needs more than one finger for balance	36 patients with chronic low back pain	κ = .83 (left) κ = .75 (right)
Active straight-leg raise test[79] ◆	The patient is supine with straight legs and feet 20 cm apart. The patient is instructed to "try to raise your legs, one after the other, above the couch without bending the knee." The patient is asked to score the maneuver on a 6-point scale ranging from "not difficult at all" to "unable to do"		κ = .70 (left) κ = .71 (right)
Active straight-leg raise test[79] ◑		50 females with lumbopelvic pain	Test-retest ICC = .83
Active straight-leg raise test[77] ◑		30 patients with low back pain	κ = .53 (.20, .84)
Posterior shear test[49] ◑	With patient standing with arms crossed over the abdomen, examiner places one hand over the patient's crossed arms while the other stabilizes the pelvis. Examiner uses the index finger to palpate the L5-S1 interspace. Examiner then applies a posterior force through the patient's crossed arms. This procedure is performed at each level. A positive test is indicated by provocation of symptoms	63 patients with current low back pain	κ = .35 (.20, .51)
Prone instability test[49] ◑			κ = .87 (.80, .94)
Prone instability test[31] ◆	The patient is prone with the edge of the torso on the plinth while the legs are over the edge and feet are resting on the floor. Examiner performs a posteroanterior pressure maneuver and notes the provocation of any symptoms. The patient then lifts the feet off the floor, and examiner again performs the posteroanterior pressure maneuver. Provocation of symptoms is reported. Test is considered positive if the patient experiences symptoms while feet are on the floor but symptoms disappear when the feet are lifted off the floor	123 patients with low back pain of less than 90 days' duration	κ = .28 (.10, .47)
Prone instability test[43] ◑		39 patients with low back pain	κ = .46 (.15, .77)
Prone instability test[77] ◑		30 patients with low back pain	κ = .67 (.29, 1.00)
Prone instability test[74] ◆		40 adults with recurrent or chronic low back pain	κ = .71 (.45, .98)

Thoracolumbar Spine

4

Reliability of Tests for Lumbar Segmental Instability—cont'd

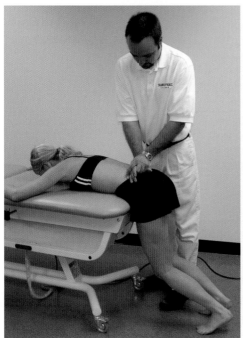 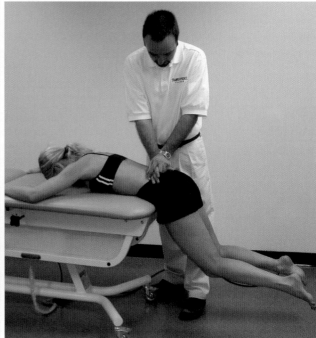

Figure 4-36
Prone instability test.

Diagnostic Utility of Tests for Lumbar Spinal Stenosis

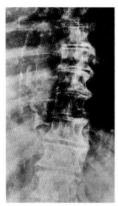

Radiograph of thoracic spine shows narrowing of intervertebral spaces and spur formation.

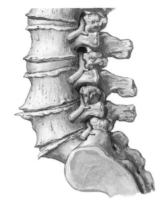

Degeneration of lumbar intervertebral discs and hypertrophic changes at vertebral margins with spur formation. Osteophytic encroachment on intervertebral foramina compresses spinal nerves.

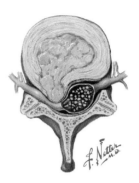

Schematic cross-section showing compression of nerve root.

Figure 4-37

Degenerative disc disease and lumbar spinal stenosis.

Test and Study Quality	Description and Positive Findings	Population	Reference Standard	Sens	Spec	+LR	−LR
Abnormal Romberg test[19] ◆	Patient stands with feet together and eyes closed for 10 seconds. Considered abnormal if compensatory movements were required to keep feet planted	93 patients with back pain with or without radiation to the lower extremities	Diagnosis of spinal stenosis by retrospective chart review and confirmed by MRI or CT	.39 (.24, .54)	.91 (.81, 1.0)	4.3	.67
Thigh pain with 30 seconds of extension[19] ◆	Patient performs hip extension for 30 seconds. Positive if patient has pain in the thigh following or during extension			.51 (.36, .66)	.69 (.53, .85)	1.6	.71
Two-stage treadmill test[20] ◉	Subjects ambulate on a level and inclined (15 degrees) treadmill for 10 minutes. The patient rests for 10 minutes while sitting upright in a chair after each treadmill test	45 subjects with low back and lower extremity pain	Diagnosis of spinal stenosis by MRI or CT scanning	Time to onset of symptoms			
				.68 (.50, .86)	.83 (.66, 1.0)	4.07 (1.40, 11.8)	.39
				Longer total walking time during the inclined test			
				.50 (.38, .63)	.92 (.78, 1.0)	6.46 (3.1, 13.5)	.54
				Prolonged recovery after level walking			
				.82 (.66 to .98)	.68 (.48, .90)	2.59 (1.3, 5.2)	.26

Thoracolumbar Spine 4

Diagnostic Utility of Tests for Radiographic Lumbar Instability

Test and Study Quality	Description and Positive Findings	Population	Reference Standard	Sens	Spec	+LR	−LR
Passive lumbar extension test[1] ◆ **2011 Systematic Review** (see Video 4-2)	With subject in the prone position, both lower extremities are passively elevated, concurrently, to a height of about 30 cm while maintaining the knees extended and gently pulling the legs. Positive with low back pain or discomfort during test	122 patients with low back pain with mean age of 68.9 years	Flexion-extension radiograph with translation motion of 5 mm	.84 (.68, .93)	.90 (.82, .96)	8.8 (4.5, 17.3)	.20 (.10, .40)
Age younger than 37 years[30] ◆	History collected prior to physical examination			.57 (.39, .74)	.81 (.60, .92)	3.0 (1.2, 7.7)	.53 (.33, .85)
Lumbar flexion greater than 53 degrees[30] ◆	Range of motion demonstrated by single inclinometer			.68 (.49, .82)	.86 (.65, .94)	4.8 (1.6, 14.0)	.38 (.21, .66)
Total extension greater than 26 degrees[30] ◆	Range of motion demonstrated by single inclinometer	49 patients with low back pain referred for flexion-extension radiographs	Radiologic findings revealed either two segments with rotational/translational instability or one segment with both rotational and translational instability	.50 (.33, .67)	.76 (.55, .89)	2.1 (.90, 4.9)	.66 (.42, 1.0)
Lack of hypomobility during intervertebral testing[30] ◆	With patient prone, examiner applies a posteroanterior force to the spinous process of each lumbar vertebra. Mobility of each segment was judged as "normal," "hypermobile," or "hypomobile"			.43 (.27, .61)	.95 (.77, .99)	9.0 (1.3, 63.9)	.60 (.43, .84)
Any hypermobility during intervertebral motion testing[30] ◆				.46 (.30, .64)	.81 (.60, .92)	2.4 (.93, 6.4)	.66 (.44, .99)
Lumbar flexion greater than 53 degrees + Lack of hypomobility during intervertebral testing[30] ◆	Combination of both factors above			.29 (.13, .46)	.98 (.91, 1.0)	12.8 (.79, 211.6)	.72 (.55, .94)
Low midline sill sign[80] ●	With patient standing, examiner observes and then palpates the lumbar spine. A positive test is both observing a capital "L" in the midline of the low back and a "sill" or "step-off" palpated at the bottom of the "L"	96 patients with low back or lumbar radicular pain seen in an interventional pain management clinic	Radiologic findings on flexion-extension lateral and oblique films of more than 4 mm translation or 10° rotation	.81 (.64, .93)	.89 (.79, .95)	7.4 (3.6, 15.2)	.21 (.10, .44)
Interspinous gap change[80] ●	The patient stands and leans forward with his or her arms on a table. A positive test is when the examiner observes and palpates an abrupt change in the width of a interspinous space during flexion and extension motion			.82 (.68, .92)	.61 (.41, .79)	2.1 (1.3, 3.4)	.29 (.15, .59)

Diagnostic Utility of Tests for Radiographic Lumbar Instability—cont'd

Fritz and colleagues[81] investigated the accuracy of the clinical examination in 49 patients with radiographically determined lumbar instability. Results revealed that two predictor variables, including lack of hypomobility of the lumbar spine and lumbar flexion greater than 53 degrees, demonstrated a +LR of 12.8 (.79, 211.6). The nomogram below represents the change in pretest probability (57% in this study) to a posttest probability of 94.3%.

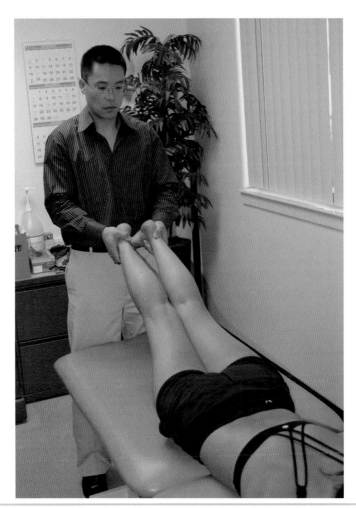

Figure 4-38
Passive lumbar extension test.

Thoracolumbar Spine

4

Diagnostic Utility of Tests for Radiographic Lumbar Instability—cont'd

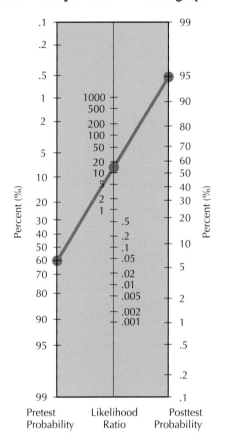

Figure 4-39
Nomogram representing the posttest probability of lumbar instability given the presence of hypomobility in the lumbar spine and lumbar flexion greater than 53 degrees. (Adapted with permission from Fagan TJ. Nomogram for Baye's theorem. *N Engl J Med.* 1975;293-257. Copyright 2005, Massachusetts Medical Society. All rights reserved.)

Reliability of Tests for Facet Joint Pain

Test and Study Quality	Description and Positive Findings	Population	Interexaminer Reliability
Unilateral local pain[82] ◆	Not specifically described	91 patients with chronic low back pain	κ = .44
Referred pain not below knee[82] ◆			κ = .62
No nerve root pain[82] ◆			κ = .29
Less pain in flexion[82] ◆			κ = .69
Pain in extension[82] ◆			κ = .59
Pain in extension with ipsilateral flexion and rotation[82] ◆			κ = .32
Ipsilateral muscle spasm[82] ◆			κ = .25
Pain with unilateral pressure on facet joint or spinous process[82] ◆			κ = .43
Limited motion or increased stiffness with unilateral pressure to facet joint[82] ◆			κ = .48
Conclusion of facet joint origin of pain[82] ◆			κ = .49

4

Thoracolumbar Spine

Diagnostic Utility of Tests for Ankylosing Spondylitis

Test and Study Quality	Description and Positive Findings	Population	Reference Standard	Sens	Spec	+LR	−LR
Measurements of chest expansion[22] ◆	Less than 7 cm (procedure not reported)	449 randomly selected patients with low back pain	The New York criteria and radiographic confirmation of ankylosing spondylitis	.63	.53	1.34	.70
	Less than 2.5 cm (procedure not reported)			.91	.99	.91	.09
Schober test less than 4 cm[22] ◆	With patient standing, examiner marks a point 5 cm below and 10 cm above S2. This distance is then measured in the upright position and then in full flexion. The difference between the two measurements is calculated and recorded to the closest centimeter			.30	.86	2.14	.81
Decreased lumbar lordosis[22] ◆	Visual observation individually judged by each examiner			.36	.80	1.8	.80
Direct tenderness over sacroiliac joint[22] ◆	Direct pressure over the joint with the patient in an upright position. Positive if patient reports pain			.27	.68	.84	1.07

Reliability of Low Back Pain Classification Systems

Test and Study Quality	Description and Positive Findings	Population	Interexaminer Reliability
McKenzie classification for low back pain[83] ◆	Therapists (of which only 32% had ever taken any form of McKenzie training) completed a McKenzie evaluation form and classified the patient as exhibiting a postural, dysfunction, or derangement syndrome. Therapists also determined if the patient presented with a lateral shift	363 patients referred to physical therapists for the treatment of low back pain	κ for classification = .26 κ for lateral shift = .26
McKenzie classification for low back pain[61] ◆	Two examiners with more than 5 years of training in the McKenzie method evaluated all patients. Therapists completed a McKenzie evaluation form and classified the patient as exhibiting a postural, dysfunction, or derangement syndrome. Therapists also determined if the patient presented with a lateral shift	39 patients with low back pain	κ for classification = .70 κ for lateral shift = .20
McKenzie evaluation[84] ◆	Examination consisted of history taking, evaluation of spinal range of motion, and specified test movements	46 consecutive patients presenting with low back pain	Classification of syndrome κ = .70 Derangement subsyndrome κ = .96 Presence of lateral shift κ = .52 Deformity of sagittal plane κ = 1.0
Movement impairment–based classification system for lumbar spine syndromes[85] ◆	Examiners used a standardized history and physical examination to assess patients and classify them into one of five lumbar spine categories	24 patients with chronic low back pain	κ for classification = .61
Treatment-based classification[31] ◆	30 examiners used a standardized history and physical examination to assess patients and classify them into one of three treatment-based categories	123 patients with low back pain for less than 90 days' duration	κ for classification = .61 (.56, .64)
Treatment-based classification[81] ◆	Examiners used a standardized history and physical examination to assess patients and classify them into one of four treatment-based categories	120 patients with low back pain	κ for classification = .56
Treatment-based classification[86] ◆	Examiners used a standardized history and physical examination to assess patients and classify them into one of four treatment-based categories after a 1-day training session	45 patients with low back pain	κ for classification = .45
Treatment-based classification[87] ◉	6 examiners experienced with TBC used a standardized history and physical examination to assess patients and classify them into one of four treatment-based categories	30 patients with low back pain	κ for classification = .62
Stabilization subgroup from treatment-based classification[77] ◉	Each examiner rated the subject's status on the stabilization subgroup based on age and the rating of aberrant movement, straight-leg raise, and prone instability test scores. If a subject presented with three or more positive tests, his or her status was considered positive	30 patients with low back pain	κ for subgroup = .86 (.65, 1.00)

4

Thoracolumbar Spine

Treatment-Based Classification Method[88]

	Subgroup Criteria	Treatment Approach
Specific Exercise Subgroup	**Extension**	
	• Symptoms distal to the buttock • Symptoms centralize with lumbar extension • Symptoms peripheralize with lumbar flexion • Directional preference for extension	• End-range extension exercises • Mobilization to promote extension • Avoidance of flexion activities
	Flexion	
	• Older age (over 50 years) • Directional preference for flexion • Imaging evidence of lumbar spine stenosis	• End-range flexion exercises • Mobilization or manipulation of the spine and/or lower extremities • Exercise to address impairments of strength or flexibility • Body weight–supported ambulation
Stabilization Subgroup	• Age (under 40 years) • Average straight-leg raise (more than 91 degrees) • Aberrant movement present • Positive prone instability test	• Exercises to strengthen large spinal muscles (erector spinae, oblique abdominals) • Exercises to promote contraction of deep spinal muscles (multifidus, transversus abdominis)
Manipulation Subgroup	• No symptoms distal to knee • Duration of symptoms less than 16 days • Lumbar hypomobility • FABQW less than 19 • Hip internal rotation range of motion of more than 35 degrees	• Manipulation techniques for the lumbopelvic region • Active lumbar range-of-motion exercises
Traction Subgroup	• Symptoms extend distal to the buttock(s) • Signs of nerve root compression are present • Peripheralization occurs with extension movement or positive findings on contralateral straight-leg raise test	• Prone mechanical traction • Extension-specific exercise activities

Rather than attempt to classify low back pain based on pathologic anatomy, the Treatment-Based Classification (TBC) system identifies subgroups of patients thought to respond to specific conservative treatment interventions. Although its initial proposal was based on experience and clinical reasoning,[89] researchers have since systematically identified many of the historical and clinical examination factors associated with each subgroup using clinical prediction rule research methodology.[2,3,90]

Diagnostic Utility of Single Factors for Identifying Patients Likely to Benefit from Spinal Manipulation

Test and Study Quality	Description and Criteria	Popula-tion	Reference Standard	Sens	Spec	+LR	−LR
Symptoms for less than 16 days' duration[2] ◆	Self-report	71 patients with low back pain	Reduction of 50% or more in back pain–related disabil-ity within 1 week as measured by the Oswestry question-naire	.56 (.39, .72)	.87 (.73, .94)	4.39 (1.83, 10.51)	Not reported
FABQ work sub-scale score less than 19[2] ◆				.84 (.68, .93)	.49 (.34, .64)	1.65 (1.17, 2.31)	
No symptoms distal to the knee[2] ◆				.88 (.72, .95)	.36 (.23, .52)	1.36 (1.04, 1.79)	
At least one hip with more than 35 degrees of internal rotation range of motion[2] ◆	With patient prone, measured with standard goniometer			.50 (.34, .66)	.85 (.70, .93)	3.25 (1.44, 7.33)	
Hypomobility in the lumbar spine[2] ◆	With patient prone, exam-iner applies a posteroante-rior force to the spinous process of each lumbar vertebra. Mobility of each segment was judged as "normal," "hy-permobile," or "hypomobile"			.97 (.84, .99)	.23 (.13, .38)	1.26 (1.05, 1.51)	

4

Thoracolumbar Spine

Diagnostic Utility of Combinations of Factors for Identifying Patients Likely to Benefit from Spinal Manipulation

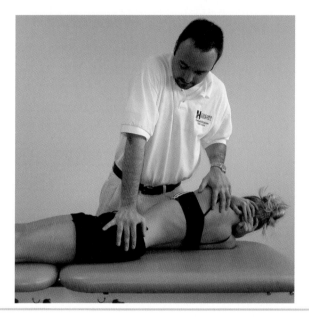

Figure 4-40
Spinal manipulation technique used by Flynn and colleagues. The patient is passively side-bent toward the side to be manipulated (away from the therapist). The therapist then rotates the patient away from the side to be manipulated (toward the therapist) and delivers a quick thrust through the anterior superior iliac spine in a posteroinferior direction. (From Flynn T, Fritz J, Whitman J, et al. A clinical prediction rule for classifying patients with low back pain who demonstrate short-term improvement with spinal manipulation. *Spine.* 2002;27:2835-2843.)

Test and Study Quality	Description and Criteria	Population	Reference Standard	Sens	Spec	+LR	−LR
Symptoms of less than 16 days' duration + No symptoms distal to the knee + Hypomobility in the lumbar spine + FABQ work subscale score less than 19 + At least one hip with more than 35 degrees of internal rotation range of motion[2] ◆	All five tests positive	71 patients with low back pain	Reduction of 50% or more in back pain–related disability within 1 week as measured by the Oswestry questionnaire	.19 (.09, .35)	1.00 (.91, 1.00)	Undefined	Not reported
	Four or more tests positive			.63 (.45 to .77)	.97 (.87 to 1.0)	24.38 (4.63 to 139.41)	
	Three or more tests positive			.94 (.80, .98)	.64 (.48, .77)	2.61 (1.78, 4.15)	
	Two or more tests positive			1.00 (.89, 1.0)	.15 (.07, .30)	1.18 (1.09, 1.42)	
	One or more tests positive			1.00 (.89, 1.0)	.03 (.005, .13)	1.03 (1.01, 1.15)	
Symptoms of less than 16 days' duration + No symptoms distal to the knee[90] ◆	Must meet both criteria	141 patients with low back pain		.56 (.43, .67)	.92 (.84, .96)	7.2 (3.2, 16.1)	

Diagnostic Utility of Single Factors and Combinations of Factors in Identifying Patients Likely to Benefit from Lumbar Stabilization Exercises

Test and Study Quality	Description and Positive Findings	Population	Reference Standard	Sens	Spec	+LR	−LR
Age younger than 40 years[3] ◆	Self-report			.61 (.39, .80)	.83 (.68, .92)	3.7 (1.6, 8.3)	.47 (.26, .85)
Average straight-leg raise test of more than 91 degrees[3] ◆	Measured with an inclinometer			.28 (.13, .51)	.92 (.78, .97)	3.3 (.90, 12.4)	.79 (.58, 1.1)
Aberrant movement present[3] ◆	Presence of any of the following during flexion range of motion: • Instability catch • Painful arc of motion • "Thigh climbing" (Gower sign) • Reversal of lumbopelvic rhythm	54 patients with low back pain with or without leg pain	Reduction of 50% or more in back pain–related disability after 8 weeks of lumbar stabilization exercises as measured by the Oswestry questionnaire	.78 (.55, .91)	.50 (.35, .66)	1.6 (1.0, 2.3)	.44 (.18, 1.1)
Positive prone instability test[3] ◆	See description under Tests for Lumbar Segmental Instability			.72 (.49, .88)	.58 (.42, .73)	1.7 (1.1, 2.8)	.48 (.22, 1.1)
Combination of any four factors above[3] ◆	Three or more tests positive			.56 (.34, .75)	.86 (.71, .94)	4.0 (1.6, 10.0)	.52 (.30, .88)
	Two or more tests positive			.83 (.61, .94)	.56 (.40, .71)	1.9 (1.2, 2.9)	.30 (.10, .88)
	One or more 1 tests positive			.94 (.74, .99)	.28 (.16, .44)	1.3 (1.0, 1.6)	.20 (.03, 1.4)

Clinical Prediction Rule to Identify Patients with Low Back Pain Likely to Benefit from Pilates-Based Exercise

Stolze and colleagues[91] developed a clinical prediction rule for identifying patients with low back pain who are likely to benefit from Pilates-based exercise. The result of their study demonstrated that if three or more of the five attributes (total trunk flexion range of motion of 70 degrees or less, duration of current symptoms of 6 months or less, no leg symptoms in the last week, body mass index of 25 kg/m^2 or greater, and left or right hip average rotation range of motion of 25 degrees or greater) were present, the +LR was 10.64 (95% CI 3.52, 32.14) and the probability of experiencing a successful outcome improved from 54% to 93%.

Thoracolumbar Spine

4

Outcome Measure	Scoring and Interpretation	Test-Retest Reliability	MCID
Oswestry Disability Index (ODI)	Users are asked to rate the difficulty of performing 10 functional tasks on a scale of 0 to 5 with different descriptors for each task. A total score out of 100 is calculated by summing each score and doubling the total. The answers provide a score between 0 and 100, with higher scores representing more disability	ICC = .91[92]	11[93]
Modified Oswestry Disability Index (modified ODI)	As above, except the modified ODI replaces the sex life question with an employment/homemaking question	ICC = .90[94]	6[94]
Roland-Morris Disability Questionnaire (RMDQ)	Users are asked to answer 23 or 24 questions (depending on the version) about their back pain and related disability. The RMDQ is scored by adding the number of items checked by the patient, with higher numbers indicating more disability	ICC = .91[95]	5[93]
Fear-Avoidance Beliefs Questionnaire (FABQ)	Users are asked to rate their level of agreement with statements concerning beliefs about the relationship between physical activity, work, and their back pain. Level of agreement is answered on a Likert-type scale ranging from 0 (completely disagree) to 7 (completely agree). The FABQ has two parts: a seven-item work subscale (FABQW) and a four-item physical activity subscale (FABQPA). Each scale is scored separately, with higher scores representing greater fear avoidance	FABQW: ICC = .82 FABQPA: ICC = .66[96]	Not available
Numeric Pain Rating Scale (NPRS)	Users rate their level of pain on an 11-point scale ranging from 0 to 10, with high scores representing more pain. Often asked as "current pain" and "least," "worst," and "average" pain in the past 24 hours	ICC = .72[97]	2[98,99]
StarT Back Tool (SBT)	Designed for screening in primary care, users answer 9 questions regarding prognostic indicators for low back pain. The tool produces 2 scores: overall scores and distress subscale scores. The overall score is used to identify the low-risk patients (≤ 3). The distress subscale is used to separate the high-risk subgroup (≥ 4) from the medium-risk subgroup (≤ 3). Patients that are deemed to be high and medium risk may need earlier and more intervention than low-risk patients	ICC = .89 (.82, .94)[100]	Not available

MCID, Minimum clinically important difference.

1. Alqarni AM, Schneiders AG, Hendrick PA. Clinical tests to diagnose lumbar segmental instability: a systematic review. *J Orthop Sports Phys Ther.* 2011;41(3):130–140.

2. Flynn T, Fritz J, Whitman J, et al. A clinical prediction rule for classifying patients with low back pain who demonstrate short-term improvement with spinal manipulation. *Spine.* 2002;27:2835–2843.

3. Hicks GE, Fritz JM, Delitto A, McGill SM. Preliminary development of a clinical prediction rule for determining which patients with low back pain will respond to a stabilization exercise program. *Arch Phys Med Rehabil.* 2005;86:1753–1762.

4. Vleeming A, Pool-Goudzwaard AL, Stoeckart R, et al. The posterior layer of the thoracolumbar fascia. Its function in load transfer from spine to legs. *Spine.* 1995;20:753–758.

5. Bogduk N. The applied anatomy of the lumbar fascia. *Spine.* 1984;9:164–170.

6. Bergmark A. Stability of the lumbar spine. A study in mechanical engineering. *Acta Orthop Scand Suppl.* 1989;230:1–54.

7. Bogduk N. *Clinical Anatomy of the Lumbar Spine and Sacrum.* London: Churchill Livingstone; 1997.

8. Evans C, Oldreive W. A study to investigate whether golfers with a history of low back pain show a reduced endurance of transversus abdominis. *J Man Manip Ther.* 2000;8:162–174.

9. Kay AG. An extensive literature review of the lumbar multifidus: biomechanics. *J Man Manip Ther.* 2001;9:17–39.

10. Norris CM. Spinal stabilisation. 1. Active lumbar stabilisation—concepts. *Physiotherapy.* 1995;81:61–78.

11. Schwarzer AC, Aprill CN, Derby R, et al. Clinical features of patients with pain stemming from the lumbar zygapophysial joints. Is the lumbar facet syndrome a clinical entity? *Spine.* 1994;19:1132–1137.

12. Schwarzer AC, Wang SC, Bogduk N, et al. Prevalence and clinical features of lumbar zygapophysial joint pain: a study in an Australian population with chronic low back pain. *Ann Rheum Dis.* 1995;54:100–106.

12a. Dreyfuss P, Tibiletti C, Dreyer SJ. Thoracic zygapophyseal joint pain patterns. A study in normal volunteers. *Spine.* 1994;19(7):807–811.

12b. Fukui S, Ohseto K, Shiotani M, et al. Distribution of referred pain from the lumbar zygapophyseal joints and dorsal rami. *Clin J Pain.* 1997;13:303–307.

13. McCombe PF, Fairbank JC, Cockersole BC, Pynsent PB. 1989 Volvo Award in clinical sciences. Reproducibility of physical signs in low-back pain. *Spine.* 1989;14:908–918.

14. Roach KE, Brown MD, Dunigan KM, et al. Test-retest reliability of patient reports of low back pain. *J Orthop Sports Phys Ther.* 1997;26:253–259.

15. Vroomen PC, de Krom MC, Knottnerus JA. Consistency of history taking and physical examination in patients with suspected lumbar nerve root involvement. *Spine.* 2000;25:91–97.

16. Van Dillen LR, Sahrmann SA, Norton BJ, et al. Reliability of physical examination items used for classification of patients with low back pain. *Phys Ther.* 1998;78:979–988.

17. Enthoven WTM, Geuze J, Scheele J, et al. Prevalence and "red flags" regarding specified causes of back pain in older adults presenting in general practice. *Phys Ther.* 2016;96(3):305–312.

18. Thiruganasambandamoorthy V, Turko E, Ansell D, et al. Risk factors for serious underlying pathology in adult emergency department nontraumatic low back pain patients. *J Emerg Med.* 2014;47(1):1–11.

19. Katz JN, Dalgas M, Stucki G, et al. Degenerative lumbar spinal stenosis. Diagnostic value of the history and physical examination. *Arthritis Rheum.* 1995;38:1236–1241.

20. Fritz JM, Erhard RE, Delitto A, et al. Preliminary results of the use of a two-stage treadmill test as a clinical diagnostic tool in the differential diagnosis of lumbar spinal stenosis. *J Spinal Disord.* 1997;10:410–416.

21. Lauder TD, Dillingham TR, Andary M, et al. Effect of history and exam in predicting electrodiagnostic outcome among patients with suspected lumbosacral radiculopathy. *Am J Phys Med Rehabil.* 2000;79:60–68. quiz 75-76.

22. Gran JT. An epidemiological survey of the signs and symptoms of ankylosing spondylitis. *Clin Rheumatol.* 1985;4:161–169.

23. Haswell K, Williams M, Hing W. Interexaminer reliability of symptom-provoking active sidebend, rotation and combined movement assessments of patients with low back pain. *J Man Manip Ther.* 2004;12:11–20.

24. Esene IN, Meher A, Elzoghby MA, et al. Diagnostic performance of the medial hamstring reflex in L5 radiculopathy. *Surg Neurol Int.* 2012;3:104.

25. Robinson HS, Mengshoel AM. Assessments of lumbar flexion range of motion: intertester reliability and concurrent validity of 2 commonly used clinical tests. *Spine.* 2014;39(4):E270–E275.

26. Lindell O, Eriksson L, Strender LE. The reliability of a 10-test package for patients with prolonged back and neck pain: could an examiner without formal medical education be used without loss of quality? A methodological study. *BMC Musculoskelet Disord.* 2007;8:31.

27. Breum J, Wiberg J, Bolton JE. Reliability and concurrent validity of the BROM II for measuring lumbar mobility. *J Manipulative Physiol Ther.* 1995;18:497–502.

28. Evans K, Refshauge KM, Adams R. Measurement of active rotation in standing: reliability of a simple test protocol. *Percept Mot Skills.* 2006;103:619–628.

Thoracolumbar Spine

4

References

29. Kolber MJ, Pizzini M, Robinson A, et al. The reliability and concurrent validity of measurements used to quantify lumbar spine mobility: an analysis of an iphone® application and gravity based inclinometry. *Int J Sports Phys Ther*. 2013;8(2):129–137.

30. Fritz JM, Piva SR, Childs JD. Accuracy of the clinical examination to predict radiographic instability of the lumbar spine. *Eur Spine J*. 2005;14:743–750.

31. Fritz JM, Brennan GP, Clifford SN, et al. An examination of the reliability of a classification algorithm for subgrouping patients with low back pain. *Spine*. 2006;31:77–82.

32. Cleland JA, Childs JD, Fritz JM, Whitman JM. Interrater reliability of the history and physical examination in patients with mechanical neck pain. *Arch Phys Med Rehabil*. 2006;87:1388–1395.

33. Kahraman T, Ozcan Kahraman B, Salik Sengul Y, Kalemci O. Assessment of sit-to-stand movement in nonspecific low back pain: A comparison study for psychometric properties of field-based and laboratory-based methods. *Int J Rehabil Res*. 2016;39(2):165–170.

34. del Pozo-Cruz B, Mocholi MH, del Pozo-Cruz J, et al. Reliability and validity of lumbar and abdominal trunk muscle endurance tests in office workers with nonspecific subacute low back pain. *J Back Musculoskelet Rehabil*. 2014;27(4):399–408.

35. Weiner DK, Sakamoto S, Perera S, Breuer P. Chronic low back pain in older adults: prevalence, reliability, and validity of physical examination findings. *J Am Geriatr Soc*. 2006;54:11–20.

36. Aartun E, Degerfalk A, Kentsdotter L, Hestbaek L. Screening of the spine in adolescents: Inter- and intra-rater reliability and measurement error of commonly used clinical tests. *BMC Musculoskelet Disord*. 2014;15:37.

37. Enoch F, Kjaer P, Elkjaer A, et al. Inter-examiner reproducibility of tests for lumbar motor control. *BMC Musculoskelet Disord*. 2011;12:114.

38. Granström H, Äng BO, Rasmussen-Barr E. Movement control tests for the lumbopelvic complex. Are these tests reliable and valid? *Physiother Theory Pract*. 2017;33(5):386–397.

39. Friedrich J, Brakke R, Akuthota V, Sullivan W. Reliability and practicality of the core score: four dynamic core stability tests performed in a physician office setting. *Clin J Sport Med*. 2017;27(4):409–414.

40. Landel R, Kulig K, Fredericson M, et al. Intertester reliability and validity of motion assessments during lumbar spine accessory motion testing. *Phys Ther*. 2008;88:43–49.

41. Qvistgaard E, Rasmussen J, Laetgaard J, et al. Intraobserver and inter-observer agreement of the manual examination of the lumbar spine in chronic low-back pain. *Eur Spine J*. 2007;16:277–282.

42. Johansson F. Interexaminer reliability of lumbar segmental mobility tests. *Man Ther*. 2006;11:331–336.

43. Schneider M, Erhard R, Brach J, et al. Spinal palpation for lumbar segmental mobility and pain provocation: an interexaminer reliability study. *J Manipulative Physiol Ther*. 2008;31:465–473.

44. Mootz RD, Keating JCJ, Kontz HP, et al. Intra- and interobserver reliability of passive motion palpation of the lumbar spine. *J Manipulative Physiol Ther*. 1989;12:440–445.

45. Keating JCJ, Bergmann TF, Jacobs GE, et al. Interexaminer reliability of eight evaluative dimensions of lumbar segmental abnormality. *J Manipulative Physiol Ther*. 1990;13:463–470.

46. Strender LE, Sjoblom A, Sundell K, et al. Interexaminer reliability in physical examination of patients with low back pain. *Spine*. 1997;22:814–820.

47. Maher CG, Latimer J, Adams R. An investigation of the reliability and validity of posteroanterior spinal stiffness judgments made using a reference-based protocol. *Phys Ther*. 1998;78:829–837.

48. Binkley J, Stratford PW, Gill C. Interrater reliability of lumbar accessory motion mobility testing. *Phys Ther*. 1995;75:786–795.

49. Hicks GE, Fritz JM, Delitto A, Mishock J. The reliability of clinical examination measures used for patients with suspected lumbar segmental instability. *Arch Phys Med Rehabil*. 2003;84:1858–1864.

50. French SD, Green S, Forbes A. Reliability of chiropractic methods commonly used to detect manipulable lesions in patients with chronic low-back pain. *J Manipulative Physiol Ther*. 2000;23:231–238.

51. Horneij E, Hemborg B, Johnsson B, Ekdahl C. Clinical tests on impairment level related to low back pain: a study of test reliability. *J Rehabil Med*. 2002;34:176–182.

52. Hidalgo B, Hall T, Nielens H, Detrembleur C. Intertester agreement and validity of identifying lumbar pain provocative movement patterns using active and passive accessory movement tests. *J Manipulative Physiol Ther*. 2014;37(2):105–115.

53. Abbott J, Mercer S. Lumbar segmental hypomobility: criterion-related validity of clinical examination items (a pilot study). *N Z J Physiother*. 2003;31:3–9.

54. Leboeuf-Yde C, van Dijk J, Franz C, et al. Motion palpation findings and self-reported low back pain in a population-based study sample. *J Manipulative Physiol Ther*. 2002;25:80–87.

55. Abbott JH, McCane B, Herbison P, et al. Lumbar segmental instability: a criterion-related validity study of manual therapy assessment. *BMC Musculoskelet Disord*. 2005;6:56.

56. Downey BJ, Taylor NF, Niere KR. Manipulative physiotherapists can reliably palpate nominated lumbar spinal levels. *Man Ther*. 1999;4:151–156.

57. Snider KT, Snider EJ, Degenhardt BF, et al. Palpatory accuracy of lumbar spinous processes using multiple bony landmarks. *J Manipulative Physiol Ther*. 2011;34(5):306–313.

58. Adelmanesh F, Jalali A, Shirvani A. The diagnostic accuracy of gluteal trigger points to differentiate radicular from nonradicular low back pain. *Clin J Pain.* 2016;32(8):666–672.

59. Kaping K, Äng BO, Rasmussen-Barr E. The abdominal drawing-in manoeuvre for detecting activity in the deep abdominal muscles: Is this clinical tool reliable and valid? *BMJ Open.* 2015;5(12).

60. Hebert JJ, Koppenhaver SL, Teyhen DS, et al. The evaluation of lumbar multifidus muscle function via palpation: reliability and validity of a new clinical test. *Spine J.* 2013. [Epub ahead of print].

61. Kilpikoski S, Airaksinen O, Kankaanpaa M, et al. Interexaminer reliability of low back pain assessment using the McKenzie method. *Spine.* 2002;27:E207–E214.

62. Fritz JM, Delitto A, Vignovic M, Busse RG. Interrater reliability of judgments of the centralization phenomenon and status change during movement testing in patients with low back pain. *Arch Phys Med Rehabil.* 2000;81:57–61.

63. Laslett M, Oberg B, Aprill CN, McDonald B. Centralization as a predictor of provocation discography results in chronic low back pain, and the influence of disability and distress on diagnostic power. *Spine J.* 2005;5:370–380.

64. Rose MJ. The statistical analysis of the intraobserver repeatability of four clinical measurement techniques. *Physiotherapy.* 1991;77:89–91.

65. Viikari-Juntura E, Takala EP, Riihimaki H, et al. Standardized physical examination protocol for low back disorders: feasibility of use and validity of symptoms and signs. *J Clin Epidemiol.* 1998;51:245–255.

66. Deville WL, van der Windt DA, Dzaferagic A, et al. The test of Lasegue: systematic review of the accuracy in diagnosing herniated discs. *Spine.* 2000;25:1140–1147.

67. Van der Windt DA, Simons E, Riphagen II, et al. Physical examination for lumbar radiculopathy due to disc herniation in patients with low-back pain. *Cochrane Database Syst Rev.* 2010;2:CD007431.

68. Majlesi J, Togay H, Unalan H, Toprak S. The sensitivity and specificity of the slump and the straight leg raising tests in patients with lumbar disc herniation. *J Clin Rheumatol.* 2008;14:87–91.

69. Ekedahl H, Jönsson B, Annertz M, Frobell RB. Accuracy of clinical tests in detecting disk herniation and nerve root compression in subjects with lumbar radicular symptoms. *Arch Phys Med Rehabil.* 2018;99(4):726–735.

70. Homayouni K, Jafari SH, Yari H. Sensitivity and specificity of modified Bragard test in patients with lumbosacral radiculopathy using electrodiagnosis as a reference standard. *J Chiropr Med.* 2018;17(1):36–43.

71. Tucker N, Reid D, McNair P. Reliability and measurement error of active knee extension range of motion in a modified slump test position: a pilot study. *J Man Manip Ther.* 2007;15:E85–E91.

72. Urban LM, MacNeil BJ. Diagnostic accuracy of the slump test for identifying neuropathic pain in the lower limb. *J Orthop Sports Phys Ther.* 2015;45(8):596–603.

73. Trainor K, Pinnington MA. Reliability and diagnostic validity of the slump knee bend neurodynamic test for upper/mid lumbar nerve root compression: a pilot study. *Physiotherapy.* 2011;97(1):59–64.

74. Alyazedi FM, Lohman EB, Wesley Swen R, Bahjri K. The inter-rater reliability of clinical tests that best predict the subclassification of lumbar segmental instability: Structural, functional and combined instability. *J Man Manip Ther.* 2015;23(4):197–204.

75. Murphy DR, Byfield D, McCarthy P, et al. Interexaminer reliability of the hip extension test for suspected impaired motor control of the lumbar spine. *J Manipulative Physiol Ther.* 2006;29:374–377.

76. Biely SA, Silfies SP, Smith SS, Hicks GE. Clinical observation of standing trunk movements: What do the aberrant movement patterns tell us? *J Orthop Sports Phys Ther.* 2014;44(4):262–272.

77. Rabin A, Shashua A, Pizem K, Dar G. The interrater reliability of physical examination tests that may predict the outcome or suggest the need for lumbar stabilization exercises. *J Orthop Sports Phys Ther.* 2013;43(2):83–90.

78. Roussel NA, Nijs J, Truijen S, et al. Low back pain: clinimetric properties of the Trendelenburg test, active straight leg raise test, and breathing pattern during active straight leg raising. *J Manipulative Physiol Ther.* 2007;30:270–278.

79. Mens JM, Vleeming A, Snijders CJ, et al. Reliability and validity of the active straight leg raise test in posterior pelvic pain since pregnancy. *Spine.* 2001;26:1167–1171.

80. Ahn K, Jhun H-J. New physical examination tests for lumbar spondylolisthesis and instability: Low midline sill sign and interspinous gap change during lumbar flexion-extension motion. *BMC Musculoskelet Disord.* 2015;16:97.

81. Fritz JM, George S. The use of a classification approach to identify subgroups of patients with acute low back pain. Interrater reliability and short-term treatment outcomes. *Spine.* 2000;25:106–114.

82. Vongsirinavarat M, Wahyuddin W, Adisaiphaopan R. Agreement of clinical examination for low back pain with facet joint origin. *Hong Kong Physiother J.* 2018;38(2):125–131.

83. Riddle DL, Rothstein JM. Intertester reliability of McKenzie's classifications of the syndrome types present in patients with low back pain. *Spine.* 1993;18:1333–1344.

84. Razmjou H, Kramer JF, Yamada R. Intertester reliability of the McKenzie evaluation in assessing patients with mechanical low-back pain. *J Orthop Sports Phys Ther.* 2000;30:368–389.

Thoracolumbar Spine

4

85. Trudelle-Jackson E, Sarvaiya-Shah SA, Wang SS. Interrater reliability of a movement impairment-based classification system for lumbar spine syndromes in patients with chronic low back pain. *J Orthop Sports Phys Ther*. 2008;38:371–376.

86. Heiss DG, Fitch DS, Fritz JM, et al. The interrater reliability among physical therapists newly trained in a classification system for acute low back pain. *J Orthop Sports Phys Ther*. 2004;34:430–439.

87. de Oliveira IO, de Vasconcelos RA, Pilz B, et al. Prevalence and reliability of treatment-based classification for subgrouping patients with low back pain. *J Man Manip Ther*. 2018;26(1):36–42.

88. Hebert J, Koppenhaver S, Fritz J, Parent E. Clinical prediction for success of interventions for managing low back pain. *Clin Sports Med*. 2008;27:463–479.

89. Delitto A, Erhard RE, Bowling RW. A treatment-based classification approach to low back syndrome: identifying and staging patients for conservative management. *Phys Ther*. 1995;75:470–489.

90. Fritz JM, Childs JD, Flynn TW. Pragmatic application of a clinical prediction rule in primary care to identify patients with low back pain with a good prognosis following a brief spinal manipulation intervention. *BMC Fam Pract*. 2005;6:29.

91. Stolze LR, Allison SC, Childs JD. Derivation of a preliminary clinical prediction rule for identifying a subgroup of patients with low back pain likely to benefit from Pilates-based exercise. *J Orthop Sports Phys Ther*. 2012;42(5):425–436.

92. Lauridsen HH, Hartvigsen J, Manniche C, et al. Danish version of the Oswestry Disability Index for patients with low back pain. Part 1: Cross-cultural adaptation, reliability and validity in two different populations. *Eur Spine J*. 2006;15:1705–1716.

93. Lauridsen HH, Hartvigsen J, Manniche C, et al. Responsiveness and minimal clinically important difference for pain and disability instruments in low back pain patients. *BMC Musculoskelet Disord*. 2006;7:82.

94. Fritz JM, Irrgang JJ. A comparison of a Modified Oswestry Disability Questionnaire and the Quebec Back Pain Disability Scale. *Phys Ther*. 2001;81:776–788.

95. Brouwer S, Kuijer W, Dijkstra PU, et al. Reliability and stability of the Roland Morris Disability Questionnaire: intraclass correlation and limits of agreement. *Disabil Rehabil*. 2004;26:162–165.

96. Grotle M, Brox JI, Vollestad NK. Reliability, validity and responsiveness of the Fear-Avoidance Beliefs Questionnaire: methodological aspects of the Norwegian version. *J Rehabil Med*. 2006;38:346–353.

97. Li L, Liu X, Herr K. Postoperative pain intensity assessment: a comparison of four scales in Chinese adults. *Pain Med*. 2007;8:223–234.

98. Farrar JT, Berlin JA, Strom BL. Clinically important changes in acute pain outcome measures: a validation study. *J Pain Symptom Manage*. 2003;25:406–411.

99. Farrar JT, Portenoy RK, Berlin JA, et al. Defining the clinically important difference in pain outcome measures. *Pain*. 2000;88:287–294.

100. Robinson HS, Dagfinrud H. Reliability and screening ability of the StarT Back screening tool in patients with low back pain in physiotherapy practice, a cohort study. *BMC Musculoskelet Disord*. 2017;18:232.

Clinical Summary and Recommendations

Patient History	
Questions	• The question "Is pain relieved by standing?" is the only question studied to demonstrate some diagnostic utility (+LR [likelihood ratio] of 3.5) for sacroiliac joint pain.
Pain Location	• Recent evidence suggests that patients with sacroiliac joint pain commonly experience the most intense pain around one or both sacroiliac joints, with or without referral into the lateral thigh.
Physical Examination	
Pain Provocation Tests	• Pain provocation tests generally demonstrate fair to moderate reliability and some exhibit moderate diagnostic utility for detecting sacroiliac joint pain. • Clusters of pain provocation tests consistently demonstrate good diagnostic utility for detecting sacroiliac joint pain. Using a cluster of four to five tests, including the *distraction test, thigh thrust test, sacral thrust test,* and *compression test* after a McKenzie-type repeated motion examination, seems to exhibit the best diagnostic utility (+LR of 6.97) and is recommended.
Motion Assessment and Static Palpation	• Motion assessment and static palpation tests generally demonstrate very poor reliability and almost no diagnostic utility for either sacroiliac joint pain or innominate torsion and, therefore, are not recommended for use in clinical practice. • Lumbar hypomobility is the one exception that, although exhibiting questionable reliability, demonstrates some diagnostic utility when used as part of a cluster to determine which patients will respond to spinal manipulation.
Interventions	• Patients with low back pain of less than 16 days' duration and no symptoms distal to the knees, and/or who meet four out of five of the Flynn and colleagues[1] criteria, should be treated with a lumbosacral manipulation.

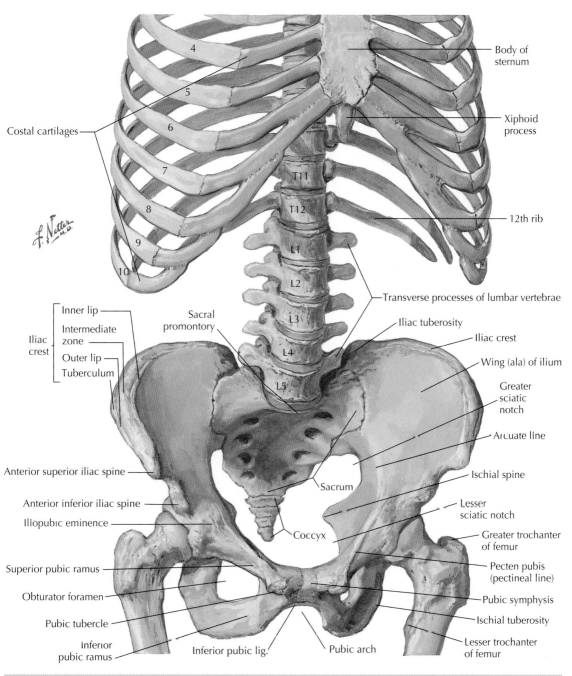

Body of
sternum

Xiphoid
process

12th rib

Costal cartilages

4

5

6

7

8

9

10

T11

T12

L1

L2

L3

L4

L5

Transverse processes of lumbar vertebrae

Sacral
promontory

Iliac tuberosity

Iliac crest

Wing (ala) of ilium

Greater
sciatic
notch

Arcuate line

Ischial spine

Lesser
sciatic notch

Greater trochanter
of femur

Pecten pubis
(pectineal line)

Pubic symphysis

Ischial tuberosity

Lesser trochanter
of femur

Inner lip

Intermediate
zone

Outer lip

Tuberculum

Iliac
crest

Anterior superior iliac spine

Anterior inferior iliac spine

Iliopubic eminence

Superior pubic ramus

Obturator foramen

Pubic tubercle

Inferior
pubic ramus

Sacrum

Coccyx

Inferior pubic lig.

Pubic arch

Figure 5-1
Bony framework of abdomen.

Sacroiliac Region

5

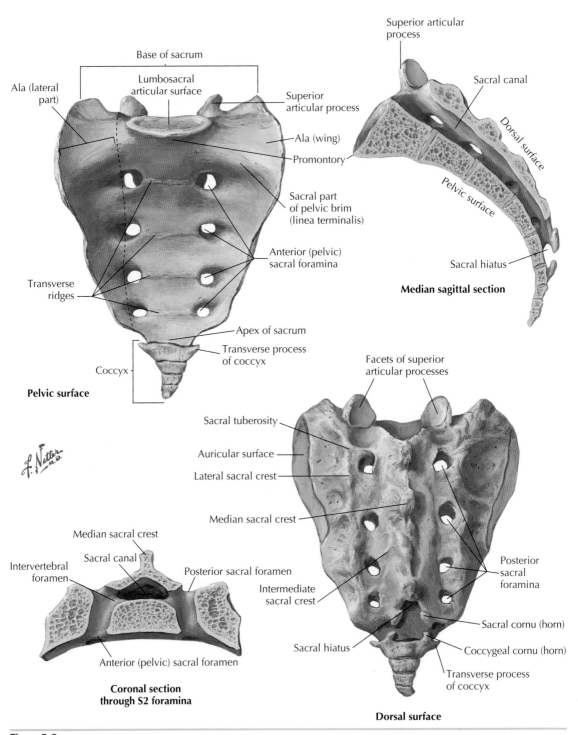

Figure 5-2
Sacrum and coccyx.

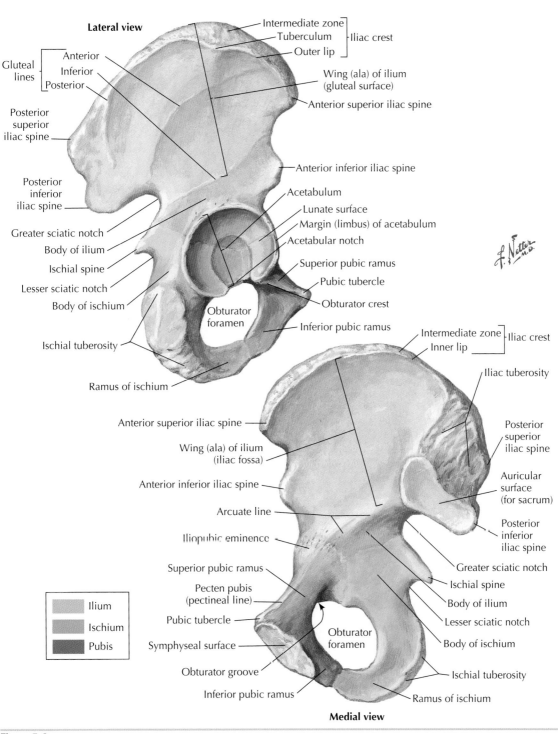

Lateral view

Gluteal lines
- Anterior
- Inferior
- Posterior

Intermediate zone
Tuberculum — Iliac crest
Outer lip

Wing (ala) of ilium
(gluteal surface)

Anterior superior iliac spine

Posterior superior iliac spine

Posterior inferior iliac spine

Greater sciatic notch

Body of ilium

Ischial spine

Lesser sciatic notch

Body of ischium

Ischial tuberosity

Ramus of ischium

Anterior inferior iliac spine

Acetabulum

Lunate surface

Margin (limbus) of acetabulum

Acetabular notch

Superior pubic ramus

Pubic tubercle

Obturator crest

Obturator foramen

Inferior pubic ramus

Intermediate zone
Inner lip — Iliac crest

Iliac tuberosity

Posterior superior iliac spine

Auricular surface (for sacrum)

Posterior inferior iliac spine

Greater sciatic notch

Ischial spine

Body of ilium

Lesser sciatic notch

Body of ischium

Ischial tuberosity

Ramus of ischium

Anterior superior iliac spine

Wing (ala) of ilium
(iliac fossa)

Anterior inferior iliac spine

Arcuate line

Iliopubic eminence

Superior pubic ramus

Pecten pubis
(pectineal line)

Pubic tubercle

Symphyseal surface

Obturator groove

Inferior pubic ramus

Obturator foramen

Ilium
Ischium
Pubis

Medial view

Figure 5-3
Hip (coxal) bone.

Sacroiliac Region

5

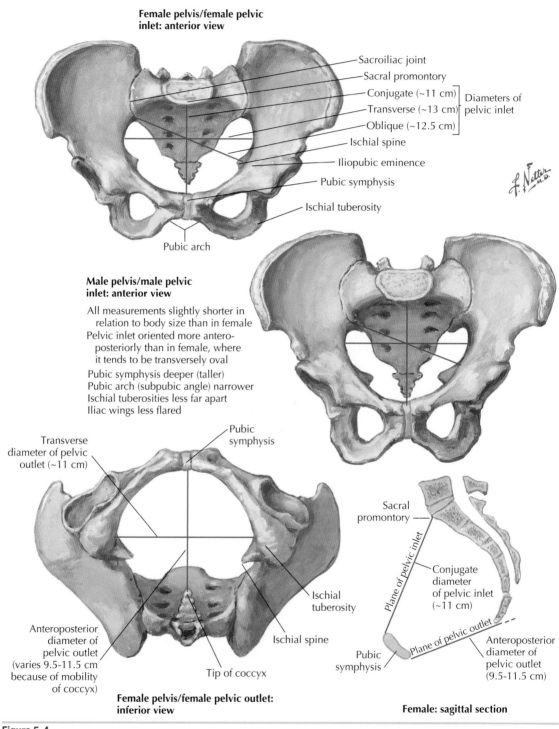

Figure 5-4
Sex differences of pelvis.

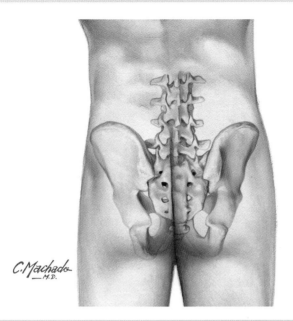

Figure 5-5
Sacroiliac joint.

Region	Joint	Type and Classification	Closed Packed Position	Capsular Pattern
Sacroiliac region	Sacroiliac joint	Plane synovial	Has not been described	Considered a capsular pattern if pain is provoked when joints are stressed
Lumbosacral region	Apophyseal joints	Plane synovial	Extension	Equal limitations of side-bending, flexion, and extension
	Intervertebral joints	Amphiarthrodial	Not applicable	Not applicable

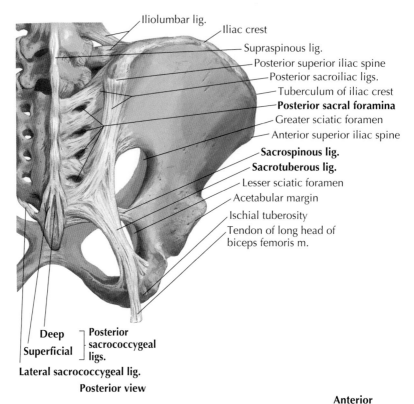

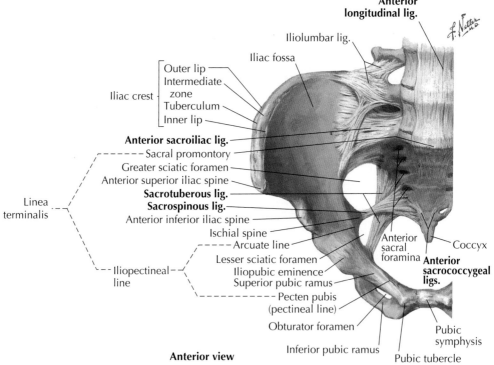

Figure 5-6
Sacroiliac region ligaments.

Sacroiliac Region Ligaments	Attachment	Function
Posterior sacroiliac	Iliac crest to tubercles of S1-S4	Limits movement of sacrum on iliac bones
Anterior sacroiliac	Anterosuperior aspect of sacrum to anterior ala of ilium	Limits movement of sacrum on iliac bones
Sacrospinous	Inferior lateral border of sacrum to ischial spine	Limits gliding and rotary movement of sacrum on iliac bones
Sacrotuberous	Middle lateral border of sacrum to ischial tuberosity	Limits gliding and rotary movement of sacrum on iliac bones
Posterior sacrococcygeal	Posterior aspect of inferior sacrum to posterior aspect of coccyx	Reinforces sacrococcygeal joint
Anterior sacrococcygeal	Anterior aspect of inferior sacrum to anterior aspect of coccyx	Reinforces sacrococcygeal joint
Lateral sacrococcygeal	Lateral aspect of inferior sacrum to lateral aspect of coccyx	Reinforces sacrococcygeal joint
Anterior longitudinal	Extends from anterior sacrum to anterior tubercle of C1. Connects anterolateral vertebral bodies and discs	Maintains stability of vertebral body joints and prevents hyperextension of vertebral column

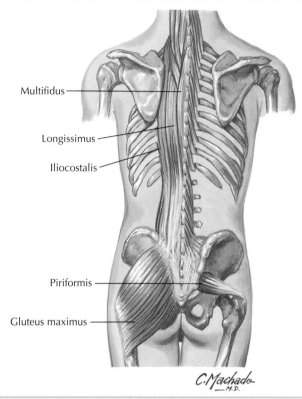

Figure 5-7
Sacroiliac region muscles. Posterior view of spine and associated musculature.

Sacroiliac Region Muscles	Proximal Attachment	Distal Attachment	Nerve and Segmental Level	Action
Gluteus maximus	Posterior border of ilium, dorsal aspect of sacrum and coccyx, and sacrotuberous ligament	Iliotibial tract of fascia lata and gluteal tuberosity of femur	Inferior gluteal nerve (L5, S1, S1)	Extension, external rotation, and some abduction of the hip joint
Piriformis	Anterior aspect of sacrum and sacrotuberous ligament	Superior greater trochanter of femur	Ventral rami of S1, S2	External rotation of extended hip, abduction of flexed hip
Multifidi	Sacrum, ilium, transverse processes of T1-T3, articular processes of C4-C7	Spinous processes of vertebrae two to four segments above origin	Dorsal rami of spinal nerves	Stabilizes vertebrae
Longissimus	Iliac crest, posterior sacrum, spinous processes of sacrum and inferior lumbar vertebrae, supraspinous ligament	Transverse processes of lumbar vertebrae	Dorsal rami of spinal nerves	Bilaterally extends vertebral column Unilaterally side-bends spinal column
Iliocostalis		Inferior surface of ribs 4-12		

Nerve	Segmental Level	Sensory	Motor
Superior gluteal	L4, L5, S1	No sensory	Tensor fasciae latae, gluteus medius, gluteus minimus
Inferior gluteal	L5, S1, S2	No sensory	Gluteus maximus
Nerve to piriformis	S1, S2	No sensory	Piriformis
Sciatic	L4, L5, S1, S2, S3	Hip joint	Knee flexors and all muscles of leg and foot
Nerve to quadratus femoris	L5, S1, S2	No sensory	Quadratus femoris, inferior gemellus
Nerve to obturator internus	L5, S1, S2	No sensory	Obturator internus, superior gemellus
Posterior cutaneous	S2, S3	Posterior thigh	No motor
Perforating cutaneous	S2, S3	Inferior gluteal region	No motor
Pudendal	S2, S3, S4	Genitals	Perineal muscles, external urethral sphincter, external anal sphincter
Nerve to levator ani	S3, S4	No sensory	Levator ani
Perineal branch	S1, S2, S3	Genitals	No motor
Anococcygeal	S4, S5, C0	Skin in the coccygeal region	No motor
Coccygeal	S3, S4	No sensory	Coccygeus
Pelvic splanchnic	S2, S3, S4	No sensory	Pelvic viscera

Sacroiliac Region

5

Schema

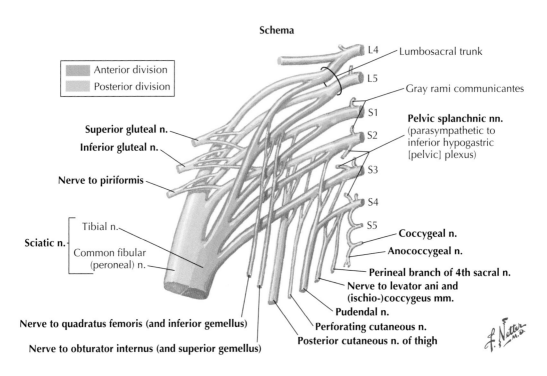

Anterior division
Posterior division

L4 — Lumbosacral trunk

L5 — Gray rami communicantes

S1

Superior gluteal n.

Inferior gluteal n.

S2 — **Pelvic splanchnic nn.**
(parasympathetic to inferior hypogastric [pelvic] plexus)

Nerve to piriformis

S3

S4

Sciatic n. — Tibial n.

Common fibular (peroneal) n.

S5 — **Coccygeal n.**

— **Anococcygeal n.**

— **Perineal branch of 4th sacral n.**

Nerve to levator ani and (ischio-)coccygeus mm.

Pudendal n.

Nerve to quadratus femoris (and inferior gemellus)

Perforating cutaneous n.

Posterior cutaneous n. of thigh

Nerve to obturator internus (and superior gemellus)

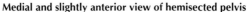

Medial and slightly anterior view of hemisected pelvis

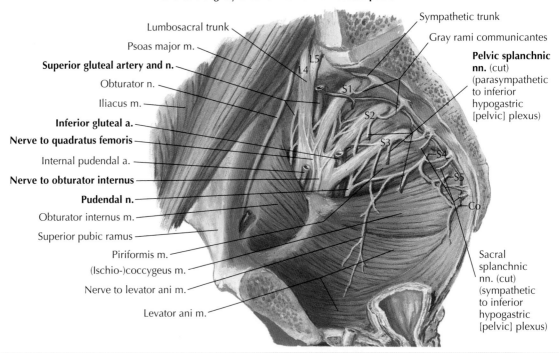

Lumbosacral trunk

Psoas major m.

Superior gluteal artery and n.

Obturator n.

Iliacus m.

Inferior gluteal a.

Nerve to quadratus femoris

Internal pudendal a.

Nerve to obturator internus

Pudendal n.

Obturator internus m.

Superior pubic ramus

Piriformis m.

(Ischio-)coccygeus m.

Nerve to levator ani m.

Levator ani m.

Sympathetic trunk

Gray rami communicantes

Pelvic splanchnic nn. (cut) (parasympathetic to inferior hypogastric [pelvic] plexus)

Sacral splanchnic nn. (cut) (sympathetic to inferior hypogastric [pelvic] plexus)

L5
L4
S1
S2
S3
S4
S5
Co

Figure 5-8
Sacroiliac region nerves.

There has been considerable controversy surrounding the contribution of the sacroiliac joint in low back pain syndromes. Recent research suggests that the sacroiliac joint can be a contributor to low back pain and disability and can certainly be a primary source of pain.[2-7] The concept of "sacroiliac joint dysfunction" is distinct from "sacroiliac joint pain" and is hypothetical at best.[3] Sacroiliac joint dysfunction is usually defined as altered joint mobility and/or malalignment,[8-10] neither of which have been consistently linked to low back or sacroiliac joint pain.

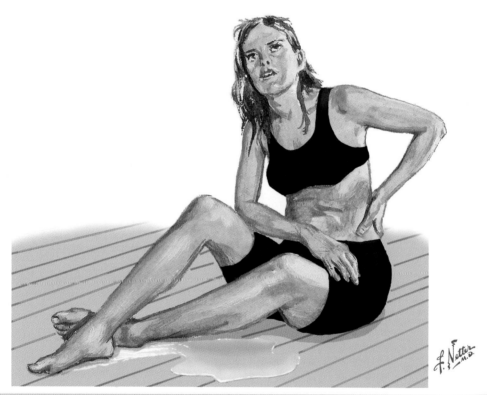

Figure 5-9
Common cause of sacroiliac injury. Falling and landing on the buttock.

Dreyfuss and colleagues[2] performed a prospective study to determine the diagnostic utility of both the history and physical examination in determining pain of sacroiliac origin. The diagnostic properties for the aggravating and easing factors and patient-reported location of pain are below.

Question and Study Quality	Population	Reference Standard	Sens	Spec	+LR	−LR
Pain relieved by standing?[2]	85 consecutive patients with low back pain referred for sacroiliac joint blocks	90% pain relief with injection of local anesthetics into sacroiliac joint	.07	.98	3.5	.95
Pain relieved by walking?[2]			.13	.77	.57	1.13
Pain relieved by sitting?[2]			.07	.80	.35	1.16
Pain relieved by lying down?[2]			.53	.49	1.04	.96
Coughing/sneezing aggravates symptoms?[2]			.45	.47	.85	1.17
Bowel movements aggravate symptoms?[2]			.38	.63	1.03	.98
Wearing heels/boots aggravates symptoms?[2]			.26	.56	.59	1.32
Job activities aggravate symptoms?[2]			.20	.74	.77	1.08
Pain aggravated by sitting in a chair?[11]	154 patients with low back pain	Unilateral buttock pain, positive Patrick or SIJ shear test, and at least 70% pain relief with analgesic SIJ injection	.65 (.45, .81)[†]	.62 (.53, .70)[†]	1.69 (1.20, 2.38)[†]	.57 (.35, .94)[†]

[†]Values calculated by book authors.

Patient Report of Pain Location and Study Quality	Population	Reference Standard	Sens	Spec	+LR	−LR
Sacroiliac joint pain[2]	85 consecutive patients with low back pain referred for sacroiliac joint blocks	90% pain relief with injection of local anesthetics into sacroiliac joint	.82*	.12*	.93	1.50
Groin pain[2]			.26*	.63*	.70	1.17
Buttock pain[2]			.78*	.18*	.95	1.22
Points to posterior superior iliac spine (PSIS) as main area of pain[2]			.71*	.47*	1.34	.62
Groin pain[11]	154 patients with low back pain	Unilateral buttock pain, positive Patrick or SIJ shear test, and at least 70% pain relief with analgesic SIJ injection	.39 (.22, .58)[†]	.78 (.70, .85)[†]	1.76 (1.01, 3.07)[†]	.79 (.58, 1.05)[†]

*Mean of chiropractor and physician sensitivity and specificity scores.

[†]Values calculated by book authors.

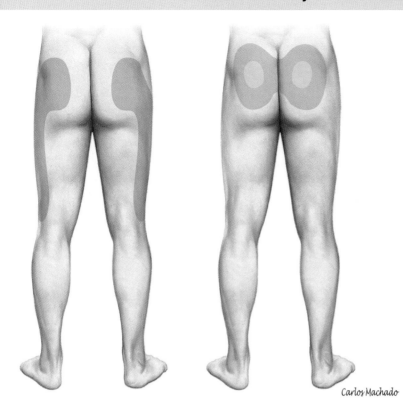

Carlos Machado

Figure 5-10

Jung and associates[12] determined the most common pain distribution patterns in patients with sacroiliac joint pain. They then prospectively tested the ability of the pain distribution patterns to diagnose the response to sacroiliac joint radiofrequency neurotomies in 160 patients with presumed sacroiliac joint pain. The pain distribution patterns with the best diagnostic utility are depicted, with colors representing pain intensity (scale, 1-5). *Left,* red = 4; *right,* blue = 5, purple = 4. (From Jung JH, Kim HI, Shin DA, et al. Usefulness of pain distribution pattern assessment in decision-making for the patients with lumbar zygapophyseal and sacroiliac joint arthropathy. *J Korean Med Sci.* 2007;22:1048-1054.)

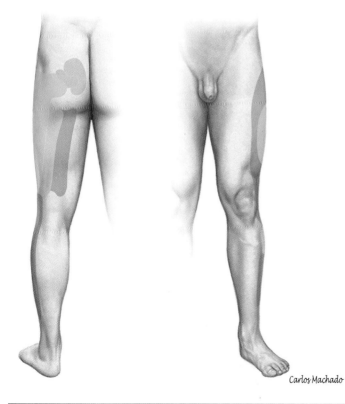

Carlos Machado

Figure 5-11

In a study similar to the one in Fig. 5-10, van der Wurff and colleagues[13] compared pain distribution maps compiled from patients who responded to double-block sacroiliac joint injections with maps from patients who did not respond. The researchers found no differences in the locations of pain distribution but did find differences in the pain intensity locations. Patients with sacroiliac joint pain reported the highest-intensity pain overlying the sacroiliac joint, as depicted, with colors representing pain intensity (scale, 1-5). *Left,* pink = 5, purple = 4, green = 3, orange = 2, red = 1; *right,* blue = 2, purple = 1. (From van der Wurff P, Buijs EJ, Groen GJ. Intensity mapping of pain referral areas in sacroiliac joint pain patients. *J Manipulative Physiol Ther.* 2006;29:190-195.)

Sacroiliac Region

5

Pain Provocation and Patient Identification of Location of Pain

Measurement and Study Quality	Population	Reference Standard	Sens	Spec	+LR	−LR
One finger test (patient points index finger to the PSIS as primary source of pain)[11] ◉	154 patients with low back pain	Unilateral buttock pain, positive Patrick or SIJ shear test, and at least 70% pain relief with analgesic SIJ injection	.77 (.59, .90)[†]	.66 (.58, .75)[†]	2.32 (1.70, 3.18)[†]	.34 (.17, .66)[†]
PSIS tenderness[11] ◉			.77 (.59, .90)[†]	.63 (.53, .71)[†]	2.07 (1.54, 2.79)[†]	.36 (.19, .70)[†]
Sacrotuberous ligament tenderness[11] ◉			.19 (.07, .37)[†]	.89 (.82, .94)[†]	1.70 (.71, 4.06)[†]	.91 (.76, 1.09)[†]
Sacral sulcus tenderness only[2] ◉	85 consecutive patients with low back pain referred for sacroiliac joint blocks 90% pain relief with injection of local anesthetics into sacroiliac joint		.89*	.14	1.03*	.79*
Sacral sulcus tenderness + Patient points to the PSIS as the main site of pain[2] ◉			.63*	.50*	1.26*	.74*
Sacral sulcus tenderness + Groin pain[2] ◉			.25*	.68*	.78*	1.10*
Patient points to PSIS as main site of pain + Patient complains of groin pain[2] ◉			.16	.85	1.07	.99
Sacral sulcus tenderness + Patient identifies PSIS as main site of pain + Groin pain[2] ◉			.13	.86	.93	1.01

*Mean of chiropractor and physician sensitivity and specificity scores.
†Values calculated by book authors.

Assessment of Symmetry of Bony Landmarks

Landmark and Study Quality	Description and Positive Findings	Population	Reliability*
Sitting PSIS[14] ◆	With patient sitting, examiner palpates right and left PSISs. Positive if one PSIS is higher than the other	62 women who were recruited from obstetrics; 42 were pregnant and had pelvic girdle pain and 20 were not pregnant and were asymptomatic	Interexaminer $\kappa = .26$
Sitting PSIS[9] ◆		65 patients with low back pain	Interexaminer $\kappa = .37$
Sitting PSIS[1] ◒			Interexaminer $\kappa = .23$
Standing PSIS[1] ◒	Same as above with patient standing		Interexaminer $\kappa = .13$
Iliac crest symmetry[1] ◒	With patient standing, examiner palpates right and left iliac crests. Positive if one crest is higher than the other	71 patients with low back pain	Interexaminer $\kappa = .23$
Prone PSIS[15] ◆	With patient prone and examiner's fingers or thumbs on landmark and dominant eye over the patient's midsagittal plane, examiner determines if the landmarks are: • Right higher than left • Left higher than right • Equal right to left	10 asymptomatic female volunteers	Intraexaminer $\kappa = .33$ Interexaminer $\kappa = .04$
Sacral inferior lateral angle[15] ◆			Intraexaminer $\kappa = .69$ Interexaminer $\kappa = .08$
Sacral sulcus[15] ◆	As above, determining if the landmarks are: • Right deeper than left • Left deeper than right • Equal right to left		Intraexaminer $\kappa = .24$ Interexaminer $\kappa = .07$
Sacral sulcus[16] ◆			Interexaminer $\kappa = .11$ (−.14, .36)
Sacral inferior lateral angle[16] ◆	As above, determining if the landmarks are: • Right more posterior than left • Left more posterior than right • Equal right to left	25 patients with low back or sacroiliac pain	Interexaminer $\kappa = .11$ (−.12, .34)
L5 transverse process[16] ◆			Interexaminer $\kappa = .17$ (−.03, .37)
Medial malleoli[16] ◆	As above, determining if the landmarks are: • Right more superior than left • Left more superior than right • Equal right to left		Interexaminer $\kappa = .28$ (−.01, .57)
Medial malleoli[17] ◆			Interexaminer $\kappa = .21$
Anterior superior iliac spine (ASIS)[17] ◒	With patient supine, evaluator palpates inferior slope of ASIS. Recorded as above	24 patients with low back pain	Interexaminer $\kappa = .15$
Sacral base[17] ◒	With patient sitting, evaluator palpates the sacral base with the patient's trunk flexed and extended. Recorded as symmetric, left-base anterior or posterior, or right-base anterior or posterior		Interexaminer $\kappa =$ [Trunk flexion] .37 [Trunk extension] .05

*Potter and Rothstein[17] also studied static palpation, but their study was excluded because they only reported the percentage of agreement.

5

Sacroiliac Region

Assessment of Symmetry of Bony Landmarks—cont'd

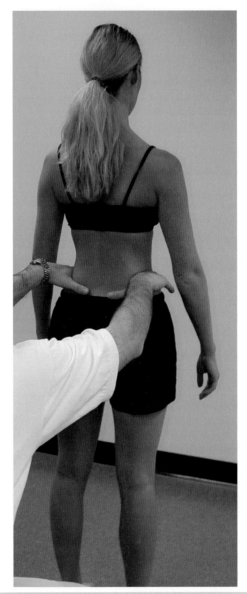

Figure 5-12
Assessment of iliac crest symmetry in standing.

Patrick Test (FABER Test)

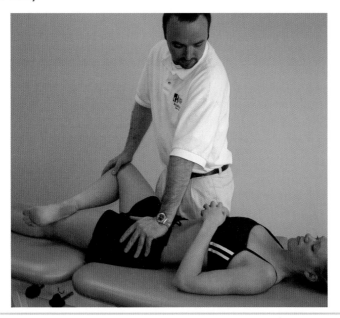

Figure 5-13
Patrick test.

Test and Study Quality	Description and Positive Findings	Population	Reliability
Patrick test[19] ◆		15 patients with ankylosing spondylitis, 30 women with postpartum pelvic pain, and 16 asymptomatic subjects	Interexaminer κ = [Right] .60 (.39, .81) [Left] .48 (.27, .69)
Patrick test[20] ◆	With patient supine, examiner brings ipsilateral knee into flexion with lateral malleolus placed over the contralateral knee, fixates the contralateral ASIS, and applies a light pressure over the ipsilateral knee. Positive if familiar pain is increased or reproduced	25 patients with asymmetric low back pain	Intraexaminer* κ = [Right] .41 (.07, .78) [Left] .40 (.03, .78) Interexaminer κ = [Right] .44 (.06, .83) [Left] .49 (.09, .89)
Patrick test[21] ◆		40 patients with chronic low back pain	Interexaminer κ = [Right] .60 (.35, .85) [Left] .43 (.15, .71)
Patrick test[22] ◆		59 patients with low back pain	Interexaminer κ = .61 (.31, −.91)
Patrick test[1] ◐		71 patients with low back pain	Interexaminer κ = .60
Patrick test[2] ◐		See diagnostic table	Interexaminer κ = .62

*Intraexaminer reliability reported for examiner #1 only.

Patrick Test (FABER Test)—cont'd

Test* and Study Quality	Description and Positive Findings	Population	Reference Standard	Sens	Spec	+LR	−LR
Patrick test[21] ◆	With patient supine, examiner brings ipsilateral knee into flexion with lateral malleolus placed over the contralateral knee, fixates the contralateral ASIS, applying a light pressure over the ipsilateral knee. Positive if familiar pain is increased or reproduced	40 patients with chronic low back pain	Sacroiliitis apparent on magnetic resonance imaging (MRI)	**Right side**			
				.66 (.30, .90)	.51 (.33, .69)	1.37 (.76, 2.48)	.64 (.24, 1.72)
				Left side			
				.54 (.24, .81)	.62 (.42, .78)	1.43 (.70, 2.93)	.73 (.36, 1.45)
Patrick test[2] ●		85 consecutive patients with low back pain referred for sacroiliac joint blocks	90% pain relief with injection of local anesthetics into sacroiliac joint	.68[†]	.29[†]	.96[†]	1.1[†]

*Broadhurst and Bond[23] also investigated this test, but the study was excluded because results for all participants were positive on the test (making sensitivity = 1 and specificity = 0).
[†]Mean of chiropractor and physician sensitivity and specificity scores.

Thigh Thrust (or Posterior Shear Test or Posterior Pelvic Provocation Test)

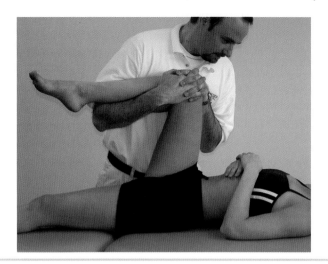

Figure 5-14
Thigh thrust test.

Test and Study Quality	Description and Positive Findings	Population	Reliability
Thigh thrust[21] ◆	Patient supine with hip flexed to 90 degrees. The examiner applies posteriorly directed force through the femur. Positive if familiar pain is increased or reproduced	See diagnostic table	Interexaminer κ = [Right] .46 (.15, .76)
Thigh thrust[19] ◆		15 patients with ankylosing spondylitis, 30 women with postpartum pelvic pain, and 16 asymptomatic subjects	Interexaminer κ = [Right] .76 (.48, .86) [Left] .74 (.57, .91)
Thigh thrust[20] ◆	Patient supine with hip flexed to 90 degrees and slightly adducted. One of the examiner's hands cups the sacrum and the other applies posteriorly directed force through the femur. Positive test is the production or increase of familiar symptoms	25 patients with asymmetric low back pain	Intraexaminer* κ = [Right] .44 (.06, .83) [Left] .40 (.00, .82) Interexaminer κ = [Right] .60 (.24, .96) [Left] .40 (.00, .82)
Thigh thrust[24] ◆		51 patients with low back pain	Interexaminer κ = .88
Thigh thrust[22] ◆		59 patients with low back pain	Interexaminer κ = .67 (.46, .88)
Thigh thrust[1] ◐		71 patients with low back pain	Interexaminer κ = .70
Thigh thrust[2] ◐		See diagnostic table	Interexaminer κ = .64

*Intraexaminer reliability reported for examiner #1 only.

Thigh Thrust (or Posterior Shear Test or Posterior Pelvic Provocation Test)—cont'd

Test* and Study Quality	Description and Positive Findings	Population	Reference Standard	Sens	Spec	+LR	−LR
Thigh thrust **2009 Meta-analysis**[26] ◆	With patient supine with hip flexed to 90 degrees and slightly adducted, one of the examiner's hands cups the sacrum and the other applies posteriorly directed force through the femur. Positive if familiar symptoms are produced or increased	Pooled from two studies[4,27]	Pooled from two studies[4,27]	.91 (.78, .97)	.66 (.53, .77)	2.68	.14
Thigh thrust[21] ◆	With patient supine with hip flexed to 90 degrees, examiner applies posteriorly directed force through the femur. Positive if familiar pain is increased or reproduced	40 patients with chronic low back pain	Sacroiliitis apparent on MRI	Right side			
				.55 (.22, .84)	.70 (.51, .85)	1.91 (.85, 4.27)	.62 (.29, 1.33)
				Left side			
				.45 (.18, .75)	.86 (.67, .95)	3.29 (1.07, 10.06)	.63 (.36, 1.09)
Thigh thrust[25]† ◐	With patient supine with hip flexed to 90 degrees and slightly adducted, one of the examiner's hands cups the sacrum and the other applies posteriorly directed force through the femur. Positive if familiar symptoms are produced or increased	454 patients with low back pain and no signs of nerve root compression	Sacroiliitis per MRI	.31 (.18, .47)	.85 (.82, .87)	2.07	.81
Thigh thrust[28] ◐	Participants in supine position with 90 degrees of flexion in the hip and knee on the side being tested. The examiner stabilized the contralateral side of the pelvis over the ASIS and applied a light manual pressure to the participant's flexed knee along the longitudinal axis of the femur. The test was positive when the patient felt a familiar well-localized pain deep in the gluteal area on the provoked side.	110 participants (57 with pelvic girdle pain and 53 with disc herniations determined by computed tomography [CT])	Participants with pelvic girdle pain determined by characteristics included in the European guidelines for pelvic girdle pain, along with pain markings in the posterior pelvic area on a pain drawing. Participants with disc herniations determined by CT.	.88‡	.89‡	8.00‡	.13‡

*Broadhurst and Bond[23] also investigated this test, but the study was excluded because results for all participants were positive on the test (making sensitivity = 1 and specificity = 0).

†Study also reported statistics by gender and found better diagnostic utility in men than in women. LRs calculated by author.

‡This study shows that the posterior pelvic pain provocation test is negative in patients with a well-defined lumbar diagnosis.

Compression Test

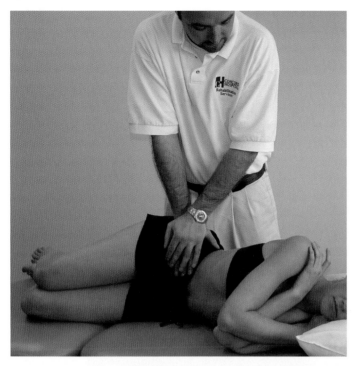

Figure 5-15
Compression test.

Test and Study Quality	Description and Positive Findings	Population	Reliability
Compression test[19] ◆	With patient side-lying, affected side up, with hips flexed approximately 45 degrees and knees flexed approximately 90 degrees, examiner applies a force vertically downward on the anterior superior iliac crest. Positive test is the production or increase of familiar symptoms	15 patients with ankylosing spondylitis, 30 women with postpartum pelvic pain, and 16 asymptomatic subjects	Interexaminer κ = [Right] .48 (.18, .78) [Left] .67 (.43, .91)
Compression test[21] ◆		40 patients with chronic low back pain	Interexaminer κ = [Right] .48 (.14, .81) [Left] .44 (.08, .79)
Compression test[24] ◆		51 patients with low back pain	Interexaminer κ = .73
Compression test[22] ◆		59 patients with low back pain	Interexaminer κ = .57 (.21, .93)
Compression test[1] ◐		71 patients with low back pain	Interexaminer κ = .26

Test and Study Quality	Description and Positive Findings	Population	Reference Standard	Sens	Spec	+LR	−LR
Compression test **2009** Metaanalysis[26] ◆	Same as below	Pooled from two studies[4,27]	Pooled from two studies[4,27]	.63 (.47, .77)	.63 (.57, .80)	1.70	.59
Compression test[21] ◆	With patient side-lying, affected side up, with hips flexed approximately 45 degrees and knees flexed approximately 90 degrees, examiner applies a force vertically downward on the anterior superior iliac crest. Positive test is the production or increase of familiar symptoms	40 patients with chronic low back pain	Sacroiliitis apparent on MRI	**Right side**			
				.22 (.03, .59)	.83 (.65, .93)	1.37 (.31, 5.94)	.92 (.64, 1.33)
				Left side			
				.27 (.07, .60)	.93 (.75, .98)	3.95 (.76, 20.57)	.78 (.54, 1.12)

Sacroiliac Region

5

Sacral Thrust Test

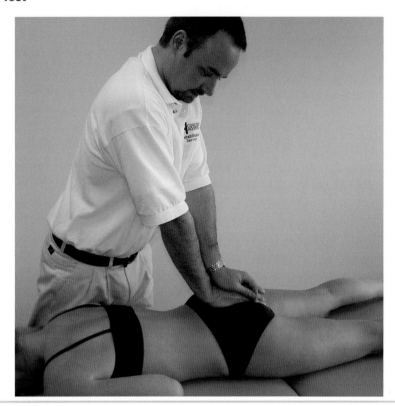

Figure 5-16
Sacral thrust test.

Test and Study Quality	Description and Positive Findings	Population	Reliability
Sacral thrust test[21] ◆		40 patients with chronic low back pain	Interexaminer κ = [Right] .87 (.70, 1.0) [Left] .69 (.40, .97)
Sacral thrust test[24] ◆	With patient prone, examiner applies a force vertically downward to the center of the sacrum. Positive test is the production or increase of familiar symptoms	51 patients with low back pain	Interexaminer κ = .56
Sacral thrust test[6] ◐		71 patients with low back pain	Interexaminer κ = .41
Sacral thrust test[2] ◐		85 patients with low back pain referred for sacroiliac joint blocks	Interexaminer κ = .30

Sacral Thrust Test—cont'd

Test and Study Quality	Description and Positive Findings	Population	Reference Standard	Sens	Spec	+LR	−LR
Sacral thrust test[21] ◆		40 patients with chronic low back pain	Sacroiliitis apparent on MRI	Right side			
				.33 (.09, .69)	.74 (.55, .87)	1.29 (.42, 3.88)	.89 (.55, 1.45)
				Left side			
	With patient prone, examiner applies a force vertically downward to the center of the sacrum. Positive test is the production or increase of familiar symptoms			.45 (.18, .75)	.89 (.71, .97)	4.39 (1.25, 15.36)	.60 (.35, 1.05)
Sacral thrust test[4] ◆		48 patients with chronic lumbopelvic pain referred for sacroiliac joint injection	80% pain relief with injection of local anesthetics into sacroiliac joint	.63 (.39, .82)	.75 (.58, .87)	2.5 (1.23, 5.09)	.50 (.24, .87)
Sacral thrust test[2] ◑		85 consecutive patients with low back pain referred for sacroiliac joint blocks	90% pain relief with injection of local anesthetics into sacroiliac joint	.52*	.38*	.84*	1.26*

*Mean of chiropractor and physician sensitivity and specificity scores.

Sacroiliac Region

5

Gaenslen Test

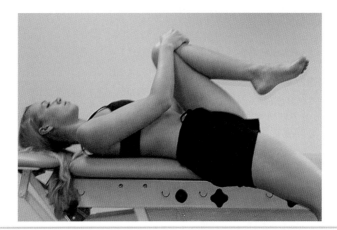

Figure 5-17
Gaenslen test.

Test and Study Quality	Description and Positive Findings	Population	Reliability
Gaenslen test[21] ◆ (see Video 5-1)	With patient supine near the edge of the table and one leg hanging over the edge of the table and the other flexed toward the patient's chest, examiner applies firm pressure to both the hanging leg and the leg flexed toward the chest. Positive test is the production or increase of familiar symptoms	40 patients with chronic low back pain	Interexaminer κ = [Right] .37 (.05, .68) [Left] .28 (0.0, .60)
Gaenslen test[24] ◆		51 patients with low back pain with or without radiation into the lower limb	Interexaminer κ = .76
Gaenslen test[22] ◆		59 patients with low back pain	Interexaminer κ = .60 (.33, .88)
Gaenslen test[1] ◐		71 patients referred to physical therapy with a diagnosis related to the lumbo-sacral spine	Interexaminer κ = .54

Gaenslen Test—cont'd

Test and Study Quality	Description and Positive Findings	Population	Reference Standard	Sens	Spec	+LR	−LR
Gaenslen test[21] ◆	With patient supine near the edge of the table and one leg hanging over the edge of the table and the other flexed toward the patient's chest, examiner applies firm pressure to both the hanging leg and the leg flexed toward the chest. Positive test is the production or increase of familiar symptoms	40 patients with chronic low back pain	Sacroiliitis apparent on MRI	Right side			
				.44 (.15, .77)	.80 (.61, .91)	2.29 (.82, 6.39)	.68 (.37, 1.25)
				Left side			
				.36 (.12, .68)	.75 (.56, .88)	1.5 (.54, 4.15)	.83 (.52, 1.33)
Gaenslen test[4] ◆		48 patients with chronic lumbopelvic pain referred for sacroiliac joint injection	80% pain relief with injection of local anesthetics into sacroiliac joint	Right side			
				.53 (.30, .75)	.71 (.53, .84)	1.84 (.87, 3.74)	.66 (.34, 1.09)
				Left side			
				.50 (.27, .73)	.77 (.60, .89)	2.21 (.95, 5.0)	.65 (.34, 1.03)
Gaenslen test[2] ◖		85 consecutive patients with low back pain referred for sacroiliac joint blocks	90% pain relief with injection of local anesthetics into sacroiliac joint	.68*	.29*	.96*	1.1*
Gaenslen test[25]† ◖		454 patients with low back pain and no signs of nerve root compression	Sacroiliitis per MRI	.13 (.05, .27)	.89 (.87, .91)	1.18	.98

*Mean of chiropractor and physician sensitivity and specificity scores.
†Study also reported statistics by gender and found better diagnostic utility in men than in women. LRs calculated by author.

Distraction Test

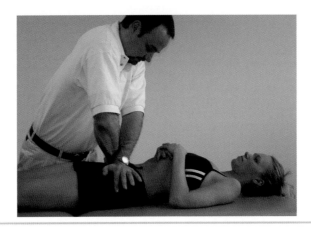

Figure 5-18
Distraction test.

Test and Study Quality	Description and Positive Findings	Population	Reliability
Distraction test[21] ◆	With patient supine, examiner applies cross-arm pressure to both anterior superior iliac spines (ASISs). Positive test is the production or increase of familiar symptoms	40 patients with chronic low back pain	Interexaminer κ = .50
Distraction test[24] ◆	With patient supine, examiner applies a posteriorly directed force to both ASISs. Positive test is the production or increase of familiar symptoms	51 patients with low back pain, with or without radiation into the lower limb	Interexaminer κ = .69
Distraction test[22] ◆		59 patients with low back pain	Interexaminer κ = .45 (.10, .78)
Distraction test[1] ●		71 patients referred to physical therapy with a diagnosis related to the lumbosacral spine	Interexaminer κ = .26

Test and Study Quality	Description and Positive Findings	Population	Reference Standard	Sens	Spec	+LR	−LR
Distraction test[21] ◆	With patient supine, examiner applies cross-arm pressure to both ASISs. Positive test is the production or increase of familiar symptoms	40 patients with chronic low back pain	Sacroiliitis apparent on MRI	.23 (.06, .54)	.81 (.61, .92)	1.24 (.35, 4.4)	.94 (.68, 1.29)
Distraction test[4] ◆	With patient supine, examiner applies a posteriorly directed force to both ASISs. Positive test is the production or increase of familiar symptoms	48 patients with chronic lumbopelvic pain referred for sacroiliac joint injection	80% pain relief with injection of local anesthetics into sacroiliac joint	.60 (.36, .80)	.81 (.65, .91)	3.20 (1.42, 7.31)	.49 (.24, .83)

Mennell Test

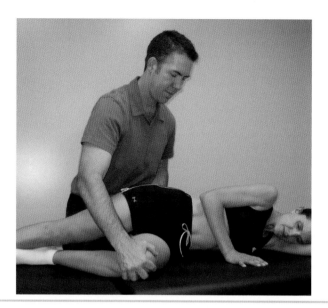

Figure 5-19
Mennell test.

5

Sacroiliac Region

Test and Study Quality	Description and Positive Findings	Population	Reliability
Mennell test[21] ◆	With patient side-lying, affected side down, with hip and knee on affected side flexed toward the abdomen, examiner puts one hand over the ipsilateral buttock and iliac crest and with the other hand grasps the semiflexed ipsilateral knee and lightly forces the leg into extension. Positive test is the production or increase of familiar symptoms	40 patients with chronic low back pain	Interexaminer κ = [Right] .54 (.26, .82) [Left] .50 (.20, .80)

Test and Study Quality	Description and Positive Findings	Population	Reference Standard	Sens	Spec	+LR	−LR
Mennell test[21] ◆	As above	40 patients with chronic low back pain	Sacroiliitis apparent on MRI	Right side			
				.66 (.30, .90)	.80 (.61, .91)	3.44 (1.49, 8.09)	.41 (.16, 1.05)
				Left side			
				.45 (.18, .75)	.86 (.67, .95)	3.29 (1.07, 10.06)	.63 (.36, 1.09)

Other Pain Provocation Tests

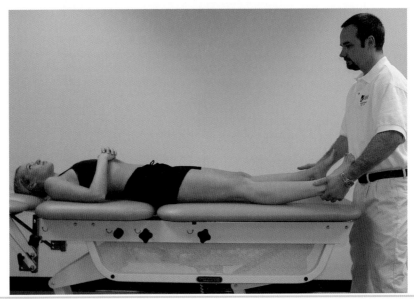

Figure 5-20
Resisted abduction of the hip.

Test* and Study Quality	Description and Positive Findings	Population	Reliability
Internal rotation of the hip[19] ◆	With patient prone, examiner maximally internally rotates one or both femurs. Positive test is the production or increase of familiar symptoms	15 patients with ankylosing spondylitis, 30 women with postpartum pelvic pain, and 16 asymptomatic subjects	Interexaminer κ = [Right] .78 (.60, .94) [Left] .88 (.75, 1.01) [Bilateral] .56 (.33, .79)
Drop test[19] ◆	With patient standing on one foot, patient lifts the heel from the floor and drops down on the heel again. Positive test is the production or increase of familiar symptoms		Interexaminer κ = [Right] .84 (.61, 1.06) [Left] .47 (.11, .83)
Resisted abduction test[20] ◆	With patient supine with legs extended and abducted 30 degrees, examiner holds the ankle and pushes medially while the patient pushes laterally. Positive test is the production or increase of familiar symptoms	25 patients with asymmetric low back pain	Intraexaminer κ = [Right] .48 (.07, .88) [Left] .50 (.06, .95) Interexaminer κ = [Right] .78 (.49, 1.07) [Left] .50 (−.02, 1.03)
Resisted abduction test[1] ◉		71 patients with low back pain	Interexaminer κ = .41
Shimpi test[30] ◉	With patient prone, examiner places palm underneath ASIS and instructs patient to extend leg so as to lift the foot just off the table. Positive test is when the ASIS lifts off table and patient reports familiar pain at SIJ	23 patients with LBP localized to the SIJ and 22 asymptomatic volunteers	Intraexaminer κ = .68 (.47, .90) Interexaminer κ = .69 (.48, .89)
Pain Pressure Threshold (PPT)[31] ◉	With patients prone, PPTs were measured using mechanical pressure algometer at 5 different points around the PSIS	31 patients with LBP localized to the SIJ and 41 asymptomatic volunteers	Interexaminer individual point ICC = .60 to .80 Mean of 5 points ICC = [Right] .79 (.65, .88) [Left] .82 (.67, .90)

*Broadhurst and Bond[23] investigated the diagnostic properties of the resisted abduction test, but the study was excluded because all participants were positive on the test (making sensitivity = 1 and specificity = 0).

Other Pain Provocation Tests—cont'd

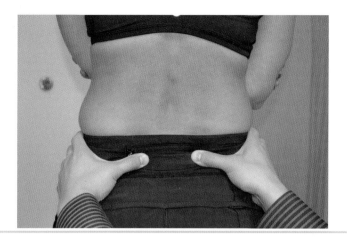

Figure 5-21
PSIS distraction test.

Test and Study Quality	Description and Positive Findings	Population	Reference Standard	Sens	Spec	+LR	−LR
PSIS distraction test[33] ● (see Video 5-2)	The examiner applies a distraction force with thumbs on each PSIS in a medial-to-lateral direction with the patient either standing or lying prone. Positive test is the reproduction of patient's symptoms	46 patients with 61 symptomatic sacroiliac joints	50% pain relief with injection of local anesthetics into sacroiliac joint	1.00	.89	9.10	0.00
Long dorsal sacro-iliac ligament test[25†] ●	Palpation of the sacroiliac ligament (just inferior to PSIS) reproduces patient's symptoms	454 patients with low back pain and no signs of nerve root compression	Sacroiliitis per MRI	.36 (.22, .51)	.72 (.69, .75)	1.29	.89

†Study also reported statistics by gender and found better diagnostic utility in men than in women. LRs calculated by author.

Sacroiliac Region

5

Gillet Test (Stork Test)

Test* and Study Quality	Description and Positive Findings	Population	Reliability
Gillet test[20] ◆	With patient standing, examiner palpates the PSIS and asks patient to flex the hip and knee on the side being tested. Positive if the PSIS fails to move posteroinferiorly	25 patients with asymmetric low back pain	Intraexaminer[†] $\kappa =$ [Right] .42 (−.01, .87) [Left] .49 (.09, .89) Interexaminer $\kappa =$ [Right] .41 (.03, .87) [Left] .34 (−.06, .70)
Gillet test[34] ◐	With patient standing, examiner palpates the following landmarks: • L5 spinous process and PSIS • S1 tubercle and PSIS • S3 tubercle and PSIS • Sacral apex and posteromedial margin of the ischium Patient is instructed to raise the ipsilateral leg of the side of palpation. Positive if the lateral landmark fails to move posteroinferiorly with respect to medial landmark	54 asymptomatic college students	Intraexaminer mean value for all tests $\kappa = .31$ Interexaminer mean value for all tests $\kappa = .02$
Gillet test[35] ◐	As above except using the following landmarks: • L5 spinous process and PSIS • S1 spinous process and PSIS • S3 spinous process and PSIS • Sacral hiatus and caudolateral just below the ischial spine	38 male students; 9 during the first testing procedure and 12 during the second had low back pain	Intraexaminer[†] $\kappa = .08$ (.01, .14) Interexaminer $\kappa = −.05$ (−.06, −.12)
Gillet test[36] ◐	With patient standing, examiner palpates the S2 spinous process with one thumb and the PSIS with the other and asks patient to flex the hip and knee on the side being tested. Rated intrapelvic motion as "cephalad," "neutral," or "caudad"	33 volunteers; 15 had pelvic girdle pain	Interexaminer $\kappa =$ [Right] .59 [Left] .59
Gillet test[17] ◐	With patient standing, examiner palpates the S2 spinous process with one thumb and the PSIS with the other and asks patient to flex the hip and knee on the side being tested. Positive if the PSIS fails to move posteroinferiorly with respect to S2	24 patients with low back pain	Interexaminer $\kappa = .27$
Gillet test[2] ◐		See diagnostic table	Interexaminer $\kappa = .22$
Gillet test[6] ◐		71 patients with low back pain	Interexaminer $\kappa = .59$

*Potter and Rothstein[18] and Herzog and colleagues[27] also studied this test, but their studies were excluded because they only reported the percentage of agreement.
[†]Intraexaminer reliability reported for examiner #1 only.

Gillet Test (Stork Test)—cont'd

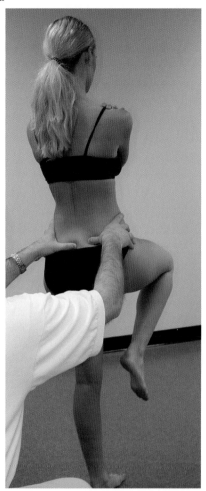

Figure 5-22
Gillet test.

Test and Study Quality	Description and Positive Findings	Population	Reference Standard	Sens	Spec	+LR	−LR
Gillet test[37] ◆	With patient standing with feet spread 12 inches apart, examiner palpates the S2 spinous process with one thumb and the PSIS with the other. The patient then flexes the hip and knee on the side being tested. The test is considered positive if the PSIS fails to move in a posteroinferior direction relative to S2	274 patients being treated for low back pain or another condition not related to the low back	Innominate torsion calculated by measured differences in pelvic landmarks	.08	.93	1.14	.99
Gillet test[2] ◉		85 consecutive patients with low back pain referred for sacroiliac joint blocks	90% pain relief with injection of local anesthetics into sacroiliac joint	.47*	.64*	1.31*	.83*

*Mean of chiropractor and physician sensitivity and specificity scores.

Spring Test (Joint Play Assessment)

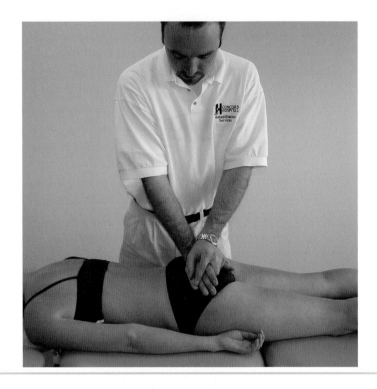

Figure 5-23
Spring test.

Test and Study Quality	Description and Positive Findings	Population	Reliability
Spring test[19] ◆	With patient prone, examiner uses one hand to lift the ilium while using the other hand to stabilize the sacrum and palpate the movement between the sacrum and ilium with the index finger. The test is positive if motion is different between the two sides.	15 patients with ankylosing spondylitis, 30 women with postpartum pelvic pain, and 16 asymptomatic subjects	Interexaminer $\kappa = -.06$

Test and Study Quality	Description and Positive Findings	Population	Reference Standard	Sens	Spec	+LR	−LR
Spring test[2] ◐	Therapist's hands are placed over the superior sacrum, and a posteroanterior thrust is applied while the therapist monitors the spring at the end range of motion. The asymptomatic side is compared with the symptomatic side	85 consecutive patients with low back pain referred for sacroiliac joint blocks	90% pain relief with injection of local anesthetics into sacroiliac joint	.66*	.42*	1.14*	.81*

*Mean of chiropractor and physician sensitivity and specificity scores.

Long-Sit Test (Supine-to-Sit Test)

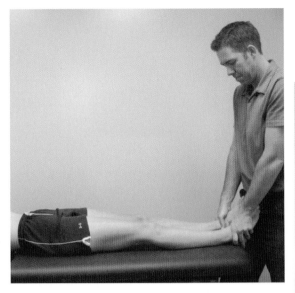
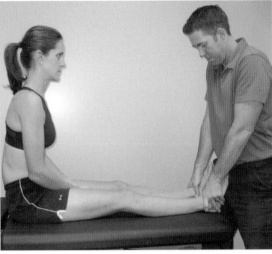

Figure 5-24
Long-sit test.

Test and Study Quality	Description and Positive Findings	Population	Reliability
Long-sit test[9] ◆	With patient supine, the lengths of the medial malleoli are compared. Patient is asked to long-sit, and the lengths of the medial malleoli are again compared. Positive if one leg appears shorter when patient is supine and then lengthens when the patient comes into the long-sitting position	65 patients with low back pain	Interexaminer κ = .19
Long-sit test[1] ◉		71 patients with low back pain	Interexaminer κ = .21

Test and Study Quality	Description and Positive Findings	Population	Reference Standard	Sens	Spec	+LR	−LR
Long-sit test[37] ◆	With patient supine, the lengths of the medial malleoli are compared. Patient is asked to long-sit, and the lengths of the medial malleoli are again compared. Positive if one leg appears shorter when patient is supine and then lengthens when the patient comes into the long-sitting position	274 patients being treated for low back pain or another condition not related to the low back	Innominate torsion calculated by measured differences in pelvic landmarks	.44	.64	1.22	.88

Standing Flexion Test

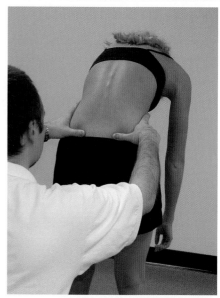

Figure 5-25
Standing flexion test.

Test* and Study Quality	Description and Positive Findings	Population	Reliability
Standing flexion test[20] ◆		25 patients with asymmetric low back pain	Intraexaminer[†] κ = [Right] .68 (.35, 1.01) [Left] .61 (.27, .96) Interexaminer κ = [Right] .51 (.08, .95) [Left] .55 (.20, .90)
Standing flexion test[9] ◆	With patient standing, examiner palpates inferior slope of PSIS. Patient is asked to forward bend completely. Positive for sacroiliac hypomobility if one PSIS moves more cranially than the PSIS on the contralateral side	65 patients currently receiving treatment for low back pain	Interexaminer κ = .32
Standing flexion test[38] ◆		14 asymptomatic graduate students	Interexaminer κ = .52
Standing flexion test[17] ◐		24 patients with low back pain	Interexaminer κ = .06
Standing flexion test 10,39 ◐		480 male construction workers; 50 had low back pain the day of the examination; 236 reported experiencing low back pain within the past 12 months	Interexaminer κ values ranged from .31 to .67
Standing flexion test[1] ◐		71 patients with low back pain	Interexaminer κ = .08

*Potter and Rothstein[18] also studied this test, but their study was excluded because they only reported the percentage of agreement.
†Intraexaminer reliability reported for examiner #1 only.

Test and Study Quality	Description and Positive Findings	Population	Reference Standard	Sens	Spec	+LR	−LR
Standing flexion test[37] ◆	With patient standing, examiner palpates inferior slope of PSIS. Patient is asked to forward bend completely. Positive for sacroiliac hypomobility if one PSIS moves more cranially than the PSIS on the contralateral side	274 patients being treated for low back pain or another condition not related to the low back	Innominate torsion calculated by measured differences in pelvic landmarks	.17	.79	.81	1.05

Sitting Flexion Test

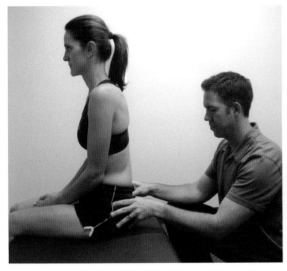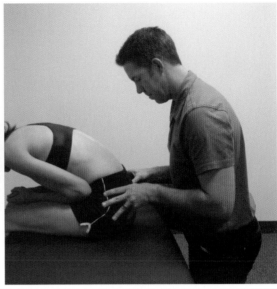

Figure 5-26
Sitting flexion test.

Test and Study Quality	Description and Positive Findings	Population	Reliability
Sitting flexion test[20] ◆	With patient sitting, examiner palpates inferior slope of PSIS. Patient is asked to forward bend completely. Positive for sacroiliac hypomobility if one PSIS moves more cranially than the PSIS on the contralateral side	25 patients with asymmetric low back pain	Intraexaminer* κ = [Right] .73 (.45, 1.01) [Left] .65 (.34, .96) Interexaminer κ = [Right] .75 (.42, 1.08) [Left] .64 (.32, .96)
Sitting flexion test[1] ◐		71 patients with low back pain	Interexaminer κ = .21
Sitting flexion test[17] ◐		24 patients with low back pain	Interexaminer κ = .06

*Intraexaminer reliability reported for examiner #1 only.

Test and Study Quality	Description and Positive Findings	Population	Reference Standard	Sens	Spec	+LR	−LR
Sitting flexion test[37] ◆	With patient seated, examiner palpates inferior aspect of each PSIS. Positive for sacroiliac joint dysfunction if inequality of the PSISs is found	274 patients being treated for low back pain or another condition not related to the low back	Innominate torsion calculated by measured differences in pelvic landmarks	.09	.93	1.29	.98

Sacroiliac Region 5

Prone Knee Bend Test

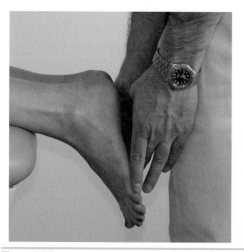
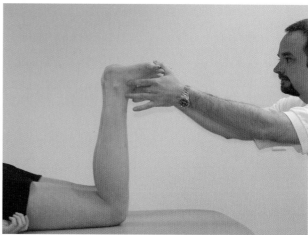

Figure 5-27
Prone knee bend test.

Test* and Study Quality	Description and Positive Findings	Population	Reliability
Prone knee bend test[20] ◆	With patient prone, examiner, looking at heels, assesses leg lengths. Knees are passively flexed to 90 degrees and leg lengths are again assessed. Considered positive if a change in leg lengths occurs between positions	25 patients with asymmetric low back pain	Intraexaminer[†] κ = [Right] .41 (.07, .78) [Left] .27 (−.22, .78) Interexaminer κ = [Right] .58 (.25, .91) [Left] .33 (−.18, .85)
Prone knee bend test[9] ◆		65 patients with low back pain	Interexaminer κ = .26
Prone knee bend test[1] ◐		71 patients with low back pain	Interexaminer κ = .21

*Potter and Rothstein[18] also studied this test, but their study was excluded because they only reported the percentage of agreement.
[†]Intraexaminer reliability reported for examiner #1 only.

Other Motion Assessment Tests

Test and Study Quality	Description and Positive Findings	Population	Reliability
Click-clack test[14] ◆	With patient sitting and examiner's thumbs on caudal PSIS, the patient rocks the pelvis forward and backward. Test is positive if one PSIS moves more slowly from cranial to caudal than the other		Interexaminer κ = .03
Heel-bank test[14] ◆	With patient sitting and examiner's thumbs on caudal PSIS, the patient raises one leg at a time and places the heel on the bench without using hands. Considered positive if the test required any effort	62 women recruited from obstetrics: 42 were pregnant and had pelvic girdle pain and 20 were not pregnant and were asymptomatic	Interexaminer κ = [Right] .32 [Left] .16
Abduction test[14] ◆	With patient side-lying with hips flexed 70 degrees and knees flexed 90 degrees, the patient is asked to lift the top leg about 20 cm. Considered positive if the test required any effort		Interexaminer κ = [Right] .61 [Left] .41

Pregnancy-Related Pelvic Girdle Pain Classification[40]

Inclusion Criteria	Classification Subgroup
All four of the following criteria must be met for subjects to be evaluated for classification: • Currently pregnant or recently pregnant (within 2 years) • Daily pain at the time of the examination (week 33 of gestation or beyond) • The ability to point out the exact area of one or more of the pelvic girdle joints as the painful area • Pain during one or more of the five selected clinical tests: active straight-leg raise test, compression test, distraction test, Gaenslen test, thigh thrust test	**Pelvic girdle syndrome:** Daily pain in all three pelvic joints confirmed by objective findings. **Symphysiolysis:** Daily pain in the pubic symphysis confirmed by objective findings. **One-sided sacroiliac syndrome:** Daily pain from one sacroiliac joint alone, confirmed by objective findings. **Double-sided sacroiliac syndrome:** Daily pain from both sacroiliac joints, confirmed by objective findings. **Miscellaneous:** Daily pain from one or more pelvic joints but inconsistent objective findings from the pelvic joints.

Reliability of Pregnancy-Related Pelvic Girdle Pain Classification

Test and Study Quality	Description and Positive Findings	Population	Reliability
Pregnancy-related pelvic girdle pain classification[40] ◆	As described in the pregnancy-related pelvic girdle pain classification above	13 female patients with pelvic girdle pain	Interexaminer κ = .78 (.64, .92)

Sacroiliac Joint Pain

Test and Study Quality	Description and Positive Findings	Population	Reference Standard	Sens	Spec	+LR	−LR
Mennell test + Gaenslen test + Thigh thrust[21] ◆	Procedures all previously described in this chapter. At least two of three tests need to be positive to indicate sacroiliitis	40 patients with chronic low back pain	Sacroiliitis apparent on MRI	**Right side**			
				.55 (.22, .84)	.83 (.65, .93)	3.44 (1.27, 9.29)	.52 (.25, 1.11)
				Left side			
				.45 (.18, .75)	.86 (.67, .95)	3.29 (1.07, 10.0)	.63 (.36, 1.09)
Distraction test + Thigh thrust + Gaenslen test + Patrick sign + Compression test[41] ◆	Procedures all previously described in this chapter. At least three of five tests need to be positive to indicate sacroiliac joint pain	60 patients with chronic low back pain referred to pain clinic	50% pain relief with injection of local anesthetics into sacroiliac joint	.85 (.72, .99)	.79 (.65, .93)	4.02 (2.04, 7.89)	.19 (.07, .47)
Distraction test + Thigh thrust + Sacral thrust + Compression test[4] ◆	Procedures all previously described in this chapter. At least two of four tests need to be positive to indicate sacroiliac joint pain	48 patients with chronic lumbopelvic pain referred for sacroiliac joint injection	80% pain relief with injection of local anesthetics into sacroiliac joint	.88 (.64, .97)	.78 (.61, .89)	4.0 (2.13, 8.08)	.16 (.04, .47)
Distraction test + Thigh thrust + Gaenslen test + Sacral thrust + Compression test[5] ◆	Procedures all previously described in this chapter. At least three of five tests need to be positive to indicate sacroiliac joint pain	48 patients with chronic lumbopelvic pain referred for diagnostic spinal injection	80% pain relief with injection of local anesthetics into sacroiliac joint	.91 (.62, −.98)	.78 (.61, .89)	4.16 (2.16, 8.39)	.12 (.02, .49)

Sacroiliac Joint Pain—cont'd

Test and Study Quality	Description and Positive Findings	Population	Reference Standard	Sens	Spec	+LR	−LR
Distraction test + Thigh thrust + Gaenslen test + Sacral thrust + Compression test[42] ◕	Procedures all previously described in this chapter. At least three of five tests need to be positive to indicate sacroiliac joint pain	81 patients with chronic lumbopelvic pain referred for diagnostic spinal injection	80% pain relief with injection of local anesthetics into sacroiliac joint	.77 (.56, .91)	.70 (.51, .85)	2.57	.33
Pooled estimate of four studies[4,5,41,42] from **2009 Systematic Review**[26] ◆	Same as above	Pooled from four studies[4,5,41,42] above	Pooled from four studies[4,5,41,42] above	.85 (.75, .92)	.76 (.68, .84)	3.54	.20
Gaenslen test + Thigh thrust test + Long dorsal sacroiliac ligament test[25†] ◕	Procedures all previously described in this chapter	454 patients with low back pain and no signs of nerve root compression	Sacroiliitis per MRI	≥1 out of 3 positive tests			
				.42 (.28, .58)	.69 (.66, .72)	1.35	.84
				≥1 out of 3 positive tests			
				.24 (.13, .40)	.86 (.83, .88)	1.71	.88
				≥1 out of 3 positive tests			
				.13 (.05, .27)	.91 (.89, .93)	1.44	.96

†Study also reported statistics by gender and found better diagnostic utility in men than in women. LRs calculated by author.

5

Sacroiliac Region

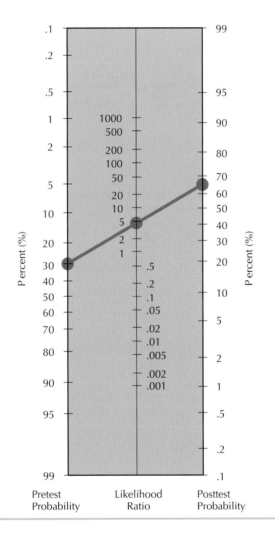

Figure 5-28
Nomogram representing the changes from pretest to posttest probability using the cluster of tests for detecting sacroiliac dysfunction. Considering a 33% pretest probability and a +LR of 4.16, the posttest probability that the patient presents with sacroiliac dysfunction is 67%. (Adapted with permission from Fagan TJ. Letter: Nomogram for Bayes theorem. *N Engl J Med.* 1975;293:257. Massachusetts Medical Society, 2005.)

Following the McKenzie Evaluation to Rule Out Discogenic Pain

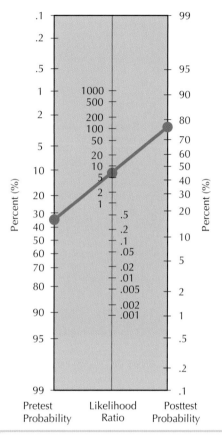

Figure 5-29

Nomagram representing the change in pretest to posttest probability of using the McKenzie method of assessment combined with the cluster of sacroiliac tests. Considering a 33% pretest probability and a +LR of 6.97, the posttest probability that the patient presents with sacroiliac dysfunction is 77%. (Adapted from Fagan TJ. Letter: Nomogram for Bayes theorem. *N Engl J Med.* 1975;293:257. Massachusetts Medical Society, 2005.)

Laslett and associates[5] assessed the diagnostic utility of the McKenzie method of mechanical assessment combined with the following sacroiliac tests: *distraction test, thigh thrust test, Gaenslen test, sacral thrust test,* and *compression test.* The McKenzie assessment consisted of flexion in standing, extension in standing, right and left side gliding, flexion in lying, and extension in lying. The movements were repeated in sets of 10, and centralization and peripheralization were recorded. If it was determined that repeated movements resulted in centralization, the patient was considered to have pain of discogenic origin. Following the use of the McKenzie method to rule out individuals presenting with discogenic pain, in terms of diagnostic utility, the cluster of these tests exhibited a sensitivity of .91 (95% CI .62, .98), specificity .87 (95% CI .68, .96), +LR of 6.97 (95% CI 2.16, 8.39), −LR .11 (95% CI .02, .44).

Sacroiliac Region

5

Identifying Patients Likely to Benefit from Spinal Manipulation

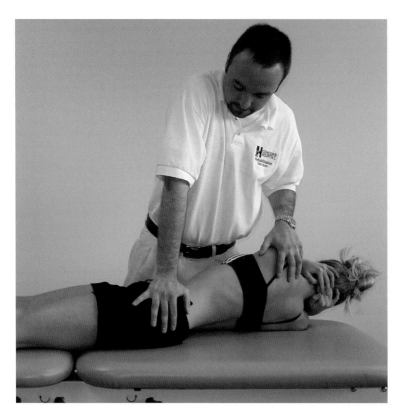

Figure 5-30
Spinal manipulation technique used by Flynn and colleagues. The patient is passively side-bent toward the side to be manipulated (away from the therapist). The therapist then rotates the patient away from the side to be manipulated (toward the therapist) and delivers a quick thrust through the ASIS in a posteroinferior direction. (From Flynn T, Fritz J, Whitman J, et al. A clinical prediction rule for classifying patients with low back pain who demonstrate short-term improvement with spinal manipulation. *Spine.* 2002;27:2835-2843.)

Flynn and colleagues[1] investigated the effects of the spinal manipulation technique in a heterogeneous population of patients with low back pain. They identified a number of variables that were associated with a successful outcome following the manipulation. A logistics regression equation was used to identify a cluster of signs and symptoms leading to a clinical prediction rule that could significantly enhance the likelihood of identifying patients who would achieve a successful outcome with spinal manipulation. Five variables form the clinical prediction rule: (1) symptoms for fewer than 16 days, (2) no symptoms distal to the knee, (3) hypomobility in the lumbar spine, (4) FABQ work subscale score of less than 19, and (5) at least one hip with more than 35 degrees of internal rotation range of motion.

Childs and colleagues[43] tested the validity of the clinical prediction rule when applied in a separate patient population and by a variety of clinicians with varying levels of clinical experience and practicing in different settings. Consecutive patients with low back pain were randomized to receive either spinal manipulation or a lumbar stabilization program. The results of the study demonstrated that patients who satisfied the clinical prediction rule and received spinal manipulation had significantly better outcomes than patients who did not meet the clinical prediction rule but still received spinal manipulation and the group who met the clinical prediction rule but received lumbar stabilization exercises.

To make use of the clinical prediction rule more practical in a primary care environment, Fritz and colleagues[44] tested an abbreviated version consisting of only the acuity and symptom location factors. Ninety-two percent of patients with low back pain who met both criteria had successful outcomes. The results of the Childs and colleagues[43] and Fritz and associates[44] studies support the findings of Flynn and colleagues[1] and significantly increase clinician confidence in using the clinical prediction rule in decision making regarding individual patients with low back pain.

Identifying Patients Likely to Benefit from Spinal Manipulation—cont'd

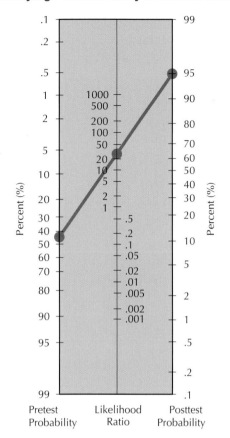

Pretest   Likelihood   Posttest
Probability   Ratio   Probability

Figure 5-31
Nomogram representing the changes from pretest to posttest likelihood that a patient with low back pain who satisfies four of five criteria for the rule will have a successful outcome following spinal manipulation. The pretest likelihood that any patient with low back pain would respond favorably to sacroiliac manipulation was determined to be 45%. However, if the patient presents with four of the five predictor variables identified by Flynn and colleagues[1] (+LR 24), then the posttest probability that the patient will respond positively to spinal manipulation increases dramatically to 95%. (Adapted from Fagan TJ. Letter: Nomogram for Bayes theorem. *N Engl J Med.* 1975;293:257. Massachusetts Medical Society, 2005.)

Test and Study Quality	Description and Criteria	Population	Reference Standard	Sens	Spec	+LR
Symptoms for less than 16 days + No symptoms distal to the knee + Hypomobility in the lumbar spine + FABQ work subscale score of less than 19 + At least one hip with more than 35 degrees of internal rotation range of motion[1] ◆	At least four of five tests needed to be positive	71 patients with low back pain	Reduction of 50% or more in back pain–related disability within 1 week as measured by the Oswestry questionnaire	.63 (.45 to .77)	.97 (.87 to 1.0)	24.38 (4.63 to 139.41)
Symptoms for less than 16 days + No symptoms distal to the knee[44] ◆	Must meet both criteria	141 patients with low back pain		.56 (.43, .67)	.92 (.84, .96)	7.2 (3.2, 16.1)

Sacroiliac Region

Outcome Measure	Scoring and Interpretation	Test-Retest Reliability	MCID
Oswestry Disability Index (ODI)	Users are asked to rate the difficulty of performing 10 functional tasks on a scale of 0 to 5 with different descriptors for each task. A total score out of 100 is calculated by summing each score and doubling the total. The answers provide a score between 0 and 100, with higher scores representing more disability	ICC = .91[45]	11[46]
Modified Oswestry Disability Index (modified ODI)	As above except replaces the sex life question with an employment/homemaking question	ICC = .90[47]	6[47]
Roland-Morris Disability Questionnaire (RMDQ)	Users are asked to answer 23 or 24 questions (depending on the version) about their back pain and related disability. The RMDQ is scored by adding up the number of items checked by the patient, with higher numbers indicating more disability	ICC = .91[48]	5[46]
Fear-Avoidance Beliefs Questionnaire (FABQ)	Users are asked to rate their level of agreement with statements concerning beliefs about the relationship between physical activity, work, and their back pain. Level of agreement is answered on a Likert-type scale ranging from 0 (completely disagree) to 7 (completely agree). The FABQ has two parts: a seven-item work subscale (FABQW) and a four-item physical activity subscale (FABQPA). Each scale is scored separately, with higher scores representing higher levels of fear avoidance	FABQW: ICC = .82 FABQPA: ICC = .66[49]	Not available
Numeric Pain Rating Scale (NPRS)	Users rate their level of pain on an 11-point scale ranging from 0 to 10, with high scores representing more pain. Often asked as current pain and least, worst, and average pain in the past 24 hours	ICCs = .72[50]	2[51,52]

MCID, Minimum clinically important difference.

1. Flynn T, Fritz J, Whitman J, et al. A clinical prediction rule for classifying patients with low back pain who demonstrate short-term improvement with spinal manipulation. *Spine*. 2002;27:2835–2843.

2. Dreyfuss P, Michaelsen M, Pauza K, et al. The value of medical history and physical examination in diagnosing sacroiliac joint pain. *Spine*. 1996;21:2594–2602.

3. Laslett M. Pain provocation tests for diagnosis of sacroiliac joint pain. *Aust J Physiother*. 2006;52:229.

4. Laslett M, Aprill CN, McDonald B, Young SB. Diagnosis of sacroiliac joint pain: validity of individual provocation tests and composites of tests. *Man Ther*. 2005;10:207–218.

5. Laslett M, Young SB, Aprill CN, McDonald B. Diagnosing painful sacroiliac joints: a validity study of a McKenzie evaluation and sacroiliac provocation tests. *Aust J Physiother*. 2003;49:89–97.

6. Maigne JY, Aivaliklis A, Pfefer F. Results of sacroiliac joint double block and value of sacroiliac pain provocation tests in 54 patients with low back pain. *Spine*. 1996;21:1889–1892.

7. Schwarzer AC, Aprill CN, Bogduk N. The sacroiliac joint in chronic low back pain. *Spine*. 1995;20:31–37.

8. Cibulka MT, Delitto A, Koldehoff RM. Changes in innominate tilt after manipulation of the sacroiliac joint in patients with low back pain. An experimental study. *Phys Ther*. 1988;68:1359–1363.

9. Riddle DL, Freburger JK. Evaluation of the presence of sacroiliac joint region dysfunction using a combination of tests: a multicenter intertester reliability study. *Phys Ther*. 2002;82:772–781.

10. Toussaint R, Gawlik CS, Rehder U, Ruther W. Sacroiliac dysfunction in construction workers. *J Manipulative Physiol Ther*. 1999;22:134–138.

11. Tonosu J, Oka H, Watanabe K, et al. Validation study of a diagnostic scoring system for sacroiliac joint-related pain. *J Pain Res*. 2018;11:1659–1663.

12. Jung JH, Kim HI, Shin DA, et al. Usefulness of pain distribution pattern assessment in decision-making for the patients with lumbar zygapophyseal and sacroiliac joint arthropathy. *J Korean Med Sci*. 2007;22:1048–1054.

13. van der Wurff P, Buijs EJ, Groen GJ. Intensity mapping of pain referral areas in sacroiliac joint pain patients. *J Manipulative Physiol Ther*. 2006;29:190–195.

14. van Kessel-Cobelens AM, Verhagen AP, Mens JM, et al. Pregnancy-related pelvic girdle pain: intertester reliability of 3 tests to determine asymmetric mobility of the sacroiliac joints. *J Manipulative Physiol Ther*. 2008;31:130–136.

15. O'Haire C, Gibbons P. Interexaminer and intra-examiner agreement for assessing sacroiliac anatomical landmarks using palpation and observation: pilot study. *Man Ther*. 2000;5:13–20.

16. Holmgren U, Waling K. Inter-examiner reliability of four static palpation tests used for assessing pelvic dysfunction. *Man Ther*. 2008;13:50–56.

17. Tong HC, Heyman OG, Lado DA, Isser MM. Inter-examiner reliability of three methods of combining test results to determine side of sacral restriction, sacral base position, and innominate bone position. *J Am Osteopath Assoc*. 2006;106:464–468.

18. Potter NA, Rothstein JM. Intertester reliability for selected clinical tests of the sacroiliac joint. *Phys Ther*. 1985;65:1671–1675.

19. Robinson HS, Brox JI, Robinson R, et al. The reliability of selected motion and pain provocation tests for the sacroiliac joint. *Man Ther*. 2007;12:72–79.

20. Arab AM, Abdollahi I, Joghataei MT, et al. Inter- and intra-examiner reliability of single and composites of selected motion palpation and pain provocation tests for sacroiliac joint. *Man Ther*. 2009;14:213–221.

21. Ozgocmen S, Bozgeyik Z, Kalcik M, Yildirim A. The value of sacroiliac pain provocation tests in early active sacroiliitis. *Clin Rheumatol*. 2008;10:1275–1282.

22. Kokmeyer DJ, van der Wurff P, Aufdemkampe G, Fickenscher TC. The reliability of multitest regimens with sacroiliac pain provocation tests. *J Manipulative Physiol Ther*. 2002;25:42–48.

23. Broadhurst NA, Bond MJ. Pain provocation tests for the assessment of sacroiliac joint dysfunction. *J Spinal Disord*. 1998;11:341–345.

24. Laslett M, Williams M. The reliability of selected pain provocation tests for sacroiliac joint pathology. *Spine*. 1994;19:1243–1249.

25. Arnbak B, Jurik A, Jensen R, et al. The diagnostic value of three sacroiliac joint pain provocation tests for sacroiliitis identified by magnetic resonance imaging. *Scand J Rheumatol*. 2017;46(2):130–137.

26. Szadek KM, van der Wurff P, van Tulder MW, et al. Diagnostic validity of criteria for sacroiliac joint pain: a systematic review. *J Pain*. 2009;10(4):354–368.

27. Herzog W, Read LJ, Conway PJ, et al. Reliability of motion palpation procedures to detect sacroiliac joint fixations. *J Manipulative Physiol Ther*. 1989;12:86–92.

28. Gutke A, Hansson ER, Zetherström G, Ostgaard HC. Posterior pelvic pain provocation test is negative in patients with lumbar herniated discs. *Eur Spine J*. 2009;18(7):1008–1012.

29. Deleted in review.

30. Shimpi A, Hatekar R, Shyam A, Sancheti P. Reliability and validity of a new clinical test for assessment of the sacroiliac joint dysfunction. *Hong Kong Physiother J*. 2018;38(1):13–22.

31. van Leeuwen RJ, Szadek K, de Vet H, et al. Pain pressure threshold in the region of the sacroiliac joint in patients diagnosed with sacroiliac joint pain. *Pain Physician*. 2016;19:147–154.

32. Adhia DB, Tumilty S, Mani R, et al. Can hip abduction and external rotation discriminate sacroiliac joint pain? *Man Ther*. 2016;21:191–197.

33. Werner CML, Hoch A, Gautier L, et al. Distraction test of the posterior superior iliac spine (PSIS) in the

diagnosis of sacroiliac joint arthropathy. *BMC Surg.* 2013;13:52.

34. Carmichael JP. Inter- and intra-examiner reliability of palpation for sacroiliac joint dysfunction. *J Manipulative Physiol Ther.* 1987;10:164–171.

35. Meijne W, van Neerbos K, Aufdemkampe G, van der Wurff P. Intraexaminer and interexaminer reliability of the Gillet test. *J Manipulative Physiol Ther.* 1999;22:4–9.

36. Hungerford BA, Gilleard W, Moran M, Emmerson C. Evaluation of the ability of physical therapists to palpate intrapelvic motion with the Stork test on the support side. *Phys Ther.* 2007;87:879–887.

37. Levangie PK. Four clinical tests of sacroiliac joint dysfunction: the association of test results with innominate torsion among patients with and without low back pain. *Phys Ther.* 1999;79:1043–1057.

38. Vincent-Smith B, Gibbons P. Inter-examiner and intra-examiner reliability of the standing flexion test. *Man Ther.* 1999;4:87–93.

39. Toussaint R, Gawlik CS, Rehder U, Ruther W. Sacroiliac joint diagnostics in the Hamburg construction workers study. *J Manipulative Physiol Ther.* 1999;22:139–143.

40. Cook C, Massa L, Harm-Ernandes I, et al. Interrater reliability and diagnostic accuracy of pelvic girdle pain classification. *J Manipulative Physiol Ther.* 2007;30(4):252–258.

41. van der Wurff P, Buijs EJ, Groen GJ. A multitest regimen of pain provocation tests as an aid to reduce unnecessary minimally invasive sacroiliac joint procedures. *Arch Phys Med Rehabil.* 2006;87:10–14.

42. Young S, Aprill C, Laslett M. Correlation of clinical examination characteristics with three sources of chronic low back pain. *Spine J.* 2003;3:460–465.

43. Childs JD, Fritz JM, Flynn TW, et al. A clinical prediction rule to identify patients with low back pain most likely to benefit from spinal manipulation: a validation study. *Ann Intern Med.* 2004;141:920–928.

44. Fritz JM, Childs JD, Flynn TW. Pragmatic application of a clinical prediction rule in primary care to identify patients with low back pain with a good prognosis following a brief spinal manipulation intervention. *BMC Fam Pract.* 2005;6:29.

45. Lauridsen HH, Hartvigsen J, Manniche C, et al. Danish version of the Oswestry Disability Index for patients with low back pain. Part 1: Cross-cultural adaptation, reliability and validity in two different populations. *Eur Spine J.* 2006;15:1705–1716.

46. Lauridsen HH, Hartvigsen J, Manniche C, et al. Responsiveness and minimal clinically important difference for pain and disability instruments in low back pain patients. *BMC Musculoskelet Disord.* 2006;7:82.

47. Fritz JM, Irrgang JJ. A comparison of a Modified Oswestry Disability Questionnaire and the Quebec Back Pain Disability Scale. *Phys Ther.* 2001;81:776–788.

48. Brouwer S, Kuijer W, Dijkstra PU, et al. Reliability and stability of the Roland Morris Disability Questionnaire: intra class correlation and limits of agreement. *Disabil Rehabil.* 2004;26:162–165.

49. Grotle M, Brox JI, Vollestad NK. Reliability, validity and responsiveness of the fear-avoidance beliefs questionnaire: methodological aspects of the Norwegian version. *J Rehabil Med.* 2006;38:346–353.

50. Li L, Liu X, Herr K. Postoperative pain intensity assessment: a comparison of four scales in Chinese adults. *Pain Med.* 2007;8:223–234.

51. Farrar JT, Berlin JA, Strom BL. Clinically important changes in acute pain outcome measures: a validation study. *J Pain Symptom Manage.* 2003;25:406–411.

52. Farrar JT, Portenoy RK, Berlin JA, et al. Defining the clinically important difference in pain outcome measures. *Pain.* 2000;88:287–294.

Hip and Pelvis 6

Clinical Summary and Recommendations

Patient History	
Complaints	• Several complaints appear to be useful in identifying specific hip pathologic conditions. A subjective complaint of "clicking in the hip" is strongly associated with acetabular labral tears. • Reports of "constant low back/buttock pain" and "ipsilateral groin pain" are moderately helpful in diagnosing osteoarthritis (OA) of the hip.

Physical Examination	
Range-of-Motion Measurements	• Measuring hip range of motion has consistently been shown to be highly reliable and when limited in three planes can be fairly useful in identifying hip OA (+LR [likelihood ratio] = 4.5 to 4.7). • Assessing pain during range-of-motion measurements can be helpful in identifying both OA and lateral tendon pathologic conditions. Lateral hip pain during passive abduction is strongly suggestive of lateral tendon pathologic disorders (+LR = 8.3), whereas groin pain during active hip abduction or adduction is moderately suggestive of OA (+LR = 5.7). • Limited hip abduction in infants can also be very helpful in identifying hip dysplasia or instability.
Strength Assessment	• Assessment of hip muscle strength has been shown to be fairly reliable, but it appears to be less helpful in identifying lateral tendon pathologic conditions than reports of pain during resisted tests, especially of the gluteus minimus and medius muscles (+LR = 3.27). • Similarly, a report of posterior pain with a squat is also fairly useful in identifying hip OA (+LR = 6.1). • Although less reliable than strength tests, the Trendelenburg test is also moderately useful in identifying both lateral tendon pathologic conditions and gluteus medius tears (+LR = 3.2 to 3.6).
Special Tests	• The FABER test in identifying the presence of hip instability (+LR = 5.4). • The patellar-pubic-percussion test is useful at detecting and ruling out hip fractures (+LR = 6.7 to 21.6, −LR = .07 to .14). • The ligamentum teres test has been found to be valuable in identifying tears of the ligamentum teres (+LR = 6, −LR = .12) • Additionally, the long-stride walking test (+LR = 6.12 and −LR = .07) and ischiofemoral impingement test (+LR = 5.35 and −LR = .21) may be useful for identifying the presence of ischiofemoral impingement. However, the wide confidence intervals should be considered.
Combinations of Findings	• Patients with at least four of five signs and symptoms (squatting aggravates symptoms, lateral pain with active hip flexion, scour test with adduction causes lateral hip or groin pain, pain with active hip extension, and passive internal rotation of 25 degrees or less) are highly likely to have hip OA.

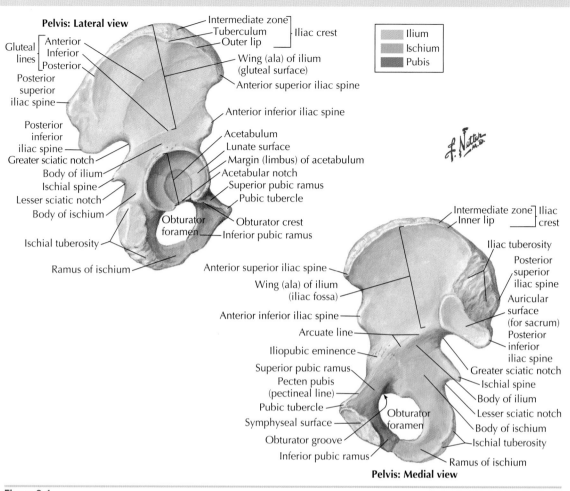

Figure 6-1
Hip (coxal) bone.

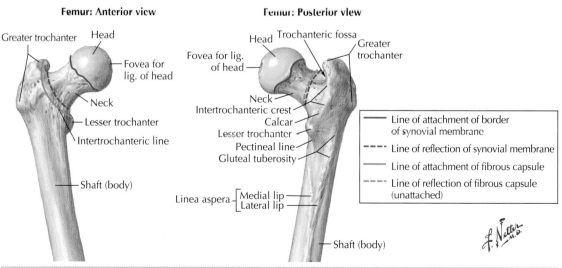

Figure 6-2
Femur.

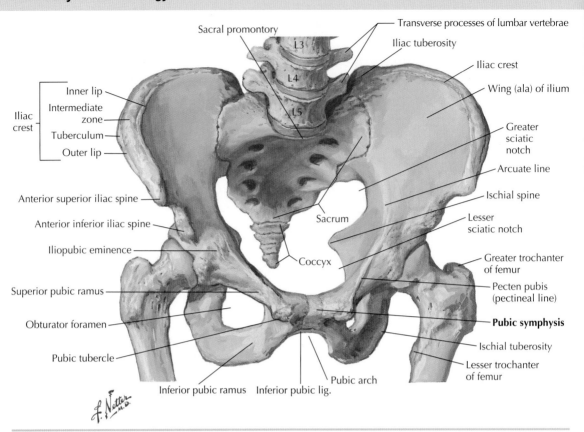

Figure 6-3
Hip and pelvis joints.

Joint	Type and Classification	Closed Packed Position	Capsular Pattern
Femoroacetabular	Synovial: Spheroidal	Full extension, some internal rotation, and abduction	Internal rotation and abduction greater than flexion and extension
Pubic symphysis	Amphiarthrodial	Not applicable	Not applicable
Sacroiliac	Synovial: Plane	Not documented	Not documented

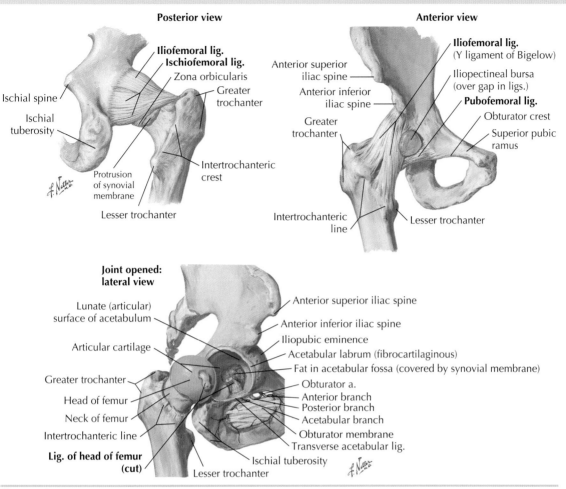

Figure 6-4
Ligaments of the hip and pelvis.

Hip Ligaments	Attachments	Function
Iliofemoral	Anterior inferior iliac spine to intertrochanteric line of femur	Limits hip extension
Ischiofemoral	Posterior inferior acetabulum to apex of greater tubercle	Limits internal rotation, external rotation, and extension
Pubofemoral	Obturator crest of pubic bone to blend with capsule of hip and iliofemoral ligament	Limits hip hyperabduction
Ligament of head of femur	Margin of acetabular notch and transverse acetabular ligament to head of femur	Carries blood supply to head of femur

Pubic Symphysis Ligaments	Attachments	Function
Superior pubic ligament	Connects superior aspects of right and left pubic crests	Reinforces superior aspect of joint
Inferior pubic ligament	Connects inferior aspects of right and left pubic crests	Reinforces inferior aspect of joint
Posterior pubic ligament	Connects posterior aspects of right and left pubic crests	Reinforces inferior aspect of joint

Posterior Muscles of Hip and Thigh

Muscle	Proximal Attachment	Distal Attachment	Nerve and Segmental Level	Action
Gluteus maximus	Posterior border of ilium, dorsal aspect of sacrum and coccyx, and sacrotuberous ligament	Iliotibial tract of fascia lata and gluteal tuberosity of femur	Inferior gluteal nerve (L5, S1, S2)	Extension, external rotation, and some abduction of the hip joint
Gluteus medius	External superior border of ilium and gluteal aponeurosis	Lateral aspect of greater trochanter of femur	Superior gluteal nerve (L5, S1)	Hip abduction and internal rotation; maintains level pelvis in single-limb stance
Gluteus minimus	External surface of ilium and margin of greater sciatic notch	Anterior aspect of greater trochanter of femur		
Piriformis	Anterior aspect of sacrum and sacrotuberous ligament	Superior greater trochanter of femur	Ventral rami of S1, S2	External rotation of extended hip, abduction of flexed hip; steadies femoral head in acetabulum
Superior gemellus	Ischial spine	Trochanteric fossa of femur	Nerve to obturator internus (L5, S1)	
Inferior gemellus	Ischial tuberosity		Nerve to quadratus femoris (L5, S1)	
Obturator internus	Internal surface of obturator membrane, border of obturator foramen		Nerve to obturator internus (L5, S1)	
Quadratus femoris	Lateral border of ischial tuberosity	Quadrate tubercle of femur	Nerve to quadratus femoris (L5, S1)	Lateral rotation of hip; steadies femoral head in acetabulum
Semitendinosus (hamstring)	Ischial tuberosity	Superomedial aspect of tibia	Tibial division of sciatic nerve (L5, S1, S2)	Hip extension, knee flexion, medial rotation of knee in knee flexion
Semimembranosus (hamstring)		Posterior aspect of medial condyle of tibia		
Biceps femoris (hamstring)	Long head: ischial tuberosity Short head: linea aspera and lateral supracondylar line of femur	Lateral aspect of head of fibula, lateral condyle of tibia	Long head: tibial division of sciatic nerve (L5, S1, S2) Short head: common fibular division of sciatic nerve (L5, S1, S2)	Knee flexion, hip extension, and knee external rotation when knee is flexed

Posterior Muscles of Hip and Thigh—cont'd

Superficial dissection　　　　　　　　**Deeper dissection**

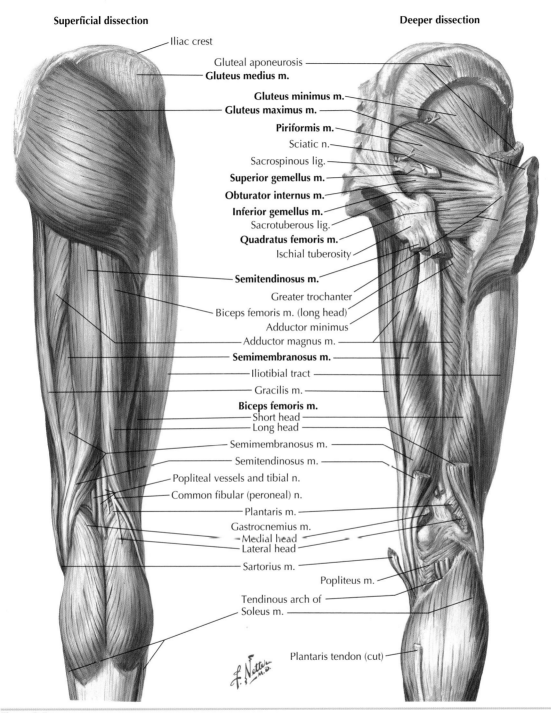

Iliac crest

Gluteal aponeurosis
Gluteus medius m.
Gluteus minimus m.
Gluteus maximus m.
Piriformis m.
Sciatic n.
Sacrospinous lig.
Superior gemellus m.
Obturator internus m.
Inferior gemellus m.
Sacrotuberous lig.
Quadratus femoris m.
Ischial tuberosity

Semitendinosus m.

Greater trochanter
Biceps femoris m. (long head)
Adductor minimus
Adductor magnus m.
Semimembranosus m.
Iliotibial tract
Gracilis m.
Biceps femoris m.
Short head
Long head
Semimembranosus m.
Semitendinosus m.
Popliteal vessels and tibial n.
Common fibular (peroneal) n.
Plantaris m.
Gastrocnemius m.
Medial head
Lateral head
Sartorius m.
Popliteus m.
Tendinous arch of
Soleus m.

Plantaris tendon (cut)

f. Netter
M.D.

Figure 6-5
Muscles of hip and thigh: posterior views.

6

Hip and Pelvis

Anterior Muscles of Hip and Thigh

Muscle	Proximal Attachment	Distal Attachment	Nerve and Segmental Level	Action
Obturator externus	Margin of obturator foramen and obturator membrane	Trochanteric fossa of femur	Obturator nerve (L3, L4)	Hip external rotation; steadies head of femur in acetabulum
Hip Flexors				
Psoas major	Lumbar transverse processes	Lesser trochanter of femur	L1-L4	Flexes the hip, assists with external rotation and abduction
Psoas minor	Lateral bodies of T12-L1	Iliopectineal eminence and arcuate line of ileum	L1-L2	Flexion of pelvis on lumbar spine
Iliacus	Superior iliac fossa, iliac crest and ala of sacrum	Lateral tendon of psoas major and distal to lesser trochanter	Femoral nerve (L1-L4)	Flexes the hip, assists with external rotation and abduction
Tensor fasciae latae	Anterior superior iliac spine and anterior aspect of iliac crest	Iliotibial tract that attaches to lateral condyle of tibia	Superior gluteal nerve (L4, L5)	Hip abduction, internal rotation and flexion; aids in maintaining knee extension
Rectus femoris	Anterior inferior iliac spine	Base of patella and through patellar ligament to tibial tuberosity	Femoral nerve (L2, L3, L4)	Hip flexion and knee extension
Sartorius	Anterior superior iliac spine and notch just inferior	Superomedial aspect of tibia	Femoral nerve (L2, L3)	Flexes, abducts, and externally rotates hip; flexes knee
Adductors				
Longus	Inferior to pubic crest	Middle third of linea aspera of femur	Obturator nerve (L2, L3, L4)	Hip adduction
Brevis	Inferior ramus of pubis	Pectineal line and proximal linea aspera of femur	Obturator nerve (L2, L3, L4)	Hip adduction and assists with hip extension
Magnus	Adductor part: inferior pubic ramus, ramus of ischium. Hamstring part: ischial tuberosity	Adductor part: gluteal tuberosity, linea aspera, medial supracondylar line. Hamstring part: adductor tubercle of femur	Adductor part: obturator nerve (L2, L3, L4). Hamstring part: tibial part of sciatic nerve (L4)	Hip adduction. Adductor part: hip flexion. Hamstring part: hip extension
Gracilis	Inferior ramus of pubis	Superomedial aspect of tibia	Obturator nerve (L2, L3)	Hip adduction and flexion; assists with hip internal rotation
Pectineus	Superior ramus of pubis	Pectineal line of femur	Femoral nerve and obturator nerve (L2, L3, L4)	Hip adduction and flexion; assists with hip internal rotation

Anterior Muscles of Hip and Thigh—cont'd

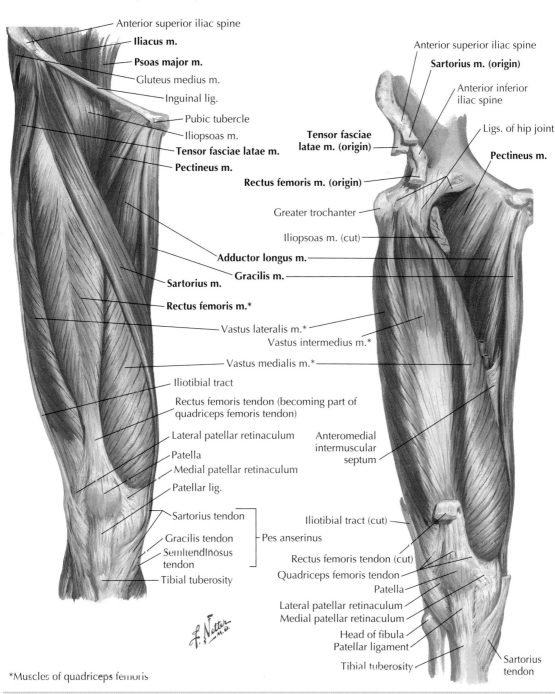

Anterior superior iliac spine
Iliacus m.
Psoas major m.
Gluteus medius m.
Inguinal lig.
Pubic tubercle
Iliopsoas m.
Tensor fasciae latae m.
Pectineus m.

Tensor fasciae latae m. (origin)

Rectus femoris m. (origin)

Greater trochanter

Iliopsoas m. (cut)

Adductor longus m.
Gracilis m.
Sartorius m.

Rectus femoris m.*

Vastus lateralis m.*
Vastus intermedius m.*

Vastus medialis m.*

Iliotibial tract

Rectus femoris tendon (becoming part of quadriceps femoris tendon)

Lateral patellar retinaculum

Patella
Medial patellar retinaculum
Patellar lig.

Sartorius tendon
Gracilis tendon
Semitendinosus tendon
Tibial tuberosity

Pes anserinus

Anterior superior iliac spine
Sartorius m. (origin)

Anterior inferior iliac spine

Ligs. of hip joint

Pectineus m.

Anteromedial intermuscular septum

Iliotibial tract (cut)

Rectus femoris tendon (cut)
Quadriceps femoris tendon
Patella
Lateral patellar retinaculum
Medial patellar retinaculum
Head of fibula
Patellar ligament
Tibial tuberosity

Sartorius tendon

*Muscles of quadriceps femoris

Figure 6-6
Muscles of thigh: anterior view.

Hip and Pelvis

6

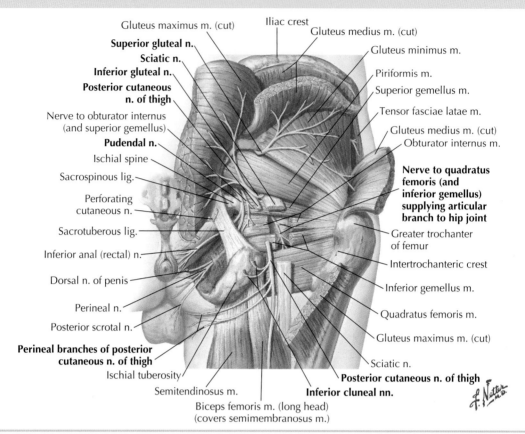

Gluteus maximus m. (cut)
Superior gluteal n.
Sciatic n.
Inferior gluteal n.
Posterior cutaneous n. of thigh
Nerve to obturator internus (and superior gemellus)
Pudendal n.
Ischial spine
Sacrospinous lig.
Perforating cutaneous n.
Sacrotuberous lig.
Inferior anal (rectal) n.
Dorsal n. of penis
Perineal n.
Posterior scrotal n.
Perineal branches of posterior cutaneous n. of thigh
Ischial tuberosity
Semitendinosus m.
Biceps femoris m. (long head) (covers semimembranosus m.)

Iliac crest
Gluteus medius m. (cut)
Gluteus minimus m.
Piriformis m.
Superior gemellus m.
Tensor fasciae latae m.
Gluteus medius m. (cut)
Obturator internus m.
Nerve to quadratus femoris (and inferior gemellus) supplying articular branch to hip joint
Greater trochanter of femur
Intertrochanteric crest
Inferior gemellus m.
Quadratus femoris m.
Gluteus maximus m. (cut)
Sciatic n.
Posterior cutaneous n. of thigh
Inferior cluneal nn.

Figure 6-7
Nerves of the hips and buttocks.

Nerve	Segmental Level	Sensory	Motor
Obturator	L2, L3, L4	Medial thigh	Adductor longus, adductor brevis, adductor magnus (adductor part), gracilis, obturator externus
Saphenous	Femoral nerve	Medial leg and foot	No motor
Femoral	L2, L3, L4	Thigh via cutaneous nerves	Iliacus, sartorius, quadriceps femoris, articularis genu, pectineus
Lateral cutaneous of thigh	L2, L3	Lateral thigh	No motor
Posterior cutaneous of thigh	S2, S3	Posterior thigh	No motor
Inferior cluneal	Dorsal rami L1, L2, L3	Buttock region	No motor
Sciatic	L4, L5, S1, S2, S3	Hip joint	Knee flexors and all muscles of lower leg and foot
Superior gluteal	L4, L5, S1	No sensory	Tensor fasciae latae, gluteus medius, gluteus minimus
Inferior gluteal	L5, S1, S2	No sensory	Gluteus maximus
Nerve to quadratus femoris	L5, S1, S2	No sensory	Quadratus femoris, inferior gemellus
Pudendal	S2, S3, S4	Genitals	Perineal muscles, external urethral sphincter, external anal sphincter

Deep dissection

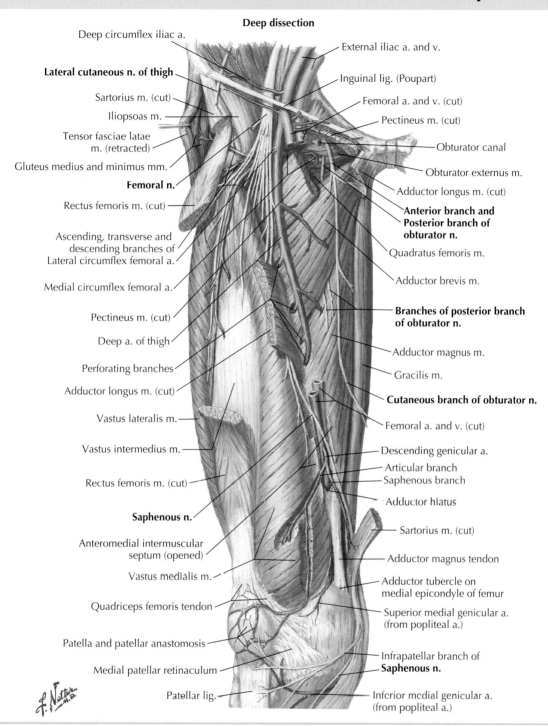

Deep circumflex iliac a.

Lateral cutaneous n. of thigh

Sartorius m. (cut)

Iliopsoas m.

Tensor fasciae latae m. (retracted)

Gluteus medius and minimus mm.

Femoral n.

Rectus femoris m. (cut)

Ascending, transverse and descending branches of Lateral circumflex femoral a.

Medial circumflex femoral a.

Pectineus m. (cut)

Deep a. of thigh

Perforating branches

Adductor longus m. (cut)

Vastus lateralis m.

Vastus intermedius m.

Rectus femoris m. (cut)

Saphenous n.

Anteromedial intermuscular septum (opened)

Vastus medialis m.

Quadriceps femoris tendon

Patella and patellar anastomosis

Medial patellar retinaculum

Patellar lig.

External iliac a. and v.

Inguinal lig. (Poupart)

Femoral a. and v. (cut)

Pectineus m. (cut)

Obturator canal

Obturator externus m.

Adductor longus m. (cut)

Anterior branch and Posterior branch of obturator n.

Quadratus femoris m.

Adductor brevis m.

Branches of posterior branch of obturator n.

Adductor magnus m.

Gracilis m.

Cutaneous branch of obturator n.

Femoral a. and v. (cut)

Descending genicular a.

Articular branch

Saphenous branch

Adductor hiatus

Sartorius m. (cut)

Adductor magnus tendon

Adductor tubercle on medial epicondyle of femur

Superior medial genicular a. (from popliteal a.)

Infrapatellar branch of **Saphenous n.**

Inferior medial genicular a. (from popliteal a.)

Figure 6-8
Nerves and arteries of thigh: anterior views.

Hip and Pelvis

6

History	Initial Hypothesis
Reports of pain at the lateral thigh. Pain exacerbated when transferring from sitting to standing	Greater trochanteric bursitis[1] Muscle strain[2]
Age over 60 years. Reports of pain and stiffness in the hip with possible radiation into the groin	OA[3]
Reports of clicking or catching in the hip joint. Pain exacerbated by full flexion or extension	Labral tear[4]
Reports of a repetitive or an overuse injury	Muscle sprain/strain[2]
Deep aching throb in the hip or groin. Possible history of prolonged steroid use	Avascular necrosis[4]
Sharp pain in groin. Often misdiagnosed by multiple providers	Femoroacetabular (anterior) impingement[5]
Pain in the gluteal region with occasional radiation into the posterior thigh and calf	Piriformis syndrome[6] Hamstring strain[2,4] Ischial bursitis[2]

Patient Complaint and Study Quality	Population	Reference Standard	Sens	Spec	+LR	−LR
Constant low back/buttock pain[8] ◆	78 patients with unilateral pain in the buttock, groin, or anterior thigh	Hip OA on radiographs using the Kellgren and Lawrence grading scale	.52 (.30, .74)	.92 (.80, .97)	6.4 (2.4, 17.4)	.52 (.33, .81)
Ipsilateral groin pain[8] ◆			.29 (.12, .52)	.92 (.80, .97)	3.6 (1.2, 11.0)	.78 (.59, 1.00)
Squatting aggravates symptoms[8] ◆			.76 (.52, .91)	.57 (.42, .70)	1.8 (1.2, 2.6)	.42 (.19, .93)
No lateral thigh pain[7] ◆	49 potential surgical patients with hip pain	Intraarticular hip pain as defined by relief of more than 50% with intraarticular anesthetic-steroid injection	.78 (.59, .89)	.36 (.2, .57)	1.2 (.84, 1.8)	.61 (.25, 1.5)
Groin pain[7] ⬤			.59 (.41, .75)	.14 (.05, .33)	.67 (.48, .98)	3.0 (.95, 9.4)
Catching[7] ⬤			.63 (.44, .78)	.54 (.35, .73)	1.39 (.81, 2.4)	.68 (.36, 1.3)
Pinching pain when sitting[7] ⬤			.48 (.31, .66)	.54 (.35, .73)	1.1 (.58, 1.9)	.95 (.56, 1.6)
Patient complains of clicking in the hip[9] ⬤	18 patients with hip pain	Acetabular labral tear as determined by magnetic resonance arthrography	1.0 (.48, 1.0)	.85 (.55, .98)	6.7	.00

6

Hip and Pelvis

Reliability of Range-of-Motion Measurements

Measurements and Study Quality	Instrumentation	Population	Interexaminer Reliability
External rotation (sitting) Internal rotation (sitting) External rotation (supine) Internal rotation (supine) Flexion Abduction Adduction Extension[10] ◆	Goniometer	6 patients with hip OA	Prestandardization/ poststandardization: ICC = .55/.80 ICC = .95/.94 ICC = .87/.80 ICC = .87/.94 ICC = .91/.91 ICC = .91/.88 ICC = .72/.56 ICC = NA/.66
Passive hip flexion[12] ◆	Gravity inclinometer	22 patients with knee OA and 17 asymptomatic subjects	ICC = .94 (.89 to .97)
Internal rotation[16] ◆	Digital inclinometer	25 healthy subjects	ICC = .93 (.84, .97)
Internal rotation External rotation Flexion Abduction Extension (knee flexed) Extension (knee unconstrained)[11] ◉	Goniometer (except rotation with inclinometer)	22 patients with hip OA	ICC = .93 (.83, .97) ICC = .96 (.91, .99) ICC = .97 (.93, .99) ICC = .94 (.86, .98) ICC = .86 (.67, .94) ICC = .89 (.72, .95)
Flexion Abduction Adduction External rotation Internal rotation Extension[8] ◉	Inclinometer	78 patients with unilateral pain in the buttock, groin, or anterior thigh	ICC = .85 (.64 to .93) ICC = .85 (.68 to .93) ICC = .54 (−.19 to .81) ICC = .77 (.53 to .89) ICC = .88 (.74 to .94) ICC = .68 (.32 to .85)
Flexion Extension Abduction Adduction External rotation Internal rotation Total hip motion[13] ◉	Goniometer	25 subjects with radiologically verified OA of the hip	ICC = .82 ICC = .94 ICC = .86 ICC = .50 ICC = .90 ICC = .90 ICC = .85
Flexion Internal rotation External rotation Abduction Extension Adduction[14] ◉	Goniometer	167 patients, 50 with no hip OA, 77 with unilateral hip OA, 40 with bilateral hip OA based on radiologic reports	ICC = .92 ICC = .90 ICC = .58 ICC = .78 ICC = .56 ICC = .62
Hip flexion, right Hip flexion, left[15] ◉	Goniometer	106 patients with OA of the hip or knee confirmed by a rheumatologist or an orthopaedic surgeon	ICC = .82 (.26, .95) ICC = .83 (.33, .96)

ICC, Intraclass correlation coefficient; NA, not applicable.

Reliability of Range-of-Motion Measurements—cont'd

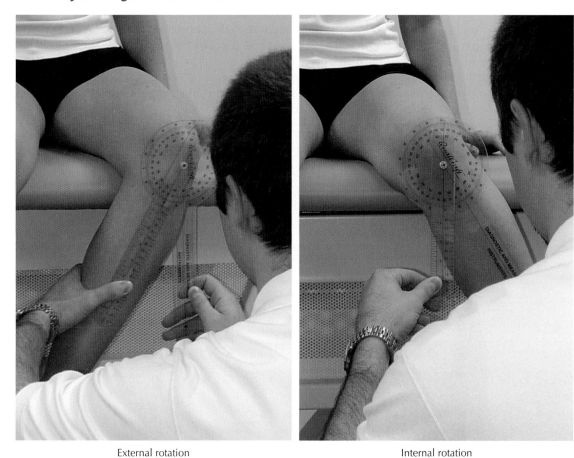

External rotation   Internal rotation

Figure 6-9
Measurement of passive range of motion.

Reliability of Determining Capsular and Noncapsular End Feels

Measurements and Study Quality	Description and Positive Finding	Population	Intraexaminer Reliability
Flexion test[8]	Maximal passive range of motion was assessed. End feels were dichotomized into "capsular" (early capsular, spasm, bone-to-bone) and "noncapsular" (soft tissue approximation, springy block, and empty) as defined by Cyriax	78 patients with unilateral pain in the buttock, groin, or anterior thigh	$\kappa = .21 \ (-.22, .64)$
Internal rotation test[8]			$\kappa = .51 \ (.19, .83)$
Scour test[8]			$\kappa = .52 \ (.08, .96)$
Patrick (FABER) test[8]			$\kappa = .47 \ (.12, .81)$
Hip flexion test[8]			$\kappa = .52 \ (.09, .96)$

Diagnostic Utility of Cyriax's Capsular Pattern for Detecting Osteoarthritis

A few studies[14,17] have investigated the diagnostic utility of Cyriax's capsular pattern (greater limitation of flexion and internal rotation than of abduction, little if any limitation of adduction and external rotation) in detecting the presence of OA of the hip. Bijl and associates[17] demonstrated that hip joints with OA had significantly lower range-of-motion values in all planes when compared with hip joints without OA. However, the magnitude of the range limitations did not follow Cyriax's capsular pattern. Similarly, Klässbo and colleagues[14] did not detect a correlation between hip OA and Cyriax's capsular pattern. In fact, they identified 138 patterns of passive range-of-motion restrictions depending on the established norms used (either the mean for symptom-free hips or Kaltenborn's published norms).

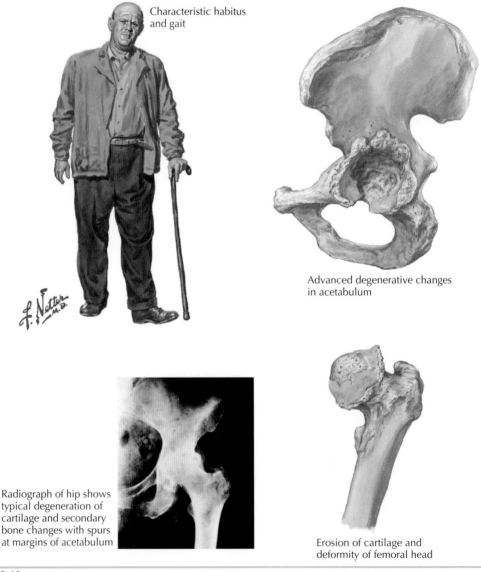

Characteristic habitus and gait

Advanced degenerative changes in acetabulum

Radiograph of hip shows typical degeneration of cartilage and secondary bone changes with spurs at margins of acetabulum

Erosion of cartilage and deformity of femoral head

Figure 6-10
Hip joint involvement in osteoarthritis.

Diagnostic Utility of Pain and Limited Range of Motion

Test and Study Quality		Population	Reference Standard	Sens	Spec	+LR	−LR
Lateral pain with active hip flexion[8] ◆		78 patients with unilateral pain in the buttock, groin, or anterior thigh	Hip OA on radiographs using the Kellgren and Lawrence grading scale	.43 (.23, .66)	.88 (.75, .95)	3.6 (1.5, 8.7)	.65 (.44, .94)
Passive internal rotation of 25 degrees or less[8] ◆				.76 (.52, .91)	.61 (.46, .74)	1.9 (1.3, 3.0)	.39 (.18, .86)
Pain with active hip extension[8] ◆				.52 (.30, .74)	.80 (.66, .90)	2.7 (1.3, 5.3)	.59 (.37, .94)
Groin pain with active abduction or adduction[8] ◆				.33 (.15, .57)	.94 (.83, .98)	5.7 (1.7, 18.6)	.71 (.52, .96)
Decreased passive hip internal rotation range of motion[18] ◆		40 patients with unilateral lateral hip pain	Lateral hip tendon pathologic condition as seen with MRI	.43 (.19, .70)	.86 (.42, .99)	3.00 (.44, 20.31)	.67 (.40, 1.10)
Pain with active hip internal rotation[18] ◆				.31 (.10, .61)	.86 (.42, .99)	2.15 (.29, 15.75)	.81 (.54, 1.22)
Pain with passive hip abduction[18] ◆				.59 (.33, .82)	.93 (.49, 1.00)	8.31 (.56, 123.88)	.44 (.24, .81)
Pain with passive hip internal rotation[18] ◆				.53 (.27, .78)	.86 (.42, .99)	3.73 (.57, 24.35)	.54 (.30, .98)
Number of planes with restricted movement[19] ◆	0	195 patients presenting with first-time episodes of hip pain	Radiographic evidence of mild to moderate OA	1.0	.00	1.0	NA
	1			.86	.54	1.87	.26
	2			.57	.77	2.48	.56
	3			.33	.93	4.71	.72
Number of planes with restricted movement[19] ◆	0		Radiographic evidence of severe OA	1.0	.00	1.0	NA
	1			1.0	.42	1.72	NA
	2			.81	.69	2.61	.28
	3			.54	.88	4.5	.52
Pain with hip passive range of motion[20] ◉		21 women diagnosed with pelvic girdle pain	Pelvic girdle pain as defined by: • Current or recent pregnancy • Daily pain • Points to the pelvic girdle joints as the painful area • Pain during one or more of the five selected clinical tests (active straight-leg raise test, Gaenslen test, sacroiliac compression test, sacroiliac distraction test, thigh thrust test)	.55	1.0	Undefined	.45

6

Hip and Pelvis

Diagnostic Utility of Pain and Limited Range of Motion—cont'd

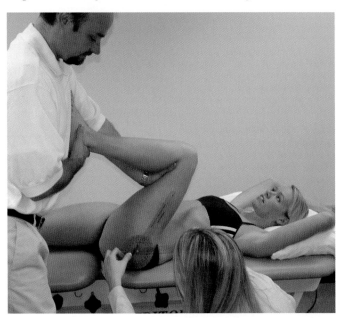

Hip flexion

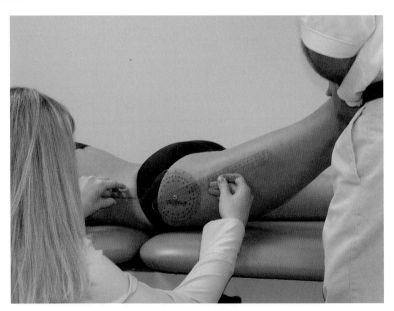

Hip extension

Figure 6-11
Passive range-of-motion measurement.

Diagnostic Utility of Limited Range of Motion for Detecting Avascular Necrosis

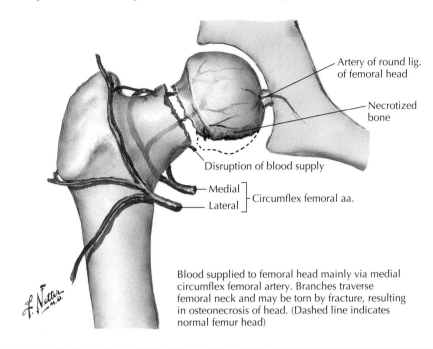

Blood supplied to femoral head mainly via medial circumflex femoral artery. Branches traverse femoral neck and may be torn by fracture, resulting in osteonecrosis of head. (Dashed line indicates normal femur head)

Figure 6-12
Osteonecrosis.

Motion and Finding and Study Quality	Population	Reference Standard	Sens	Spec	+LR	−LR
Passive range-of-motion extension of less than 15 degrees[21]	176 asymptom- atic HIV-infected patients	MRI confirmation of avascular ne- crosis of the hip. Ten had avascular necrosis	.19 (.00, .38)	.92 (.89, .95)	2.38	.88
Passive range-of-motion abduction of less than 45 degrees[21]			.31 (.09, .54)	.85 (.82, .89)	2.07	.81
Passive range-of-motion internal rotation of less than 15 degrees[21]			.50 (.26, .75)	.67 (.62, .72)	1.52	.75
Passive range-of-motion external rotation of less than 60 degrees[21]			.38 (.14, .61)	.73 (.68, .77)	.48	.85
Pain with internal rota- tion[21]			.13 (.00, .29)	.86 (.83, .89)	.93	1.01

HIV, Human immunodeficiency virus; MRI, magnetic resonance imaging.

Diagnostic Utility of Limited Hip Abduction for Detecting Developmental Dysplasia in Infants

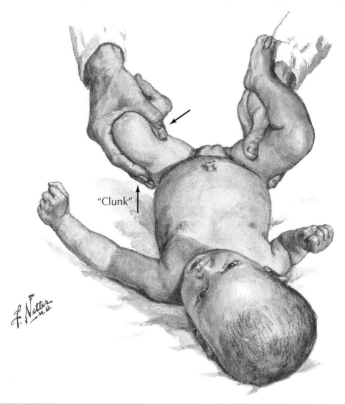

"Clunk"

Figure 6-13
Recognition of congenital dislocation of the hip.

Test and Study Quality		Description and Positive Findings	Popula-tion	Reference Standard	Sens	Spec	+LR	−LR
Limited hip abduction test[22]	Unilateral limitation	Passive abduction of the hips performed with both hips flexed 90 degrees. Considered positive if abduction is more than 20 degrees greater than on the contralateral side	1107 infants	Ultrasound verification of clinical instability of the hip	.70 (.60, .69)	.90 (.88, .92)	7.0	.33
	Bilateral limitation				.43 (.50, .64)	.90 (.88, .92)	4.3	.63
Limited hip abduction[23]		As above, except considered positive if either (1) abduction is less than 60 degrees or (2) there is asymmetry in abduction of 20 degrees compared to contralateral side	683 infants	Hip dysplasia as detected by ultrasound	.69	.54	1.5	.57

Diagnostic Utility of the Clinical Exam in Identifying Hip Instability

Test and Study Quality	Description and Positive Findings	Population	Reference Standard	Sens	Spec	+LR	−LR
FABER test[24] ⬤	The participant was supine, and the investigator passively moved the hip into a combination of flexion, adduction, and external rotation until the end of the range of motion was achieved. Pain or discomfort was considered a positive test	199 patients with lateral groin or hip pain	Plain film radiographs	.54	.90	5.4	.5
Foot progression angle walking test[24] ⬤	Patient was asked to ambulate with his or her normal gait pattern for 20 feet. The examiner categorized the foot progression angle as neutral, out-toeing, or in-toeing. The patient was next instructed to internally rotate his or her foot from baseline and again walk 20 feet. Patient is then asked to walk the 20 feet with his or her foot in 15 degrees of external rotation. Pain during the internal rotation or external rotation was considered a positive finding for femoracetabular impingement			.67	.70	2.2	.5

Hip and Pelvis

6

Reliability of Detecting Pain or Weakness during Resisted Tests

Test and Study Quality	Description and Positive Findings	Population	Reliability	
			Intraexaminer	**Interexaminer**
Abduction strength[10] ◆	With patient sitting, the patient abducts bilateral hips into examiner's hands. Strength graded on scale of 0 to 2	6 patients with hip OA	Interexaminer prestandardization/post-standardization: κ = .90/.86	
Adduction strength[10] ◆	As above, except the patient adducts bilateral hips	6 patients with hip OA	Interexaminer prestandardization/post-standardization: κ = .87/.86	
Flexion strength (sitting)[10] ◆	With patient sitting, the patient lifts one knee against examiner's hand. Strength graded on scale of 0 to 2	6 patients with hip OA	Interexaminer prestandardization/post-standardization: κ = .83/.95	
Flexion strength (supine)[10] ◆	As above, except the patient is supine with knees bent 90 degrees	6 patients with hip OA	Interexaminer prestandardization/post-standardization: κ = NA/.90	
Extension strength[10] ◆	Patient side-lying with tested leg up. Bottom leg with hip flexed 45 degrees and knee flexed 90 degrees. Patient pushes top leg posteriorly into examiner with knee extended. Strength graded on scale of 0 to 2	6 patients with hip OA	Interexaminer prestandardization/post-standardization: κ = .85/.86	
Abduction strength[25] ◐	With patient supine, the patient exerts maximal isometric hip abduction force into a handheld dynamometer placed just proximal to the knee	29 football players	ICC (right/left) = .81/.84	ICC (right/left) = .73/.58
Abduction strength[26] ◐	With patient sitting, the patient exerts maximal isometric hip abduction force into a handheld dynamometer placed 5 cm above the lateral malleolus	37 patients with hip OA	ICC (most symptomatic limb) = .85	Not tested
Adduction strength[25] ◐	With patient supine, the patient exerts maximal isometric hip adduction force into a sphygmomanometer placed between the knees	29 football players	ICC = .81 to .94 (depending on knee angle)	ICC = .80 to .83 (depending on knee angle)
Adduction strength[26] ◐	With patient sitting, the patient exerts maximal isometric hip abduction force into a handheld dynamometer placed 5 cm above the medial malleolus	37 patients with hip OA	ICC (most symptomatic limb) = .86	Not tested
Internal rotation[25] ◐	With subject supine and tested knee flexed to 90 degrees, patient exerts maximal isometric rotational force into a handheld dynamometer placed just proximal to the lateral malleolus	29 football players	ICC (right/left) = .67/.57	ICC (right/left) = .40/.54
Internal rotation[26] ◐	With patient sitting, the patient exerts maximal isometric hip abduction force into a handheld dynamometer placed 5 cm above the lateral malleolus	37 patients with hip OA	ICC (most symptomatic limb) = .83	Not tested
External rotation[25] ◐	With patient supine and the tested knee flexed to 90 degrees, the patient exerts maximal isometric rotational force into a handheld dynamometer placed just proximal to the medial malleolus	29 football players	ICC (right/left) = .55/.64	ICC (right/left) = .60/.63

Reliability of Detecting Pain or Weakness during Resisted Tests—cont'd

Test and Study Quality	Description and Positive Findings	Population	Reliability	
			Intraexaminer	Interexaminer
External rotation[26]	With patient sitting, the patient exerts maximal isometric hip abduction force into a handheld dynamometer placed 5 cm above the medial malleolus	37 patients with hip OA	ICC (most symptomatic limb) = .78	Not tested
Flexion strength (sitting)[26]	With patient sitting, the patient exerts maximal isometric hip abduction force into a handheld dynamometer placed 5 cm above the patella	37 patients with hip OA	ICC (most symptomatic limb) = .85	
Hip abductor strength[27]	Patient side-lying with the limb to be tested on top. The knee of the test limb was in full extension. Hip abductor strength was then tested with the hip in no extension, flexion, or rotation	210 individuals postunilateral total knee arthroplasty	Test-retest reliability ICC = .95 (95% CI: .86, .98)	

Hip and Pelvis

6

Reliability of Detecting Pain or Weakness during Resisted Tests—cont'd

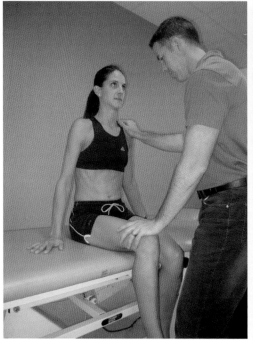

Assessing hip flexion strength

Assessing hip abduction strength

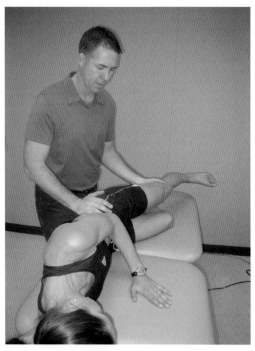

Assessing hip extension strength

Figure 6-14
Assessing hip strength.

Diagnostic Utility of Pain or Weakness for Identifying Lateral Hip Tendon Pathologic Conditions

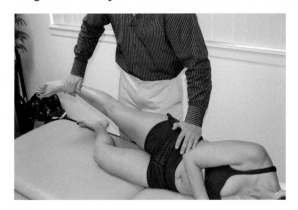

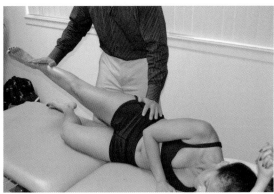

Figure 6-15
Gluteus minimus and medius manual muscle test.

Test and Study Quality	Description and Positive Findings	Population	Reference Standard	Sens	Spec	+LR	−LR
Pain with resisted gluteus minimus[18] ◆	Tested isometrically as described by Kendal and colleagues. Positive if there is reproduction of pain	40 patients with unilateral lateral hip pain	Lateral hip tendon pathologic condition as seen with MRI	.47 (.22, .73)	.86 (.42, .99)	3.27 (.49, 21.70)	.62 (.37, 1.05)
Pain with resisted gluteus minimus and medius[18] ◆				.47 (.22, .73)	.86 (.42, .99)	3.27 (.49, 21.70)	.62 (.37, 1.05)
Gluteus minimus and medius weakness[18] ◆	Tested isometrically as described by Kendal and colleagues. Positive if five or fewer signs or symptoms are seen			.80 (.51, .95)	.71 (.30, .95)	2.80 (.85, 9.28)	.28 (.09, .86)
Gluteus minimus weakness[18] ◆				.80 (.51, .95)	.57 (.20, .88)	1.87 (.76, 4.55)	.35 (.10, 1.19)
Pain with resisted abduction[28] ◆	With patient supine and affected hip at 45 degrees, positive if symptoms over the greater trochanter are reproduced on resisted abduction	24 patients with lateral hip pain and tenderness over the greater trochanter	Gluteus medius tendon tear via MRI	.73	.46	1.35	.59
Pain with resisted internal rotation[28] ◆	With patient supine and affected hip at 45 degrees and maximal external rotation, positive if symptoms over the greater trochanter are replicated on internal rotation			.55	.69	1.77	.65

Hip and Pelvis

6

Reliability of the Trendelenburg Test

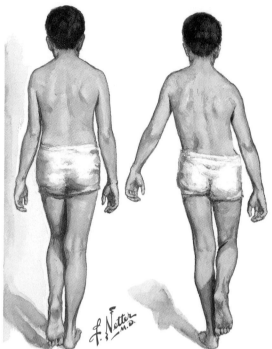

Left: patient demonstrates negative Trendelenburg test of normal right hip. Right: positive test of involved left hip. When weight is on affected side, normal hip drops, indicating weakness of left gluteus medius muscle. Trunk shifts left as patient attempts to decrease biomechanical stresses across involved hip and thereby maintain balance

Figure 6-16
Trendelenburg test.

Test and Study Quality	Description and Positive Findings	Population	Intraexaminer Reliability
Positive Trendelenburg test[10] ◆	Standing patient raises one foot 10 cm off the ground while examiner inspects for change in level of pelvis. Positive if pelvis drops on the unsupported side or trunk shifts to the stance side	6 patients with hip OA	κ = .36 (prestandardization) κ = .06 (poststandardization)
Positive Trendelenburg test[28] ◉	Assessed in two ways. Pelvic tilt was assessed in single-leg stance on the affected leg. Pelvic movement was assessed during gait. A positive test was defined as clearly abnormal pelvic tilt during both stance and gait	24 patients with lateral hip pain and tenderness over the greater trochanter	κ = .67 (.27, 1.08)

Diagnostic Utility of the Trendelenburg Test for Identifying Lateral Hip Tendon Pathology

Test and Study Quality	Description and Positive Findings	Population	Reference Standard	Sens	Spec	+LR	−LR
Positive Trendelenburg test[18] ◆	Patient lifts one foot off the ground at a time while standing. Positive if the patient is unable to elevate his or her pelvis on the nonstance side and hold the position for at least 30 seconds	40 patients with unilateral lateral hip pain	Lateral hip tendon pathologic condition as seen with MRI	.23 (.05, .57)	.94 (.53, 1.00)	3.64 (.20, 65.86)	.82 (.59, 1.15)
Positive Trendelenburg test[28] ◆	Assessed in two ways. Pelvic tilt was assessed in single-leg stance on the affected leg. Pelvic movement was assessed during gait. A positive test was defined as clearly abnormal pelvic tilt during both stance and gait	24 patients with lateral hip pain and tenderness over the greater trochanter	Gluteus medius tendon tear via MRI	.73	.77	3.17	.35

6

Hip and Pelvis

Reliability of Tests for Iliotibial Band Length

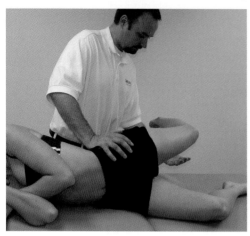

Ober test

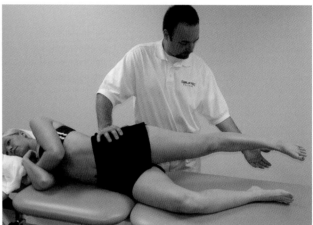

Modified Ober test

Figure 6-17
Tests for iliotibial band length.

Measurements and Study Quality	Test Procedure	Population	Reliability
Ober test[10] ◆	With patient side-lying with examined leg up, examiner flexes patient's knee to 90 degrees and abducts and extends the hip until the hip is in line with the trunk. Examiner allows gravity to adduct hip as much as possible. Positive if unable to adduct to horizontal position	6 patients with hip OA	κ = .38 (prestandardization) κ = .80 (poststandardization)
Ober test[30] ◆	As above, except an inclinometer is used on the distal lateral thigh to measure hip adduction angle	61 asymptomatic individuals	Intraexaminer ICC = .90
Ober test[29] ●		30 patients with patellofemoral pain syndrome	Interexaminer ICC = .97 (.93, .98)
Modified Ober test[31] ●	As above, but with test knee fully extended	10 patients experiencing anterior knee pain	Interexaminer ICC = .73 Intraexaminer ICC = .94
Modified Ober test[31] ●		61 asymptomatic individuals	Intraexaminer ICC = .91

Reliability of the Thomas Test for Hip Flexor Contracture

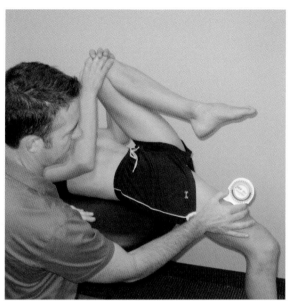

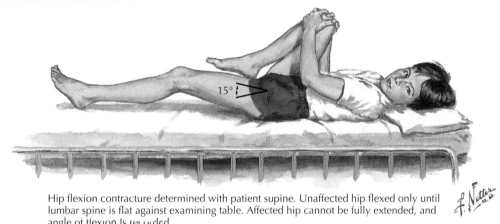

Hip flexion contracture determined with patient supine. Unaffected hip flexed only until lumbar spine is flat against examining table. Affected hip cannot be fully extended, and angle of flexion is recorded

Figure 6-18
Thomas test.

Measurements and Study Quality	Test Procedure	Population	Reliability
Modified Thomas test[32] ◆	With the patient sitting as close to the edge of the table as possible and holding the nontested thigh, the patient rolls back into supine position and flexes the untested hip until the lumbar lordosis is flattened. The tested limb is allowed to hang into extension and is measured with an inclinometer or goniometer	42 asymptomatic individuals	ICC = .92 (goniometer) ICC = .89 (inclinometer)
Thomas test[10] ◆	With patient supine with both hips flexed and maintaining one hip in flexion, the tested hip is extended. Positive if unable to touch posterior thigh with examination table	6 patients with hip OA	κ = .60 (prestandardization) κ = .88 (poststandardization)

Reliability of Assessing Muscle Length

Test and Study Quality	Description and Positive Findings	Population	Reliability	
			Intraexaminer	Interexaminer
Bent knee fall-out (adductors)[25] ◑	With patient supine and knees flexed to 90 degrees, the patient lets knees fall out while keeping feet together. The distance from the fibular head to the table is measured with a tape measure	29 football players	ICC (right/left) = .90/.89	ICC (right/left) = .93/.91
External rotators of the hip[25] ◑	With patient prone and knees flexed to 90 degrees, the patient lets feet fall outward while keeping knees together. Examiner passively flexes knee 90 degrees. Internal rotation measurement is taken with an inclinometer		ICC (right/left) = .97/.96	ICC (right/left) = .89/.93
Internal rotators of the hip[25] ◑	With patient supine with nontested hip flexed and the test leg hanging over the end of the table, passive external rotation is measured with an inclinometer		ICC (right/left) = .82/.80	ICC (right/left) = .64/.77
Short hip extensors[33] ◑	With patient supine, examiner brings hip passively into flexion while palpating posterior superior iliac spine on ipsilateral side. As soon as the posterior superior iliac spine moves posteriorly, the movement is ceased and the measurement is recorded with an inclinometer	11 asymptomatic individuals	Intraexaminer ICC = .87	
Short hip flexors[33] ◑	With patient supine, lower limbs over the plinth, and both hips flexed, examiner slowly lowers the side being tested. When limb ceases to move, measurement is recorded with an inclinometer		Intraexaminer ICC = .98	
External rotators of the hip[33] ◑	With patient prone, examiner passively flexes knee 90 degrees. Examiner palpates contralateral posterior superior iliac spine and passively internally rotates limb. When rotation of pelvis occurs, measurement is taken with an inclinometer		Intraexaminer ICC = .99	
Internal rotators of the hip[33] ◑	Same as above, except examiner takes hip into external rotation		Intraexaminer ICC = .98	

Reliability of Assessing Muscle Length—cont'd

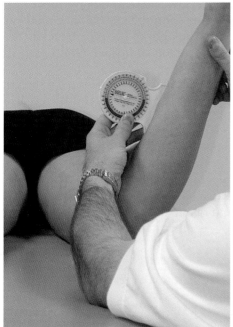

Measurement of the length of external
rotators of the hip

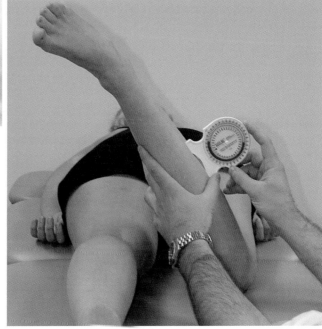

Measurement of the length of internal
rotators of the hip

Figure 6-19
Measurement of muscle length with a bubble inclinometer.

Hip and Pelvis

6

Forward Step-Down Test

The forward step-down test[34] is a functional task used to assess lower extremity movement quality involving weight-bearing stress as well as dynamic muscular control. Subjects with moderate movement quality have been shown to have significantly less strength of the hip abductors, less hip adduction range of motion, and less knee flexion range of motion compared with those with good movement quality.

The subject stands on a 20-cm step, with the foot of the tested limb close to the edge of the step and the nontested limb positioned in front of the step, with the knee straight and the ankle at maximum dorsiflexion. The subject is asked to keep the trunk straight and the hands on the waist and to bend the knee on the tested side until the heel of the nontested limb touches the floor. The subject is asked not to apply any weight on the heel of the nontested limb once it reaches the floor and to immediately reextend the knee of the tested limb to return to the starting position. The examiner rates the performance of the subject across five repetitions. A total score of 0 or 1 is classified as good movement quality, a total score of 2 or 3 is classified as moderate movement quality, and a total score of 4 or more is classified as poor movement quality.

Criteria	Description	Scoring
Arm strategy	Patient removes the hands from the waist (interpreted as a strategy to recover balance)	1 point is given
Trunk movement	Patient leans the trunk to either side (interpreted as a strategy to recover balance)	1 point is given
Pelvic plane	If one side of the pelvis is rotated in the transverse plane or elevated in the frontal plane compared with the other side	1 point is given
Knee position (only one score is given from this category)	If the knee of the tested limb moves medially in the frontal plane and the tibial tuberosity crossed an imaginary vertical line positioned directly over the second toe of the tested foot, 1 point was given	1 point is given
	If the knee moves medially and the tibial tuberosity crossed an imaginary vertical line positioned directly over the medial border of the tested foot, 2 points were given	2 points are given
Maintenance of a steady unilateral stance	Subject has to support body weight on the nontested limb, or the foot of the tested limb moved during testing	1 point is given

Reliability of the Forward Step-Down Test

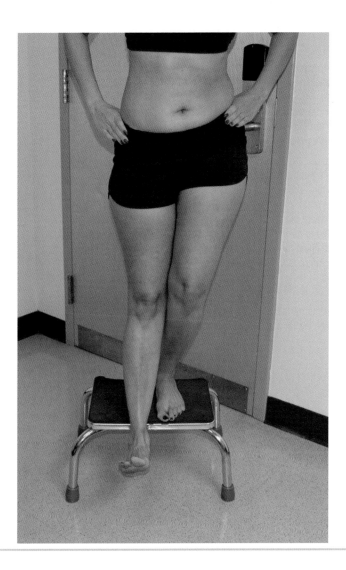

Figure 6-20
Forward step-down test.

Test and Study Quality	Description and Positive Findings	Population	Intraexaminer Reliability
Forward step-down test[34] ◆	As described on previous page	26 asymptomatic female subjects	κ = .80 (.57, 1.00)

Reliability of Movement Control Tests for the Hip

Test and Study Quality	Description	Positive Findings	Population	Reliability (95% CI)
Small squat up to 30 degrees[35] ◆	Patient is instructed to perform 4 small knee bends. On the 4th repetition the patient is instructed to remain in the bent knee position for 10 seconds	1. The performance of the movement should come from the knee, not the hip. 2. The vertical axis of the leg should remain straight. Rated as correct, almost correct, or incorrect		Intertester: κ = .52 (.17, .86) Intratester: κ = .55 (.21, .88) to .76 (.62, .91)
Squat up to 90 degrees[35] ◆	Patient was instructed to take 4 stationary steps followed by 4 small knee bends. The patient was then instructed to perform 4 squats, remaining in the squat on the 4th repetition for 4 seconds	1. Movement should come initially from the hip joint. Knees can move only slightly forwards. 2. The vertical axis of the leg should remain straight. 3. The spine should be kept in a neutral position. Rated as correct, almost correct, or incorrect		Intertester: κ = .71 (.53, .89) Intratester: κ = .35 (.07, .63) to .80 (.63, .96)
One leg stand[35] ◆	The patient is instructed to stand on one leg for 10 seconds	1. The hip should remain stable in rotation, abduction, and extension. Pelvis position should not change. 2. The vertical axis of the leg should remain straight. 3. The need for upper extremity support would be considered incorrect. Rated as correct, almost correct, or incorrect	16 patients with hip osteoarthritis and 14 individuals with no hip pain	Intertester: κ = .68 (.44, .92) Intratester: κ = .55 (.33, .76) to .87 (.75, .99)
Small single leg squat[35] ◆	From the single leg stance position patient is asked to perform 4 small knee bends. On the 4th knee bend patient is asked to remain in that position for 10 seconds	1. The performance of the movement should come from the knee not the hip. 2. The hip should remain stable in rotation, abduction, and extension. Pelvis position should not change. 3. The vertical axis of the leg should remain straight. 4. The need for upper extremity support would be considered incorrect. Rated as correct, almost correct, or incorrect		Intertester: κ = .66 (.46 .86) Intratester: κ = .61 (.40, .82) to .78 (.64, .93)
Step up Yellow[35] ◆	Patient is standing in front of a step and asked to step up and down with the same leg 4 times while the therapist observes	1. The hip should remain stable in rotation, abduction, and extension. Pelvis position should not change. 2. The vertical axis of the leg should remain straight. Rated as correct, almost correct, or incorrect		Intertester: κ = .52 (.21, .81) Intratester: κ = .55 (.34, .76) to .56 (.32, .80)

Diagnostic Utility of Pain with Functional Movement Assessments

Test and Study Quality	Description and Positive Findings	Population	Reference Standard	Sens	Spec	+LR	−LR
Posterior pain with squat[8] ◆	Patient squats as low as possible with feet 20 cm apart, trunk upright, and hands on hips	78 patients with unilateral pain in the buttock, groin, or anterior thigh	Hip OA on x-rays using the Kellgren and Lawrence grading scale	.24 (.09, .48)	.96 (.85, .99)	6.1 (1.5, 25.6)	.79 (.62, 1.00)
Step-up test[20]	No details given	21 women with pelvic girdle pain	Pelvic girdle pain defined by: • Current or recent pregnancy	.29	1.0	Undefined	.71
Single-leg stance[20]			• Daily pain	.35	.67	1.1	.97
Lunge[20]			• Points to the pelvic girdle joints as the painful area	.44	.83	2.6	.68
Sit to stand[20]			• Pain during one or more of the six selected clinical tests (active straight-leg raise test, Gaenslen test, sacroiliac compression test, sacroiliac distraction test, thigh thrust test, palpation of pubic symphysis)	.13	1.0	Undefined	.88
Deep squat[20]				.24	1.0	Undefined	.88

Hip and Pelvis — 6

Reliability of Pain with Palpation

Test and Study Quality	Description and Positive Findings	Population	Interexaminer Reliability
Trochanteric tenderness[10] ◆	With patient supine, firm pressure is applied to the greater trochanter. Test positive if patient's symptoms are reproduced	6 patients with hip OA	κ = .40 (prestandardization) κ = .68 (poststandardization)
Trochanteric tenderness[36] ◆		70 patients with hip pain	κ = .66 (.48, .84)

Diagnostic Utility of Pain with Palpation for Intraarticular Hip Pain

Patient Complaint and Study Quality	Description and Positive Findings	Population	Reference Standard	Sens	Spec	+LR	−LR
Trochanteric tenderness[7]	With patient supine, firm pressure is applied to the greater trochanter. Test positive if patient's symptoms are reproduced	49 potential surgical patients with hip pain	Intraarticular hip pain as defined by relief of more than 50% with intraarticular anesthetic-steroid injection	.57 (.39, .74)	.45 (.27, .65)	1.1 (.36, 3.6)	.93 (.49, 1.8)

Reliability of the Patrick (FABER) Test

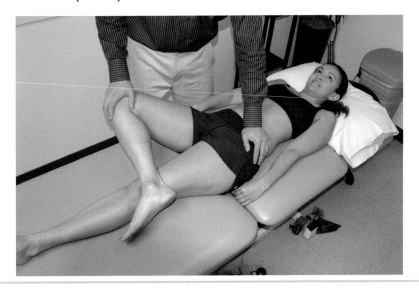

Figure 6-21
Patrick test.

Test and Study Quality	Description and Positive Findings	Population	Reliability
Patrick test[36] ◆	With patient supine, examiner flexes, abducts, and externally rotates the involved hip so that the lateral ankle is placed just proximal to the contralateral knee. While stabilizing the anterior superior iliac spine, the involved leg is lowered toward the table to end range. Test is positive if it reproduces the patient's symptoms	70 patients with hip pain	Intraexaminer κ = .63 (.43, .83)
Patrick test[10] ◆	As above, except test is considered positive if the patient has inguinal pain	6 patients with hip OA	Interexaminer κ = .78 (prestandardization) κ = .75 (poststandardization)
Patrick test[8] ●	As above, except inclinometer is used 2.5 cm proximal to the patient's flexed knee	78 patients with unilateral pain in the buttock, groin, or anterior thigh	Intraexaminer ICC = .90 (.78 to .96)

Diagnostic Utility of the Patrick (FABER) Test

Test and Study Quality	Description and Positive Findings	Population	Reference Standard	Sens	Spec	+LR	−LR
Patrick test less than 60 degrees[8] ◆	As below, but also uses inclinometer 2.5 cm proximal to the patient's flexed knee	78 patients with unilateral pain in the buttock, groin, or anterior thigh	Hip OA on radiographs using the Kellgren and Lawrence grading scale	.57 (.34, .77)	.71 (.56, .82)	1.9 (1.1, 3.4)	.61 (.36, 1.00)
Patrick test[7] ● (see Video 6-1)	With patient supine, examiner flexes, abducts, and externally rotates the involved hip so that the lateral ankle is placed just proximal to the contralateral knee. While stabilizing the anterior superior iliac spine, the involved leg is lowered toward the table to end range. Test is positive if it reproduces the patient's symptoms	49 potential surgical patients with hip pain	Intraarticular hip pain as defined by relief of more than 50% with intraarticular anesthetic-steroid injection	.60 (.41, .77)	.18 (.07, .39)	.73 (.50, 1.1)	2.2 (.80, 6.0)

Reliability of Special Tests for Detecting Intraarticular Pathologic Conditions

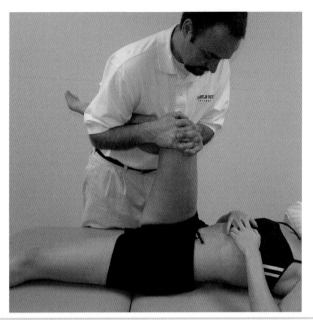

Figure 6-22
Internal rotation–flexion–axial compression maneuver.

Test and Study Quality	Description and Positive Findings	Population	Interexaminer Reliability
Flexion–internal rotation–adduction (FADIR) impingement test[36] ◆	With patient supine, examiner flexes, adducts, and internally rotates the involved hip to end range. Test is positive if it reproduces the patient's symptoms		κ = .58 (.29, .87)
Log roll[36] ◆	With patient supine with greater trochanters in the maximally prominent position, examiner places both hands on the patient's midthigh and passively externally rotates each hip maximally. Test is positive if greater external rotation is noted on the symptomatic side	70 patients with hip pain	κ = .61 (.41, .81)

Diagnostic Utility of Special Tests for Detecting Intraarticular Pathologic Conditions

Test and Study Quality	Description and Positive Findings	Population	Reference Standard	Sens	Spec	+LR	−LR
Scour test with adduction causes lateral hip or groin pain[8] ◆	With patient supine, examiner passively flexes the symptomatic hip to 90 degrees and then moves the knee toward the opposite shoulder and applies an axial load to the femur	78 patients with unilateral pain in the buttock, groin, or anterior thigh	Hip OA on radiographs using the Kellgren and Lawrence grading scale	.62 (.39, .81)	.75 (.60, .85)	2.4 (1.4, 4.3)	.51 (.29, .89)
FADIR test[37] ◆	The participant was supine and the investigator passively moved the hip into a combination of flexion, adduction, and internal rotation until the end of the range of motion was achieved	74 youth ice hockey players	Magnetic resonance imaging indication of cam or pincer femoroacetabular impingement	.41 (95% CI: .18, .67)	.47 (95% CI: .34, .61)	.78 (95% CI: .42, 1.45)	1.24 (95% CI: .77, 2.0)
Squat test[38] ◆	Patients were instructed to stand with their feet shoulder width apart and perform a maximal squat. Pain during the squat was considered a positive test for femoracetabular impingement	76 patients with hip pain referred to an outpatient orthopaedic clinic	Magnetic resonance imaging and magnetic resonance image arthrogram indication of cam type femoroacetabular impingement	.75 (95% CI: .57, .89)	.41 (95% CI: .27, .57)	1.3 (95% CI: .9, 1.7)	.6 (95% CI: .3, 1.2)
FADIR impingement test[7] ● (see Video 6-2)	With patient supine, examiner flexes, adducts, and internally rotates the involved hip to end range. Test is positive if it reproduces the patient's symptoms	49 potential surgical patients with hip pain	Intraarticular hip pain as defined by relief of more than 50% with intraarticular anesthetic-steroid injection	.78 (.59, .89)	.10 (.03, .29)	.86 (.67, 1.1)	2.3 (.52, 10.4)
Internal rotation–flexion–axial compression maneuver[9] ●	With patient supine, examiner flexes and internally rotates the hip and then applies an axial compression force through the femur. Provocation of pain is considered positive	18 patients with hip pain	Acetabular labral tear as determined by magnetic resonance arthrography	.75 (.19, .99)	.43 (.18, .72)	1.32	.58

Diagnostic Utility of Special Tests for Detecting Intraarticular Pathologic Conditions—cont'd

Test and Study Quality	Description and Positive Findings	Population	Reference Standard	Sens	Spec	+LR	−LR
FADIR test[24]	The participant was supine, and the investigator passively moved the hip into a combination of flexion, adduction, and internal rotation until the end of the range of motion was achieved. Pain or discomfort was considered a positive test			.96	.11	1.1	.4
Foot progression angle walking test[24]	Patient was asked to ambulate with his or her normal gait pattern for 20 feet. The examiner categorized the foot progression angle as neutral, out-toeing, or in-toeing. The patient was next instructed to internally rotate his or her foot from baseline and again walk 20 feet. Patient is then asked to walk the 20 feet with his or her foot in 15 degrees of external rotation. Pain during the internal rotation or external rotation was considered a positive finding for femoracetabular impingement	199 patients with lateral groin or hip pain	Plain film radiograph indication of femoroacetabular impingement	.61	.56	1.4	.7

Hip and Pelvis

6

Diagnostic Utility of Tests for Identifying Intraarticular Pathology of Tears of the Ligamentum Teres

Test and Study Quality	Description and Positive Findings	Population	Reference Standard	Sens (95% CI)	Spec (95% CI)	+LR	−LR
Ligamentum teres test[39] ◆	The patient is supine, and the examiner flexes the knee to 90 degrees and hip to 70 degrees. The hip is then abducted as far as the patient will tolerate. The hip is then adducted until it is 30 degrees short of full abduction then fully internally and externally rotated. Pain in either internal or external rotation is considered positive	75 patients undergoing hip arthroscopy	Arthroscopy	.90 (.39, .56)	.85 (.75, .92)	6*	.12*

*Values were calculated by the authors of this text.

Diagnostic Utility of Tests for Detecting Ischiofemoral Impingement

Test and Study Quality	Description and Positive Findings	Population	Reference Standard	Sens (95% CI)	Spec (95% CI)	+LR (95% CI)	−LR (95% CI)
Long-stride walking test[40] ⬤	Patient is asked to walk with long strides. Pain at terminal extension is considered positive. Pain with hip extension in neutral or adducted with pain relieved when abducted is considered positive	564 patients who had previously undergone hip surgery were retrospectively reviewed	Magnetic resonance imaging or computed tomography	.94 (.69, .99)	.85 (.54, .97)	6.12 (1.7, 22.1)	0.07 (0.01, 0.48)
Ischiofemoral impingement test[40] ⬤	The patient is side lying with the affected leg on top. The examiner passively extends the hip			.82 (.56, .95)	.85 (.54, .97)	5.35 (1.47, 19.52)	.21 (.07, .60)

Diagnostic Utility of the Patellar-Pubic-Percussion Test for Detecting Hip Fractures

Percussion test

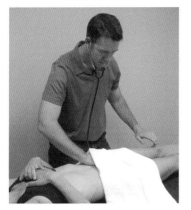

Intertrochanteric Fracture of Femur

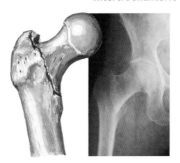

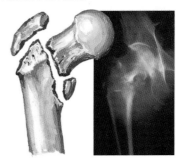

I. Nondisplaced fracture   II. Comminuted displaced fracture

Fracture of Shaft Femur

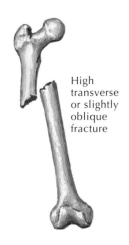

High
transverse
or slightly
oblique
fracture

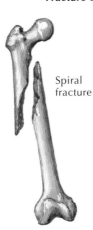

Spiral
fracture

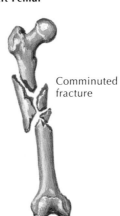

Comminuted
fracture

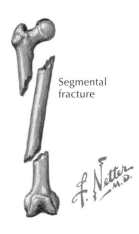

Segmental
fracture

Figure 6-23
Percussion test and hip fractures.

Test and Study Quality	Description and Positive Findings	Population	Reference Standard	Sens	Spec	+LR	−LR
Patellar-pubic-percussion test[41] ●	With patient supine, examiner percusses (taps) one patella at a time while auscultating the pubic symphysis with a stethoscope. A positive test is a diminution of the percussion note on the affected side	290 patients with suspected radiologically occult hip fractures	Hip fracture seen on repeat radiographs, bone scintigraphy, MRI, or computed tomography (CT)	.96 (.87, .99)	.86 (.49, .98)	6.73	.14

Reliability of Balance Tests

Test and Study Quality	Description and Positive Findings	Population	Reliability	
			Intraexaminer (95% CI)	**Interexaminer (95% CI)**
Four-square step test[42] ◆	Four walking sticks are placed on the floor at right angles to each other with handles outward so that they form four squares. The participant starts in square 1, facing square 2, and remains facing in this direction for the duration of the test. The participant steps forward with both feet as quickly as possible into square 2, then sideways to the right into square 3, then backward into square 4, and finally sideways to the left back into square 1. The participant then reverses the sequence back to the starting position. The trial is recorded to the nearest 10th of a second		ICC = .83 (.57, .93)	ICC = .86 (.72, .93)
Step test[42] ◆	A step that is 15 cm high is used with a cardboard template 5 cm wide positioned on the floor along the edge of the step to provide a standardized starting position. As the test is performed, the participant remains on the stance leg the entire time while moving the other leg back and forth from the step to the floor (i.e., the participant places the stepping foot flat up onto the step and then back down flat onto the ground) as many times as possible in 15 seconds without moving the stance leg from the starting position. The number of whole steps (up onto the step and back down to a flat position on the floor) performed in 15 seconds is recorded for each stance leg. If the participant overbalances, the test is concluded and the number of completed steps and the time taken are recorded	30 patients with hip OA	ICC = .81 (.42, .93)	ICC = .85 (.71, .93)
Timed single-leg stance test[42] ◆	The participant starts with hands on hips and stands on one leg for as long as possible up to a maximum of 30 seconds. The nonstance hip remains in a neutral position with the knee flexed so that the foot is positioned behind and is not permitted to touch the stance leg. The participant is encouraged to look at a nonmoving target 1 to 3 meters ahead. The test is stopped if the participant moves his or her hands off the hips, touches the nonstance foot down on the floor, or touches the stance leg with the nonstance leg. The longest time, up to a maximum of 30 seconds, is recorded		ICC = .82 (.64, .91)	ICC = .89 (.78, .95)
Forward reach test[42] ◆	The participant starts in a normal relaxed stance with the dominant arm facing side-on, but not touching, a wall. A leveled measuring tape is mounted on the wall at acromion height. The participant makes a fist with the dominant hand and elevates the arm to shoulder level. The position of the third knuckle along the tape is recorded as the starting point. Keeping the contralateral arm by the side and both heels on the floor, the participant reaches as far forward as possible to maintain a maximal reach position for 3 seconds without losing balance. The final reach position of the third knuckle along the tape is recorded as the finishing point. The mean difference between the starting point and the finishing point across three trials is recorded to the nearest millimeter as the test score		ICC = .68 (.42, .84)	ICC = .68 (.29, .85)

Reliability of Balance Tests—cont'd

Test and Study Quality	Description and Positive Findings	Population	Reliability	
			Intraexaminer (95% CI)	Interexaminer (95% CI)
Four square step test[43] ◆	Four walking sticks were placed on the floor to form 4 squares. Participants started in square 1, facing square 2, and remained facing this direction for the duration of the test. Participants were asked to step forward with both feet as quickly as possible into square 2, then sideways to the right into square 3, then backward into square 4, and finally sideways to the left back into square 1. They were then asked to reverse the sequence back to the starting position. The patient performed this twice with the fastest time recorded		ICC = .83 (.57, .93)	ICC = .86 (.72, .93)
Step test[43] ◆	The patient repeatedly placed the stepping leg onto a 15 cm high step as many times as possible in 15 seconds. The number of whole steps performed in 15 seconds was recorded for each standing leg	30 people with hip osteoar-thritis	Involved limb: ICC = .81 (.42, .93) Uninvolved limb: ICC = .91 (.77, .96)	Involved limb: ICC = .94 (.88, .97) Uninvolved limb: ICC = .85 (.71, .93)
Functional reach test forward[43] ◆	Participants reached as far forward as possible to maintain a maximal reach position for 3 seconds without losing balance. The mean difference between the starting and finishing points was recorded to the nearest mil-limeter		ICC = .68 (.42, .84)	ICC = .68 (.29, .85)
Functional reach test lateral[43] ◆	Participants were standing with their back toward a wall without touching it. They were instructed to reach as far lateral as able while keeping both heels on the ground. The mean difference between the starting and finishing points was recorded to the nearest millimeter		ICC = .64 (.35, .82)	ICC = .62 (.34, .80)
Timed single-leg stance[43] ◆	Participants placed their hands on their hips and stood on 1 leg for as long as possible up to a maximum of 30 seconds. The longest time of 2 trials was recorded		Involved: ICC = .82 (.64, .91) Uninvolved: ICC = .91 (.81, .96)	Involved: ICC = .89 (.78, .95) Uninvolved: ICC = .90 (.80, .95)

6

Hip and Pelvis

Diagnostic Utility of Combinations of Tests for Osteoarthritis

Test and Study Quality	Number of Variables Present	Population	Reference Standard	Sens	Spec	+LR	−LR
Squatting aggravates symptoms + Lateral pain with active hip flexion + Scour test with adduction causes lateral hip or groin pain + Pain with active hip extension + Passive internal rotation of 25 degrees or less[8] ◆	Five of five	78 patients with unilateral pain in the buttock, groin, or anterior thigh	Hip OA on radiograph using the Kellgren and Lawrence grading scale	.14 (.04, .37)	.98 (.88, 1.0)	7.3 (1.1, 49.1)	.87 (.73, 1.1)
	Four or more of five			.48 (.26, .70)	.98 (.88, 1.0)	24.3 (4.4, 142.1)	.53 (.35, .80)
	Three or more of five			.71 (.48, .88)	.86 (.73, .94)	5.2 (2.6, 10.9)	.33 (.17, .66)
	Two or more of five			.81 (.57, .94)	.61 (.46, .74)	2.1 (1.4, 3.1)	.31 (.13, .78)
	One or more of five			.95 (.74, 1.0)	.18 (.09, .31)	1.2 (.99, 1.4)	.27 (.04, 2.0)

Interventions

Clinical Prediction Rule to Identify Patients with Primary Hip Osteoarthritis Likely to Benefit from Physical Therapy Intervention

Wright and colleagues[44] developed a clinical prediction rule for identifying patients with primary hip OA who are likely to benefit from physical therapy interventions. The result of their study demonstrated that if two or more of the five attributes (unilateral hip pain, age 58 years or younger, score of 6/10 or higher on the numeric pain rating scale, 40-meter self-paced walk test score of 25.9 seconds or less, and duration of symptoms 1 year or less) were present, the +LR was 3.99 (95% CI 2.66, 4.48) and the probability of experiencing a successful outcome improved from 22% to 65%.

Outcome Measure	Scoring and Interpretation	Test-Retest Reliability and Study Quality	MCID
Lower Extremity Functional Scale (LEFS)	Users are asked to rate the difficulty of performing 20 functional tasks on a Likert-type scale ranging from 0 (extremely difficult or unable to perform activity) to 4 (no difficulty). A total score out of 80 is calculated by summing each score. The answers provide a score between 0 and 80, with lower scores representing more disability	ICC = .92[45] ●	9[46]
Western Ontario and McMaster Universities Osteoarthritis Index (WOMAC)	The WOMAC consists of three subscales: pain (5 items), stiffness (2 items), and physical function (17 items). Users answer the 24 condition-specific questions on a numeric rating scale ranging from 0 (no symptoms) to 10 (extreme symptoms), or alternatively on a Likert-type scale from 0 to 4. Scores from each subscale are summed, with higher scores indicating more pain, stiffness, and disability	ICC = .90[45] ●	6.7% for improvement and 12.9% for worsening[47]
Numeric Pain Rating Scale (NPRS)	Users rate their level of pain on an 11-point scale ranging from 0 to 10, with high scores representing more pain. Often asked as "current pain" and "least," "worst," and "average pain" in the past 24 hours	ICC = .72[48] ●	2[49,50]

MCID, Minimum clinically important difference.

Hip and Pelvis

6

References

1. Hertling D, Kessler RM. *Management of Common Musculoskeletal Disorders: Physical Therapy Principles and Methods.* 3rd ed. Philadelphia: Lippincott; 1996.

2. Pecina MM, Bojanic I. *Overuse Injuries of the Musculoskeletal System.* Boca Raton, Florida: CRC Press; 1993.

3. Altman R, Alarcon G, Appelrouth D, et al. The American College of Rheumatology criteria for the classification and reporting of osteoarthritis of the hip. *Arthritis Rheum.* 1991;34:505–514.

4. Hartley A. *Practical Joint Assessment.* St Louis: Mosby; 1995.

5. Clohisy JC, Knaus ER, Hunt DM, et al. Clinical presentation of patients with symptomatic anterior hip impingement. *Clin Orthop Relat Res.* 2009;467:638–644.

6. Fishman LM, Dombi GW, Michaelsen C, et al. Piriformis syndrome: diagnosis, treatment, and outcome—a 10-year study. *Arch Phys Med Rehabil.* 2002;83:295–301.

7. Martin RL, Irrgang JJ, Sekiya JK. The diagnostic accuracy of a clinical examination in determining intra-articular hip pain for potential hip arthroscopy candidates. *Arthroscopy.* 2008;24:1013–1018.

8. Sutlive TG, Lopez HP, Schnitker DE, et al. Development of a clinical prediction rule for diagnosing hip osteoarthritis in individuals with unilateral hip pain. *J Orthop Sports Phys Ther.* 2008;38:542–550.

9. Narvani AA, Tsiridis E, Kendall S, et al. A preliminary report on prevalence of acetabular labrum tears in sports patients with groin pain. *Knee Surg Sports Traumatol Arthrosc.* 2003;11:403–408.

10. Cibere J, Thorne A, Bellamy N, et al. Reliability of the hip examination in osteoarthritis: effect of standardization. *Arthritis Rheum.* 2008;59:373–381.

11. Pua YH, Wrigley TV, Cowan SM, Bennell KL. Intrarater test-retest reliability of hip range of motion and hip muscle strength measurements in persons with hip osteoarthritis. *Arch Phys Med Rehabil.* 2008;89:1146–1154.

12. Cliborne AV, Wainner RS, Rhon DI, et al. Clinical hip tests and a functional squat test in patients with knee osteoarthritis: reliability, prevalence of positive test findings, and short-term response to hip mobilization. *J Orthop Sports Phys Ther.* 2004;34:676–685.

13. Holm I, Bolstad B, Lutken T, et al. Reliability of goniometric measurements and visual estimates of hip ROM in patients with osteoarthrosis. *Physiother Res Int.* 2000;5:241–248.

14. Klässbo M, Harms-Ringdahl K, Larsson G. Examination of passive ROM and capsular patterns in the hip. *Physiother Res Int.* 2003;8:1–12.

15. Lin YC, Davey RC, Cochrane T. Tests for physical function of the elderly with knee and hip osteoarthritis. *Scand J Med Sci Sports.* 2001;11:280–286.

16. Krause DA, Hollman JH, Krych AJ, et al. Reliability of hip internal rotation range of motion measurement using a digital inclinometer. *Knee Surg Sports Traumatol Arthrosc.* 2014. [Epub ahead of print].

17. Bijl D, Dekker J, van Baar ME, et al. Validity of Cyriax's concept capsular pattern for the diagnosis of osteoarthritis of hip and/or knee. *Scand J Rheumatol.* 1998;27:347–351.

18. Woodley SJ, Nicholson HD, Livingstone V, et al. Lateral hip pain: findings from magnetic resonance imaging and clinical examination. *J Orthop Sports Phys Ther.* 2008;38:313–328.

19. Birrell F, Croft P, Cooper C, et al. Predicting radiographic hip osteoarthritis from range of movement. *Rheumatology (Oxford).* 2001;40:506–512.

20. Cook C, Massa L, Harm-Ernandes I, et al. Interrater reliability and diagnostic accuracy of pelvic girdle pain classification. *J Manipulative Physiol Ther.* 2007;30:252–258.

21. Joe G, Kovacs J, Miller K, et al. Diagnosis of avascular necrosis of the hip in asymptomatic HIV-infected patients: clinical correlation of physical examination with magnetic resonance imaging. *J Back Musculoskeletal Rehabil.* 2002;16:135–139.

22. Jari S, Paton RW, Srinivasan MS. Unilateral limitation of abduction of the hip. A valuable clinical sign for DDH? *J Bone Joint Surg Br.* 2002;84:104–107.

23. Castelein RM, Korte J. Limited hip abduction in the infant. *J Pediatr Orthop.* 2001;21:668–670.

24. Ranawat AS, Gaudiani MA, Slullitel PA, et al. Foot progression angle walking test. A dynamic diagnostic assessment for femoroacetabular impingement and hip stability. *Orthop J Sports Med.* 2017;5:1–5.

25. Malliaras P, Hogan A, Nawrocki A, et al. Hip flexibility and strength measures: reliability and association with athletic groin pain. *Br J Sports Med.* 2009;43(10):739–744.

26. Bieler T, Magnusson SP, Kjaer M, Beyer N. Intrarater reliability and agreement of muscle strength, power and functional performance measures in patients with hip osteoarthritis. *J Rehabil Med.* 2014;46(10):997–1005.

27. Alnahdi AH, Zeni JA, Snyder-Mackler L. His abductor strength reliability and association with physical function after unilateral total knee arthroplasty: a cross sectional study. *Phys Ther.* 2014;94:1154–1162.

28. Bird PA, Oakley SP, Shnier R, Kirkham BW. Prospective evaluation of magnetic resonance imaging and physical examination findings in patients with greater trochanteric pain syndrome. *Arthritis Rheum.* 2001;44:2138–2145.

29. Piva SR, Fitzgerald K, Irrgang JJ, et al. Reliability of measures of impairments associated with patellofemoral pain syndrome. *BMC Musculoskelet Disord.* 2006;7:33.

30. Reese NB, Bandy WD. Use of an inclinometer to measure flexibility of the iliotibial band using the Ober test and the modified Ober test: differences in magnitude and reliability of measurements. *J Orthop Sports Phys Ther.* 2003;33:326–330.

31. Melchione WE, Sullivan MS. Reliability of measurements obtained by use of an instrument designed

to indirectly measure iliotibial band length. *J Orthop Sports Phys Ther*. 1993;18:511–515.

32. Clapis PA, Davis SM, Davis RO. Reliability of inclinometer and goniometric measurements of hip extension flexibility using the modified Thomas test. *Physiother Theory Pract*. 2008;24:135–141.

33. Bullock-Saxton JE, Bullock MI. Repeatability of muscle length measures around the hip. *Physiother Can*. 1994;46:105–109.

34. Park K-M, Cynn H-S, Choung S-D. Musculoskeletal predictors of movement quality for the forward step-down test in asymptomatic women. *J Orthop Sports Phys Ther*. 2013;43(7):504–510.

35. Lenzlinger-Asprion R, Keller N, Meichtry A, Luomajoki H. Intertester and intratester reliability of movement control tests on the hip for patients with hip osteoarthritis. *BMC Musculoskelet Disord*. 2017;18:55.

36. Martin RL, Sekiya JK. The interrater reliability of 4 clinical tests used to assess individuals with musculoskeletal hip pain. *J Orthop Sports Phys Ther*. 2008;38(2):71–77.

37. Casartelli NC, Brunner R, Maffiuletti NA, et al. The FADIR test for accuracy for screening can and pincer morphology in youth ice hockey players. *J Sci Med Sport*. 2018;21:134–138.

38. Ayeni O, Chu R, Hetaimish B, et al. A painful squat test provides limited diagnostic utility in CAM-type femoroacetabular impingement. *Knee Surg Sports Traumatol Arthrosc*. 2014;22:806–811.

39. O'Donnell J, Economopoulos K, Singh P, et al. The ligamentum teres test. A novel and effective test in diagnosing tera of the ligamentum teres. *Am J Sports Med*. 2013;42.138–143.

40. Gomez-Hoyos J, Martin RL, Schroder R, et al. Accuracy of 2 clinical tests for ischiofemoral impingement in patients with posterior hip pain and endoscopically confirmed diagnosis. *Arthroscopy*. 2016;32:1279–1284.

41. Tiru M, Goh SH, Low BY. Use of percussion as a screening tool in the diagnosis of occult hip fractures. *Singapore Med J*. 2002;43:467–469.

42. Choi YM, Dobson F, Martin J, et al. Interrater and intrarater reliability of common clinical standing balance tests for people with hip osteoarthritis. *Phys Ther*. 2014;94(5):696–704.

43. Ming Choi Y, Dobson F, Martin J, et al. Interrater and intrarater reliability of common clinical standing balance tests for people with hip osteoarthritis. *Phys Ther*. 2014;94:696–704.

44. Wright AA, Cook CE, Flynn TW, et al. Predictors of response to physical therapy intervention in patients with primary hip osteoarthritis. *Phys Ther*. 2011;91(4):510–524.

45. Pua YH, Cowan SM, Wrigley TV, Bennell KL. The lower extremity functional scale could be an alternative to the Western Ontario and McMaster Universities osteoarthritis index physical function scale. *J Clin Epidemiol*. 2009;62(10):1103–1111.

46. Binkley JM, Stratford PW, Lott SA, Riddle DL. The Lower Extremity Functional Scale (LEFS): scale development, measurement properties, and clinical application. North American Orthopaedic Rehabilitation Research Network. *Phys Ther*. 1999;79:371–383.

47. Angst F, Aeschlimann A, Stucki G. Smallest detectable and minimal clinically important differences of rehabilitation intervention with their implications for required sample sizes using WOMAC and SF-36 quality of life measurement instruments in patients with osteoarthritis of the lower extremities. *Arthritis Rheum*. 2001;45:384–391.

48. Li L, Liu X, Herr K. Postoperative pain intensity assessment: a comparison of four scales in Chinese adults. *Pain Med*. 2007;8:223–234.

49. Farrar JT, Berlin JA, Strom BL. Clinically important changes in acute pain outcome measures: a validation study. *J Pain Symptom Manage*. 2003;25:406–411.

50. Farrar JT, Portenoy RK, Berlin JA, et al. Defining the clinically important difference in pain outcome measures. *Pain*. 2000;88:287–294.

6

Hip and Pelvis

Clinical Summary and Recommendations

Patient History

Complaints

- Little is known about the utility of subjective complaints with knee pain.
- The absence of "weight bearing during trauma" may help rule out a meniscal tear (likelihood ratio [LR] = .40).
- Symptoms in combination with examination findings may be optimized to identify patients at increased risk of knee joint effusion. Self-noticed knee swelling in combination with self-reported pain with leg straightening may help in ruling in the presence of medium/large knee joint effusion (+LR = 2.9 to 9.7).

Physical Examination

Screening

- The Ottawa Knee Rule for Radiography is highly sensitive for knee fractures in both adults and children. When patients are younger than 55 years, can bear weight and flex the knee to 90 degrees, and have no tenderness on the patella or fibular head, providers can confidently rule out a knee fracture (−LR = .05 to .07).

Range-of-Motion and Strength Assessment

- Measuring knee range of motion has consistently been shown to be highly reliable but is of unknown diagnostic utility. The assessment of "end feel" during range-of-motion measurements, however, is unreliable, especially between different examiners.
- Assessing strength with manual muscle testing has been shown to accurately detect side-to-side knee extension strength deficits, at least in patients in an acute rehabilitation hospital setting.

Special Tests

- Several systematic reviews with metaanalysis have examined special tests of the knee.
- The Thessaly test, McMurray test, and "joint line tenderness" consistently show moderate utility in detecting and ruling out meniscal tears.
- Although the anterior drawer test and pivot shift test are good at identifying anterior cruciate ligament (ACL) tears (+LR = 1.5 to 36.5), the Lachman test is best at ruling them out (−LR = .10 to .24).
- Varus and valgus testing, while not particularly reliable, is fairly good at ruling out medial collateral ligament (MCL) tears (−LR = .20 to .30).
- The "moving patellar apprehension test" seems to show very good diagnostic utility in both identifying and ruling out patellar instability (+LR = 8.3, −LR = .00).

Combinations of Findings

- Generally, the clinical examination and/or combinations of findings seem to be very good at identifying and ruling out various knee pathologic conditions, including meniscal tears, ACL tears, and symptomatic plica.
- Presence of joint line tenderness and a positive McMurray test seems to show good diagnostic utility in both identifying and ruling out meniscal tears (+LR = 10.1 to 75, −LR = .10 to .25).
- Presence of joint line tenderness and a positive Thessaly test also seems to show good diagnostic utility in both identifying and ruling out meniscal tears (+LR = 11.6 to 78, −LR = .08 to .22).
- Clinical prediction rules for both identifying and ruling out symptomatic meniscal tear (+LR = 3.99 to 10.39, −LR = .03 to .31), patellofemoral pain (+LR = 5.2 to 14.58, −LR = .06 to .27), and knee osteoarthritis (+LR = 6.53 to 28.41, −LR = .06 to .20) have been developed and show good initial diagnostic utility.

Interventions

- In patients with patellofemoral pain syndrome, a combination of factors (age over 25 years, height less than 65 inches, worst pain visual analog scale less than 53 mm, and a difference in midfoot width from non−weight bearing to weight bearing of more than 11 mm) seems to predict a favorable response to foot orthoses (+LR = 8.8 if three of four factors present).
- Similarly, several factors have been identified that predict which patients with knee osteoarthritis (OA) may benefit from hip mobilizations.

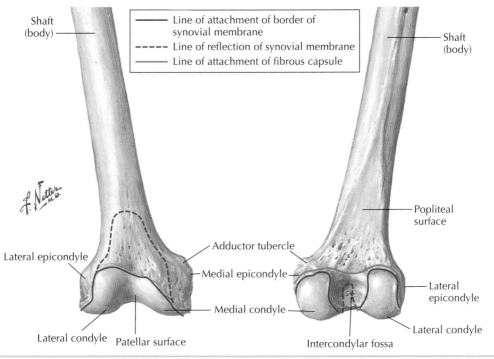

Line of attachment of border of
synovial membrane

--- Line of reflection of synovial membrane

Line of attachment of fibrous capsule

Shaft
(body)

Shaft
(body)

Popliteal
surface

Adductor tubercle

Lateral epicondyle

Medial epicondyle

Lateral
epicondyle

Medial condyle

Lateral condyle Patellar surface

Lateral condyle

Intercondylar fossa

Figure 7-1
Femur.

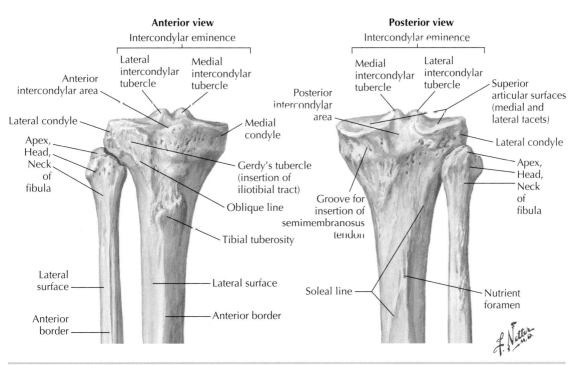

Anterior view

Intercondylar eminence

Posterior view

Intercondylar eminence

Lateral
intercondylar
tubercle

Medial
intercondylar
tubercle

Medial
intercondylar
tubercle

Lateral
intercondylar
tubercle

Superior
articular surfaces
(medial and
lateral facets)

Anterior
intercondylar area

Posterior
intercondylar
area

Lateral condyle

Medial
condyle

Lateral condyle

Apex,
Head,
Neck
of
fibula

Apex,
Head,
Neck
of
fibula

Gerdy's tubercle
(insertion of
iliotibial tract)

Oblique line

Groove for
insertion of
semimembranosus
tendon

Tibial tuberosity

Lateral
surface

Lateral surface

Soleal line

Nutrient
foramen

Anterior
border

Anterior border

Figure 7-2
Tibia and fibula.

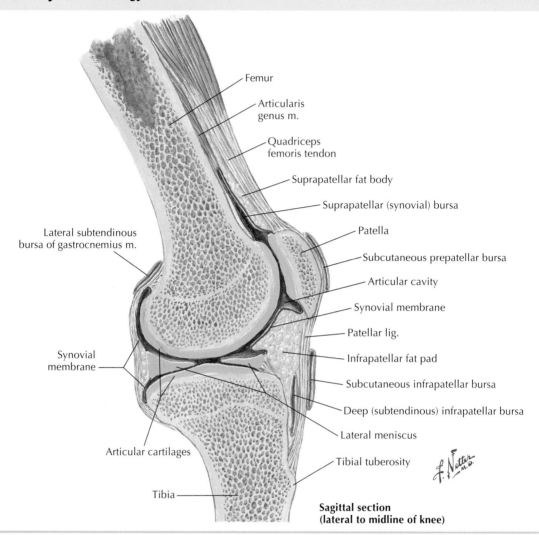

Femur

Articularis genus m.

Quadriceps femoris tendon

Suprapatellar fat body

Suprapatellar (synovial) bursa

Patella

Subcutaneous prepatellar bursa

Articular cavity

Synovial membrane

Patellar lig.

Infrapatellar fat pad

Subcutaneous infrapatellar bursa

Deep (subtendinous) infrapatellar bursa

Lateral meniscus

Tibial tuberosity

Lateral subtendinous bursa of gastrocnemius m.

Synovial membrane

Articular cartilages

Tibia

Sagittal section (lateral to midline of knee)

Figure 7-3
Sagittal knee.

Joints	Type and Classification	Closed Packed Position	Capsular Pattern
Tibiofemoral	Double condyloid	Full extension	Flexion restricted greater than extension
Proximal tibiofibular	Synovial: plane	Not reported	Not reported
Patellofemoral	Synovial: plane	Full flexion	Not reported

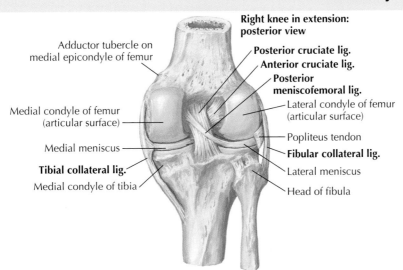

Right knee in extension: posterior view

Adductor tubercle on medial epicondyle of femur

Posterior cruciate lig.

Anterior cruciate lig.

Posterior meniscofemoral lig.

Lateral condyle of femur (articular surface)

Medial condyle of femur (articular surface)

Medial meniscus

Popliteus tendon

Fibular collateral lig.

Tibial collateral lig.

Lateral meniscus

Medial condyle of tibia

Head of fibula

Figure 7-4

Posterior ligaments of knee.

Ligaments	Attachments	Function
Posterior meniscofemoral	Lateral meniscus to posterior cruciate ligament (PCL) and medial femoral condyle	Reinforces posterior lateral meniscal attachment
Oblique popliteal	Posterior aspect of medial tibial condyle to posterior aspect of fibrous capsule	Strengthens posterior portion of joint capsule
Arcuate popliteal	Posterior fibular head over tendon of popliteus to posterior capsule	Strengthens posterior portion of joint capsule
Posterior ligament of fibular head	Posterior fibular head to inferior lateral tibial condyle	Reinforces posterior joint capsule
Anterior cruciate	Anterior intracondylar aspect of tibial plateau to posteromedial side of lateral femoral condyle	Prevents posterior translation of femur on tibia and anterior translation of tibia on femur
Posterior cruciate	Posterior intracondylar aspect of tibial plateau to anterolateral side of medial femoral condyle	Prevents anterior translation of femur on tibia and posterior translation of tibia on femur
Fibular collateral	Lateral epicondyle of femur to lateral aspect of fibular head	Protects joint from varus stress
Tibial collateral	Femoral medial epicondyle to medial condyle of tibia	Protects the joint from valgus stress
Transverse ligament of knee	Anterior edges of menisci	Allows menisci to move together during knee movement

7

Knee

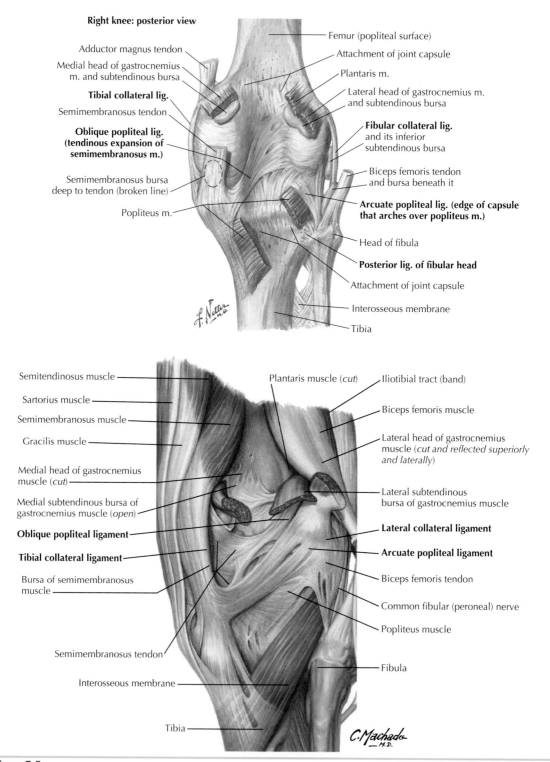

Right knee: posterior view

Adductor magnus tendon

Medial head of gastrocnemius m. and subtendinous bursa

Tibial collateral lig.

Semimembranosus tendon

Oblique popliteal lig. (tendinous expansion of semimembranosus m.)

Semimembranosus bursa deep to tendon (broken line)

Popliteus m.

Femur (popliteal surface)

Attachment of joint capsule

Plantaris m.

Lateral head of gastrocnemius m. and subtendinous bursa

Fibular collateral lig. and its inferior subtendinous bursa

Biceps femoris tendon and bursa beneath it

Arcuate popliteal lig. (edge of capsule that arches over popliteus m.)

Head of fibula

Posterior lig. of fibular head

Attachment of joint capsule

Interosseous membrane

Tibia

Semitendinosus muscle

Sartorius muscle

Semimembranosus muscle

Gracilis muscle

Medial head of gastrocnemius muscle (*cut*)

Medial subtendinous bursa of gastrocnemius muscle (*open*)

Oblique popliteal ligament

Tibial collateral ligament

Bursa of semimembranosus muscle

Semimembranosus tendon

Interosseous membrane

Tibia

Plantaris muscle (*cut*)

Iliotibial tract (band)

Biceps femoris muscle

Lateral head of gastrocnemius muscle (*cut and reflected superiorly and laterally*)

Lateral subtendinous bursa of gastrocnemius muscle

Lateral collateral ligament

Arcuate popliteal ligament

Biceps femoris tendon

Common fibular (peroneal) nerve

Popliteus muscle

Fibula

Figure 7-5

Posterior ligaments of knee (continued).

Right knee in flexion: anterior view

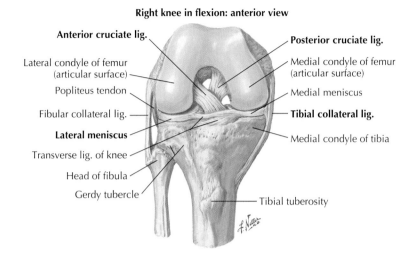

Anterior cruciate lig.

Lateral condyle of femur
(articular surface)

Popliteus tendon

Fibular collateral lig.

Lateral meniscus

Transverse lig. of knee

Head of fibula

Gerdy tubercle

Posterior cruciate lig.

Medial condyle of femur
(articular surface)

Medial meniscus

Tibial collateral lig.

Medial condyle of tibia

Tibial tuberosity

Inferior view

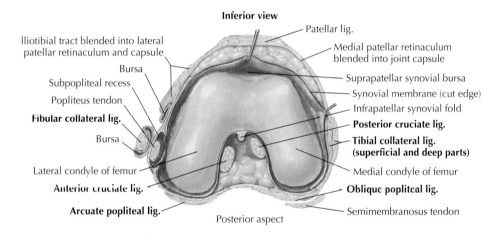

Iliotibial tract blended into lateral
patellar retinaculum and capsule

Bursa

Subpopliteal recess

Popliteus tendon

Fibular collateral lig.

Bursa

Lateral condyle of femur

Anterior cruciate lig.

Arcuate popliteal lig.

Patellar lig.

Medial patellar retinaculum
blended into joint capsule

Suprapatellar synovial bursa

Synovial membrane (cut edge)

Infrapatellar synovial fold

Posterior cruciate lig.

**Tibial collateral lig.
(superficial and deep parts)**

Medial condyle of femur

Oblique popliteal lig.

Semimembranosus tendon

Posterior aspect

Superior view

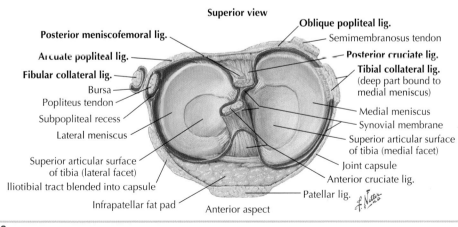

Posterior meniscofemoral lig.

Arcuate popliteal lig.

Fibular collateral lig.

Bursa

Popliteus tendon

Subpopliteal recess

Lateral meniscus

Superior articular surface
of tibia (lateral facet)

Iliotibial tract blended into capsule

Infrapatellar fat pad

Oblique popliteal lig.

Semimembranosus tendon

Posterior cruciate lig.

Tibial collateral lig.
(deep part bound to
medial meniscus)

Medial meniscus

Synovial membrane

Superior articular surface
of tibia (medial facet)

Joint capsule

Anterior cruciate lig.

Patellar lig.

Anterior aspect

Figure 7-6

Inferior, anterior, and superior views of ligaments of knee.

7

Kree

Muscles	Proximal Attachments	Distal Attachments	Nerve and Segmental Level	Action
Quadriceps *Rectus femoris*	Anterior inferior iliac spine and ileum just superior to acetabulum	Base of patella and by patellar ligament to tibial tuberosity	Femoral nerve (L2, L3, L4)	Extends knee; rectus femoris also flexes hip and stabilizes head of femur in acetabulum
Vastus lateralis	Greater trochanter and linea aspera of femur			
Vastus medialis	Intertrochanteric line and linea aspera			
Vastus intermedius	Anterolateral aspect of shaft of femur			
Articularis genu	Anteroinferior aspect of femur	Synovial membrane of knee joint	Femoral nerve (L3, L4)	Pulls synovial membrane superiorly during knee extension to prevent pinching of membrane
Hamstrings *Semimembranosus*	Ischial tuberosity	Medial aspect of superior tibia	Tibial branch of sciatic nerve (L4, L5, S1, S2)	Flexes and medially rotates knee, extends and medially rotates hip
Semitendinosus	Ischial tuberosity	Posterior aspect of medial condyle of tibia		
Biceps femoris *Short head*	Lateral linea aspera and proximal two thirds of supracondylar line of femur	Lateral head of fibula and lateral tibial condyle	Fibular branch of sciatic nerve (L5, S1, S2)	Flexes and laterally rotates knee
Long head	Ischial tuberosity		Tibial branch of sciatic nerve (L5, S1-S3)	Flexes and laterally rotates knee, extends and laterally rotates hip
Gracilis	Body and inferior ramus of pubis	Medial aspect of superior tibia	Obturator nerve (L2, L3)	Adducts hip, flexes and medially rotates knee
Sartorius	Anterior superior iliac spine and anterior iliac crest	Superomedial aspect of tibia	Femoral nerve (L2, L3)	Flexes, abducts, and externally rotates hip, flexes knee
Gastrocnemius *Lateral head* *Medial head*	Lateral femoral condyle Superior aspect of medial femoral condyle	Posterior calcaneus	Tibial nerve (S1, S2)	Plantarflexes ankle and flexes knee
Popliteus	Lateral femoral condyle and lateral meniscus	Superior to soleal line on posterior tibia	Tibial nerve (L4, L5, S1)	Weak knee flexion and unlocking of knee joint
Plantaris	Lateral supracondylar line of femur and oblique popliteal ligament	Posterior calcaneus	Tibial nerve (S1, S2)	Weak assist in knee flexion and ankle plantarflexion

Right knee in extension

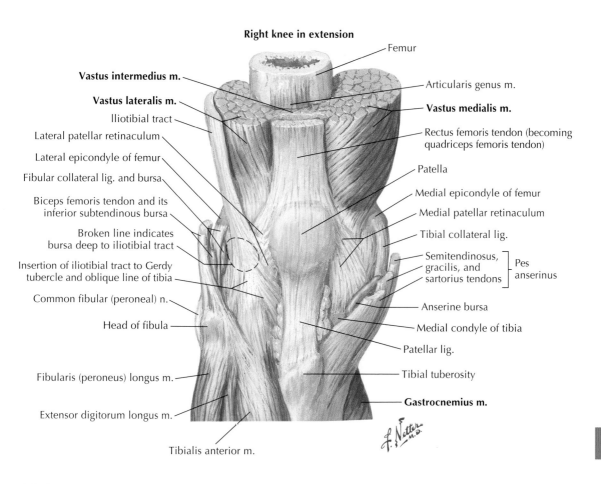

Vastus intermedius m.

Vastus lateralis m.

Iliotibial tract

Lateral patellar retinaculum

Lateral epicondyle of femur

Fibular collateral lig. and bursa

Biceps femoris tendon and its inferior subtendinous bursa

Broken line indicates bursa deep to iliotibial tract

Insertion of iliotibial tract to Gerdy tubercle and oblique line of tibia

Common fibular (peroneal) n.

Head of fibula

Fibularis (peroneus) longus m.

Extensor digitorum longus m.

Tibialis anterior m.

Femur

Articularis genus m.

Vastus medialis m.

Rectus femoris tendon (becoming quadriceps femoris tendon)

Patella

Medial epicondyle of femur

Medial patellar retinaculum

Tibial collateral lig.

Semitendinosus, gracilis, and sartorius tendons — Pes anserinus

Anserine bursa

Medial condyle of tibia

Patellar lig.

Tibial tuberosity

Gastrocnemius m.

Right leg

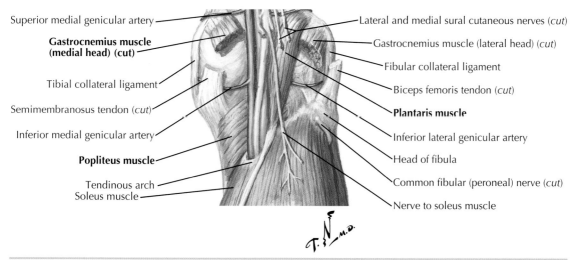

Superior medial genicular artery

Gastrocnemius muscle (medial head) (cut)

Tibial collateral ligament

Semimembranosus tendon (cut)

Inferior medial genicular artery

Popliteus muscle

Tendinous arch

Soleus muscle

Lateral and medial sural cutaneous nerves (cut)

Gastrocnemius muscle (lateral head) (cut)

Fibular collateral ligament

Biceps femoris tendon (cut)

Plantaris muscle

Inferior lateral genicular artery

Head of fibula

Common fibular (peroneal) nerve (cut)

Nerve to soleus muscle

Figure 7-7
Anterior and posterior muscles of knee.

7

Knee

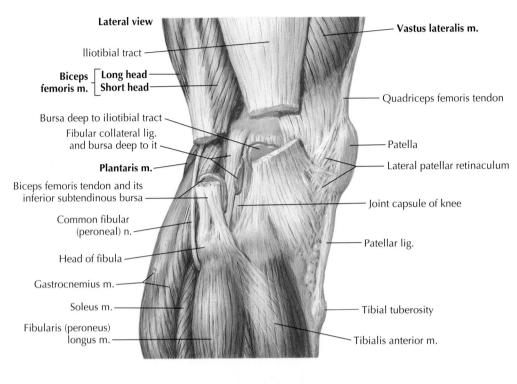

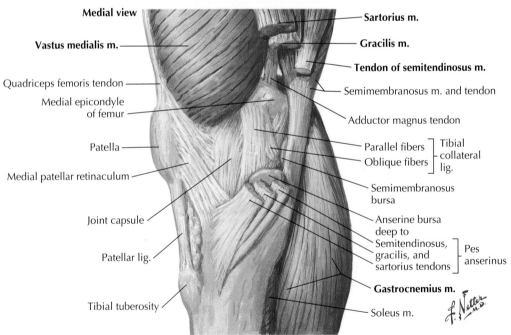

Figure 7-8
Lateral and medial muscles of knee.

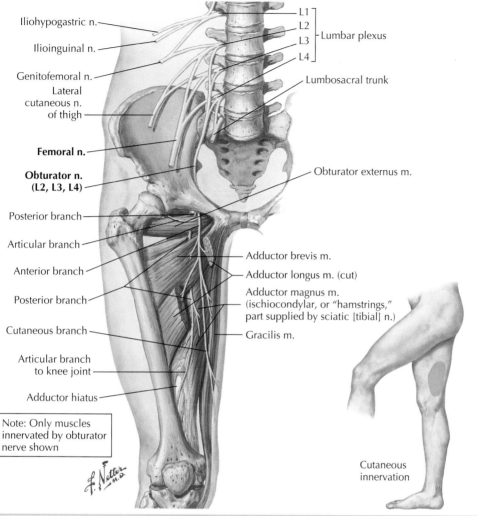

Iliohypogastric n.
Ilioinguinal n.
Genitofemoral n.
Lateral cutaneous n. of thigh
Femoral n.
Obturator n. (L2, L3, L4)
Posterior branch
Articular branch
Anterior branch
Posterior branch
Cutaneous branch
Articular branch to knee joint
Adductor hiatus

L1
L2
L3
L4
— Lumbar plexus

Lumbosacral trunk

Obturator externus m.

Adductor brevis m.
Adductor longus m. (cut)
Adductor magnus m. (ischiocondylar, or "hamstrings," part supplied by sciatic [tibial] n.)
Gracilis m.

Note: Only muscles innervated by obturator nerve shown

Cutaneous innervation

Knee
7

Figure 7-9
Obturator nerve.

Nerves	Segmental Level	Sensory	Motor
Femoral	L2, L3, L4	Thigh via cutaneous nerves	Iliacus, sartorius, quadriceps femoris, articularis genu, pectineus
Obturator	L2, L3, L4	Medial thigh	Adductor longus, adductor brevis, adductor magnus (adductor part), gracilis, obturator externus
Saphenous	L2, L3, L4	Medial leg and foot	No motor
Tibial nerve	L4, L5, S1, S2, S3	Posterior heel and plantar surface of foot	Semitendinosus, semimembranosus, biceps femoris, adductor magnus, gastrocnemius, soleus, plantaris, flexor hallucis longus, flexor digitorum longus, tibialis posterior
Common fibular nerve	L4, L5, S1, S2	Lateral posterior leg	Biceps femoris

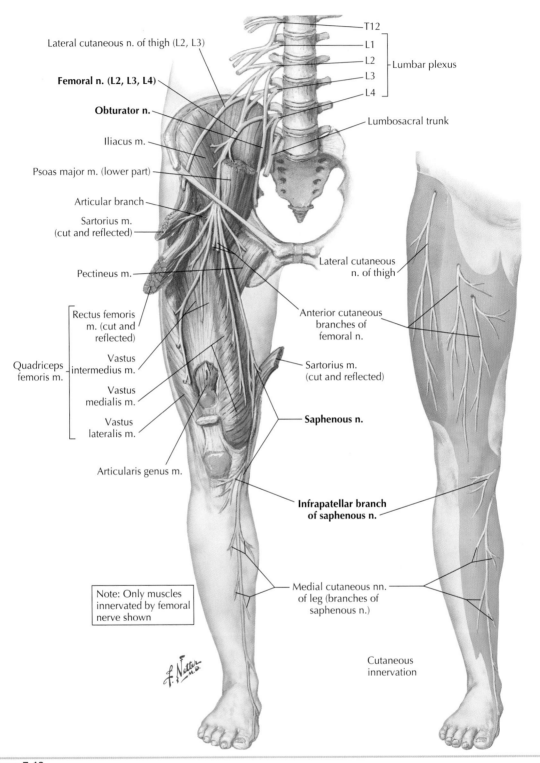

Lateral cutaneous n. of thigh (L2, L3)

Femoral n. (L2, L3, L4)

Obturator n.

Iliacus m.

Psoas major m. (lower part)

Articular branch

Sartorius m.
(cut and reflected)

Pectineus m.

Rectus femoris
m. (cut and
reflected)

Quadriceps
femoris m.

Vastus
intermedius m.

Vastus
medialis m.

Vastus
lateralis m.

Articularis genus m.

Note: Only muscles
innervated by femoral
nerve shown

T12

L1

L2

L3

L4

Lumbar plexus

Lumbosacral trunk

Lateral cutaneous
n. of thigh

Anterior cutaneous
branches of
femoral n.

Sartorius m.
(cut and reflected)

Saphenous n.

**Infrapatellar branch
of saphenous n.**

Medial cutaneous nn.
of leg (branches of
saphenous n.)

Cutaneous
innervation

Figure 7-10
Femoral nerve and lateral femoral cutaneous nerves.

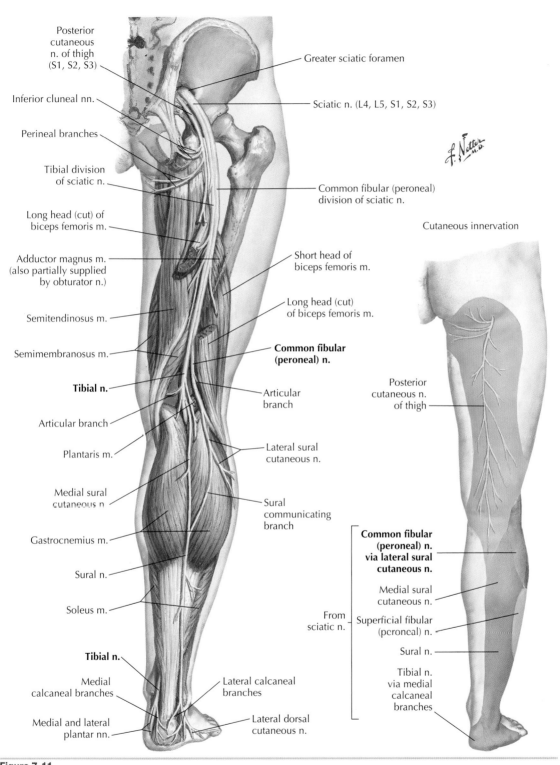

Posterior cutaneous n. of thigh (S1, S2, S3)

Inferior cluneal nn.

Perineal branches

Tibial division of sciatic n.

Long head (cut) of biceps femoris m.

Adductor magnus m. (also partially supplied by obturator n.)

Semitendinosus m.

Semimembranosus m.

Tibial n.

Articular branch

Plantaris m.

Medial sural cutaneous n.

Gastrocnemius m.

Sural n.

Soleus m.

Tibial n.

Medial calcaneal branches

Medial and lateral plantar nn.

Greater sciatic foramen

Sciatic n. (L4, L5, S1, S2, S3)

F. Netter
M.D.

Common fibular (peroneal) division of sciatic n.

Short head of biceps femoris m.

Long head (cut) of biceps femoris m.

Common fibular (peroneal) n.

Articular branch

Lateral sural cutaneous n.

Sural communicating branch

From sciatic n.

Lateral calcaneal branches

Lateral dorsal cutaneous n.

Cutaneous innervation

Posterior cutaneous n. of thigh

Common fibular (peroneal) n. via lateral sural cutaneous n.

Medial sural cutaneous n.

Superficial fibular (peroneal) n.

Sural n.

Tibial n. via medial calcaneal branches

7

Knee

Figure 7-11
Sciatic nerve and posterior femoral cutaneous nerve.

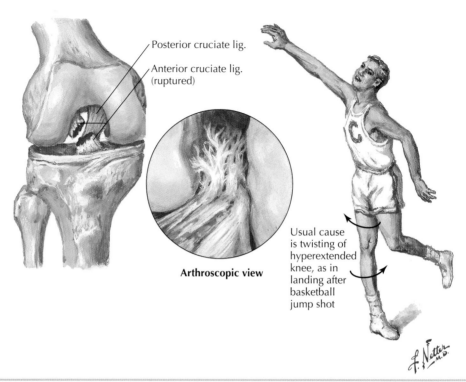

Figure 7-12
Anterior cruciate ligament ruptures.

Patient Reports	Initial Hypothesis
Patient reports a traumatic onset of knee pain that occurred during jumping, twisting, or changing directions with foot planted	Possible ligamentous injury (ACL)[1,2] Possible patellar subluxation[2] Possible quadriceps rupture Possible meniscal tear
Patient reports traumatic injury that resulted in a posteriorly directed force to tibia with knee flexed	Possible PCL injury[3]
Patient reports traumatic injury that resulted in a varus or valgus force exerted on knee	Possible collateral ligament injury (lateral collateral ligament [LCL] or MCL)[3]
Patient reports anterior knee pain with jumping and full knee flexion	Possible patellar tendinitis[2,4] Possible patellofemoral pain syndrome[5,6]
Patient reports swelling in knee with occasional locking and clicking	Possible meniscal tear[7] Possible loose body within knee joint
Patient reports pain with prolonged knee flexion, during squats, and while going up and down stairs	Possible patellofemoral pain syndrome[5,6]
Patient reports pain and stiffness in morning that diminishes after a few hours	Possible OA[8,9]

Progressive stages in joint pathology

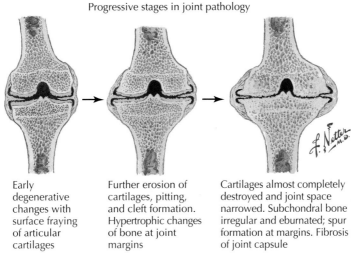

Early degenerative changes with surface fraying of articular cartilages

Further erosion of cartilages, pitting, and cleft formation. Hypertrophic changes of bone at joint margins

Cartilages almost completely destroyed and joint space narrowed. Subchondral bone irregular and eburnated; spur formation at margins. Fibrosis of joint capsule

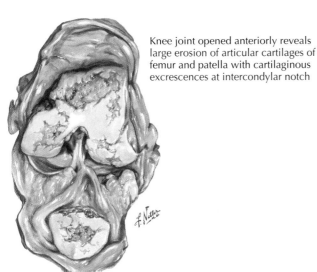

Knee joint opened anteriorly reveals large erosion of articular cartilages of femur and patella with cartilaginous excrescences at intercondylar notch

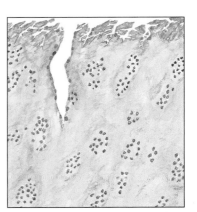

Section of articular cartilage shows fraying of surface and deep cleft. Hyaline cartilage abnormal with clumping of chondrocytes

Figure 7-13
Osteoarthritis of the knee.

History and Study Quality	Population	Interexaminer Reliability
Acute injury[10]		$\kappa = .21 (.03, .39)$
Swelling[10]		$\kappa = .33 (.17, .49)$
Giving way[10]		$\kappa = .12 (-.04, .28)$
Locking[10]		$\kappa = .44 (.26, .62)$
Pain, generalized[10]	152 patients with OA of knee	$\kappa = -.03 (.15, .21)$
Pain at rest[10]		$\kappa = .16 (.00, .32)$
Pain rising from chair[10]		$\kappa = .25 (.05, .45)$
Pain climbing stairs[10]		$\kappa = .21 (.06, .48)$

History and Study Quality	Population	Interexaminer Reliability
Clicking: "Do you feel a clicking sensation or hear a clicking noise when you move your knee?"[11] ●		$\kappa = .80\ (.58, 1.0)$
Catching: "Do you feel that sometimes something is caught in your knee that momentarily prevents movement?"[11] ●		$\kappa = .65\ (.37, .93)$
Giving way: "Do you sometimes feel that your knee will give out and not support your weight?"[11] ●	30 patients with meniscal tear	$\kappa = .80\ (.58, 1.0)$
Localized pain: "Is your knee pain centered to one spot on the knee that you can point to with your finger?"[11] ●		$\kappa = .84\ (.63, 1.0)$

Patient History • *Diagnostic Utility of Meniscal Symptom Index in Patients with Meniscal Tears*

Patient Report and Study Quality*	Population	Reference Standard	Sens	Spec	+LR	−LR
Clicking: "Do you feel a clicking sensation or hear a clicking noise when you move your knee?"[11]	300 patients with knee pain	Physician's impression, supported by magnetic resonance imaging (MRI) findings	.65 (.56, .73)	.50 (.43, .58)	1.3	0.7
Catching: "Do you feel that sometimes something is caught in your knee that momentarily prevents movement?"[11]			.59 (.50, .67)	.75 (.68, .80)	2.4	5.5
Giving way: "Do you sometimes feel that your knee will give out and not support your weight?"[11]			.69 (.60, .77)	.53 (.45, .60)	1.5	5.9
Localized pain: "Is your knee pain centered to one spot on the knee that you can point to with your finger?"[11]			.74 (.65, .81)	.49 (.31, .56)	1.5	5.3

*Among patients with none of these symptoms, 16% (95% CI: 2% to 30%) had symptomatic meniscal tear, while among those with all four symptoms, 76% (95% CI: 63% to 88%) had symptomatic meniscal tear.

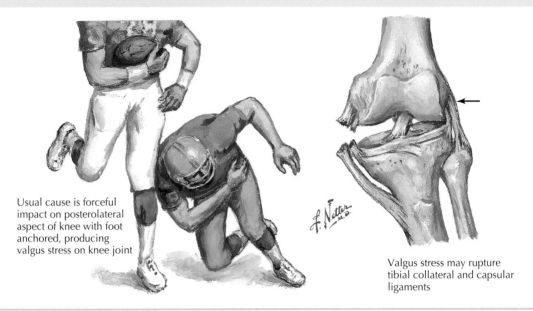

Usual cause is forceful impact on posterolateral aspect of knee with foot anchored, producing valgus stress on knee joint

Valgus stress may rupture tibial collateral and capsular ligaments

Figure 7-14
Medial collateral ligament rupture.

Patient Report and Study Quality	Population	Reference Standard	Sens	Spec	+LR	−LR
Self-noticed swelling[12] ◆		Knee joint effusion per MRI	.80 (.68, .92)	.45 (.35, .39)	1.5 (1.1, 1.9)	.40 (.20, .90)
Trauma by external force to the leg[13] ◆		MCL tear per MRI	.21 (.07, .35)	.89 (.83, .96)	2.0 (.80, 4.8)	.90 (.70, 1.1)
Rotational trauma[13] ◆	134 patients with traumatic knee complaints		.62 (.41, .83)	.63 (.51, .74)	1.7 (1.1, 2.6)	.60 (.30, 1.1)
Age over 40 years[14] ◆		Meniscal tear per MRI	.70 (.57, .83)	.64 (.54, .74)	2.0 (1.4, 2.8)	.50 (.30, .70)
Continuation of activity impossible[1] ◆			.64 (.49, .78)	.55 (.45, .66)	1.4 (1.0, 2.0)	.70 (.40, 1.0)
Weight bearing during trauma[14] ◆			.85 (.75, .96)	.35 (.24, .46)	1.3 (1.1, 1.6)	.40 (.20, .90)

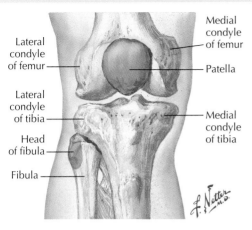

Lateral
condyle
of femur

Lateral
condyle
of tibia

Head
of fibula

Fibula

Medial
condyle
of femur

Patella

Medial
condyle
of tibia

Stiell and colleagues[66,67] identified a clinical prediction rule to determine the need to order radiographs following knee trauma. If one of five variables identified was present, radiographs were required. The five variables included an age ≥55 years, isolated patellar tenderness without other bone tenderness, tenderness of the fibular head, inability to flex knee to 90°, inability to bear weight immediately after injury and in the emergency room (unable to transfer weight onto each lower extremity, regardless of limping). This rule has been validated in numerous studies in adult[14,67,71] and pediatric[72,74] populations. The interexaminer agreement between clinicians for identification of predictor variables exhibited a kappa value of .77 with a 95% confidence interval of .65 to .89.[67]

Types of distal femur fractures

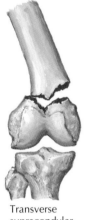

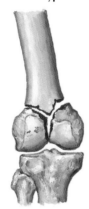

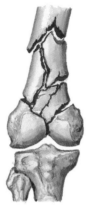

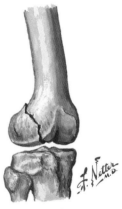

Transverse
supracondylar
fracture

Intercondylar (T or Y)
fracture

Comminuted fracture
extending into shaft

Fracture of single
condyle (may occur in
frontal or oblique plane)

Figure 7-15
Identifying the need to order radiographs following acute knee trauma.

7

Knee

Reliability of the Ottawa Knee Rule for Radiography

Test and Study Quality	Description and Positive Findings	Population	Interexaminer Reliability
Ottawa Knee Rule for Radiography in Adults[15] ◆	Knee x-rays ordered when patients exhibited any of the following: (1) Age 55 years or older (2) Isolated patellar tenderness without other bone tenderness (3) Tenderness of the fibular head (4) Inability to flex knee to 90 degrees (5) Inability to bear weight immediately after injury and in the emergency department	90 patients 18 to 79 years old visiting the emergency department of a general hospital with a knee injury that had occurred within the prior 7 days	κ = .51 (.32, .71)

Diagnostic Utility of the Ottawa Knee Rule for Radiography

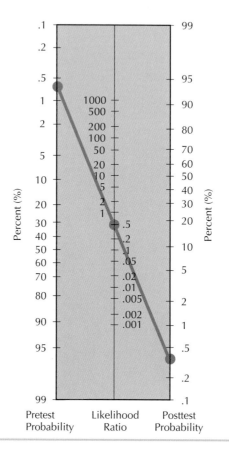

Figure 7-16

Nomogram. Assuming a fracture prevalence of 7% (statistically pooled from Bachmann and colleagues), an adult seen in the emergency department with an acute injury whose finding was negative on the Ottawa Knee Rule would have a 0.37% (95% CI: 0.15% to 1.48%) chance of having a knee fracture. (Adapted from Fagan TJ. Letter: Nomogram for Bayes theorem. *N Engl J Med.* 1975;293:257. Copyright 2005, Massachusetts Medical Society. See also Bachmann LM, Haberzeth S, Steurer J, ter Riet G. The accuracy of the Ottawa Knee Rule to rule out knee fractures: a systematic review. *Ann Intern Med.* 2004;140:121-124.)

Test and Study Quality	Description and Positive Findings	Population	Reference Standard	Sens	Spec	+LR	−LR
Ottawa Knee Rule for Radiography in Adults[16] ◆ **2004 Metaanalysis**		Statistically pooled data from six high-quality studies involving 4249 adults		.99 (.93, 1.0)	.49 (.43, .51)	1.9	.05 (.02, .23)
Ottawa Knee Rule for Radiography in Children[17] ◆ **2009 Metaanalysis**	As above	Statistically pooled data from three high-quality studies involving 1130 children	X-rays	.99 (.94, 1.0)	.46 (.43, .49)	1.9 (1.6, 2.4)	.07 (.02, .29)

Reliability of the Pittsburgh Decision Rule for Radiography

Test and Study Quality	Description and Positive Findings	Population	Interexaminer Reliability
Pittsburgh Rule for Radiography[15] ◆	Knee x-rays ordered when patients exhibited any of the following: (1) Fall or blunt trauma mechanism (2) Age older than 12 years or younger than 50 years or (1) Fall or blunt trauma mechanism (2) Age between 12 and 50 years (3) Inability to walk four weight-bearing steps in emergency department	90 patients 18 to 79 years old visiting the emergency department of a general hospital with a knee injury that had occurred within the prior 7 days	$\kappa = .71$ (.57, .86)

Diagnostic Utility of the Pittsburgh Decision Rule for Radiography

Test and Study Quality	Description and Positive Findings	Popula-tion	Reference Standard	Sens	Spec	+LR	−LR
Pittsburgh Rule for Radiography[15] ◆	As above	As above	X-rays	.86 (.57, .96)	.51 (.44, .59)	1.76	.28

Reliability of Clinical Assessments for Knee Osteoarthritis (OA)

Test and Study Quality	Description and Positive Findings	Population	Interexaminer Reliability
Bony Enlargement[18] ◆	With the patient's knees extended, observation and palpation of the distal end of femur and the proximal end of tibia was made for the presence of enlargement, assessed as either present, absent, or unsure		Interobserver κ = .66 (.32, 1.00) Intraobserver κ = .98 (.93, 1.00)
Quadriceps Wasting[18] ◆	With the patient's knee extended, observation was made by comparing it with the opposite leg for any apparent reduced muscle bulk of the quadriceps over the anterior aspect of the thigh proximal to the base of the patella, assessed as either present, unsure, or absent		Interobserver κ = .78 (.40, 1.00) Intraobserver κ = .83 (.72, .95)
Knee Joint Crepitus[18] ◆	Patient's knee flexed and extended with the examiner's hand over the anterior aspect of the knee joint and feeling for the presence of any palpatory/audible crepitus anywhere within the knee joint, assessed as present (palpable), present (audible), absent, or unsure		Interobserver κ = .78 (.36, 1.00) Intraobserver κ = .78 (.55, 1.00)
Medial Tibiofemoral Joint Tenderness[18] ◆	With the knee flexed to about 90°, firm thumb pressure was used to palpate for any tenderness along the tibiofemoral joint line, differentiating tenderness on the medial and lateral side of the joint, assessed as present or absent medial tenderness and present or absent lateral tenderness		Interobserver κ = .76 (.50, 1.00) Intraobserver κ = 64 (.49, .80)
Lateral Tibiofemoral Joint Tenderness[18] ◆		Interobserver Reliability = 25 subjects with symptomatic knee OA	Interobserver κ = 1.00 (1.00, 1.00) Intraobserver κ = .60 (.39, .80)
Patellofemoral Joint Tenderness[18] ◆	With the knee extended, firm thumb pressure was used to palpate along the medial, lateral, superior, and inferior borders of the patella for any tenderness, assessed as present or absent	Intraobserver Reliability = 88 subjects with symptomatic knee OA	Interobserver κ = .53 (.16, .89) Intraobserver κ = .66 (.60, .92)
Anserine Tenderness[18] ◆	With the knee flexed to about 90°, firm thumb pressure was used to palpate the area of the pes anserine bursa over the anteromedial superior aspect of tibia, about 3 to 4 fingers distal to the medial joint line, assessed as present or absent		Interobserver κ = .49 (.09, .87) Intraobserver κ = .73 (.61, .99)
Effusion: Bulge Sign[18] ◆	With the knee extended, starting at the medial gutter, the examiner stroked upward 2 to 3 times toward the suprapatellar pouch and then stroked downward on the lateral aspect of the knee joint from the suprapatellar pouch toward the lateral joint line and observed for any wave of fluid reappearing on the medial side of the knee. Graded from 0 to 3 (0 = no wave produced on downstroke; 1 = larger bulge on medial side with downstroke; 2 = spontaneously returned to medial side after upstroke, 3 = so much fluid that it was not possible to move the effusion out of the medial aspect of the knee)		Interobserver κ = .78 (.55, 1.00) Intraobserver κ = .83 (.73, .94)
Effusion: Ballottement Test[18] ◆	With the knee extended, using one hand to apply pressure over the suprapatellar pouch squeezing fluid downward while the thumb and index finger of the opposite hand applied anteroposterior pressure onto the patella, assessed as present without click, present with click (tap), or absent		Interobserver κ = .73 (.45, 1.00) Intraobserver κ = .77 (.60, .95)

Reliability of Detecting Inflammation

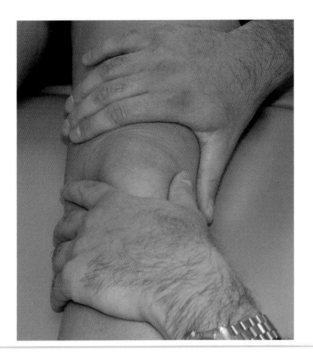

Figure 7-17
Fluctuation test.

Test and Study Quality	Description and Positive Findings	Population	Interexaminer Reliability
Observation of swelling[19]	Not described	53 patients with knee pain	$\kappa = -.02$ to .65
Palpation for warmth[19]			$\kappa = -.18$
Palpation for swelling[19]			$\kappa = -.11$ to .11
Fluctuation test[20]	With patient supine, examiner places thumb and finger around patella while pushing any fluid from suprapatellar pouch with other hand. Positive if finger and thumb are pushed apart	152 patients with unilateral knee dysfunction	$\kappa = .37$
Patellar tap test[20]	With patient supine, examiner presses suprapatellar pouch and then taps on patella. Patella remains in contact with femur if no swelling is present		$\kappa = .21$
Palpation for warmth[20]	Examiner palpates anterior aspect of knee. Results compared with uninvolved knee		$\kappa = .66$
Visual inspection for redness[20]	Examiner visually inspects involved knee for redness and compares it with uninvolved side		$\kappa = .21$

Reliability of the Stroke Test for Identifying Knee Joint Effusion

Test and Study Quality	Description and Positive Findings	Population	Interexaminer Reliability
Stroke test[21]	Patient is supine and has knee in full extension. Starting at the medial tibiofemoral joint line, the examiner strokes upward two or three times toward the suprapatellar pouch in an attempt to move the swelling within the joint capsule to the suprapatellar pouch. The examiner then strokes downward on the distal lateral thigh, just superior to the suprapatellar pouch, toward the lateral joint line. Positive if fluid is observed on the medial side of the knee and quantified using a 5-point scale	75 patients referred to an outpatient physical therapy clinic for treatment of knee dysfunction for which effusion testing was deemed appropriate by the treating therapist	$\kappa = .64$ (.54, .81)

Stroke Test Grading Scale[21]

Grade	Test Result
Zero	No wave produced on downstroke
Trace	Small wave on medial side with downstroke
1+	Larger bulge on medial side with downstroke
2+	Effusion spontaneously returns to medial side after upstroke (no downstroke necessary)
3+	So much fluid that it is not possible to move the effusion out of the medial aspect of the knee

Diagnostic Utility of Tests for Identifying Knee Joint Effusion

Test and Study Quality	Description and Positive Findings	Population	Reference Standard	Sens	Spec	+LR	−LR
Ballottement test[12] ◆	Examiner quickly pushes the patient's patella posteriorly with two or three fingers. Positive if patella bounces off trochlea with a distinct impact	134 patients with traumatic knee complaints	Knee joint effusion per MRI	.83 (.71, .94)	.49 (.39, .59)	1.6 (1.3, 2.1)	.30 (.20, .70)
Self-noticed knee swelling + Ballottement test[12] ◆	Combination of two findings			.67 (.52, .81)	.82 (.73, .90)	3.6 (2.2, 5.9)	.40 (.30, .60)
Bulge sign[106] ◆	Examiner uses the flat of the hand to sweep upward from the lower medial side of the knee with sustained moderate pressure and then sweeps the hand downward on the lateral side of the knee. Positive if bulge appeared in the medial recess	312 participants (344 knees) with early knee OA		.38 (.26, .52)	.88 (.83, .93)	3.08 (1.8, 4.9)	0.71 (0.55, 0.86)
Patellar tap test[22] ◆	Fluid in the suprapatellar pouch is pushed into the knee joint and held with sustained hand pressure. Positive if the patella is felt to abruptly stop as it contacted the underlying femoral condyles			.10 (.02, .19)	.96 (.93, .98)	2.25 (0.5, 6.3)	0.94 (0.84, 1.02)
Self-noticed knee swelling[22] ◆	Patient reports knee swelling			.49 (.35, .62)	.86 (.81, .90)	3.35 (2.3, 5.1)	0.60 (0.44, 0.76)
Self-reported pain with leg straightening[22] ◆	Patient reports pain with leg straightening			.56 (.43, .70)	.80 (.76, .85)	2.87 (2.0, 4.1)	0.54 (0.37, 0.71)
Self-noticed knee swelling + Self-reported pain with leg straightening[22] ◆	Combination of two findings			.36 (.23, .50)	.93 (.90, .96)	5.19 (2.9, 9.7)	0.69 (0.54, 0.83)

7

Knee

Reliability of Range-of-Motion Measurements

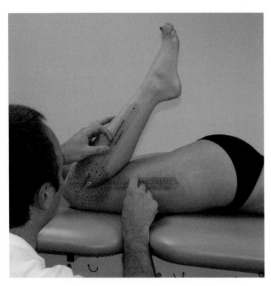

Figure 7-18
Measurement of active knee flexion range of motion.

Measurements and Study Quality	Instrumentation	Population	Reliability			
Active flexion sitting[23] ◆	Standard goniometer	30 patients 3 days after total knee arthroplasty	Interexaminer ICC = .86 (.64, .94)			
Passive flexion sitting[23] ◆			Interexaminer ICC = .88 (.69, .95)			
Active flexion supine[23] ◆			Interexaminer ICC = .89 (.78, .95)			
Passive flexion supine[23] ◆			Interexaminer ICC = .88 (.77, .94)			
Active extension[23] ◆			Interexaminer ICC = .64 (.38, .81)			
Passive extension[23] ◆			Interexaminer ICC = .62 (.28, .80)			
Passive flexion Passive extension[24] ◆	Standard goniometer	25 patients with knee OA	Interexaminer ICC = .87 (.73, .94) Interexaminer ICC = .69 (.41, .85)			
Passive flexion and extension[25] ◆	Three standard goniometers (metal, large plastic, and small plastic)	24 patients referred for physical therapy	Intraexaminer ICC			
				Flexion	Extension	
			Metal	.97	.96	
			Large	.99	.91	
			Small	.99	.97	
Passive flexion Passive extension[27] ◆	Standard goniometer	43 patients referred for physical therapy where examination would normally include passive range-of-motion measurements of knee	Intraexaminer ICC		Interexaminer ICC	
			Flexion	.99	Flexion	.90
			Extension	.98	Extension	.86
Passive flexion Passive extension[27] ◆	Visual estimation		Interexaminer ICC = .83 Interexaminer ICC = .82			
Passive flexion[19] ◖	Standard goniometer	53 patients with knee pain	Intraexaminer ICC = .82 Interexaminer ICC = .68			
Passive flexion[26] ◖	Standard goniometer	30 asymptomatic subjects	Interexaminer ICC = .99			

Reliability of Range-of-Motion Measurements—cont'd

Measurements and Study Quality	Instrumentation	Population	Reliability			
Active flexion Active extension[28]	Standard goniometer	20 asymptomatic subjects	Intraexaminer ICC = .95 Intraexaminer ICC = .85			
Active flexion[29]	Universal goniometer	60 healthy university students	Intraexaminer ICC = .86 to .97 Interexaminer ICC = .62 to 1.0			
Passive flexion Passive extension[20]	Standard goniometer	152 patients with unilateral knee dysfunction	Interexaminer ICC			
			Involved knee		Uninvolved knee	
			Flexion	.97	Flexion	.80
			Extension	.94	Extension	.72

ICC, Intraclass correlation coefficient.

Reliability of Determining Capsular and Noncapsular End Feels

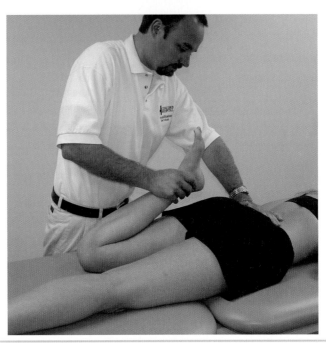

Figure 7-19
Assessment of end feel for knee flexion.

Test and Study Quality	Description and Positive Findings	Population	Reliability
Flexion end feel Extension end feel[24] ◆	End feel is assessed at end of passive range of motion and categorized as "normal," "empty," "stiff," or "loose"	25 patients with knee OA	Interexaminer ICC = .31 (−.53, 1.15) Interexaminer ICC = .25 (−.18, .68)
Flexion end feel Extension end feel[30] ◆	End feel is assessed at end of passive range of motion and graded on an 11-point scale with "capsular at end of normal range," "capsular early in range," "capsular," "tissue approximation," "springy block," "bony," "spasm," or "empty"	40 patients with unilateral knee pain	Intraexaminer κ = .76 (.55, .97) Interexaminer κ = −.01 (−.36, .35) Intraexaminer κ = 1.0 (1.0, 1.0) Interexaminer κ = .43 (−.06, .92)
End-feel assessment during Lachman test[31] ◆	Examiners asked to grade end feel during Lachman test. End feel graded as "hard" or "soft"	35 patients referred to physical therapy clinics for rehabilitation of knee joint	Intraexaminer κ = .33
End feel of adduction stress applied to knee[32] ◆	Examiner places knee in 0 degrees and 30 degrees of flexion and applies valgus force through knee. End feel graded as "soft" or "firm"	50 patients referred to an outpatient orthopaedic clinic who would normally undergo valgus stress tests directed at knee	Interexaminer 0 degrees of flexion κ = .00 30 degrees of flexion κ = .33

Reliability of Assessing Pain during Range-of-Motion Movements

Test and Study Quality	Description and Positive Findings	Population	Reliability
Pain resistance sequence: Passive flexion[29] ◆	Pain sequence is assessed during passive range of motion of knee. Pain is graded on a 4-point scale as "no pain," "pain occurs after resistance is felt," "pain occurs at the same time as resistance is felt," or "pain occurs before resistance is felt"	40 patients with unilateral knee pain	Intraexaminer κ = .78 (.68, .87) Interexaminer κ = .51
Pain resistance sequence: Passive extension[30] ◆			Intraexaminer κ = .85 (.75, .95) Interexaminer κ = .42
Assessment of pain during adduction stress applied to knee[32] ◆	Examiner places knee in 0 degrees and 30 degrees of flexion and applies valgus force through knee. Pain responses recorded	50 patients referred to outpatient orthopaedic clinic who would normally undergo valgus stress tests directed at knee	Interexaminer 0 degrees of flexion κ = .40 30 degrees of flexion κ = .33
Pain resistance sequence: Passive flexion[20] ◐	Examiner passively flexes knee. Subject is directed to report when pain is above baseline levels. Examiner reports if pain occurs before, during, or after passive range-of-motion limitation has occurred	152 patients with unilateral knee dysfunction	Interexaminer κ = .28

7

Knee

Reliability of Strength Assessment

Measurements and Study Quality	Instrumentation	Population	Reliability
Determination of one repetition maximum (1RM) knee extension[33] ●	With patient sitting in leg extension machine, patient performs slow knee extension from 100 degrees to 0 degrees. Amount of weight is systematically increased until patient can no longer complete lift. 1RM defined as the heaviest resistance that could be lifted once	27 asymptomatic adults	Interday (same examiner) ICC = .90 Interexaminer ICC = .96
Isometric extensor strength[19] ●	Against inflated sphygmomanometer cuff	53 patients with knee pain	Intraexaminer ICC = .85 Interexaminer ICC = .83
Isometric flexor strength[19] ●			Intraexaminer ICC = .89 Interexaminer ICC = .70

Diagnostic Utility of Manual Muscle Testing for Detecting Strength Deficits

Test and Study Quality	Description and Positive Findings	Population	Reference Standard	Sens	Spec	+LR	−LR
Manual muscle testing of knee extension strength[34] ●	Patient extends knee as forcefully as possible into examiner's hand. Strength graded on a scale of 0 to 5	107 patients from an acute rehabilitation hospital	Side-to-side difference with a handheld dynamometer of: 15%	.63	.89	5.7	.42
			20%	.68	.88	5.7	.36
			25%	.72	.83	4.2	.34
			30%	.72	.77	3.1	.36

Reliability of Assessing Muscle Length

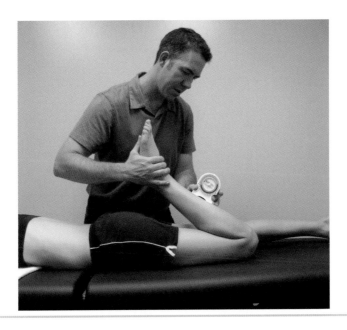

Figure 7-20
Quadriceps length.

Test and Study Quality	Description and Positive Findings	Population	Interexaminer Reliability
Quadriceps length[24] ◆	Assessed with Thomas test	25 patients with knee OA	Result: $\kappa = .18$ (−.17, .53) Pain: $\kappa = .39$ (.14, .64)
Quadriceps length[35] ◆	Passive knee flexion test with inclinometer	14 asymptomatic participants	Intraexaminer ICC = .73 to .90 Interexaminer ICC = .81 to .95
Hamstring length[35] ◆	Passive knee extension test with inclinometer	14 asymptomatic participants	Intraexaminer ICC = .88 to .97 Interexaminer ICC = .88 to .97
Hamstring length[36] ◉	Active knee extension test with goniometer	16 asymptomatic participants	ICC = .81 (.41, .94)
Hamstring length[37] ◉	Straight-leg raise test with inclinometer		ICC = .92 (.82, .96)
Iliotibial band/tensor fasciae latae complex length[37] ◉	Ober test with inclinometer		ICC = .97 (.93, .98)
Quadriceps length[37] ◉	Quadriceps femoris muscle angle with inclinometer	30 patients with patellofemoral pain syndrome	ICC = .91 (.80, .96)
Gastrocnemius length[37] ◉	Dorsiflexion with knee extended and inclinometer		ICC = .92 (.83, .96)
Soleus length[37] ◉	Dorsiflexion with knee flexed 90 degrees and inclinometer		ICC = .86 (.71, .94)

7

Knee

Reliability of Assessment of Mediolateral Patellar Tilt

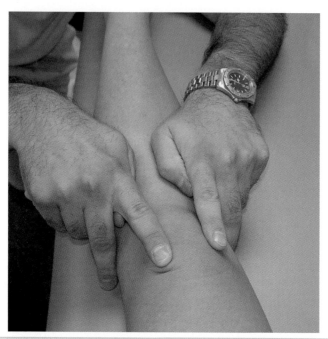

Figure 7-21
Examination of mediolateral patellar tilt.

Test and Measure Quality	Procedure	Determination of Positive Finding	Population	Reliability
Mediolateral tilt[38] ◆	Examiner estimates patellar alignment while palpating medial and lateral aspects of patella	Patellar orientation graded using an ordinal scale extending from −2 to +2, with −2 representing a lateral tilt, 0 no appreciable tilt, and +2 a medial tilt	27 asymptomatic subjects	Intraexaminer κ = .57 Interexaminer κ = .18
Mediolateral tilt[39] ●	Examiner palpates medial and lateral borders of patella with thumb and index finger	If digit palpating the medial border is higher than the lateral border, then patella is considered laterally tilted. If digit palpating the lateral border is higher than the patella, then patella is medially tilted	66 patients referred for physical therapy who would normally undergo an evaluation of patellofemoral alignment	Interexaminer κ = .21
Mediolateral tilt[40] ●	Examiner attempts to palpate posterior surface of medial and lateral patellar borders	Scored 0, 1, or 2. Score is 0 if examiner palpates posterior border on both medial and lateral sides. Score is 1 if more than 50% of lateral border can be palpated but posterior surface cannot. Score is 2 if less than 50% of lateral border can be palpated	56 subjects, 25 of whom had symptomatic knees	Intraexaminer κ = .28 to .33 Interexaminer κ = .19
Patellar tilt test[40] ●	Examiner lifts lateral edge of patella from lateral femoral epicondyle	Graded as having positive, neutral, or negative angle with respect to horizontal plane	99 knees, of which 26 were symptomatic	Intraexaminer κ = .44 to .50 Interexaminer κ = .20 to .35

Reliability of Assessment of Patellar Orientation

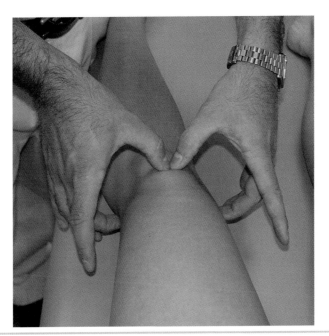

Figure 7-22
Examination of mediolateral patellar orientation.

Test and Measure Quality	Procedure	Determination of Positive Finding	Population	Reliability
Mediolateral position[38] ◆	Examiner visually estimates patellar alignment while palpating sides of lateral epicondyles with index fingers and patella midline with thumbs	Patellar orientation graded using an ordinal scale extending from −2 to +2, with −2 representing a lateral displacement and +2 a medial displacement	27 asymptomatic subjects	Intraexaminer κ = .40 Interexaminer κ = .03
Mediolateral orientation[41] ●	With patient's knee supported in 20 degrees of flexion, examiner identifies medial and lateral epicondyle of femur and midline of patella. Examiner then marks medial and lateral epicondyle and patella midline with tape	Distances between patella midline and medial and lateral condyles are measured	20 healthy physiotherapy students	Interexaminer Medial distance: ICC = .91 Lateral distance: ICC = .94
Mediolateral orientation[42] ●	As described above	As described above	15 asymptomatic subjects	Interexaminer ICC = .60 to .75

Reliability of Assessment of Patellar Orientation—cont'd

Test and Measure Quality	Procedure	Determination of Positive Finding	Population	Reliability
Mediolateral displacement[39] ●	Examiner palpates medial and lateral epicondyles with index fingers while simultaneously palpating midline of patella with thumbs	Distance between index fingers and thumbs should be same. When distance between index finger palpating lateral epicondyle is less, patella is laterally displaced. When distance between index finger palpating medial epicondyle is less, patella is medially displaced	66 patients referred for physical therapy who would normally undergo evaluation of patellofemoral alignment	Interexaminer κ = .10
Mediolateral glide[40] ●	Examiner uses a tape measure to record distance from medial and lateral femoral condyles to midpatella	Scored 0 or 1. Score is 0 if the distance from medial epicondyle to midpatella equals distance from lateral epicondyle to midpatella. Score is 1 if the distance from medial epicondyle to midpatella is 0.5 cm greater than from lateral condyle to midpatella	56 subjects, 25 of whom had symptomatic knees	Intraexaminer κ = .11 to .35 Interexaminer κ = .02

Reliability of Assessing Superoinferior Patellar Tilt

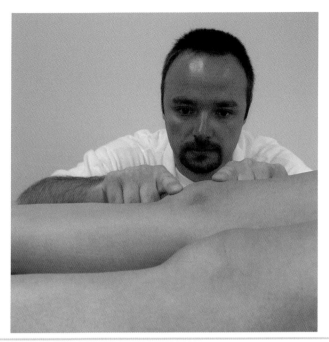

Figure 7-23
Examination of anteroposterior patellar tilt.

Test and Measure Quality	Procedure	Determination of Positive Finding	Population	Reliability
Superoinferior tilt[38] ◆	Examiner visually estimates patellar alignment while palpating superior and inferior patellar poles	Patellar orientation graded using an ordinal scale extending from −2 to +2, with −2 representing inferior patellar pole below superior pole and +2 representing inferior patellar pole above superior pole	27 asymptomatic subjects	Intraexaminer κ = .50 Interexaminer κ = .30
Anterior tilt[39]	Examiner palpates inferior patellar pole	If examiner easily palpates inferior pole, no anterior tilt exists. If downward pressure on superior pole is required to palpate inferior pole, it is considered to have an anterior tilt	66 patients referred for physical therapy who would normally undergo evaluation of patellofemoral alignment	Interexaminer κ = .24
Anteroposterior tilt component[40]	Examiner palpates inferior and superior patellar poles	Scored 0, 1, or 2. Score is 0 if inferior patellar pole is as easily palpable as superior pole. Score is 1 if inferior patellar pole is not as easily palpable as superior pole. Score is 2 if inferior pole is not clearly palpable compared with superior pole	56 subjects, 25 of whom had symptomatic knees	Intraexaminer κ = .03 to .23 Interexaminer κ = .04

Reliability of Assessing Patellar Rotation

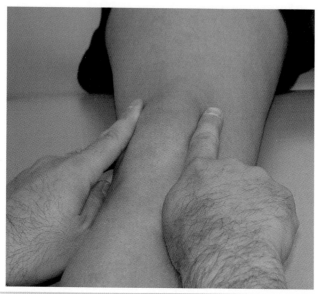

Figure 7-24
Examination of patellar rotation.

Test and Measure Quality	Procedure	Determination of Positive Finding	Population	Reliability
Rotation[38] ◆	Examiner positions index fingers along longitudinal axes of patella and estimates acute angle formed	Graded using ordinal scale extending from −2 to +2. −2 represents longitudinal axis of patella being more lateral than axis of femur. +2 represents patella being more medial than axis of femur	27 asymptomatic subjects	Intraexaminer κ = .41 Interexaminer κ = −.03
Patellar rotation[39] ●		Longitudinal axis of patella should be in line with anterior superior iliac spine. If distal end of patella is medial, it is considered to be medially rotated. If distal end is lateral, it is considered to be laterally rotated	66 patients referred for physical therapy who would normally undergo evaluation of patellofemoral alignment	Interexaminer κ = .36
Patellar rotation component[40] ●	Examiner determines relationship between longitudinal axis of patella and femur	Scored as −1, 0, or +1. Score is 0 when patellar long axis is parallel to long axis of femur. Score is 1 when inferior patellar pole is lateral to axis of femur and classified as a lateral patellar rotation. Score is −1 when inferior pole is medial to axis of femur and classified as medial patellar rotation	56 subjects, 25 of whom had symptomatic knees	Intraexaminer κ = −.06 to .00 Interexaminer κ = −.03

Reliability of Patellar Mobility in Patients with Patellofemoral Pain Syndrome

Test and Measure Quality	Procedure	Determination of Positive Finding	Population	Reliability
Superior-inferior mobility[43] ●	Examiner translates patella inferiorly	Patellar mobility graded as diminished or nondiminished	82 patients with anterior knee pain of more than 4 weeks' duration	Interexaminer κ = .55 (−.37, .69)
Medial-lateral mobility[43] ●	Examiner translates patella laterally			Interexaminer κ = .59 (.42, .72)
Inferior pole tilt[43] ●	Examiner applies a posterior force with index finger on superior pole of patella and observes for tilting of inferior pole of patella			Interexaminer κ = .48 (−.28, .61)
Patellar tendon mobility[43] ●	Examiner stabilizes the patella with one hand while translating the patellar tendon medially with the other hand			Interexaminer κ = .45 (−.27, .56)

Diagnostic Utility of Patellar Mobility in Identifying Patients with Patellofemoral Pain Syndrome

Test and Study Quality	Description and Positive Findings	Population	Reference Standard*	Sens	Spec	+LR	−LR
Superior-inferior mobility[43] ●	Examiner translates patella inferiorly. Patellar mobility graded as diminished or nondiminished	82 patients with anterior knee pain of more than 4 weeks' duration	Physician diagnosis of patellofemoral pain syndrome	.63 (.56, .69)	.56 (.39, .72)	1.4 (.90, 2.5)	.70 (.40, 1.1)
Medial-lateral mobility[43] ●	Examiner translates patella laterally. Patellar mobility graded as diminished or nondiminished			.54 (.47, .59)	.69 (.52, 83)	1.8 (.90, 3.6)	.70 (.50, 1.0)
Inferior pole tilt[43] ●	Examiner applies a posterior force with index finger on superior pole of patella and observes for tilting of inferior pole of patella. Patellar mobility graded as diminished or nondiminished			.19 (.13, .22)	.83 (.68, .93)	1.1 (.40, 3.0)	.90 (.80, 1.3)
Patellar tendon mobility[43] ●	Examiner stabilizes the patella with one hand while translating the patellar tendon medially with the other hand. Patellar mobility graded as diminished or nondiminished			.49 (.43, .53)	.83 (.66, .93)	2.8 (1.3, 7.3)	.60 (.50, .90)

*Note: There is currently no definitive reference standard for patellofemoral pain syndrome. The disorder is a clinical diagnosis often made by ruling out other potential disorders.

7

Knee

Reliability of Assessing Quadriceps Angle Measurements

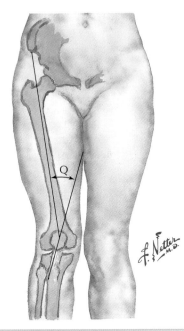

Q-angle formed by intersection of lines from anterior superioriliac spine and from tibial tuberosity through midpoint of patella. Large Q-angle predisposes to patellar subluxation

Figure 7-25
Quadriceps angle.

Test and Measure Quality	Procedure	Population	Reliability ICC	
Q angle[45] ◆	As below. Measure with knee in 10 degrees of flexion	18 asymptomatic subjects	Short-arm goniometer	
			Intraexaminer ICC = .78 (.67, .86)	Interexaminer ICC = .56 (.28, .75)
			Long-arm goniometer	
			Intraexaminer ICC = .92 (.88, .95)	Interexaminer ICC = .88 (.77, .93)
Q angle[38] ◆	Proximal arm of goniometer is aligned with anterior superior iliac spine, distal arm is aligned with tibial tubercle, and fulcrum is positioned over patellar midpoint	27 asymptomatic subjects	Intraexaminer ICC = .63 Interexaminer ICC = .23	
Q angle[37] ●		30 patients with patellofemoral pain syndrome	Interexaminer ICC = .70 (.46, .85)	
Q angle[44] ●	As above. Measure with knee fully extended and in 20 degrees of flexion	50 asymptomatic knees	Interexaminer at full extension	
			Right ICC = .14 to .21	Left ICC = .08 to .11
			Interexaminer at 20 degrees of knee flexion	
			Right ICC = .04 to .08	Left ICC = .13 to .16

Reliability of Assessing the Angle between the Longitudinal Axis of the Patella and the Patellar Tendon (A Angle)

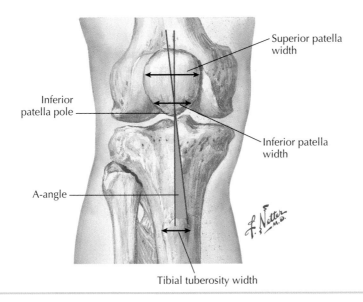

Figure 7-26
The A angle.

Test and Measure Quality	Procedure	Population	Reliability
A angle[38] ◆	Proximal and distal goniometer arms are aligned with middle of superior patellar pole and tibial tubercle. Fulcrum is positioned over midpoint of inferior patellar pole. Angle recorded in degrees	27 asymptomatic subjects	Intraexaminer ICC = .61 Interexaminer ICC = .49
A angle[46] ◉	Superior patellar pole, superior patellar width, inferior patellar width, inferior patellar pole, and tibial tuberosity are identified. The A angle is then measured with a goniometer. Angle recorded in degrees	36 asymptomatic subjects	Intraexaminer ICC = .20 to .32 Interexaminer ICC = −.01

Reliability of the Lateral Pull Test to Assess Patellar Alignment

Test and Study Quality	Description and Positive Findings	Population	Reliability
Lateral pull test[47] ◆	With patient supine and knee extended, examiner asks patient to perform isometric quadriceps contraction. Examiner observes patellar tracking during contraction. Positive if patella tracks more laterally than superiorly. Negative if superior displacement is equal to lateral displacement	99 knees, 26 of which were symptomatic	Intraexaminer κ = .39 to .47 Interexaminer κ = .31

Reliability of Pain during Palpation

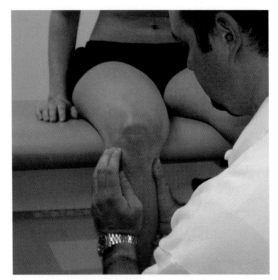

Palpation of lateral joint line

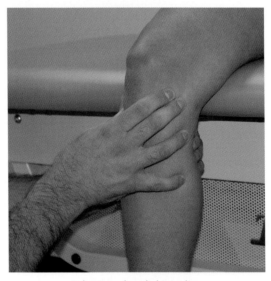

Palpation of medial joint line

Figure 7-27
Palpation of joint lines.

Physical Finding and Study Quality	Population	Reliability
Posterior joint line tenderness[48] ◆	71 patients with knee pain	Interexaminer κ = .48
Palpation for tenderness[19] ●	53 patients with knee pain	Interexaminer κ = .10 to .30
Tenderness at medial joint line[10] ●	152 patients with OA of knee	Interexaminer κ = .21 (.01, .41)
Tenderness at lateral joint line[10] ●		Interexaminer κ = .25 (.07, .43)

Diagnostic Utility of Joint Line Tenderness

Test and Study Quality	Description and Positive Findings	Population	Reference Standard	Sens	Spec	+LR	−LR
Joint line tenderness[49] ◆ 2010 Metaanalysis	Depended on study, but generally: Examiner palpates joint line with patient's knee in 90 degrees of flexion. Positive if test reproduces pain	Pooled estimates from 13 studies*	Meniscal tears via arthroscopy, arthrotomy, or MRI	.64 (.62, .66)	.61 (.59, .63)	1.6 (1.5, 1.8)	.59 (.54, .65)
Joint line tenderness[50] ◆ 2008 Metaanalysis		Pooled, quality-adjusted estimates from eight studies*	Meniscal tears via arthroscopy or arthrotomy	.76 (.73, .80)	.77 (.64, .87)	3.3	.31
Joint line tenderness[51] ◆ 2007 Metaanalysis		Pooled estimates from 14 studies*	Meniscal tears via arthroscopy, arthrotomy, or MRI	.63 (.61, .66)	.77 (.76, .79)	2.7	.48

*Some of the included studies would not have met our QUADAS quality criterion for inclusion.

Diagnostic Utility of Joint Line Fullness

Test and Study Quality	Description and Positive Findings	Population	Reference Standard	Sens	Spec	+LR	−LR
Joint line fullness[52] ◆	With patient supine, the examiner palpates along the joint line to identify palpable fullness in comparison with the normal knee. The lateral compartment of the knee was examined at 30 to 45 degrees of knee flexion to relax the iliotibial band and the medial compartment, at 70 to 90 degrees of flexion to relax the medial collateral ligament. Any joint line fullness causing a loss of normal joint compression was a positive result	100 patients undergoing routine knee arthroscopy (18 for lateral compartment pathologic condition, 70 for medial compartment pathologic condition, 12 for unknown intraarticular knee pathologic condition)	Meniscal tears via arthroscopy	.70	.82	3.89	.37

7

Knee

Reliability of the Lachman Test

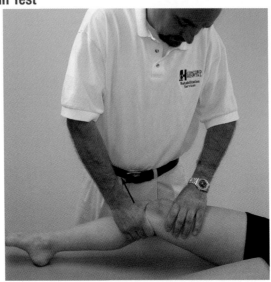

Figure 7-28
Lachman test (see Fig. 7-29 for prone Lachman test).

Test and Measure Quality	Procedure	Determination of Positive Finding	Population	Reliability
Lachman test[53] ◆	Patient in supine with knee flexed 20 to 30 degrees. Examiner's upper hand stabilized the unsupported distal thigh, while the lower hand, with the thumb on the anterior joint line, and the fingers feeling to ensure that the hamstrings were relaxed, pulled the tibia forward with approximately 30 lbs of force	Examiner provided a translational (numerical) grade and an endpoint (letter) grade based on the following operation definition: I (<5 mm translation), II (5–10 mm translation), III (>10 mm translation) A (firm, sudden endpoint to passive anterior translation), B (absent, ill-defined, or softened endpoint to passive anterior translation)	45 patients referred from the emergency room to orthopaedic surgery/sports medicine for definitive evaluation of a painful knee	For translational (numerical) grade
				Interexaminer κ = .42 (.16, .66)
				For endpoint (letter) grade
				Interexaminer κ = .72 (.50, .95)
Lachman test[31] ◆	Examiners perform Lachman test as they would in practice	Results are graded as "positive" or "negative." Examiners also grade amount of anterior tibial translation as 0, 1+, 2+, or 3+. Score of 0 represents no difference in tibial translation between unaffected and affected knees	35 patients referred to physical therapy clinics for rehabilitation of knee joint	For positive or negative findings
				Intraexaminer κ = .51 Interexaminer κ = .19
				For grading of tibial translation
				Intraexaminer κ = .44 to .60 Interexaminer κ = .02 to .61

Reliability of the Lachman Test—cont'd

Test and Measure Quality	Procedure	Determination of Positive Finding	Population	Reliability
Prone Lachman test[54]◆ (see Video 7-1)	Patient in prone position with lower extremity fully relaxed and small towel roll placed under distal end of the involved thigh. The examiner places the distal hand on the anterior proximal tibia, with the index finger and long finger positioned on each side of the patellar tendon, resting on the anterior joint line. The examiner's thigh is placed under the patient's shin to support the patient's knee in 10 to 30 degrees of flexion. The heel of the examiner's proximal hand is placed over the posterocentral aspect of the proximal tibia, with the fingers lightly resting on the medial gastrocnemius, and is used to direct an anterior force on the posterior tibia, while the fingers of the distal hand apply slight pressure directed posteriorly and simultaneously palpate the amount of anterior tibial translation relative to the femur	The test is positive if there is absence of end feel or a perception of greater than 3 mm anterior translation on the injured side as compared with the uninvolved side	52 patients referred from the emergency room of a hospital to orthopaedic surgery for definitive evaluation of a painful knee	Interexaminer κ = .60
Lachman test[10] ◍	Not specified	Not specified	152 patients with OA of knee	Interexaminer κ = −.08 (−.12, .04)

Diagnostic Utility of the Lachman Test in Identifying Anterior Cruciate Ligament Tears

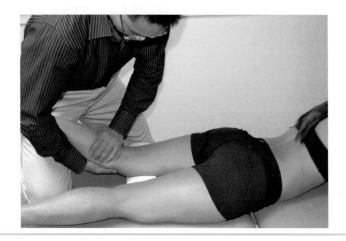

Figure 7-29
Prone Lachman test.

Test and Study Quality	Description and Positive Findings	Population	Reference Standard	Sens	Spec	+LR	−LR
Lachman test (without anesthesia)[55] ◆ **2013 Metaanalysis**	Depended on study, but generally: With patient supine and knee joint flexed between 10 and 20 degrees, examiner stabilizes femur with one hand. With other hand, examiner translates tibia anteriorly. Positive if lack of end point for tibial translation or subluxation is positive	Pooled estimates from 1579 patients from 17 studies*	ACL tears via arthroscopy, arthrotomy, or MRI	.81	.81	4.26	.24
Lachman test (with anesthesia)[55] ◆ **2013 Metaanalysis**		Pooled estimates from 1189 patients from 12 studies*		.91	.78	4.14	.12
Lachman test (without anesthesia)[56] ◆ **2006 Metaanalysis**		Pooled estimates from 2276 patients from 21 studies*		.85 (.83, .87)	.94 (.92, .95)	1.2 (4.6, 22.7)	.20 (.10, .30)
Lachman test (with anesthesia)[56] ◆ **2006 Metaanalysis**		Pooled estimates from 1174 patients from 15 studies*		.97 (.96, .98)	.93 (.89, .96)	12.9 (1.5, 108.5)	.10 (.00, .30)
Prone Lachman test[54] ◆	As described for the prone Lachman test above	52 patients referred from the emergency room of a hospital to orthopaedic surgery for definitive evaluation of a painful knee	ACL tears via arthroscopy or MRI	.70 (.40, .89)	.80 (.38, .96)	3.5 (5.8, 21.2)	.57 (.32, .69)

*Some of the included studies would not have met our QUADAS quality criterion for inclusion.

Reliability of the Anterior Drawer Test

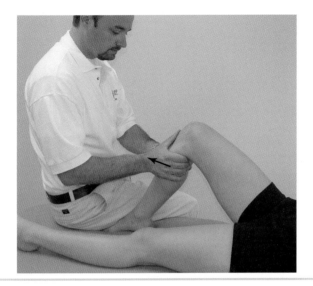

Figure 7-30
Anterior drawer test.

Test and Study Quality	Description and Positive Finding	Population	Interexaminer Reliability
Anterior drawer test[19] ●	Not specified	53 patients with knee pain	κ = .34

Diagnostic Utility of the Anterior Drawer Test in Identifying Anterior Cruciate Ligament Tears

Test and Study Quality	Description and Positive Findings	Population	Reference Standard	Sens	Spec	+LR	−LR
Anterior drawer test (without anesthesia)[55] ◆ **2013 Metaanalysis**	Depended on study, but generally: With patient's knee flexed between 60 and 90 degrees with foot on examination table, examiner draws tibia anteriorly. Positive if there is anterior subluxation of more than 5 mm	Pooled estimates from 934 patients from 13 studies*		.38	.81	2	.77
Anterior drawer test (without anesthesia)[55] ◆ **2013 Metaanalysis**		Pooled estimates from 826 patients from 10 studies*	ACL tears via arthroscopy, arthrotomy, or MRI	.63	.91	7	.41
Anterior drawer test (without anesthesia)[56] ◆ **2006 Metaanalysis**		Pooled estimates from 1809 patients from 20 studies*		.55 (.52, .58)	.92 (.90, .94)	7.3 (3.5, 15.2)	.50 (.40, .60)
Anterior drawer test (with anesthesia)[56] ◆ **2006 Metaanalysis**		Pooled estimates from 1306 patients from 15 studies*		.77 (.82, .91)	.87 (.82, .91)	5.9 (.90, 38.2)	.40 (.20, .80)

*Some of the included studies would not have met our QUADAS quality criterion for inclusion.

Diagnostic Utility of the Pivot Shift Test in Identifying Anterior Cruciate Ligament Tears

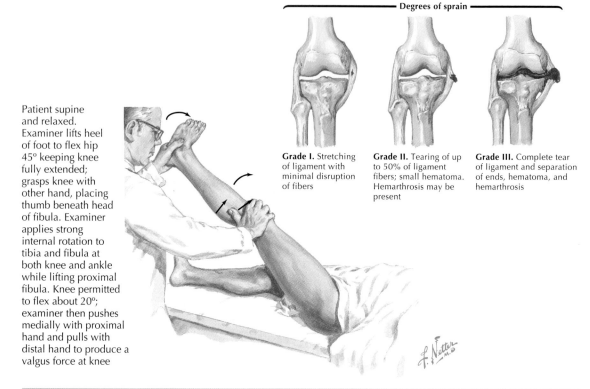

Patient supine and relaxed. Examiner lifts heel of foot to flex hip 45° keeping knee fully extended; grasps knee with other hand, placing thumb beneath head of fibula. Examiner applies strong internal rotation to tibia and fibula at both knee and ankle while lifting proximal fibula. Knee permitted to flex about 20°; examiner then pushes medially with proximal hand and pulls with distal hand to produce a valgus force at knee

Degrees of sprain

Grade I. Stretching of ligament with minimal disruption of fibers

Grade II. Tearing of up to 50% of ligament fibers; small hematoma. Hemarthrosis may be present

Grade III. Complete tear of ligament and separation of ends, hematoma, and hemarthrosis

Figure 7-31
Pivot shift test.

Test and Study Quality	Description and Positive Findings	Population	Reference Standard	Sens	Spec	+LR	−LR
Pivot shift test (without anesthesia)[55] ◆ **2013 Meta-analysis**	Depended on study, but generally: Patient's knee is placed in 10 to 20 degrees of flexion, and tibia is rotated internally while examiner applies valgus force. Positive if lateral tibial plateau subluxes anteriorly	Pooled estimates from 1192 patients from 12 studies*	ACL tears via arthroscopy, arthrotomy, or MRI	.28	.81	1.47	.89
Pivot shift test (with anesthesia)[55] ◆ **2013 Meta-analysis**		Pooled estimates from 1094 patients from 10 studies*		.73	.98	36.5	.28
Pivot shift test (without anesthesia)[56] ◆ **2006 Meta-analysis**		Pooled estimates from 1431 patients from 15 studies*		.24 (.21, .27)	.98 (.96, .99)	8.5 (4.7, 15.5)	.90 (.80, 1.0)
Pivot shift test (with anesthesia)[56] ◆ **2006 Meta-analysis**		Pooled estimates from 1077 patients from 13 studies*		.74 (.71, .77)	.99 (.96, 1.0)	2.9 (2.8, 156.2)	.30 (.10, .70)

*Some of the included studies would not have met our QUADAS quality criterion for inclusion.

Reliability of the Lever Sign

Test and Study Quality	Description and Positive Finding	Population	Interexaminer Reliability
Lever sign[57] ◔	See table below	94 patients at least 16 years old who suffered from knee trauma and had indications for knee arthroscopic surgery	$\kappa = .82$

Diagnostic Utility of the Lever Sign in Identifying Anterior Cruciate Ligament Tears

Test and Study Quality	Description and Positive Findings	Population	Reference Standard	Sens	Spec	+LR	−LR
Lever Sign[58] ◆ **2018 Meta-analysis**	Patient is supine with knees fully extended. The examiner stands at the side of the injured knee and places a closed fist under the calf at a proximal distance of one third of the lower leg to keep the knee joint in a slightly flexed position. With the other hand, the examiner applies moderate downward force to the distal third part of the patient's femur. The test is conducted only once. Positive if the knee joint does not extend and the heel stays on the table. Negative if the knee joint moves into full extension and the patient's heel rises up from the examination table	Pooled data from 6 studies	ACL tears via arthroscopy	.55 (.22, .84)	.89 (.44, .99)	9.2 (.70, 46.1)	.58 (.18, 1.28)

7

Knee

Diagnostic Utility of the Loss-of-Extension Test in Identifying Anterior Cruciate Ligament Tears

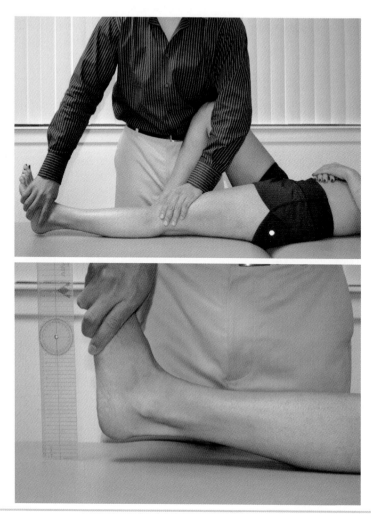

Figure 7-32
Loss-of-extension test.

Test and Study Quality	Description and Positive Findings	Population	Reference Standard	Sens	Spec	+LR	−LR
Loss-of-extension test[59] ◆ (see Video 7-2)	The examiner stabilizes the thigh of the affected knee with one hand with the patella facing forward, while the other hand extends the knee into maximum passive extension. A second examiner measures the distance between the patient's heel and the bed. The test is positive when the affected knee extends less than the healthy knee	196 patients with unilateral knee pathologic findings	ACL tears via MRI or surgical findings	.78	.95	15.6	.23

Reliability of Tests for Posterolateral Instability

Test and Study Quality	Description and Positive Finding	Population	Interex-aminer Reliabil-ity
Dial test at 30°[60] ●	Patient is in prone position with knee flexed at 30° and 90°. Examiner places both hands on the patient's feet, cupping the heels and applies external rotation to the knee joint. Positive if side-to-side difference of ≥10° of external rotation	52 patients between 18 and 50 years with strong suspicion or MRI evidence of ACL injury	κ = .29 (.01, .56)
Dial test at 90°[60] ●			κ = .38 (.10, .66)
Frog-leg test[61] ●	Patient in supine with both knees abducted and flexed 90 degrees bringing the soles of the feet together. Examiner faces patient with hypothenar eminence of each hand on the anteromedial aspect of patient's tibia. A varus stress is then applied simultaneously to both knees while the index or middle finger of each hand palpates the respective lateral joint line to assess for the amount of lateral compartment gapping and for comparison between knees. Positive if lateral compartment gapping of one knee is increased compared with the contralateral knee	12 subjects with chronic instability of the knee and posterolateral corner injury diagnosed by intraopera-tive findings and 9 subjects without posterolateral corner injury (used as controls)	κ = .86 (.72, 1.00)

Diagnostic Utility of Tests for Posterolateral Instability

Test and Study Quality	Description and Positive Findings	Population	Reference Standard	Sens	Spec	+LR	−LR
Frog-leg test[61]◆	Patient in supine with both knees abducted and flexed 90 degrees bringing the soles of the feet together. Examiner faces patient with hypothenar eminence of each hand on the anteromedial aspect of patient's tibia. A varus stress is then applied simultaneously to both knees while the index or middle finger of each hand palpates the respective lateral joint line to assess for the amount of lateral compartment gapping and for comparison between knees. Positive if lateral compartment gapping of one knee is increased compared with the contralat-eral knee	12 subjects with chronic instability of the knee and posterolateral corner injury diag-nosed by intraoper-ative findings and 9 subjects without posterolateral corner injury (used as controls)	MRI and in-traoperative findings	.92	.95	18.4*	.08*

*Values were calculated by the authors of this text.

Reliability of Varus and Valgus Stress Tests

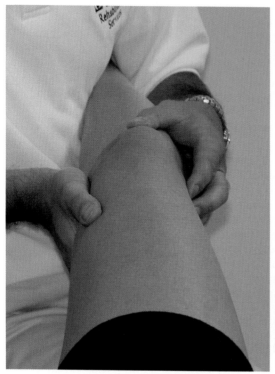

Varus stress test

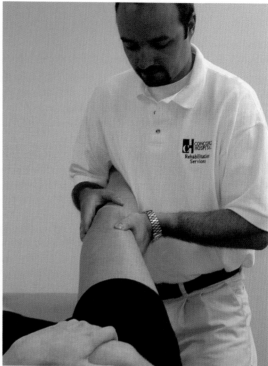

Valgus stress test

Figure 7-33
Varus and valgus stress tests.

Test and Study Quality	Description and Positive Finding	Population	Interexaminer Reliability
Varus test[19] ●		53 patients with knee pain	(Laxity) κ = .24 (Pain) κ = .18
Valgus test[19] ●	Not specified		(Laxity) κ = .48 (Pain) κ = .37
Varus test[10] ●		152 patients with OA of knee	κ = 0 (−.18, .18)
Valgus test[10] ●			κ = .05 (−.13, 2.3)

Diagnostic Utility of Valgus Stress for Identifying Medial Collateral Ligament Tears

Test and Study Quality	Description and Positive Findings	Population	Reference Standard	Sens	Spec	+LR	−LR
Pain with valgus stress at 30 degrees of knee flexion[13] ◆	Not specifically described	134 patients with traumatic knee complaint	MCL tears per MRI	.78 (.64, .92)	.67 (.57, .76)	2.3 (1.7, 3.3)	.30 (.20, .60)
Laxity with valgus stress at 30 degrees of knee flexion[13] ◆				.91 (.81, 1.0)	.49 (.39, .59)	1.8 (1.4, 2.2)	.20 (.10, .60)

Reliability of Tests for Identifying Meniscal Tears

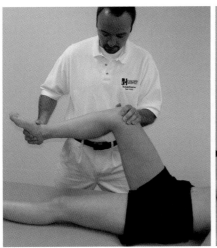
With internal rotation of tibia

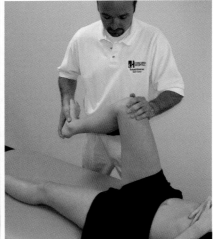
With external rotation of tibia

Figure 7-34
McMurray test.

Test and Study Quality	Description and Positive Finding	Population	Reliability
Deep squat test[62] ◆	Patient stands flatfooted on the floor and squats as deeply as possible while the examiner holds the patient's hands for balance. Positive if the patient experiences internal knee pain during flexion or a sense of locking		Interexaminer κ = .46 (.26, .65)
Thessaly test[62] ◆	Patient stands flatfooted on the affected limb, with the knee in 20° of flexion. With the examiner holding the patient's hands, the patient rotates the knee and body 3 times in each direction, while keeping the knee in 20° of flexion. Positive if the patient experiences medial or lateral joint line discomfort or has a sense of locking or catching	88 patients suspected of having internal derangement of the knee of less than 6 months in duration	Interexaminer κ = .54 (.37, .72)
Joint line tenderness test[62] ◆	With patient's knee joint in 90° of flexion, examiner systematically palpates the tibiofemoral joint line for the presence of tenderness. A positive test result is defined as a local area of tenderness that exceeds normal discomfort when compared to the unaffected knee		Interexaminer κ = .17 (−.02, .36)
McMurray test[10] ◉	Knee is passively flexed, externally rotated, and axially loaded while brought into extension. Test is repeated in internal rotation. Positive if a palpable or audible click or pain occurs during rotation	152 patients with osteoarthritis of knee	Interexaminer κ = .16 (−.01, .33)

Diagnostic Utility of the McMurray Test

Test and Study Quality	Description and Positive Findings	Population	Reference Standard	Sens	Spec	+LR	−LR
McMurray test[63] ◆ **2015 Meta-analysis**		Pooled estimates from 9 studies*	Arthroscopy, arthrotomy, or MRI	.61 (.45, .74)	.84 (.69, .92)	3.2 (1.7, 5.9)	.52 (.34, .81)
McMurray test[49] ◆ **2010 Metaanalysis**		Pooled estimates from 13 studies*	Arthroscopy, arthrotomy, or MRI	.51 (.48, .53)	.78 (.77, .80)	2.3 (2.1, 2.6)	.63 (.59, .68)
McMurray test[50] ◆ **2008 Metaanalysis**	Depended on study	Pooled, quality-adjusted estimates from eight studies*	Arthroscopy or arthrotomy	.55 (.50, .60)	.77 (.62, .87)	2.4	.58
McMurray test[51] ◆ **2007 Metaanalysis**		Pooled estimates from 14 studies*	Arthroscopy, arthrotomy, or MRI	.71 (.67, .73)	.71 (.69, .73)	2.5	.41
McMurray test[64] ◆	The examiner grasps the patient's heel and flexes the knee to end range with one hand, while using the other hand to hold the distal femur. For testing the medial meniscus, the examiner places the knee into external rotation and adduction while extending the knee to about 90°. To test the lateral meniscus, the examiner flexes the knee but now internally rotates and abducts the patient's knee. Positive if the patient experiences pain or when a click is felt by the examiner	590 patients with a knee pathology possibly due to a meniscal tear, who were referred for an arthroscopic examination	Arthroscopy	.69 (.65, .74)	.37 (.30, .44)	1.09 (.96, 1.24)	.84 (.71, .99)
				.72 (.64, .79)	.34 (.30, .39)	1.09 (.97, 1.23)	.83 (.63, 1.08)

*Some of the included studies would not have met our QUADAS quality criterion for inclusion.

Diagnostic Utility of the Apley Test

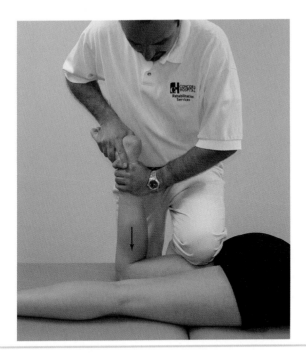

Figure 7-35
Apley grinding test.

Test and Study Quality	Description and Positive Findings	Population	Reference Standard	Sens	Spec	+LR	−LR
Apley test[49] ◆ **2010 Metaanalysis**	Depended on study, but generally: Patient is prone with knee flexed to 90 degrees. Examiner places downward pressure on foot, compressing knee, while internally and externally rotating tibia	Pooled estimates from seven studies*	Arthroscopy	.38 (.36, .41)	.84 (.82, 86)	2.4 (2.0, 3.0)	.73 (.68, .78)
Apley test[50] ◆ **2008 Metaanalysis**		Pooled, quality-adjusted estimates from three studies*	Arthroscopy or arthrotomy	.22 (.17, .28)	.88 (.72, .96)	1.8	.89
Apley test[51] ◆ **2007 Meta-analysis**		Pooled estimates from seven studies*	Arthroscopy, arthrotomy, or MRI	.61 (.56, .66)	.70 (.68, .72)	2.0	.56

*Some of the included studies would not have met our QUADAS quality criterion for inclusion.

Diagnostic Utility of Other Tests for Identifying Meniscal Tears

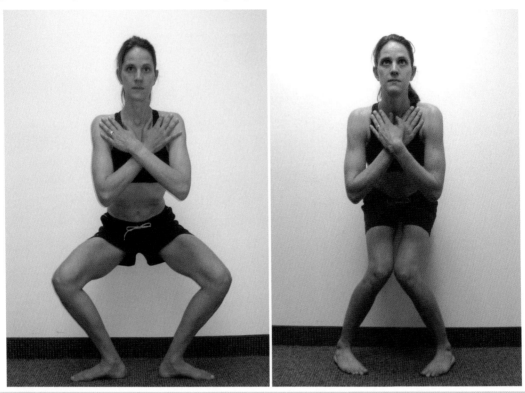

Figure 7-36
Ege test.

Test and Study Quality	Description and Positive Findings	Population	Reference Standard	Sens	Spec	+LR	−LR
Deep squat test[62] ◆	Patient stands flatfooted on the floor and squats as deeply as possible while the examiner holds the patient's hands for balance. Positive if the patient experiences internal knee pain during flexion or a sense of locking	117 patients suspected of having internal derangement of the knee of less than 6 months in duration	MRI	.75 (.61, .85)	.42 (.31, .54)	1.29 (.97, 1.68)	.60 (.35, 1.04)
Pain with passive knee flexion[14] ◆	Not described	134 patients with traumatic knee complaint	Meniscal tear per MRI	.77 (.64, .89)	.41 (.31, .52)	1.3 (1.0, 1.7)	.60 (.30, 1.0)
Ege test[65] ●	Patient stands with feet 30 to 40 cm apart. To detect medial meniscal tears, the patient performs a full squat with legs maximally externally rotated. To detect lateral meniscal tears, the patient performs a full squat with legs maximally internally rotated. Positive when the patient feels pain and/or a click in the joint line	150 consecutive patients with knee symptoms related to intraarticular knee pathologic conditions	Knee arthroscopy	**Medial** .67 **Lateral** .64	.81 .90	3.5 6.4	.41 .40

Diagnostic Utility of the Thessaly Test for Identifying Meniscal Tears

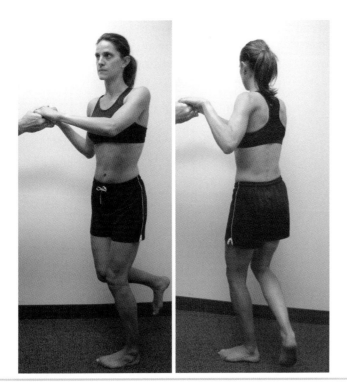

Figure 7-37
Thessaly test.

Test and Study Quality	Description and Positive Findings	Population	Reference Standard	Sens	Spec	+LR	−LR
Thessaly test [63] ◆ **2015 Meta-analysis**	Depended on study but generally same as below	Pooled estimates from 9 studies*	Arthroscopy, arthrotomy, or MRI	.75 (.53, .89)	.87 (.65, .96)	5.6 (1.5, 21.0)	.28 (.11, .71)
Thessaly test [62] ◆	Patient stands flatfooted on the affected limb, with the knee in 20° of flexion. With the examiner holding the patient's hands, the patient rotates the knee and body 3 times in each direction, while keeping the knee in 20° of flexion. Positive if the patient experiences medial or lateral joint line discomfort or has a sense of locking or catching	117 patients suspected of having internal derangement of the knee of less than 6 months in duration	MRI	.67 (.53, .78)	.38 (.27, .50)	1.07 (.82, 1.41)	.88 (.54, 1.45)

Diagnostic Utility of the Thessaly Test for Identifying Meniscal Tears—cont'd

Test and Study Quality	Description and Positive Findings	Population	Reference Standard	Sens	Spec	+LR	−LR
Thessaly test[64] ◆	Same as above	589 patients with a knee pathology possibly due to a meniscal tear, who were referred for an arthroscopic examination	Arthroscopy	.64 (.59, .69) MMT	.45 (.37, .52) MMT	1.16 (1.00, 1.35) MMT	.81 (.70, .93) MMT
				.64 (.56, .72) LMT	.40 (.35, .44) LMT	1.06 (.92, 1.22) LMT	.91 (.73, 1.14) LMT

LMT, Lateral meniscal tear; MMT, medial meniscal tear.

Diagnostic Utility of Tests for Identifying Patellar Instability

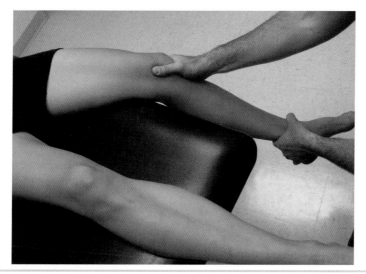

Figure 7-38
Moving patellar apprehension test.

Test and Study Quality	Description and Positive Findings	Population	Reference Standard	Sens	Spec	+LR	−LR
Reversed dynamic patellar apprehension test[60] ◆	Patient is supine with knee flexed to 120 degrees. The knee extended while the patella is translated laterally with the examiner's thumb as far as possible. The maneuver is stopped at the first onset of a subjective apprehensive reaction. Positive if apprehensive reaction occurs before the knee is fully extended	78 consecutive patients with recurrent lateral patellar instability and 35 controls	MRI findings fulfilling the criteria for lateral patellar dislocations	.94 (.86, .90)	.88 (.73, .97)	7.83*	.07*
Moving patellar apprehension test[69] ◕	With patient supine with ankle off examination table and knee fully extended, examiner flexes the knee to 90 degrees and back to extension while holding the patella in lateral translation. The procedure is then repeated with medial translation. Positive if patient exhibits apprehension and/or quadriceps contraction during lateral glide and no apprehension during medial glide	51 patients who had had knee surgery and in whom patellar instability was suspected	Ability to dislocate the patella when examined under anesthesia	1.0	.88	8.3	.00

*Values were calculated by the authors of this text.

Diagnostic Utility of Combinations of Tests for Diagnosing Meniscal Tears

Test and Study Quality	Description and Positive Findings	Population	Reference Standard	Sens	Spec	+LR	−LR
Both pain and laxity with valgus stress at 30 degrees + Trauma by external force to the leg or rotational trauma[13] ◆	Self-reported trauma and physical examination of valgus stress	134 patients with traumatic knee complaint	MRI	.56 (.33, .79)	.91 (.85, .98)	6.4 (2.7, 15.2)	.50 (.30, .80)
Age older than 40 years + Continuation of activity impossible + Weight bearing during trauma + Pain with passive knee flexion[14] ◆	All four factors positive	134 patients with traumatic knee complaint	MRI	.15 (.05, .25)	.97 (.94, 1.0)	5.8 (1.3, 26.8)	.90 (.80, 1.0)
Tenderness to palpation of joint line + Bohler test + Steinmann test + Apley grinding test + Payr test + McMurray test[7] ◆	If two tests are positive, then patient is considered to have meniscal lesion	36 patients scheduled to undergo arthroscopic surgery	Arthroscopic visualization	.97	.87	7.5	.03
Tenderness to palpation of joint line + Apley test + McMurray test[70] ●	If two tests are positive, then patient is considered to have meniscal lesion	80 patients with a history of knee trauma, preoperative RX, and MRI	Arthroscopy	Lateral meniscus: .86 Medial meniscus: .91	Lateral meniscus: .90 Medial meniscus: .87	Lateral meniscus: 8.6* Medial meniscus: 7.0*	Lateral meniscus: .16* Medial meniscus: .10*

*Values were calculated by the authors of this text.

Diagnostic Utility of Combinations of Tests for Diagnosing Meniscal Tears—cont'd

Test and Study Quality	Description and Positive Findings	Population	Reference Standard	Sens	Spec	+LR	−LR
Joint line tenderness + McMurray test[73] ◆	Both tests positive	109 patients with history or symptoms suggestive of meniscal tear	Meniscal tears via arthroscopy	Medial meniscus			
				.91	.91	10.1	.10
				Lateral meniscus			
				.75	.99	75.0	.25
Joint line tenderness + Thessaly test (20 degrees of knee flexion)[73] ◆				Medial meniscus			
				.93	.92	11.6	.08
				Lateral meniscus			
				.78	.99	78.0	.22
Combined historical and physical examination[71] ◒	Physical examination includes assessment of joint effusion and joint line tenderness, McMurray test, hyperflexion test, and squat test. Exact procedures of each test not defined	100 consecutive patients who underwent arthroscopic surgery of knee	Arthroscopic visualization	.86	.83	5.06	.17
Patient history + Joint line tenderness + McMurray test + Steinmann test + Modified Apley test[72] ◒	Conclusion of examiner	50 patients with clinical diagnosis of meniscal tears and/or ACL rupture	Knee arthroscopy	Medial			
				.87	.68	2.7	.19
				Lateral			
				.75	.95	15.0	.26

7

Knee

Diagnostic Utility of Combinations of Tests for Diagnosing Meniscal Tears—cont'd

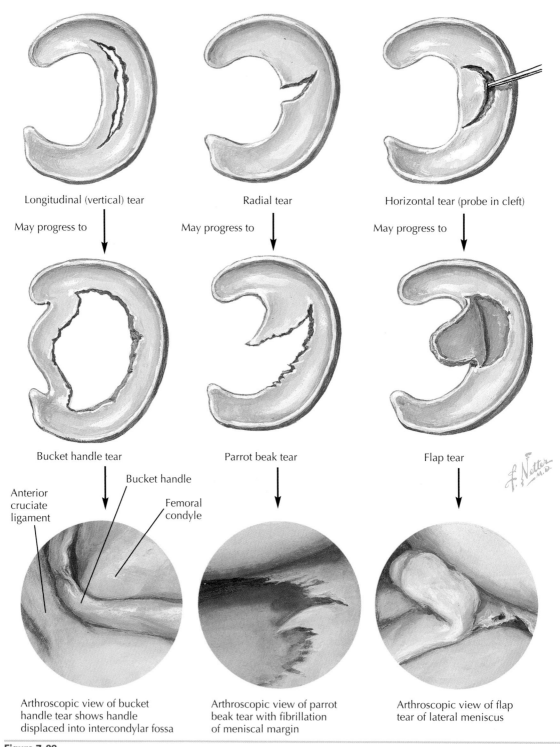

Longitudinal (vertical) tear

Radial tear

Horizontal tear (probe in cleft)

May progress to

May progress to

May progress to

Bucket handle tear

Parrot beak tear

Flap tear

Anterior cruciate ligament

Bucket handle

Femoral condyle

Arthroscopic view of bucket handle tear shows handle displaced into intercondylar fossa

Arthroscopic view of parrot beak tear with fibrillation of meniscal margin

Arthroscopic view of flap tear of lateral meniscus

Figure 7-39
Types of meniscal tears.

Diagnostic Utility of Combinations of Tests for Diagnosing Pathologic Conditions of the Knee Other Than Meniscal Tears

Test and Study Quality	Description and Positive Findings	Population	Reference Standard	Sens	Spec	+LR	−LR
Clinical examination[74]	Retrospective review of clinical examination and clinical diagnosis	698 patients who had undergone knee arthroscopy	Medial meniscal tear via arthroscopy	.92	.79	4.4	.10
			OA via arthroscopy	.75	.97	25.0	.26
			ACL tear via arthroscopy	.86	.98	43.0	.14
			Lateral meniscal tear via arthroscopy	.54	.96	13.5	.48
			Loose body via arthroscopy	.94	.98	47.0	.06
			Tight lateral retinaculum via arthroscopy	1.0	1.0	UD	.00
			Synovitis via arthroscopy	.57	1.0	UD	.43
			Lateral meniscal cyst via arthroscopy	1.0	.99	100.0	.00
Patient history + Anterior drawer test + Lachman test + Pivot shift test[72]	Conclusion of examiner	50 patients with clinical diagnosis of meniscal tears and/ or ACL rupture	ACL rupture via arthroscopy	1.0	1.0	UD	.00
History of anteromedial knee pain + Pain primarily over the medial femoral condyle + Visible or palpable plica + Exclusion of other causes of anteromedial knee pain[75]	Meet all four criteria	48 patients with anteromedial knee pain that was clinically suspected of being caused by pathologic medial plica	Pathologic medial plica via arthroscopy	1.0 (.92, 1.0)	.00	1.0	UD

UD, Undefined.

Patellofemoral Pain: Clinical Prediction Rule

Décary and colleagues[76] developed clinical prediction rules that combined history elements and physical examination tests to diagnose or exclude patellofemoral pain (PFP). In the study, 279 patients consulting a physician for a current knee compliant in an outpatient orthopaedic clinic or primary care family medicine clinic were evaluated, and diagnostic clusters were identified through recursive partitioning. The diagnostic clusters to rule in PFP demonstrated a +LR of 8.70 (95% CI: 5.20, 14.58) (Fig. 7-40). The diagnostic clusters to rule out PFP demonstrated a –LR of .12 (95% CI: .06, .27) (Fig. 7-41).

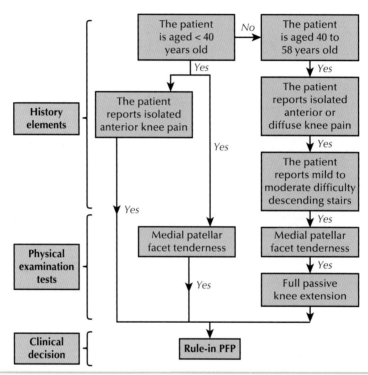

Figure 7-40

Diagnostic cluster to rule in PFP. (From Décary S, Pierre Frémont P, Pelletier B, et al. Validity of Combining History Elements and Physical Examination Tests to Diagnose Patellofemoral Pain. Archives of Physical Medicine and Rehabilitation. Volume 99, Issue 4, April 2018, Pages 607-614.)

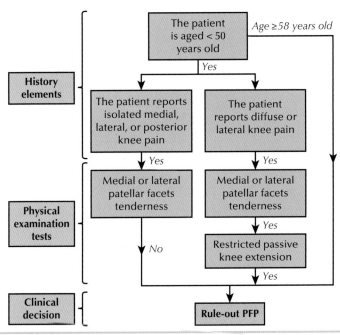

Figure 7-41
Diagnostic cluster to rule out PFP. (From Décary S, Pierre Frémont P, Pelletier B, et al. Validity of Combining History Elements and Physical Examination Tests to Diagnose Patellofemoral Pain. Archives of Physical Medicine and Rehabilitation. Volume 99, Issue 4, April 2018, Pages 607-614.)

Symptomatic Knee Osteoarthritis: Clinical Prediction Rule

Décary and colleagues[77] developed clinical prediction rules that combined history elements and physical examination tests to diagnose or exclude symptomatic knee osteoarthritis (SOA). In the study, 279 patients consulting a physician for a current knee compliant in an outpatient orthopaedic clinic or primary care family medicine clinic were evaluated, and diagnostic clusters were identified through recursive partitioning. The diagnostic clusters to rule in SOA demonstrated a +LR of 13.62 (95% CI: 6.53, 28.41) (Fig. 7-42). The diagnostic clusters to rule out SOA demonstrated a −LR of .11 (95% CI: .06, .20) (Fig. 7-43).

7

Knee

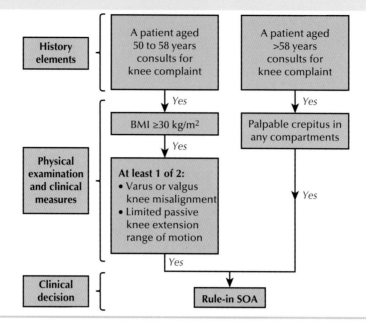

Figure 7-42

Diagnostic cluster to rule in symptomatic knee osteoarthritis. (From Décary S, Feldman D, Frémont P, et al. Initial derivation of diagnostic clusters combining history elements and physical examination tests for symptomatic knee osteoarthritis. Musculoskeletal Care. 2018;16(3):370-379.)

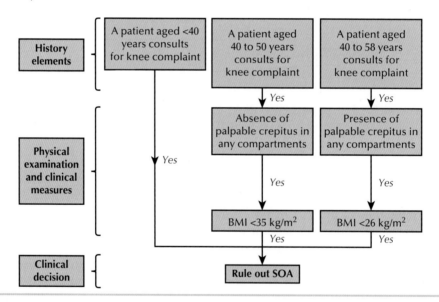

Figure 7-43

Diagnostic cluster to rule out symptomatic knee osteoarthritis. (From Décary S, Feldman D, Frémont P, et al. Initial derivation of diagnostic clusters combining history elements and physical examination tests for symptomatic knee osteoarthritis. Musculoskeletal Care. 2018;16(3):370-379.)

Symptomatic Meniscal Tear: Clinical Prediction Rule

Décary and colleagues[78] developed clinical prediction rules that combined history elements and physical examination tests to diagnose or exclude symptomatic meniscal tear (SMT). In the study, 279 patients consulting a physician for a current knee compliant in an outpatient orthopaedic clinic or primary care family medicine clinic were evaluated, and diagnostic clusters were identified through recursive partitioning. The diagnostic clusters to rule in SMT demonstrated a +LR of 6.44 (95% CI: 3.99, 10.39) (Fig. 7-44). The diagnostic clusters to rule out SMT demonstrated a –LR of .10 (95% CI: .03, .31) (Fig. 7-45).

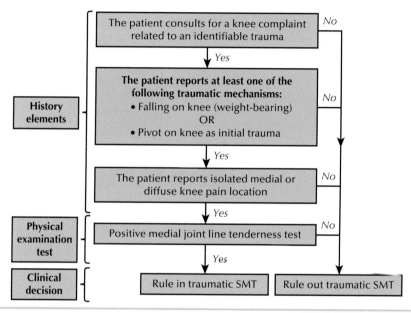

Figure 7-44

Diagnostic cluster to rule in symptomatic meniscal tear. (From Décary S, Fallaha M, Frémont P, et al. Diagnostic Validity of Combining History Elements and Physical Examination Tests for Traumatic and Degenerative Symptomatic Meniscal Tears. PM R. 2018 May;10(5):472-482.)

Knee

7

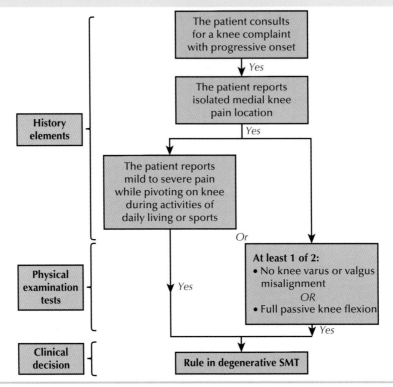

Figure 7-45

Diagnostic cluster to rule out symptomatic meniscal tear. (From Décary S, Fallaha M, Frémont P, et al. Diagnostic Validity of Combining History Elements and Physical Examination Tests for Traumatic and Degenerative Symptomatic Meniscal Tears. PM R. 2018 May;10(5):472-482.)

Diagnostic Utility of History and Physical Examination Findings for Predicting a Favorable Response to Foot Orthoses and Activity Modification

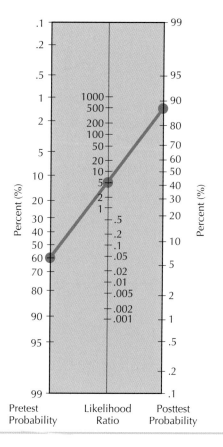

Pretest Probability   Likelihood Ratio   Posttest Probability

Figure 7-46

Nomogram. Considering a pretest probability of success of 60% (as determined in the Sutlive et al. study), 2 degrees or more of forefoot valgus or 78 degrees or less of great toe extension results in a posttest probability of 85%. This means that if a patient presented with one of the two aforementioned variables, the likelihood of achieving a successful outcome with off-the-shelf orthotics and activity modification would be 85%. (Adapted from Fagan TJ. Letter: Nomogram for Bayes theorem. *N Engl J Med.* 1975;293:257. Copyright 2005, Massachusetts Medical Society. See also Sutlive TG, Mitchell SD, Maxfield SN, et al. Identification of individuals with patellofemoral pain whose symptoms improved after a combined program of foot orthosis use and modified activity: a preliminary investigation. *Phys Ther.* 2004;84:49-61.)

Sutlive and colleagues[79] have developed a clinical prediction rule that identifies individuals with patellofemoral pain who are likely to improve with an off-the-shelf foot orthosis and modified activity. The study identified a number of predictor variables.

Test and Study Quality	Population	Reference Standard	Sens	Spec	+LR	−LR
2 degrees or more of forefoot valgus[79] ◆			.13 (.04, .24)	.97 (.90, 1.0)	4.0 (.70, 21.9)	.90
78 degrees or less of great toe extension[79] ◆			.13 (.04, .24)	.97 (.90, 1.0)	4.0 (.70, 21.9)	.90
3 mm or less of navicular drop[79] ◆		Decrease in pain of more than 50% after 3 weeks of wearing off-the-shelf foot orthoses and activity modification	.47 (.32, .61)	.80 (.67, .93)	2.4 (1.3, 4.3)	.66
5 degrees or less of valgus and any varus of relaxed calcaneal stance[79] ◆	50 patients with patellofemoral pain syndrome		.36 (.17, .55)	.81 (.71, .92)	1.9 (1.0, 3.6)	.79
Tight hamstring muscles as measured by 90/90 straight-leg raise test[79] ◆			.68 (.55, .80)	.56 (.37, .75)	1.5 (1.0, 2.3)	.57
Reports of difficulty walking[79] ◆			.71 (.55, .86)	.48 (.33, .62)	1.4 (1.0, 1.8)	.60

Diagnostic Utility of History and Physical Examination Findings for Predicting a Favorable Short-Term Response to Hip Mobilizations

Test and Study Quality	Population	Reference Standard	Sens	Spec	+LR	−LR
Ipsilateral anterior thigh pain[24] ◆	60 patients with knee OA	Decrease in pain of more than 30% or Global Rating of Change scale rated as "moderately better" 2 days after hip mobilizations	.27 (.13, .40)	.95 (.85, 1.05)	5.1 (.71, 36.7)	.77 (.62, .96)
Intermittent hip or groin pain[24] ◆			.15 (.05, .26)	.98 (.91, 1.04)	6.2 (.40, 104.7)	.87 (.75, 1.00)
Strengthening exercises aggravate knee pain[24] ◆			.20 (.04, .37)	.96 (.85, 1.07)	4.9 (.30, 83.7)	.83 (.65, 1.06)
Location of hip or groin pain bilaterally[24] ◆			.18 (.06, .29)	.98 (.91, 1.04)	7.1 (.40, 119.0)	.84 (.72, .99)
Side-to-side difference in hip internal rotation range of motion[24] ◆			.98 (.93, 1.02)	.11 (−.03, .24)	1.1 (.90, 1.3)	.23 (.02, 2.40)
Empty end feel on ipsilateral hip flexion range of motion[24] ◆			.13 (.03, .23)	.98 (.91, 1.04)	5.2 (.30, 9.2)	.89 (.78, 1.02)
Pain with ipsilateral hip distraction[24] ◆			.13 (.03, .23)	.98 (.91, 1.04)	5.2 (.30, 9.2)	.89 (.78, 1.02)
Pain at knee on ipsilateral hip extension range of motion[24] ◆			.11 (.01, .20)	.98 (.91, 1.04)	4.3 (.20, 75.8)	.92 (.81, 1.04)
Ipsilateral knee flexion passive range of motion of less than 122 degrees[24] ◆			.32 (.17, .46)	.95 (.85, 1.05)	6.0 (.90, 42.8)	.72 (.57, .91)
Ipsilateral hip internal rotation passive range of motion of less than 17 degrees[24] ◆			.32 (.17, .45)	.95 (.85, 1.05)	6.0 (.90, 42.8)	.72 (.57, .91)
Pain or paresthesia in ipsilateral hip or groin[24] ◆			.20 (.08, .32)	.98 (.91, 1.04)	8.1 (.50, 133.4)	.82 (.09, .97)

7

Knee

Diagnostic Utility of History and Physical Examination Findings for Predicting a Favorable Short-Term Response to Hip Mobilizations—cont'd

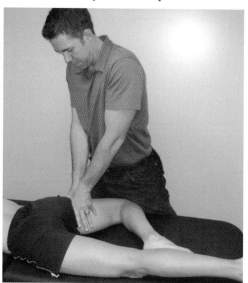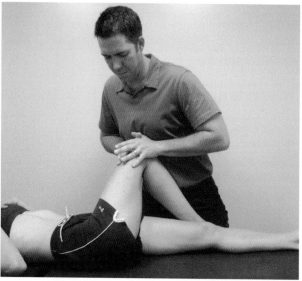

Figure 7-47

Hip mobilization technique used in the management of patients with knee OA. Patients were treated with one session of four different hip mobilizations, including (1) posteroanterior glide with flexion, abduction, and lateral rotation (depicted left), (2) caudal glide, (3) anteroposterior glide (depicted right), and (4) posteroanterior glide.

Clinical Prediction Rule to Identify Patients with Patellofemoral Pain Likely to Benefit from Foot Orthoses

Vicenzino and colleagues[80] developed a clinical prediction rule for identifying patients with patellofemoral pain who are likely to benefit from foot orthoses. The result of their study demonstrated that if three or more of the four attributes (age older than 25 years, height less than 65 inches, worst pain visual analog scale of less than 53 mm, and a difference in midfoot width from non–weight bearing to weight bearing of more than 11 mm) were present, the +LR was 8.8 (95% CI: 1.2 to 66.9) and the probability of experiencing a successful outcome improved from 40% to 86%.

Outcome Measure	Scoring and Interpretation	Test-Retest Reliability and Study Quality	MCID
Lower Extremity Functional Scale (LEFS)	Users rate the difficulty of performing 20 functional tasks on a Likert-type scale ranging from 0 (extremely difficult or unable to perform activity) to 4 (no difficulty). A total score out of 80 is calculated by summing each score. The answers provide a score between 0 and 80, with lower scores representing more disability	ICC = .92[81]	9[82]
Western Ontario and McMaster Universities Osteoarthritis Index (WOMAC)	The WOMAC consists of three subscales: pain (5 items), stiffness (2 items), and physical function (17 items). Users answer the 24 condition-specific questions on a numeric rating scale ranging from 0 (no symptoms) to 10 (extreme symptoms), or alternatively on a Likert-type scale from 0 to 4. Scores from each subscale are summed, with higher scores indicating more pain, stiffness, and disability	ICC = .90[81]	6.7% for improvement 12.9% for worsening[83]
Knee Outcome Survey (KOS) Activity of Daily Living Scale (ADLS)	The KOS ADLS consists of one section on symptoms and one section on functional disability. Users rate the eight symptom items on a Likert-type scale from 5 (never have) to 0 (prevent me from all daily activity) and the eight functional items from 5 (not difficult at all) to 0 (unable to do). Scores are summed and divided by 80 to get a percentage. Higher scores represent fewer symptoms and higher function	ICC = .93[84]	7.1%[85]
Numeric Pain Rating Scale (NPRS)	Users rate their level of pain on an 11-point scale ranging from 0 to 10, with high scores representing more pain. Often asked as "current pain" and "least," "worst," and "average" pain in the past 24 hours	ICC = .72[86]	2[87,88]

MCID, Minimum clinically important difference.

7

Knee

References

1. Greenfield B, Tovin BJ. Knee. In: *Current Concepts of Orthopedic Physical Therapy (11.2.11). La Crosse, Wisconsin: Orthopaedic Section,* American Physical Therapy Association; 2001.

2. Hartley A. *Practical Joint Assessment.* St Louis: Mosby; 1995.

3. DeHaven KE. Diagnosis of acute knee injuries with hemarthrosis. *Am J Sports Med.* 1980;8:9–14.

4. Cook JL, Khan KM, Kiss ZS, et al. Reproducibility and clinical utility of tendon palpation to detect patellar tendinopathy in young basketball players. Victorian Institute of Sport tendon study group. *Br J Sports Med.* 2001;35:65–69.

5. Cleland JA, McRae M. Patellofemoral pain syndrome: a critical analysis of current concepts. *Phys Ther Rev.* 2002;7:153–161.

6. Grelsamer RP, McConnell J. *The Patella: A Team Approach.* Gaithersburg, Maryland: Aspen Publishers; 1998.

7. Muellner T, Weinstabl R, Schabus R, et al. The diagnosis of meniscal tears in athletes. A comparison of clinical and magnetic resonance imaging investigations. *Am J Sports Med.* 1997;25:7–12.

8. Cibere J, Bellamy N, Thorne A, et al. Reliability of the knee examination in osteoarthritis: effect of standardization. *Arthritis Rheum.* 2004;50:458–468.

9. Jones A, Hopkinson N, Pattrick M, et al. Evaluation of a method for clinically assessing osteoarthritis of the knee. *Ann Rheum Dis.* 1992;51:243–245.

10. Dervin GF, Stiell IG, Wells GA, et al. Physicians' accuracy and interrator reliability for the diagnosis of unstable meniscal tears in patients having osteoarthritis of the knee. *Can J Surg.* 2001;44:267–274.

11. Niu NN, Losina E, Martin SD, et al. Development and preliminary validation of a meniscal symptom index. *Arthritis Care Res (Hoboken).* 2011;63(2):208–215.

12. Kastelein M, Luijsterburg PA, Wagemakers HP, et al. Diagnostic value of history taking and physical examination to assess effusion of the knee in traumatic knee patients in general practice. *Arch Phys Med Rehabil.* 2009;90:82–86.

13. Kastelein M, Wagemakers HP, Luijsterburg PA, et al. Assessing medial collateral ligament knee lesions in general practice. *Am J Med.* 2008;121:982–988.

14. Wagemakers HP, Heintjes EM, Boks SS, et al. Diagnostic value of history-taking and physical examination for assessing meniscal tears of the knee in general practice. *Clin J Sport Med.* 2008;18:24–30.

15. Cheung TC, Tank Y, Breederveld RS, et al. Diagnostic accuracy and reproducibility of the Ottawa Knee Rule vs the Pittsburgh Decision Rule. *Am J Emerg Med.* 2013;31(4):641–645.

16. Bachmann LM, Haberzeth S, Steurer J, ter Riet G. The accuracy of the Ottawa Knee Rule to rule out knee fractures: a systematic review. *Ann Intern Med.* 2004;140:121–124.

17. Vijayasankar D, Boyle AA, Atkinson P. Can the Ottawa Knee Rule be applied to children? A systematic review and meta-analysis of observational studies. *Emerg Med J.* 2009;26:250–253.

18. Maricar N, Callaghan MJ, Parkes MJ, et al. Interobserver and intraobserver reliability of clinical assessments in knee osteoarthritis. *J Rheumatol.* 2016;43(12):2171–2178.

19. Wood L, Peat G, Wilkie R, et al. A study of the non-instrumented physical examination of the knee found high observer variability. *J Clin Epidemiol.* 2006;59:512–520.

20. Fritz JM, Delitto A, Erhard RE, Roman M. An examination of the selective tissue tension scheme, with evidence for the concept of a capsular pattern of the knee. *Phys Ther.* 1998;78:1046–1056. discussion 1057-1061.

21. Sturgill LP, Snyder-Mackler L, Manal TJ, Axe MJ. Interrater reliability of a clinical scale to assess knee joint effusion. *J Orthop Sports Phys Ther.* 2009;39(12):845–849.

22. Berlinberg A, Ashbeck EL, Roemer FW, et al. Diagnostic performance of knee physical exam and participant-reported symptoms for MRI-detected effusion-synovitis among participants with early or late stage knee osteoarthritis: data from the Osteoarthritis Initiative. *Osteoarthr Cartil.* 2019;27(1):80–89.

23. Lenssen AF, van Dam EM, Crijns YH, et al. Reproducibility of goniometric measurement of the knee in the in-hospital phase following total knee arthroplasty. *BMC Musculoskelet Disord.* 2007;8:83.

24. Currier LL, Froehlich PJ, Carow SD, et al. Development of a clinical prediction rule to identify patients with knee pain and clinical evidence of knee osteoarthritis who demonstrate a favorable short-term response to hip mobilization. *Phys Ther.* 2007;87:1106–1119.

25. Rothstein JM, Miller PJ, Roettger RF. Goniometric reliability in a clinical setting. Elbow and knee measurements. *Phys Ther.* 1983;63:1611–1615.

26. Gogia PP, Braatz JH, Rose SJ, Norton BJ. Reliability and validity of goniometric measurements at the knee. *Phys Ther.* 1987;67:192–195.

27. Watkins MA, Riddle DL, Lamb RL, Personius WJ. Reliability of goniometric measurements and visual estimates of knee range of motion obtained in a clinical setting. *Phys Ther.* 1991;71:90–97.

28. Clapper MP, Wolf SL. Comparison of the reliability of the Orthoranger and the standard goniometer for assessing active lower extremity range of motion. *Phys Ther.* 1988;68:214–218.

29. Brosseau L, Tousignant M, Budd J, et al. Intratester and intertester reliability and criterion validity of the parallelogram and universal goniometers for active knee flexion in healthy subjects. *Physiother Res Int.* 1997;2:150–166.

30. Hayes KW, Petersen CM. Reliability of assessing end-feel and pain and resistance sequence in subjects

with painful shoulders and knees. *J Orthop Sports Phys Ther*. 2001;31:432–445.

31. Cooperman JM, Riddle DL, Rothstein JM. Reliability and validity of judgments of the integrity of the anterior cruciate ligament of the knee using the Lachman's test. *Phys Ther*. 1990;70:225–233.

32. McClure PW, Rothstein JM, Riddle DL. Intertester reliability of clinical judgments of medial knee ligament integrity. *Phys Ther*. 1989;69:268–275.

33. Tagesson SK, Kvist J. Intra- and interrater reliability of the establishment of one repetition maximum on squat and seated knee extension. *J Strength Cond Res*. 2007;21:801–807.

34. Bohannon RW. Manual muscle testing: does it meet the standards of an adequate screening test? *Clin Rehabil*. 2005;19:662–667.

35. Gnat R, Kuszewski M, Koczar R, Dziewońska A. Reliability of the passive knee flexion and extension tests in healthy subjects. *J Manipulative Physiol Ther*. 2010;33(9):659–665.

36. Hamid MS, Ali MR, Yusof A. Interrater and intrarater reliability of the active knee extension (AKE) test among healthy adults. *J Phys Ther Sci*. 2013;25:957–961.

37. Piva SR, Fitzgerald K, Irrgang JJ, et al. Reliability of measures of impairments associated with patellofemoral pain syndrome. *BMC Musculoskelet Disord*. 2006;7:33.

38. Tomsich DA, Nitz AJ, Threlkeld AJ, Shapiro R. Patellofemoral alignment: reliability. *J Orthop Sports Phys Ther*. 1996;23:200–208.

39. Fitzgerald GK, McClure PW. Reliability of measurements obtained with four tests for patellofemoral alignment. *Phys Ther*. 1995;75:84–92.

40. Watson CJ, Propps M, Galt W, et al. Reliability of McConnell's classification of patellar orientation in symptomatic and asymptomatic subjects. *J Orthop Sports Phys Ther*. 1999;29:378–393.

41. Herrington LC. The inter-tester reliability of a clinical measurement used to determine the medial-lateral orientation of the patella. *Man Ther*. 2002;7:163–167.

42. Sacco ICN, Onodera AN, Butugan MK, et al. Inter- and intra-tester reliability of clinical measurement to determine medio-lateral patellar position using a pachymeter or visual assessment. *Knee*. 2010;17(1):92–95.

43. Sweitzer BA, Cook C, Steadman JR, et al. The interrater reliability and diagnostic accuracy of patellar mobility tests in patients with anterior knee pain. *Phys Sportsmed*. 2010;38(3):90–96.

44. Greene CC, Edwards TB, Wade MR, Carson EW. Reliability of the quadriceps angle measurement. *Am J Knee Surg*. 2001;14:97–103.

45. Draper CE, Chew KTL, Wang R, et al. Comparison of quadriceps angle measurements using short-arm and long-arm goniometers: correlation with MRI. *PM R*. 2011;3(2):111–116.

46. Ehrat M, Edwards J, Hastings D, Worrell T. Reliability of assessing patellar alignment: the A angle. *J Orthop Sports Phys Ther*. 1994;19:22–27.

47. Watson CJ, Leddy HM, Dynjan TD, Parham JL. Reliability of the lateral pull test and tilt test to assess patellar alignment in subjects with symptomatic knees: student raters. *J Orthop Sports Phys Ther*. 2001;31:368–374.

48. Wadey VM, Mohtadi NG, Bray RC, Frank CB. Positive predictive value of maximal posterior joint-line tenderness in diagnosing meniscal pathology: a pilot study. *Can J Surg*. 2007;50:96–100.

49. Ockert B, Haasters F, Polzer H, et al. [Value of the clinical examination in suspected meniscal injuries. A meta-analysis]. *Unfallchirurg*. 2010;113(4):293–299.

50. Meserve BB, Cleland JA, Boucher TR. A meta-analysis examining clinical test utilities for assessing meniscal injury. *Clin Rehabil*. 2008;22:143–161.

51. Hegedus EJ, Cook C, Hasselblad V, et al. Physical examination tests for assessing a torn meniscus in the knee: a systematic review with meta-analysis. *J Orthop Sports Phys Ther*. 2007;37:541–550.

52. Couture J-F, Al-Juhani W, Forsythe ME, et al. Joint line fullness and meniscal pathology. *Sports Health*. 2012;4(1):47–50.

53. Mulligan EP, McGuffie DQ, Coyner K, Khazzam M. The reliability and diagnostic accuracy of assessing the translation endpoint during the Lachman test. *Int J Sports Phys Ther*. 2015;10(1):52–61.

54. Mulligan EP, Harwell JL, Robertson WJ. Reliability and diagnostic accuracy of the Lachman test performed in a prone position. *J Orthop Sports Phys Ther*. 2011;41(10):749–757.

55. Van Eck CF, van den Bekerom MPJ, Fu FH, et al. Methods to diagnose acute anterior cruciate ligament rupture: a meta-analysis of physical examinations with and without anaesthesia. *Knee Surg Sports Traumatol Arthrosc*. 2013;21(8):1895–1903.

56. Benjaminse A, Gokeler A, van der Schans CP. Clinical diagnosis of an anterior cruciate ligament rupture: a meta-analysis. *J Orthop Sports Phys Ther*. 2006;36:267–288.

57. Lichtenberg MC, Koster CH, Teunissen LPJ, et al. Does the Lever sign test have added value for diagnosing anterior cruciate ligament ruptures?. *Orthop J Sports Med*. 2018;6(3):2325967118759631.

58. Reiman MP, Reiman CK, Décary S. Accuracy of the Lever sign to diagnose anterior cruciate ligament tear: A systematic review with meta-analysis. *Int J Sports Phys Ther*. 2018;13(5):774–788.

59. Salvi M, Caputo F, Piu G, et al. The loss of extension test (LOE test): a new clinical sign for the anterior cruciate ligament insufficient knee. *J Orthop Traumatol*. 2013;14(3):185–191.

60. Slichter ME, Wolterbeek N, Auw Yang KG, et al. Rater agreement reliability of the dial test in the ACL-deficient knee. *J Exp Orthop*. 2018;5(1):18.

7

Knee

References

61. Ellera Gomes JL, Leie MA, Ramirez E, Gomes TE. Frog-leg test maneuver for the diagnosis of injuries to the posterolateral corner of the knee: A diagnostic accuracy study. *Clin J Sport Med.* 2016;26(3):216–220.

62. Snoeker BAM, Lindeboom R, Zwinderman AH, et al. Detecting meniscal tears in primary care: Reproducibility and accuracy of 2 weight-bearing tests and 1 non-weight-bearing test. *J Orthop Sports Phys Ther.* 2015;45(9):693–702.

63. Smith BE, Thacker D, Crewesmith A, Hall M. Special tests for assessing meniscal tears within the knee: a systematic review and meta-analysis. *Evid Based Med.* 2015;20(3):88–97.

64. Goossens P, Keijsers E, van Geenen RJC, et al. Validity of the Thessaly test in evaluating meniscal tears compared with arthroscopy: a diagnostic accuracy study. *J Orthop Sports Phys Ther.* 2015;45(1):18–24, B1.

65. Akseki D, Ozcan O, Boya H, Pinar H. A new weight-bearing meniscal test and a comparison with Mc-Murray's test and joint line tenderness. *Arthroscopy.* 2004;20:951–958.

66. Karachalios T, Hantes M, Zibis AH, et al. Diagnostic accuracy of a new clinical test (the Thessaly test) for early detection of meniscal tears. *J Bone Joint Surg Am.* 2005;87:955–962.

67. Harrison BK, Abell BE, Gibson TW. The Thessaly test for detection of meniscal tears: validation of a new physical examination technique for primary care medicine. *Clin J Sport Med.* 2009;19:9–12.

68. Zimmermann F, Liebensteiner MC, Balcarek P. The reversed dynamic patellar apprehension test mimics anatomical complexity in lateral patellar instability. *Knee Surg Sports Traumatol Arthrosc.* 2019;27:604–610.

69. Ahmad CS, McCarthy M, Gomez JA, et al. The moving patellar apprehension test for lateral patellar instability. *Am J Sports Med.* 2009;37:791–796.

70. Antinolfi P, Crisitiani R, Manfreda F, et al. Relationship between clinical, MRI, and arthroscopic findings: A guide to correct diagnosis of meniscal tears. *Joints.* 2017;5(3):164–167.

71. Bonamo JJ, Shulman G. Double contrast arthrography of the knee. A comparison to clinical diagnosis and arthroscopic findings. *Orthopedics.* 1988;11:1041–1046.

72. Kocabey Y, Tetik O, Isbell WM, et al. The value of clinical examination versus magnetic resonance imaging in the diagnosis of meniscal tears and anterior cruciate ligament rupture. *Arthroscopy.* 2004;20:696–700.

73. Konan S, Rayan F, Haddad FS. Do physical diagnostic tests accurately detect meniscal tears? *Knee Surg Sports Traumatol Arthrosc.* 2009;17(7):806–811.

74. Nickinson R, Darrah C, Donell S. Accuracy of clinical diagnosis in patients undergoing knee arthroscopy. *Int Orthop.* 2010;34(1):39–44.

75. Shetty VD, Vowler SL, Krishnamurthy S, Halliday AE. Clinical diagnosis of medial plica syndrome of the knee: a prospective study. *J Knee Surg.* 2007;20:277–280.

76. Décary S, Frémont P, Pelletier B, et al. Validity of combining history elements and physical examination tests to diagnose patellofemoral pain. *Arch Phys Med Rehabil.* 2018;99(4):607–614. e1.

77. Décary S, Feldman D, Frémont P, et al. Initial derivation of diagnostic clusters combining history elements and physical examination tests for symptomatic knee osteoarthritis. *Musculoskeletal Care.* 2018;16(3):370–379.

78. Décary S, Fallaha M, Frémont P, et al. Diagnostic validity of combining history elements and physical examination tests for traumatic and degenerative symptomatic meniscal tears. *PM R.* 2018;10(5):472–482.

79. Sutlive TG, Mitchell SD, Maxfield SN, et al. Identification of individuals with patellofemoral pain whose symptoms improved after a combined program of foot orthosis use and modified activity: a preliminary investigation. *Phys Ther.* 2004;84:49–61.

80. Vicenzino B, Collins N, Cleland J, McPoil T. A clinical prediction rule for identifying patients with patellofemoral pain who are likely to benefit from foot orthoses: a preliminary determination. *Br J Sports Med.* 2010;44(12):862–866.

81. Pua YH, Cowan SM, Wrigley TV, Bennell KL. The Lower Extremity Functional Scale could be an alternative to the Western Ontario and McMaster Universities Osteoarthritis Index physical function scale. *J Clin Epidemiol.* 2009;62(10):1103–1111.

82. Binkley JM, Stratford PW, Lott SA, Riddle DL. The Lower Extremity Functional Scale (LEFS): scale development, measurement properties, and clinical application. North American Orthopaedic Rehabilitation Research Network. *Phys Ther.* 1999;79:371–383.

83. Angst F, Aeschlimann A, Stucki G. Smallest detectable and minimal clinically important differences of rehabilitation intervention with their implications for required sample sizes using WOMAC and SF-36 quality of life measurement instruments in patients with osteoarthritis of the lower extremities. *Arthritis Rheum.* 2001;45:384–391.

84. Marx RG, Jones EC, Allen AA, et al. Reliability, validity, and responsiveness of four knee outcome scales for athletic patients. *J Bone Joint Surg Am.* 2001;83A:1459–1469.

85. Piva SR, Gil AB, Moore CG, Fitzgerald GK. Responsiveness of the activities of daily living scale of the knee outcome survey and numeric pain rating scale in patients with patellofemoral pain. *J Rehabil Med.* 2009;41:129–135.

86. Li L, Liu X, Herr K. Postoperative pain intensity assessment: a comparison of four scales in Chinese adults. *Pain Med.* 2007;8:223–234.

87. Farrar JT, Berlin JA, Strom BL. Clinically important changes in acute pain outcome measures: a validation study. *J Pain Symptom Manage.* 2003;25:406–411.

88. Farrar JT, Portenoy RK, Berlin JA, et al. Defining the clinically important difference in pain outcome measures. *Pain.* 2000;88:287–294.

Clinical Summary and Recommendations

Patient History	
Complaints	• No studies of acceptable quality have assessed either the reliability or diagnostic utility of items from the subjective history in patients with foot and ankle problems.

Physical Examination	
Screening	• The Ottawa Ankle Rule for Radiography is highly sensitive for ankle and midfoot fractures in both adults and children. When patients can bear weight and have no tenderness on the malleoli, navicular bone, or base of the fifth metatarsal, providers can confidently rule out foot and ankle fractures ($-LR$ [likelihood ratio] = .09–.14).
Range-of-Motion and Strength Assessment	• Measuring ankle range of motion has consistently been shown to be highly reliable when one person does the measuring, but it is much less reliable when different people do the measuring. • Calf strength can be reliably assessed using repeated calf raises. The paper grip test is a simple yet accurate method to measure toe plantarflexion strength.
Other Assessments	• Assessments of static foot alignment, sensation, swelling, proprioception, and dynamic performance have all been shown to be adequately reliable but are of unknown diagnostic utility. Dynamic assessments of hindfoot motion during gait are likely too unreliable to be clinically useful.
Special Tests	• The Thompson test seems to show very good diagnostic utility in both identifying and ruling out subcutaneous tears of the Achilles tendon ($+LR$ = 13.47, $-LR$ = .04). • The impingement sign seems to show very good diagnostic utility in both identifying and ruling out anterolateral ankle impingement ($+LR$ = 7.9, $-LR$ = .06). • The triple compression test seems to show good diagnostic utility in ruling out tarsal tunnel syndrome ($-LR$ = .14). • Clinical examination seems to show poor diagnostic utility for detecting syndesmotic injuries in acute ankle sprains.

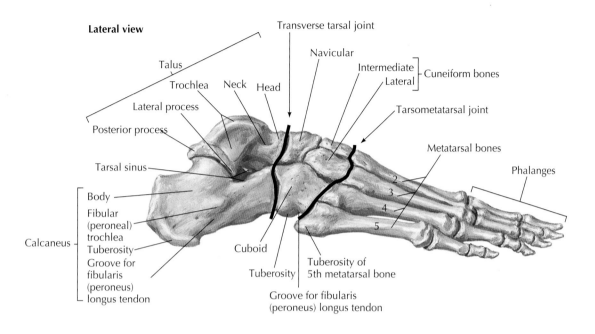

Lateral view

Transverse tarsal joint

Navicular

Talus

Intermediate
Lateral — Cuneiform bones

Trochlea   Neck   Head

Lateral process

Tarsometatarsal joint

Posterior process

Metatarsal bones

Tarsal sinus

Phalanges

Body

Fibular
(peroneal)
trochlea

Cuboid

Tuberosity

Tuberosity of
5th metatarsal bone

Calcaneus

Groove for
fibularis
(peroneus)
longus tendon

Groove for fibularis
(peroneus) longus tendon

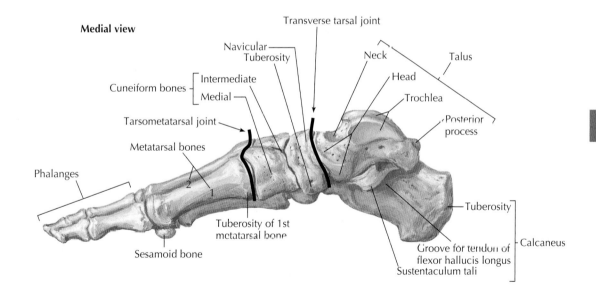

Medial view

Transverse tarsal joint

Navicular
Tuberosity

Neck

Talus

Cuneiform bones — Intermediate
Medial

Head

Trochlea

Tarsometatarsal joint

Posterior
process

Metatarsal bones

Phalanges

Tuberosity

Tuberosity of 1st
metatarsal bone

Calcaneus

Sesamoid bone

Groove for tendon of
flexor hallucis longus

Sustentaculum tali

Figure 8-1
Bones of the foot.

Foot and Ankle

8

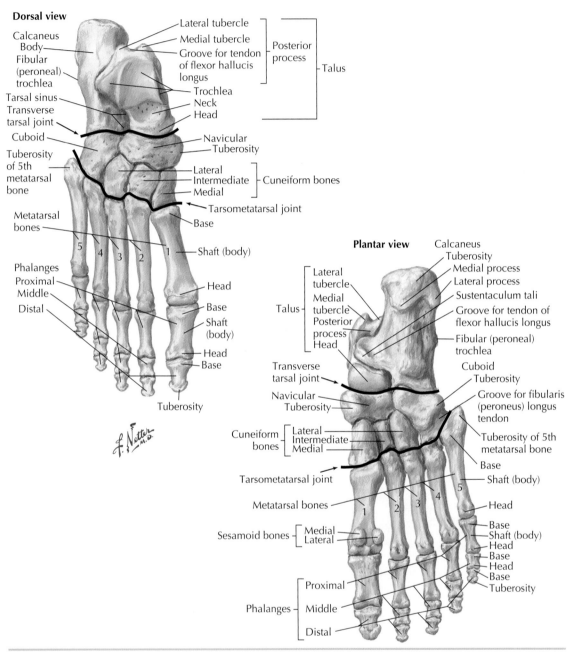

Dorsal view

Calcaneus
Body
Fibular
(peroneal)
trochlea

Lateral tubercle
Medial tubercle
Groove for tendon
of flexor hallucis
longus

Posterior
process

Talus

Tarsal sinus
Transverse
tarsal joint
Cuboid
Tuberosity
of 5th
metatarsal
bone

Trochlea
Neck
Head

Navicular
Tuberosity

Lateral
Intermediate
Medial

Cuneiform bones

Tarsometatarsal joint
Base

Metatarsal
bones

5   4   3   2   1

Shaft (body)

Phalanges
Proximal
Middle
Distal

Head
Base
Shaft
(body)

Head
Base

Tuberosity

f. Netter

Plantar view

Calcaneus
Tuberosity
Medial process
Lateral process
Sustentaculum tali
Groove for tendon of
flexor hallucis longus
Fibular (peroneal)
trochlea

Lateral
tubercle
Medial
tubercle
Posterior
process
Head

Talus

Transverse
tarsal joint
Navicular
Tuberosity

Cuboid
Tuberosity
Groove for fibularis
(peroneus) longus
tendon
Tuberosity of 5th
metatarsal bone
Base

Cuneiform
bones

Lateral
Intermediate
Medial

Tarsometatarsal joint

Shaft (body)

Metatarsal bones

1   2   3   4   5

Head

Sesamoid bones

Medial
Lateral

Base
Shaft (body)
Head
Base
Head
Base
Tuberosity

Phalanges

Proximal
Middle
Distal

Figure 8-2
Bones of the foot.

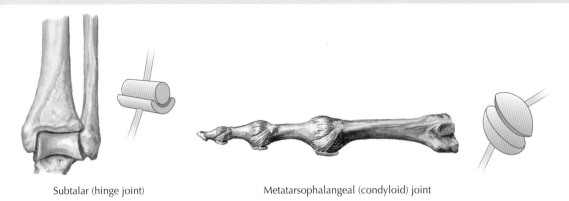

Subtalar (hinge joint)   Metatarsophalangeal (condyloid) joint

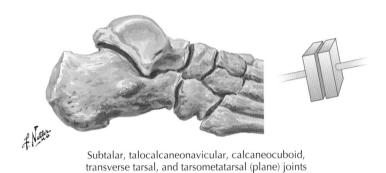

Subtalar, talocalcaneonavicular, calcaneocuboid,
transverse tarsal, and tarsometatarsal (plane) joints

Figure 8-3
Talocrural (hinge) joint.

Joint	Type and Classification	Closed Packed Position	Capsular Pattern
Talocrural	Synovial: hinge	Dorsiflexion	Plantarflexion slightly more limited than dorsiflexion
Distal tibiofibular	Syndesmosis	Not available	Not available
Subtalar	Synovial: plane	Supination	Inversion greatly restricted; eversion not restricted
Talocalcaneonavicular	Synovial: plane	Supination	Supination more limited than pronation
Calcaneocuboid	Synovial: plane	Supination	
Transverse tarsal	Synovial: plane	Supination	
Tarsometatarsal	Synovial: plane	Supination	Not available
Metatarsophalangeal (MTP)	Synovial: condyloid	Extension	Great toe: extension more limited than flexion MTP joints 2 to 5: variable
Interphalangeal (IP)	Synovial: hinge	Extension	Extension more limited than flexion

8

Foot and Ankle

Posterior Ankle Ligaments

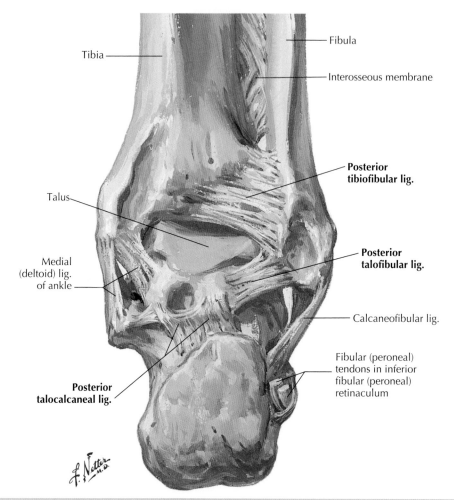

Figure 8-4
Calcaneus: posterior view with ligaments.

Ligaments	Attachments	Function
Posterior talocalcaneal	Superior body of calcaneus to posterior process of talus	Limits posterior separation of talus from calcaneus
Posterior tibiofibular	Distal posterior tibia to distal posterior fibula	Maintains distal tibiofibular joint
Posterior talofibular	Posterior talus to posterior lateral malleolus	Limits separation of fibula from talus
Interosseous membrane	Continuous connection between tibia and fibula	Reinforces approximation between tibia and fibula

Lateral Ankle Ligaments

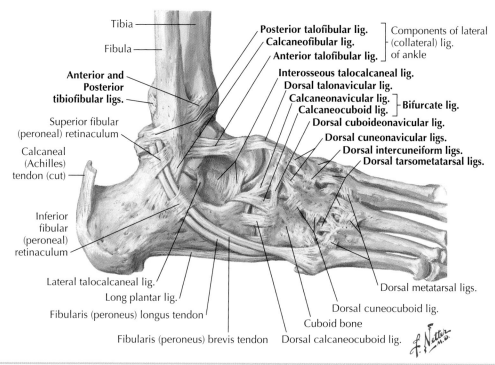

Figure 8-5
Ligaments of ankle: lateral view of right foot.

Ligaments	Attachments	Function
Anterior tibiofibular	Anterior aspect of lateral malleolus to inferior border of medial tibia	Reinforces anterior tibiofibular joint
Lateral collateral *Posterior talofibular* *Calcaneofibular* *Anterior talofibular*	Lateral malleolus to lateral talus Lateral malleolus to lateral calcaneus Lateral malleolus to talus	Limits ankle inversion
Interosseous talocalcaneal	Inferior aspect of talus to superior aspect of calcaneus	Limits separation of talus from calcaneus
Dorsal talonavicular	Dorsal aspect of talus to dorsal aspect of navicular	Limits separation of navicular from talus
Bifurcate *Calcaneonavicular* *Calcaneocuboid*	Distal calcaneus to proximal navicular Distal calcaneus to proximal cuboid	Limits separation of navicular and cuboid from calcaneus
Dorsal cubonavicular	Lateral aspect of cuboid to dorsal aspect of navicular	Limits separation of navicular from cuboid
Dorsal cuneonavicular	Navicular to three cuneiforms	Limits separation of cuneiforms from navicular
Dorsal intercuneiform	Joining of three cuneiforms	Limits separation of cuneiforms
Dorsal tarsometatarsal	Dorsal tarsal bones to corresponding metatarsal bones	Reinforces tarsometatarsal joints

8

Foot and Ankle

Medial Ankle Ligaments

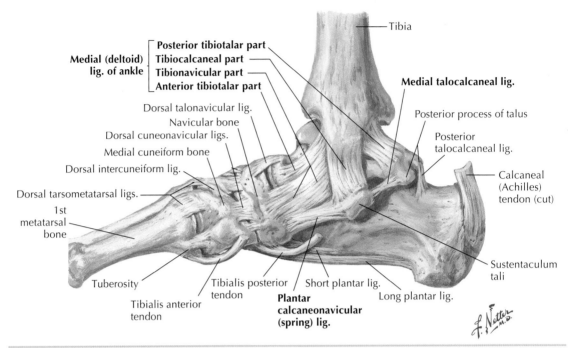

Figure 8-6
Ligaments of ankle: medial view of right foot.

Ligaments	Attachments	Function
Medial (deltoid)		
Posterior tibiotalar	Medial malleolus to medial talus	Limits ankle eversion
Tibiocalcaneal	Anterior distal medial malleolus to sustentaculum tali	
Tibionavicular	Medial malleolus to proximal aspect of navicular	
Anterior tibiotalar	Medial malleolus to talus	
Medial talocalcaneal	Sustentaculum tali to talus	Limits posterior separation of talus on calcaneus
Plantar calcaneonavicular (spring)	Sustentaculum tali to posteroinferior navicular	Maintains longitudinal arch of foot

Plantar Foot Ligaments

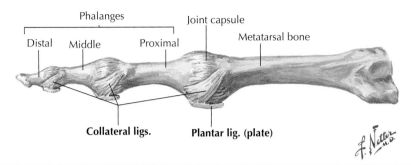

Phalanges

Distal   Middle   Proximal

Joint capsule

Metatarsal bone

Collateral ligs.   **Plantar lig. (plate)**

Figure 8-7
Capsules and ligaments of metatarsophalangeal and interphalangeal joints: lateral view.

Ligaments	Attachments	Function
Long plantar	Plantar of calcaneus to cuboid	Maintains arches of foot
Plantar calcaneocuboid (short plantar)	Anteroinferior aspect of calcaneus to inferior aspect of cuboid	Maintains arches of foot
Plantar calcaneonavicular (spring)	Sustentaculum tali to posteroinferior aspect of talus	Maintains longitudinal arch of foot
Plantar cubonavicular	Inferior navicular to inferomedial cuboid	Limits separation of cuboid from navicular and supports arch
Plantar tarsometatarsal	Connects metatarsals 1 to 5 to corresponding tarsal on plantar aspect	Limits separation of metatarsals from corresponding tarsal bones
Collateral	Distal aspect of proximal phalanx to proximal aspect of distal phalanx	Reinforces capsule of IP joints
Plantar plate	Thickening of plantar aspect of joint capsule	Reinforces plantar aspect of IP joint
Deep transverse metatarsal	MTP joints on plantar aspect	Limits separation of MTP joints

8

Foot and Ankle

Plantar Foot Ligaments—cont'd

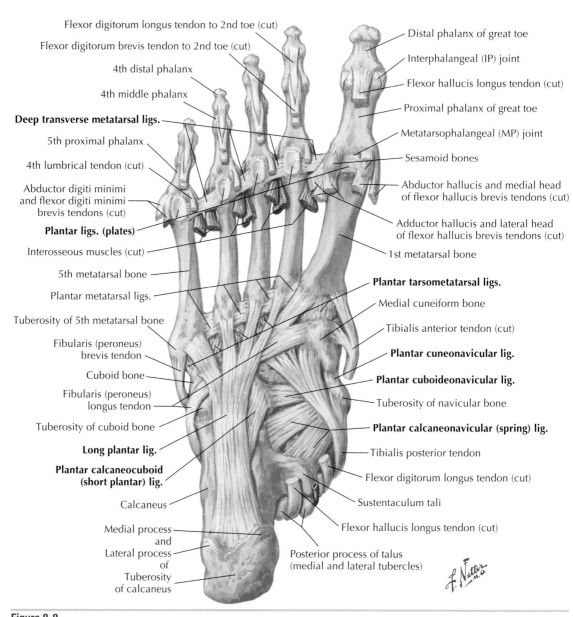

Flexor digitorum longus tendon to 2nd toe (cut)

Flexor digitorum brevis tendon to 2nd toe (cut)

4th distal phalanx

4th middle phalanx

Deep transverse metatarsal ligs.

5th proximal phalanx

4th lumbrical tendon (cut)

Abductor digiti minimi and flexor digiti minimi brevis tendons (cut)

Plantar ligs. (plates)

Interosseous muscles (cut)

5th metatarsal bone

Plantar metatarsal ligs.

Tuberosity of 5th metatarsal bone

Fibularis (peroneus) brevis tendon

Cuboid bone

Fibularis (peroneus) longus tendon

Tuberosity of cuboid bone

Long plantar lig.

Plantar calcaneocuboid (short plantar) lig.

Calcaneus

Medial process and Lateral process of Tuberosity of calcaneus

Distal phalanx of great toe

Interphalangeal (IP) joint

Flexor hallucis longus tendon (cut)

Proximal phalanx of great toe

Metatarsophalangeal (MP) joint

Sesamoid bones

Abductor hallucis and medial head of flexor hallucis brevis tendons (cut)

Adductor hallucis and lateral head of flexor hallucis brevis tendons (cut)

1st metatarsal bone

Plantar tarsometatarsal ligs.

Medial cuneiform bone

Tibialis anterior tendon (cut)

Plantar cuneonavicular lig.

Plantar cuboideonavicular lig.

Tuberosity of navicular bone

Plantar calcaneonavicular (spring) lig.

Tibialis posterior tendon

Flexor digitorum longus tendon (cut)

Sustentaculum tali

Flexor hallucis longus tendon (cut)

Posterior process of talus (medial and lateral tubercles)

Figure 8-8
Ligaments and tendons of foot: plantar view.

Lateral Muscles of Leg

Muscles	Proximal Attachments	Distal Attachments	Nerve and Segmental Level	Action
Gastrocnemius	Lateral head: lateral femoral condyle Medial head: popliteal surface of femur	Posterior aspect of calcaneus	Tibial nerve (S1, S2)	Plantarflexes ankle and flexes knee
Soleus	Posterior aspect of head of fibula, fibular soleal line, and medial aspect of tibia	Posterior aspect of calcaneus	Tibial nerve (S1, S2)	Plantarflexes ankle
Fibularis longus	Superolateral surface of fibula	Base of first metatarsal and medial cuneiform	Superficial fibular nerve (L5, S1, S2)	Everts foot and assists in plantarflexion
Fibularis brevis	Distal aspect of fibula	Tuberosity of base of fifth metatarsal	Superficial fibular nerve (L5, S1, S2)	Everts foot and assists in plantarflexion
Fibularis tertius	Anteroinferior aspect of fibula and interosseus membrane	Base of fifth metatarsal	Deep fibular nerve (L5, S1)	Dorsiflexes ankle and everts foot
Extensor digitorum longus	Lateral condyle of tibia, medial surface of fibula	Middle and distal phalanges of digits 2 to 5	Deep fibular nerve (L5, S1)	Extends digits 2 to 5 and assists with ankle dorsiflexion
Extensor hallucis longus	Anterior fibula and interosseous membrane	Dorsal base of distal phalanx of great toe	Deep fibular nerve (L5, S1)	Extends great toe and assists with ankle dorsiflexion
Extensor digitorum brevis	Superolateral aspect of calcaneus, extensor retinaculum	Dorsal base of middle phalanx of digits 2 to 5	Deep fibular nerve (L5, S1)	Extends digits 2 to 4 at MTP joints
Tibialis anterior	Lateral condyle and anterior surface of tibia	Inferomedial aspect of medial cuneiform and base of first metatarsal	Deep fibular nerve (L4, L5)	Ankle dorsiflexion and foot inversion

8

Foot and Ankle

Lateral Muscles of Leg—cont'd

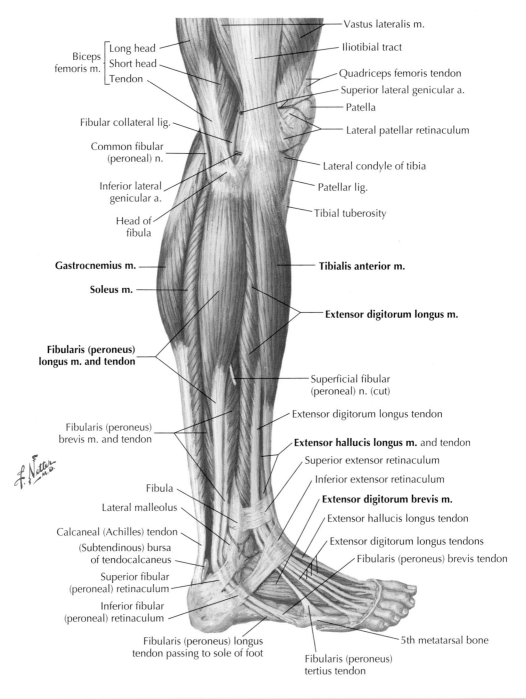

Vastus lateralis m.

Iliotibial tract

Quadriceps femoris tendon

Superior lateral genicular a.

Patella

Lateral patellar retinaculum

Lateral condyle of tibia

Patellar lig.

Tibial tuberosity

Biceps femoris m.
- Long head
- Short head
- Tendon

Fibular collateral lig.

Common fibular (peroneal) n.

Inferior lateral genicular a.

Head of fibula

Gastrocnemius m.

Soleus m.

Fibularis (peroneus) longus m. and tendon

Fibularis (peroneus) brevis m. and tendon

Tibialis anterior m.

Extensor digitorum longus m.

Superficial fibular (peroneal) n. (cut)

Extensor digitorum longus tendon

Extensor hallucis longus m. and tendon

Superior extensor retinaculum

Inferior extensor retinaculum

Extensor digitorum brevis m.

Extensor hallucis longus tendon

Extensor digitorum longus tendons

Fibularis (peroneus) brevis tendon

Fibula

Lateral malleolus

Calcaneal (Achilles) tendon

(Subtendinous) bursa of tendocalcaneus

Superior fibular (peroneal) retinaculum

Inferior fibular (peroneal) retinaculum

Fibularis (peroneus) longus tendon passing to sole of foot

Fibularis (peroneus) tertius tendon

5th metatarsal bone

Figure 8-9
Muscles of foot and ankle: lateral view.

Posterior Muscles of Leg

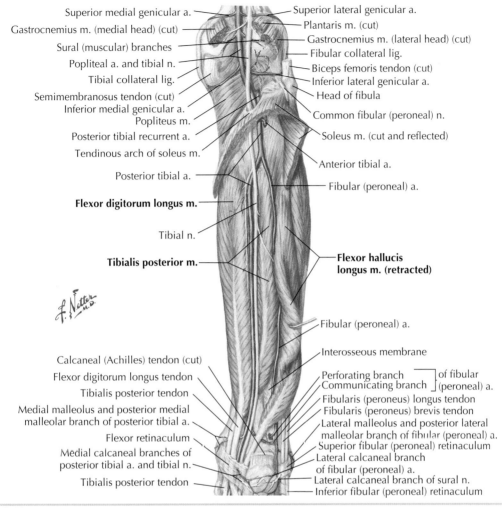

Superior medial genicular a.
Gastrocnemius m. (medial head) (cut)
Sural (muscular) branches
Popliteal a. and tibial n.
Tibial collateral lig.
Semimembranosus tendon (cut)
Inferior medial genicular a.
Popliteus m.
Posterior tibial recurrent a.
Tendinous arch of soleus m.
Posterior tibial a.
Flexor digitorum longus m.
Tibial n.
Tibialis posterior m.

Superior lateral genicular a.
Plantaris m. (cut)
Gastrocnemius m. (lateral head) (cut)
Fibular collateral lig.
Biceps femoris tendon (cut)
Inferior lateral genicular a.
Head of fibula
Common fibular (peroneal) n.
Soleus m. (cut and reflected)
Anterior tibial a.
Fibular (peroneal) a.
Flexor hallucis longus m. (retracted)

Calcaneal (Achilles) tendon (cut)
Flexor digitorum longus tendon
Tibialis posterior tendon
Medial malleolus and posterior medial malleolar branch of posterior tibial a.
Flexor retinaculum
Medial calcaneal branches of posterior tibial a. and tibial n.
Tibialis posterior tendon

Fibular (peroneal) a.
Interosseous membrane
Perforating branch ⎤ of fibular
Communicating branch ⎦ (peroneal) a.
Fibularis (peroneus) longus tendon
Fibularis (peroneus) brevis tendon
Lateral malleolus and posterior lateral malleolar branch of fibular (peroneal) a.
Superior fibular (peroneal) retinaculum
Lateral calcaneal branch of fibular (peroneal) a.
Lateral calcaneal branch of sural n.
Inferior fibular (peroneal) retinaculum

Figure 8-10
Muscles of leg: posterior view.

Muscles	Proximal Attachments	Distal Attachments	Nerve and Segmental Level	Action
Tibialis posterior	Interosseous membrane, posteroinferior aspect of tibia, and posterior fibula	Navicular tuberosity, cuneiform, cuboid, and bases of metatarsals 2 to 4	Tibial nerve (L4, L5)	Plantarflexes ankle and inverts foot
Flexor hallucis longus	Posteroinferior fibula and interosseous membrane	Base of distal phalanx of great toe	Tibial nerve (S2, S3)	Flexes great toe and assists with ankle plantarflexion
Flexor digitorum longus	Posteroinferior tibia	Bases of distal phalanges 2 to 5	Tibial nerve (S2, S3)	Flexes lateral four digits, plantarflexes ankle, supports longitudinal arch of foot

Foot and Ankle

8

Muscles of Dorsum of Foot

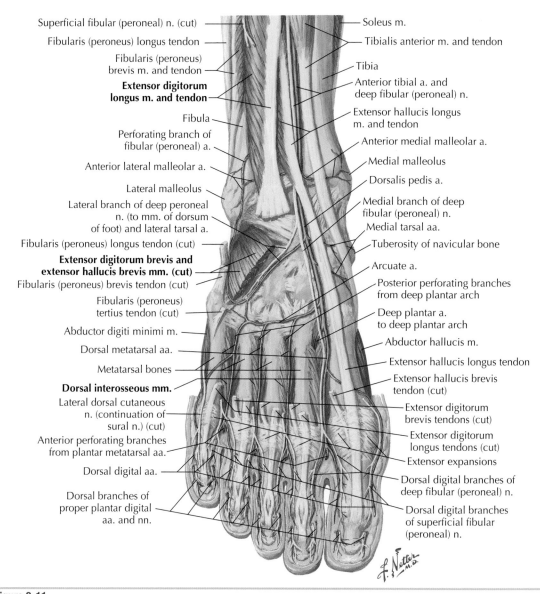

Superficial fibular (peroneal) n. (cut)

Fibularis (peroneus) longus tendon

Fibularis (peroneus) brevis m. and tendon

Extensor digitorum longus m. and tendon

Fibula

Perforating branch of fibular (peroneal) a.

Anterior lateral malleolar a.

Lateral malleolus

Lateral branch of deep peroneal n. (to mm. of dorsum of foot) and lateral tarsal a.

Fibularis (peroneus) longus tendon (cut)

Extensor digitorum brevis and extensor hallucis brevis mm. (cut)

Fibularis (peroneus) brevis tendon (cut)

Fibularis (peroneus) tertius tendon (cut)

Abductor digiti minimi m.

Dorsal metatarsal aa.

Metatarsal bones

Dorsal interosseous mm.

Lateral dorsal cutaneous n. (continuation of sural n.) (cut)

Anterior perforating branches from plantar metatarsal aa.

Dorsal digital aa.

Dorsal branches of proper plantar digital aa. and nn.

Soleus m.

Tibialis anterior m. and tendon

Tibia

Anterior tibial a. and deep fibular (peroneal) n.

Extensor hallucis longus m. and tendon

Anterior medial malleolar a.

Medial malleolus

Dorsalis pedis a.

Medial branch of deep fibular (peroneal) n.

Medial tarsal aa.

Tuberosity of navicular bone

Arcuate a.

Posterior perforating branches from deep plantar arch

Deep plantar a. to deep plantar arch

Abductor hallucis m.

Extensor hallucis longus tendon

Extensor hallucis brevis tendon (cut)

Extensor digitorum brevis tendons (cut)

Extensor digitorum longus tendons (cut)

Extensor expansions

Dorsal digital branches of deep fibular (peroneal) n.

Dorsal digital branches of superficial fibular (peroneal) n.

Figure 8-11
Muscles, arteries, and nerves of front of ankle and dorsum of foot: deeper dissection.

Muscles of Dorsum of Foot—cont'd

Muscles	Proximal Attachments	Distal Attachments	Nerve and Segmental Level	Action
Extensor digitorum brevis	Superolateral aspect of calcaneus and extensor retinaculum	Dorsal base of middle phalanx of digits 2 to 5	Deep fibular nerve (L5, S1)	Extends digits 2 to 4 at MTP joints
Extensor hallucis brevis	Superolateral aspect of calcaneus and extensor retinaculum	Dorsal base of proximal phalanx of great toe	Deep fibular nerve (L5, S1)	Extends great toe at MTP joints
Dorsal interossei	Sides of metatarsals 1 to 5	First: medial aspect of proximal phalanx of second digit Second to fourth: lateral aspect of digits 2 to 4	Lateral plantar nerve (S2, S3)	Abducts digits 2 to 4 and flexes MTP joints

8

Foot and Ankle

First Layer of Muscles: Sole of Foot

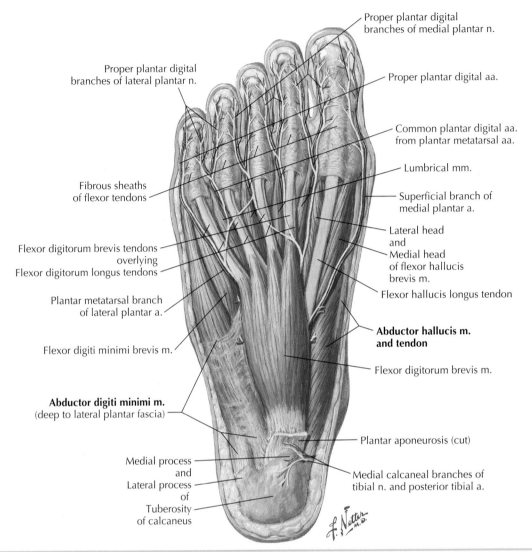

Proper plantar digital
branches of medial plantar n.

Proper plantar digital
branches of lateral plantar n.

Proper plantar digital aa.

Common plantar digital aa.
from plantar metatarsal aa.

Lumbrical mm.

Fibrous sheaths
of flexor tendons

Superficial branch of
medial plantar a.

Lateral head
and
Medial head
of flexor hallucis
brevis m.

Flexor digitorum brevis tendons
overlying
Flexor digitorum longus tendons

Flexor hallucis longus tendon

Plantar metatarsal branch
of lateral plantar a.

Abductor hallucis m.
and tendon

Flexor digiti minimi brevis m.

Flexor digitorum brevis m.

Abductor digiti minimi m.
(deep to lateral plantar fascia)

Plantar aponeurosis (cut)

Medial process
and
Lateral process
of
Tuberosity
of calcaneus

Medial calcaneal branches of
tibial n. and posterior tibial a.

Figure 8-12
Muscles of sole of foot: first layer.

Muscles	Proximal Attachments	Distal Attachments	Nerve and Segmental Level	Action
Abductor hallucis longus	Medial calcaneal tuberosity, flexor retinaculum, and plantar aponeurosis	Base of proximal phalanx of first digit	Medial plantar nerve (S2, S3)	Abducts and flexes great toe
Flexor digitorum brevis	Medial calcaneal tuberosity and plantar aponeurosis	Sides of middle phalanges of digits 2 to 5	Medial plantar nerve (S2, S3)	Flexes digits 2 to 5
Abductor digiti minimi	Medial and lateral calcaneal tuberosities	Lateral aspect of base of proximal phalanx of fifth metatarsal	Lateral plantar nerve (S2, S3)	Abducts and flexes fifth digit

Second Layer of Muscles: Sole of Foot

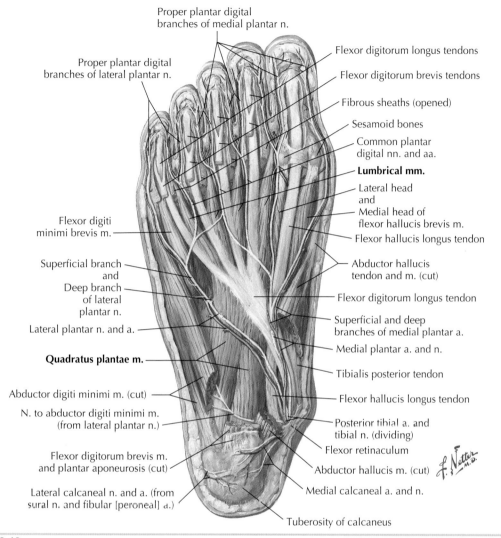

Proper plantar digital branches of medial plantar n.

Proper plantar digital branches of lateral plantar n.

Flexor digitorum longus tendons

Flexor digitorum brevis tendons

Fibrous sheaths (opened)

Sesamoid bones

Common plantar digital nn. and aa.

Lumbrical mm.

Lateral head and Medial head of flexor hallucis brevis m.

Flexor hallucis longus tendon

Flexor digiti minimi brevis m.

Superficial branch and Deep branch of lateral plantar n.

Lateral plantar n. and a.

Quadratus plantae m.

Abductor digiti minimi m. (cut)

N. to abductor digiti minimi m. (from lateral plantar n.)

Flexor digitorum brevis m. and plantar aponeurosis (cut)

Lateral calcaneal n. and a. (from sural n. and fibular [peroneal] a.)

Abductor hallucis tendon and m. (cut)

Flexor digitorum longus tendon

Superficial and deep branches of medial plantar a.

Medial plantar a. and n.

Tibialis posterior tendon

Flexor hallucis longus tendon

Posterior tibial a. and tibial n. (dividing)

Flexor retinaculum

Abductor hallucis m. (cut)

Medial calcaneal a. and n.

Tuberosity of calcaneus

Figure 8-13
Muscles of sole of foot: second layer.

Muscles	Proximal Attachments	Distal Attachments	Nerve and Segmental Level	Action
Lumbricals	Tendons of flexor digitorum longus	Medial aspect of expansion over lateral four digits	Lateral three: lateral plantar nerve (S2, S3) Medial one: medial plantar nerve (S2, S3)	Flexes proximal phalanges and extends middle and distal phalanges of digits 2 to 5
Quadratus plantae	Medial and plantar aspect of calcaneus	Posterolateral aspect of tendon of flexor digitorum longus	Lateral plantar nerve (S2, S3)	Assists in flexing digits 2 to 5

8

Foot and Ankle

Third Layer of Muscles: Sole of Foot

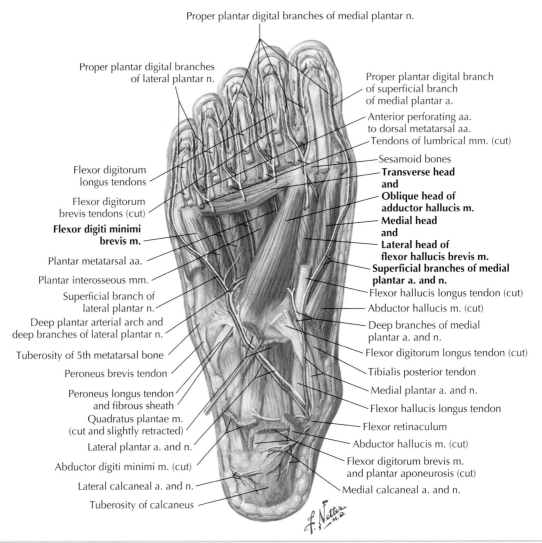

Figure 8-14
Muscles of sole of foot: third layer.

Muscles	Proximal Attachments	Distal Attachments	Nerve and Segmental Level	Action
Flexor digiti minimi brevis	Base of fifth metatarsal	Base of proximal phalanx of fifth metatarsal	Superficial branch of lateral plantar nerve	Flexes proximal phalanx of fifth digit
Adductor hallucis (transverse head)	Plantar ligaments of MTP joints	Lateral base of proximal phalanx of great toe	Deep branch of lateral plantar nerve (S2, S3)	Adducts great toe
Adductor hallucis (oblique head)	Bases of metatarsals 2 to 4			
Flexor hallucis brevis	Plantar cuboid and lateral cuneiforms	Sides of proximal phalanx of great toe	Medial plantar nerve (S2, S3)	Flexes proximal phalanx of great toe

Deep Interosseous Muscles: Sole of Foot

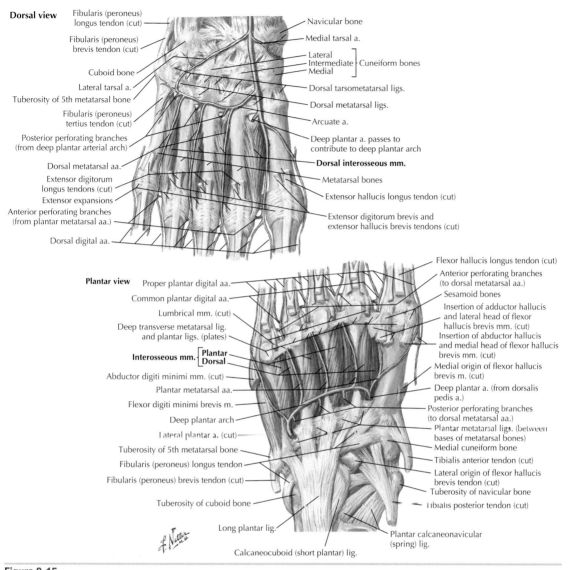

Figure 8-15
Interosseous muscles and plantar arterial arch.

Muscles	Proximal Attachments	Distal Attachments	Nerve and Segmental Level	Action
Plantar interosseous	Bases of metatarsals 3 to 5	Medial bases of proximal phalanges 3 to 5	Lateral plantar nerve (S2, S3)	Adducts digits 2 to 4 and flexes MTP joints
Dorsal interosseous	Sides of metatarsals 1 to 5	First: medial aspect of proximal phalanx of second digit Second to fourth: Lateral aspect of digits 2 to 4	Lateral plantar nerve (S2, S3)	Abducts digits 2 to 4 and flexes MTP joints

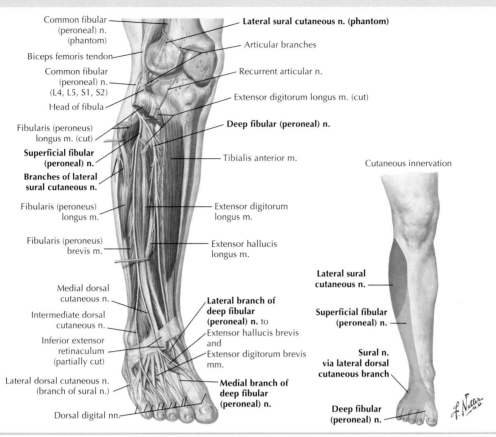

Figure 8-16
Tibial and fibular nerves: anterior view.

Nerves	Segmental Levels	Sensory	Motor
Sural	S1, S2	Posterior and lateral leg and lateral foot	No motor
Tibial	L4, L5, S1, S2, S3	Posterior heel and plantar surface of foot	Semitendinosus, semimembranosus, biceps femoris, adductor magnus, gastrocnemius, soleus, plantaris, flexor hallucis longus, flexor digitorum longus, tibialis posterior
Medial plantar	S2, S3	Medial 3½ digits	Flexor hallucis brevis, abductor hallucis, flexor digitorum brevis, lumbricales
Lateral plantar	S2, S3	Lateral 1½ digits	Adductor hallucis, abductor digiti minimi, quadratus plantae, lumbricales, flexor digiti minimi brevis, interossei
Saphenous	L2, L3, L4	Medial leg and foot	No motor
Deep fibular	L4, L5, S1	First interdigital cleft	Tibialis anterior, extensor digitorum longus, extensor hallucis longus, fibularis tertius, extensor digitorum brevis, extensor hallucis brevis
Superficial fibular	L5, S1, S2	Distal anterior leg and dorsum of foot	Fibularis longus, fibularis brevis

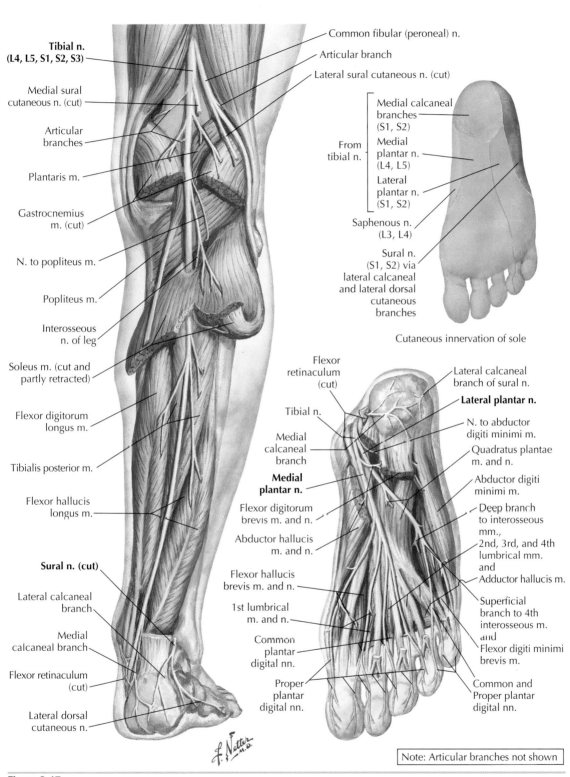

Tibial n.
(L4, L5, S1, S2, S3)

Medial sural
cutaneous n. (cut)

Articular
branches

Plantaris m.

Gastrocnemius
m. (cut)

N. to popliteus m.

Popliteus m.

Interosseous
n. of leg

Soleus m. (cut and
partly retracted)

Flexor digitorum
longus m.

Tibialis posterior m.

Flexor hallucis
longus m.

Sural n. (cut)

Lateral calcaneal
branch

Medial
calcaneal branch

Flexor retinaculum
(cut)

Lateral dorsal
cutaneous n.

Common fibular (peroneal) n.

Articular branch

Lateral sural cutaneous n. (cut)

Medial calcaneal
branches
(S1, S2)

From
tibial n.

Medial
plantar n.
(L4, L5)

Lateral
plantar n.
(S1, S2)

Saphenous n.
(L3, L4)

Sural n.
(S1, S2) via
lateral calcaneal
and lateral dorsal
cutaneous
branches

Cutaneous innervation of sole

Flexor
retinaculum
(cut)

Tibial n.

Medial
calcaneal
branch

**Medial
plantar n.**

Flexor digitorum
brevis m. and n.

Abductor hallucis
m. and n.

Flexor hallucis
brevis m. and n.

1st lumbrical
m. and n.

Common
plantar
digital nn.

Proper
plantar
digital nn.

Lateral calcaneal
branch of sural n.

Lateral plantar n.

N. to abductor
digiti minimi m.

Quadratus plantae
m. and n.

Abductor digiti
minimi m.

Deep branch
to interosseous
mm.,
2nd, 3rd, and 4th
lumbrical mm.
and
Adductor hallucis m.

Superficial
branch to 4th
interosseous m.
and
Flexor digiti minimi
brevis m.

Common and
Proper plantar
digital nn.

Note: Articular branches not shown

Figure 8-17
Tibial and fibular nerves: posterior view.

Foot and Ankle

8

Patient Reports	Initial Hypothesis
Patient reports a traumatic incident resulting in either forced inversion or eversion	Possible ankle sprain[1,2] Possible fracture Possible peroneal nerve involvement (if mechanism of injury is inversion)[3-5]
Patient reports trauma to ankle that included tibial rotation on a planted foot	Possible syndesmotic sprain[1]
Patient notes tenderness of anterior shin and may exhibit excessive pronation. Symptoms may be exacerbated by repetitive weight-bearing activities	Possible medial tibial stress syndrome[6]
Patient reports traumatic event resulting in inability to plantarflex ankle	Possible Achilles tendon rupture
Patient reports pain with stretch of calf muscles and during gait (toe push off)	Possible Achilles tendonitis[7] Possible Sever disease[1]
Patient reports pain at heel with first few steps out of bed after prolonged periods of walking	Possible plantar fasciitis
Patient reports pain or paresthesias in plantar surface of foot	Possible tarsal tunnel syndrome[1] Possible sciatica Possible lumbar radiculopathy
Patient reports pain on plantar surface of foot between third and fourth metatarsals. Might also state that pain is worse when walking with shoes compared with barefoot	Possible Morton neuroma[7] Possible metatarsalgia

Evaluation Following Acute Ankle Trauma

Test and Study Quality	Description and Positive Findings	Population	Interexaminer Reliability
Ability to bear weight[8]			$\kappa = .83$
Bone tenderness at base of fifth metatarsal[8]			$\kappa = .78$
Bone tenderness at posterior edge of lateral malleolus[8]			$\kappa = .75$
Bone tenderness at tip of medial malleolus[8]			$\kappa = .66$
Bone tenderness at proximal fibula[8]	Tenderness calculated as tender or not. Swelling and range-of-motion limitations dichotomized as "none-minimal" or "moderate-marked"	100 patients having sustained acute ankle trauma	$\kappa = -.01$
Combinations of bone tenderness[8]			$\kappa = .76$
Soft tissue tenderness[8]			$\kappa = .41$
Degree of swelling in area of anterior talofibular ligament[8]			$\kappa = .18$
Ecchymosis[8]			$\kappa = .39$
Range-of-motion restrictions present[8]			$\kappa = .33$
Palpation of anterior inferior tibiofibular ligament[9] ●	Tenderness on palpation over the anterior inferior tibiofibular ligament		$\kappa = .61$
Palpation of proximal fibula[9] ●	Tenderness on palpation over the proximal fibula	100 consecutive patients with an acute ankle sprain examined within 24 hours after injury	$\kappa = .66$
Palpation of deltoid ligament[9] ●	Tenderness on palpation over the deltoid ligament		$\kappa = .65$
Palpation of anterior talofibular[9] ●	Tenderness on palpation over the anterior talofibular		$\kappa = .39$
Palpation of calcaneo-fibular ligament[9] ●	Tenderness on palpation over the calcaneo-fibular ligament		$\kappa = .46$

8

Foot and Ankle

Evaluation Following Acute Ankle Trauma—cont'd

Test and Study Quality	Description and Positive Findings	Population	Interexaminer Reliability
Palpation test[1]	Examiner palpates over anterior talofibular ligament. Positive if pain is reproduced		$\kappa = .36$
External rotation test[1]	Patient sitting over edge of plinth. Passive external rotation stress is applied to foot and ankle. Positive if pain is reproduced over syndesmotic ligaments		$\kappa = .75$
Squeeze test[1]	Patient sitting over edge of plinth. Examiner manually compresses fibula and tibia over calf midpoint. Positive if pain is reproduced over syndesmotic ligaments	53 patients presenting for treatment of ankle injury	$\kappa = .50$
Dorsiflexion-compression test[1]	Patient is standing. Patient actively dorsi-flexes ankle while bearing weight. Examiner applies manual compression around mal-leoli while in dorsiflexed position. Positive if significant increase in ankle dorsiflexion or reduction in pain with compression		$\kappa = .36$

Test and Study Quality	Description	Positive Findings	Population	Reference Standard	Sens	Spec	+LR	−LR
Crossed leg test[9] ◆	The patient sits and crosses the affected leg over the opposite knee. Pressure is then applied to the proximal fibula of the affected leg	A positive test is pain in the distal ankle	100 consecutive patients with an acute ankle sprain examined within 24 hours after injury	MRI	.14	.83	.82*	1.04*

*Values were calculated by the authors of this text.

Diagnostic Utility of the Ottawa Ankle Rule for Radiography

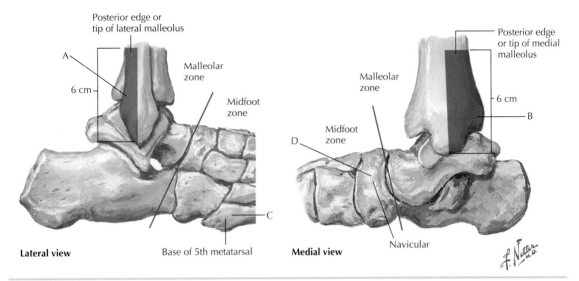

Figure 8-18
Ottawa Ankle Rules.

Test and Study Quality	Description and Positive Findings	Population	Reference Standard	Sens	Spec	+LR	−LR
Ottawa Ankle Rule for Radiography[10] **2017 Meta-analysis ◆**	Ankle x-ray series ordered when a patient had bone tenderness (exhibited at *A, B, C,* or *D* in Fig. 8.18) or if the patient could not bear weight immediately after the injury or during the examination (four steps regardless of limping)	Statistically pooled data from 9 high-quality studies involving 2185 adults and children	Ankle or midfoot fracture on x-rays	.94	.46	1.73 (1.41. 2.11)	.14 (0.07, .28)
Ottawa Ankle Rule for Radiography[11] **2017 Meta-analysis ◆**	As above	Statistically pooled data from 31 high-quality studies involving adults and children	Ankle or midfoot fracture on x-rays	.97 (.96, .98)	.35 (.27, .43)	1.5 (1.30, 1.68)	.09 (.06, .13)

8

Foot and Ankle

Diagnostic Utility of the Ottawa Ankle Rule for Radiography—cont'd

Test and Study Quality	Description and Positive Findings	Population	Reference Standard	Sens	Spec	+LR	−LR
Ottawa Ankle Rule for Radiography[3] **2003 Meta-analysis** ◆	As above	Statistically pooled data from 27 high-quality studies involving 15,581 adults and children		.98 (.97, .99)	.20	1.23	.10 (.06, .16)
Bernese Ankle Rules[10] **2017 Meta-analysis** ◆	Ankle x-ray series ordered when patients had pain with any of the following: (1) indirect fibular stress applied by compressing the tibia and fibula proximal to the malleoli (2) direct medial malleolar stress with examiner's thumb (3) compression stress of the midfoot and hindfoot applied simultaneously	Statistically pooled data from 4 high-quality studies involving 1519 adults	Ankle or midfoot fracture on x-rays	.69	.81	3.54 (1.73, 7.260)	.39 (.21, .79)
Adding tuning fork to Ottawa Ankle Rule for Radiography[12] ◐	Base of a vibrating tuning fork placed on tip of lateral malleolus. Positive if report of discomfort or pain	49 patients reporting to emergency department after inversion ankle injury		1.0	.61	2.59	.00
	As above, but placed on distal fibular shaft			1.0	.95	22.00	.00

Diagnostic Utility of the Ottawa Ankle Rule for Radiography—cont'd

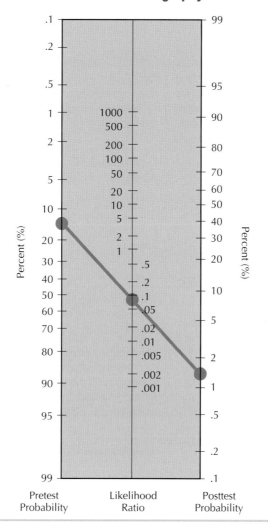

Figure 8-19

Nomogram. Assuming a fracture prevalence of 15% (statistically pooled from Bachmann et al[10]), an adult seen in the emergency department with an acute injury whose findings were negative on the Ottawa Ankle Rule would have a 1.4% (95% CI: 0.15% to 1.48%) chance of having an ankle and/or midfoot fracture. (From Fagan TJ. Nomogram for Bayes' theorem. *N Engl J Med.* 1975;293-257. Copyright 2005, Massachusetts Medical Society. See also Bachmann LM, Kolb E, Koller MT, et al. Accuracy of Ottawa ankle rules to exclude fractures of the ankle and mid-foot: systematic review. *BMJ.* 2003;326:417.)

Foot and Ankle

8

Reliability of Range-of-Motion Measurements

Measurements and Study Quality	Instrumentation	Population	Reliability	
			Intraexaminer	**Interexaminer**
Weight-bearing lunge test for ankle dorsiflexion[13] **2015 Systematic Review** ◆	Digital inclinometer used to measure angle of tibia between vertical position and calf stretch position with knee extended	Based on 9 studies for intrarater reliability and 12 studies for interrater reliability	ICC = .65 to .99	ICC = .80 to .99
Active range of motion (sitting) Subtalar joint inversion Subtalar joint eversion[15] ◆	Plastic goniometer	31 asymptomatic subjects	ICC = .91 to .96 ICC = .82 to .93	ICC = .73 (.61, .82) ICC = .62 (.49, .74)
Active range of motion (prone) Subtalar joint inversion Subtalar joint eversion[15] ◆	Plastic goniometer	31 asymptomatic subjects	ICC = .94 (.91, .96) ICC = .83 to .94	ICC = .54 (.33, .70) ICC = .41 (.25, .56)
Active range of motion Ankle dorsiflexion Ankle plantarflexion[16] ◆	Plastic goniometer	38 patients with orthopaedic disorders of ankle or knee	ICC = .89 ICC = .91	ICC = .28 ICC = .25
Passive range of motion Subtalar joint neutral Subtalar joint inversion Subtalar joint eversion Plantarflexion Dorsiflexion[17] ◆	Plastic goniometer	43 patients with orthopaedic or neurologic disorders where measurements of foot and ankle would be appropriate in a clinical setting	ICC = .77 ICC = .62 ICC = .59 ICC = .86 ICC = .90	ICC = .25 ICC = .15 ICC = .12 ICC = .72 ICC = .50
Passive range of motion Pronation Supination Ankle dorsiflexion First-ray plantarflexion First-ray dorsiflexion[18] ◉	Inclinometer	30 healthy subjects	ICC = .89 to .97 ICC = .90 to .95 ICC = .86 to .97 ICC = .72 to .97 ICC = .90 to .98	ICC = .46 to .49 ICC = .28 to .40 ICC = .26 to .31 ICC = .21 to .91 ICC = .14 to .16
First-ray mobility[7] ◉	Manual assessment. Graded as hypomobile, normal, or hypermobile	30 asymptomatic subjects	Not tested	κ = .08 to .20
Dorsiflexion in a modified lunge test[14] ◉	During lunge, inclinometer used to take measurements of angle formed by fibular head and lateral malleolus	31 subjects 76 to 87 years of age recruited from general population	ICC = .87 (.74, .94)	Not tested
Open kinetic chain: Resting subtalar joint Subtalar joint neutral[19] ◉	Inclinometer	30 asymptomatic subjects	ICC = .85 ICC = .85	ICC = .68 ICC = .79
Passive dorsiflexion[20] ◉	Standard goniometer	63 healthy naval reserve officers	ICC = .74	ICC = .65

Reliability of Range-of-Motion Measurements—cont'd

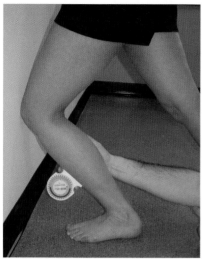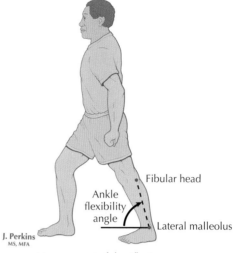

Weight-bearing lunge measurement
of ankle dorsiflexion

Measurement of dorsiflexion
with modified lunge test

Fibular head

Ankle
flexibility
angle

Lateral malleolus

J. Perkins
MS, MFA

Figure 8-20
Lunge measurements.

Reliability of Range-of-Motion Measurements of Calcaneal Position

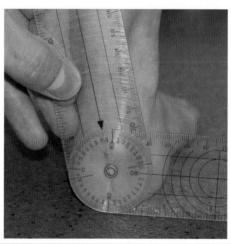

Figure 8-21
Measurement of relaxed calcaneal stance.

Measurements and Study Quality	Instrumentation	Population	Reliability	
			Intraexaminer	**Interexaminer**
Relaxed calcaneal stance position[21] ◐	Standard goniometer	212 healthy subjects: 88 adults and 124 children	ICC = .61 to .90	Not tested
Relaxed calcaneal stance Neutral calcaneal stance[18] ◐	Gravity goniometer	30 healthy subjects	ICC = .95 to .97 ICC = .87 to .93	ICC = .61 to .62 ICC = .21 to .31
Rearfoot angle[20] ◐	Standard goniometer	63 healthy naval reserve officers	ICC = .88	ICC = .86

Foot and Ankle

8

Reliability of Strength Assessment

Test or Measure and Study Quality	Description	Population	Interexaminer Reliability
Ankle plantarflexion strength and endurance[22] ◐	Children asked to perform as many single-leg heel rises as possible at a rate of one every 2 seconds while the examiner counts the repetitions	95 children 7 to 9 years old	ICC = .99

Diagnostic Utility of the Paper Grip Test for Detecting Toe Plantarflexion Strength Deficits

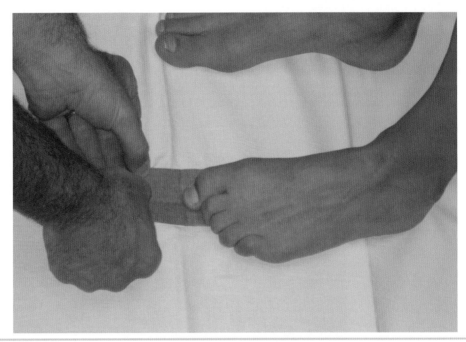

Figure 8-22
Paper grip test.

Test and Study Quality	Description and Positive Findings	Population	Reference Standard	Sens	Spec	+LR	−LR
Paper grip test[23] ◐	Patient is sitting with hips, knees, and ankles at 90 degrees and toes on a piece of cardboard. While stabilizing the feet, the examiner attempts to slide cardboard away from the patient's toes. Positive if patient cannot maintain cardboard under toes	80 asymptomatic adults	Toe plantarflexion strength as measured by a force plate system	.80	.79	3.8	.25

Measurement of Navicular Height

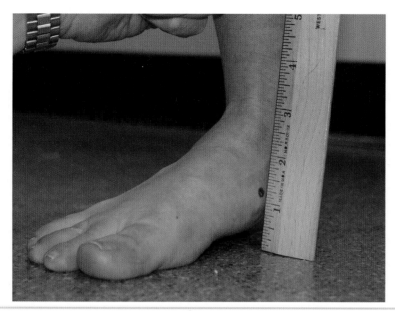

Figure 8-23
Measurement of navicular height.

Test or Measure and Study Quality	Description	Population	Reliability	
			Intraexaminer	**Interexaminer**
Navicular height[14] ◐	Navicular tuberosity is marked while patient is in weight-bearing position. Distance from ground to navicular tuberosity is measured	31 subjects 76 to 87 years of age recruited from general population	ICC = .64 (.38, .81)	Not tested
Navicular drop test[24] ◐	Navicular tuberosity is marked. Examiner measures height of navicular tuberosity	30 patients with patellofemoral pain syndrome	Not tested	ICC = .93 (.84, .97)
Navicular height technique[19] ◐	(1) as patient's foot rests on the ground, weight bearing is mostly on contralateral lower extremity, and examiner maintains the subtalar joint in neutral position and (2) as the patient's foot is in relaxed bilateral stance with full weight bearing. The two measurements are recorded	30 asymptomatic subjects	ICC = .83	ICC = .73
Navicular height[25] ◐	Height of navicular tuberosity is calculated with a digital caliper	100 consecutive patients presenting to an orthopaedic foot and ankle clinic	ICC = .90	ICC = .74

8

Foot and Ankle

Assessment of Medial Arch Height

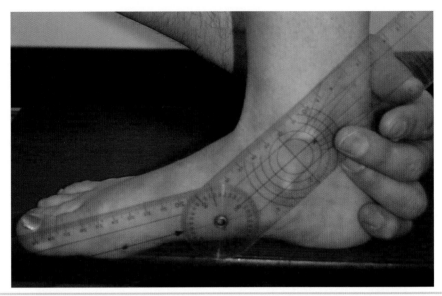

Figure 8-24
Measurement of arch angle.

Test or Measure and Study Quality	Description	Population	Reliability	
			Intraexaminer	Interexaminer
Arch angle[20] ●	Patient is in weight-bearing position. Examiner measures angle formed by line connecting medial malleolus and navicular tuberosity and angle from tuberosity to medial aspect of first metatarsal head with standard goniometer	63 healthy naval reserve officers	ICC = .90	ICC = .81
Arch height test[25] ●	Highest point of soft tissue margin along medial longitudinal arch is recorded with a digital caliper	100 consecutive patients presenting to an orthopaedic foot and ankle clinic	ICC = .91	ICC = .76

Measuring Forefoot Position

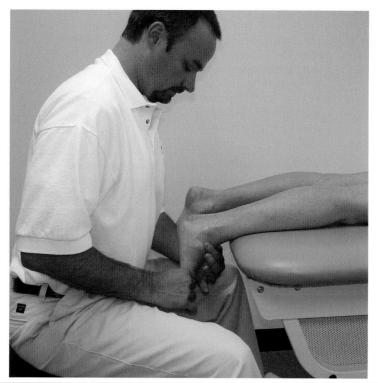

Figure 8-25
Determination of forefoot varus/valgus.

Test or Measure and Study Quality	Description	Population	Reliability	
			Intraexaminer	**Interexaminer**
Forefoot varus[18] ◑	Patient is prone with foot over edge of table. Examiner palpates medial and lateral talar head and then grasps fourth and fifth metatarsals and takes up slack in midtarsal joints. Subtalar neutral is position in which medial and lateral talar head is palpated equally[26]	30 healthy subjects	ICC = .95 to .99	ICC = .61

Foot and Ankle

8

Reliability of Assessing Balance and Proprioception

Test and Study Quality	Description	Population	Reliability
Single-leg balance test[28] ◆	Participant is asked to stand on one foot, without shoes on, and with the contralateral leg bent and not touching the tested limb. Test is positive if participant is unable to remain balanced or if participant reports a sense of imbalance	240 healthy athletes	Interexaminer $\kappa = .90$
Single-leg balance test[27] ●	Participant is asked to stand on one foot, without shoes on, on a polyfoam mat with the eyes closed and the contralateral leg bent for 1 minute. Number of errors (e.g., surface contact with contralateral foot or movement of the test foot) is counted by the examiner	24 male recreational athletes with functional ankle instability	Test-retest ICC = .94
Threshold for perception of passive movement[29] ●	Examiner collects measurements with potentiometer	24 healthy adult subjects	Test-retest ICC = .95
Active-to-active reproduction of joint position[29] ●			Test-retest ICC = .83
Reproduction of movement velocity[29] ●			Test-retest ICC = .79
Reproduction of torque[29] ●			Test-retest ICC = (Dorsiflexion) .86 (Plantarflexion) .72

Reliability of Assessing Dynamic Performance

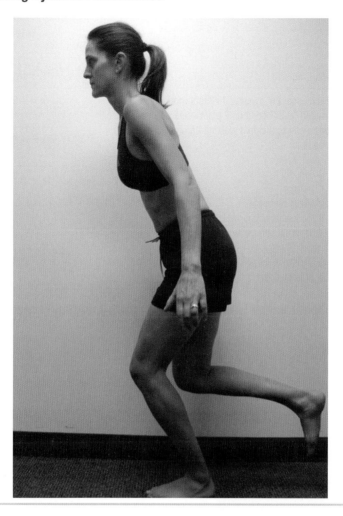

Figure 8-26
Single-leg hop test.

Test or Measure and Study Quality	Description	Population	Reliability
Single-leg hopping course[27] ●	Course consists of eight squares, some of which are inclined, declined, or have a lateral inclination. Patient is asked to jump on each square on one leg as quickly as possible. Performance is indicated by the number of seconds taken	24 male recreational athletes with functional ankle instability	Test-retest ICC = .97
Single-leg hop for distance[27] ●	Patient is asked to hop once or three times as far as possible on one leg. Performance is indicated by distance covered		Test-retest ICC = .97
Triple hop for distance[27] ●			Test-retest ICC = .98
6-meter hop for time[27] ●	Patient is asked to hop, in a straight line or crosswise over a line, for 6 meters on one leg as quickly as possible. Performance is indicated by the number of seconds taken		Test-retest ICC = .95
Cross 6-meter hop for time[27] ●			Test-retest ICC = .94

8

Foot and Ankle

Reliability of Assessing Hindfoot Motion during Gait

Test or Measure and Study Quality	Description	Population	Interexaminer Reliability	
			5-Point Scale	2-Point Scale
Duration of hindfoot motion[30] ⬤	Each aspect of dynamic hindfoot motion is graded on a 2-point or 5-point scale while observing participant walking barefoot on a treadmill. *5-point scale:* (1) Less than normal (2) Normal (3) Mildly abnormal (4) Moderately abnormal (5) Severely abnormal *2-point scale:* (1) Normal or less than normal (2) Greater than normal	24 healthy participants	κ = −.03 to .01	κ = .14 to .24
Velocity of hindfoot motion[30] ⬤			κ = −.04 to .01	κ = .02 to .20
Timing of hindfoot motion[30] ⬤			κ = .15 to .20	κ = .19 to .20
Maximum degree of hindfoot motion[30] ⬤			κ = .13 to .18	κ = .27 to .48
Range of hindfoot motion[30] ⬤			κ = .06 to .19	κ = .15 to .28

Accuracy of the Functional Hallux Limitus Test to Predict Abnormal Excessive Midtarsal Function during Gait

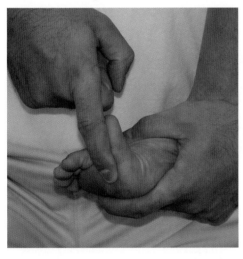

Figure 8-27
Functional hallux limitus test.

Test and Study Quality	Description and Positive Findings	Population	Reference Standard	Sens	Spec	+LR	−LR
Functional hallux limitus test[31] ⬤	With the patient in a non–weight-bearing position, the examiner uses one hand to maintain the subtalar joint in a neutral position while maintaining the first ray in dorsiflexion. The other hand is used to dorsiflex the proximal phalanx of the hallux. The test is considered positive if the examiner notes immediate plantarflexion of the first metatarsal upon dorsiflexion of the proximal phalanx	46 asymptomatic students (86 feet) with no significant orthopaedic or structural deformities of the foot	Abnormal midtarsal motion by observing if the navicular moved in a plantar direction or was adducted when the heel began to lift off the ground	.72	.66	2.1	.42

Reliability of Measuring Ankle Joint Swelling

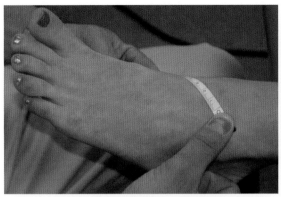

Start of figure-of-eight measurement

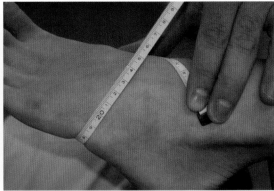

Figure-of-eight measurement continued

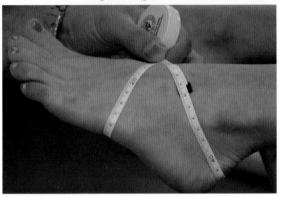

Completed figure-of-eight measurement

Figure 8-28
Figure-of-eight measurement.

Test and Study Quality	Description	Population	Reliability	
			Intraexaminer	**Interexaminer**
Figure-of-eight method[32] ●	In open kinetic chain, examiner places tape measure midway between tibialis anterior tendon and lateral malleolus. Tape is then drawn medially and placed just distal to navicular tuberosity. Tape is then pulled across arch and just proximal to base of fifth metatarsal. Tape is then pulled across anterior tibialis tendon and around ankle joint just distal to medial malleolus. Tape is finally pulled across Achilles tendon and placed just distal to lateral malleolus and across start of tape	30 postoperative patients with ankle edema	ICC = .99 to 1.0	ICC = .99 to 1.0
Figure-of-eight method[33] ●		50 healthy subjects	ICC = .99	ICC = .99
Figure-of-eight method[33] ●		29 individuals with ankle swelling	ICC = .98	ICC = .98
Water volumetrics[33] ●	Water displacement is measured with patient's foot in a volumeter with toe tips touching front wall		ICC = .99	ICC = .99

8

Foot and Ankle

Detecting Subcutaneous Tears of the Achilles Tendon

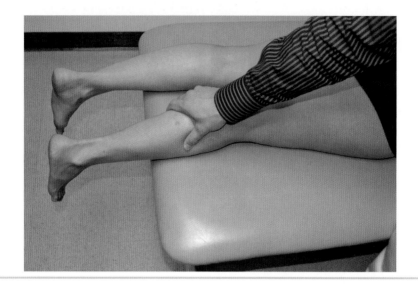

Figure 8-29
Thompson test.

Test and Study Quality	Description	Positive Findings	Population	Reference Standard	Sens	Spec	+LR	−LR
Thompson test[34] ●	Patient positioned prone while examiner gently squeezes the patient's calf muscles with the palm of his or her hand	If the Achilles tendon is intact, plantarflexion occurs in the ankle. If the Achilles tendon is torn, the ankle either remains still or only minimal plantarflexion occurs	174 patients with suspected Achilles tendon tear referred to orthopaedic clinic	Surgical confirmation for subjects with the diagnosis; magnetic resonance imaging (MRI) and ultrasound for subjects without the diagnosis	.96 (.91, .99)	.93 (.75, .99)	13.47 (3.54, 51.25)	.04 (.02, .10)
Achilles palpation[34] ●	Patient positioned prone while examiner gently palpates the course of the tendon	The gap is classified as present or absent			.73 (.64, .80)	.89 (.71, .97)	6.81 (2.32, 19.93)	.30 (.23, .40)

Reliability of Tests for Detecting Syndesmotic Injury

Test and Study Quality	Description	Population	Reliability	
			Intraexaminer	Interexaminer
Squeeze test[9] ⬤	With patient sitting over the side of the bed, a passive external rotation stress to the involved foot and ankle with the knee held at 90° and the ankle in a neutral position. Positive if pain produced over the area of the syndesmotic ligaments	100 consecutive patients with an acute ankle sprain examined within 24 hours after injury	Unknown	$\kappa = .45$
External rotation test[9] ⬤	With patient sitting over the side of the bed, examiner manually compresses the fibula to the tibia above the midpoint of the calf. Positive if pain produced over the area of the syndesmotic ligaments		Unknown	$\kappa = .40$
Cotton test[9] ⬤	Distal tibia stabilized and lateral force applied to the foot. Positive with increased lateral translation of the talus from medial to lateral compared with contralateral side		Unknown	$\kappa = .52$
Crossed leg test[9] ⬤	The patient sits and crosses the affected leg over the opposite knee. Pressure is then applied to the proximal fibula of the affected leg. A positive test is pain in the distal ankle		Unknown	$\kappa = .44$

8

Foot and Ankle

Detecting Syndesmotic Injury

Test and Study Quality	Description	Positive Findings	Population	Reference Standard	Sens	Spec	+LR	−LR
Crossed leg test[9] ◆	The patient sits and crosses the affected leg over the opposite knee. Pressure is then applied to the proximal fibula of the affected leg	A positive test is pain in the distal ankle	100 consecutive patients with an acute ankle sprain examined within 24 hours after injury	MRI	.14	.83	.82*	1.04*
Cotton test[9] ◆	Distal tibia stabilized and lateral force applied to the foot	Positive with increased lateral translation of the talus from medial to lateral compared with contralateral side			.31	.68	.97*	1.01*
External rotation test[9] ◆	With patient sitting over the side of the bed, examiner manually compresses the fibula to the tibia above the midpoint of the calf	Positive if pain produced over the area of the syndesmotic ligaments			.56	.48	1.08*	.92*
External rotation test[35] ◆	Clinician applies external rotation of patient's foot with leg stabilized and ankle in neutral position	Pain elicited at anterolateral ankle	56 patients with lateral ankle sprain referred to orthopaedic clinic	MRI	.20 (.04, .56)	.85 (.71, .93)	1.31 (.32, 5.41)	.94 (.69, 1.30)
Dorsiflexion–external rotation test[36] ◆	Leg is stabilized in 90 degrees of knee flexion, and the ankle is in maximal dorsiflexion; an external rotation stress is applied to the injured foot and ankle	Reproduction of anterolateral pain over the syndesmosis area	87 patients with an acute ankle injury	MRI	.71 (.55, .83)	.63 (.49, .75)	1.93 (1.28, 2.94)	.46 (.27, .79)
Dorsiflexion lunge with compression test[36] ◆	Patient lunges forward on the injured leg as far as possible. The lunge is repeated with manual compression provided by the examiner across the ankle syndesmosis	Increase in the ankle range of motion or decreased pain when compression added			.69 (.53, .82)	.41 (.28, .56)	1.18 (.86, 1.64)	.74 (.41, 1.35)

Detecting Syndesmotic Injury—cont'd

Test and Study Quality	Description	Positive Findings	Population	Reference Standard	Sens	Spec	+LR	−LR
Squeeze test[9] ◆	With patient sitting over the side of the bed, a passive external rotation stress to the involved foot and ankle with the knee held at 90° and the ankle in a neutral position	Positive if pain produced over the area of the syndesmotic ligaments	100 consecutive patients with an acute ankle sprain examined within 24 hours after injury	MRI	.44	.56	1.00*	1.00*
Syndesmosis squeeze test[35] ◆	Clinician applies lateromedial compression at the transition between the middle and distal third of the patient's leg	Pain elicited at distal syndesmosis	56 patients with lateral ankle sprain referred to orthopaedic clinic	MRI	.30 (.08, .65)	.93 (.81, .98)	4.60 (1.08, 19.55)	.75 (.50, 1.13)
Syndesmosis squeeze test[36] ◆	Patient sitting over the side of the bed. Compression of the fibula to the tibia about the midpoint of the calf using one or both hands	Replication of pain in the area of the ankle syndesmosis	87 patients with an acute ankle injury	MRI	.26 (.15, .42)	.88 (.76, .94)	2.15 (.86, 5.39)	.84 (.68, 1.04)
Syndesmosis ligament palpation[36] ◆	Palpation of anterior and posterior inferior tibiofibular ligament Palpation between the tibia and fibula	Report of pain after pressing the ligament or membrane		MRI	.92 (.79, .97)	.29 (.18, .42)	1.29 (1.06, 1.58)	.28 (.09, .89)
Anterior inferior tibiofibular ligament palpation[9] ◆	Palpation of anterior inferior tibiofibular ligament	Tenderness on palpation over the anterior inferior tibiofibular ligament			.42	.53	.89*	1.09*
Proximal fibula palpation[9] ◆	Palpation of proximal fibula	Tenderness on palpation over the proximal fibula	100 consecutive patients with an acute ankle sprain examined within 24 hours after injury	MRI	.01	.94	.17*	1.05*
Deltoid ligament palpation[9] ◆	Palpation of deltoid ligament	Tenderness on palpation over the deltoid ligament			.33	.70	1.1*	.96*
Anterior talofibular palpation[9] ◆	Palpation of anterior talofibular	Tenderness on palpation over the anterior talofibular			.78	.27	1.07*	.81*
Calcaneofibular ligament palpation[9] ◆	Palpation of calcaneo-fibular ligament	Tenderness on palpation over the calcaneofibular ligament			.61	.48	1.17*	.81*

*Values were calculated by the authors of this text.

Foot and Ankle

8

Detecting Syndesmotic Injury—cont'd

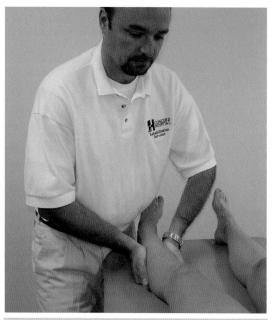

Figure 8-30
Squeeze test.

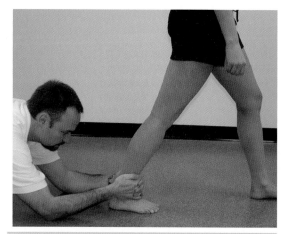

Figure 8-31
Dorsiflexion-compression test.

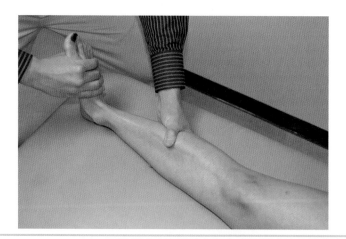

Figure 8-32
External rotation test.

Detecting Anterolateral Ankle Impingement

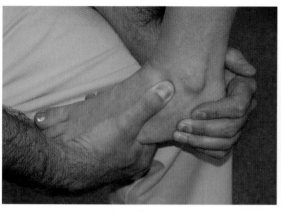
Plantarflexion

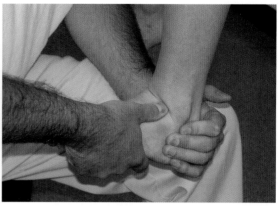
Dorsiflexion

Figure 8-33
Impingement sign.

Test and Study Quality	Description	Positive Findings	Population	Reference Standard	Sens	Spec	+LR	−LR
Impingement sign[37] (see Video 8-1) ◉	Patient is seated. Examiner grasps calcaneus with one hand and uses other hand to grasp forefoot and bring it into plantarflexion. Examiner uses thumb to place pressure over anterolateral ankle. Foot is then brought from plantarflexion to dorsiflexion while thumb pressure is maintained	Positive if pain provoked with pressure from examiner's thumb is greater in dorsiflexion than plantarflexion	73 patients with ankle pain	Arthroscopic visualization	.95	.88	7.91	.06
History and clinical examination[38] ◉	Examiner records aggravating factors and reports loss of motion. Examination includes observation of swelling, passive forced ankle dorsiflexion and eversion, active range of motion and double-leg and single-leg squats	Positive if five or more findings are positive: (1) Anterolateral ankle joint tenderness (2) Anterolateral ankle joint swelling (3) Pain with forced dorsiflexion and eversion (4) Pain with single-leg squat (5) Pain with activities (6) Ankle instability	22 patients undergoing arthroscopic surgery for complaints of chronic ankle pain	Arthroscopic visualization	.94	.75	3.76	.08

8

Foot and Ankle

Detecting Joint Instability after Lateral Ankle Sprain

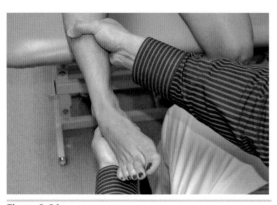

Figure 8-34
Medial talar tilt stress test.

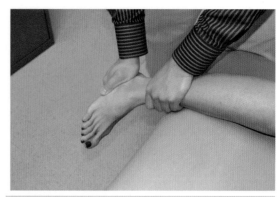

Figure 8-35
Medial subtalar glide test.

Test and Study Quality	Description	Positive Findings	Population	Reference Standard	Sens	Spec	+LR	−LR
Anterior drawer test[16] ◆	Clinician stabilizes patient's distal leg and grasps the calcaneus to impart an anteriorly directed force in an attempt to move the talus; patient is seated with ankle in 10 to 20 degrees of plantarflexion	Clinician-assessed grades of 3 and above on a 4-point laxity scale	66 patients with history of lateral ankle sprain and 20 healthy controls	Ultrasound	.33 (.18, .53)	.73 (.59, .85)	1.27 (.59, 2.72)	.90 (.64, 1.26)
Anterior drawer test[39] (see Video 8-2) ◍	Manual examination for anterior displacement of the talus within the mortise	Anterior displacement of the talus within the mortise graded on a 4-point laxity scale			.58 (.29, .84)	1.00 (.60, 1.00)	Undefined	.42 (.21, .81)
Medial talar tilt stress test[39] (see Video 8-3) ◍	Manual examination for excessive inversion of the talus within the mortise	Inversion of the talus within the mortise graded on a 4-point laxity scale	12 subjects with history of lateral ankle sprain and 8 healthy controls	Stress fluoroscopy	.50 (.22, .78)	.88 (.47, .99)	4.00 (.59, 27.25)	.57 (.31, 1.04)
Medial subtalar glide test[39] ◍	Examiner holds the talus in subtalar neutral position with one hand and glides the calcaneus medially on the fixed talus with the other hand	Examiner assesses the end feel of the glide graded on a 4-point laxity scale			.58 (.29, .84)	.88 (.47, .99)	4.67 (.70, 31.04)	.48 (.24, .96)

Detecting Joint Instability after Lateral Ankle Sprain—cont'd

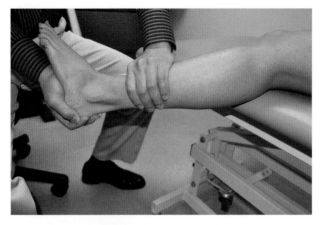

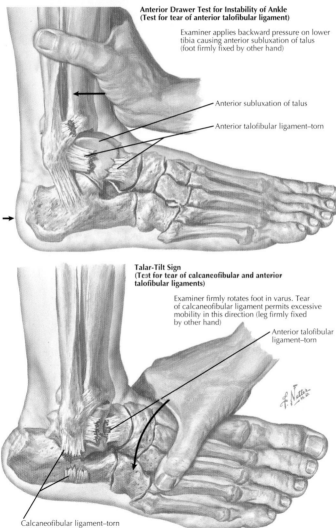

Anterior Drawer Test for Instability of Ankle
(Test for tear of anterior talofibular ligament)

Examiner applies backward pressure on lower tibia causing anterior subluxation of talus (foot firmly fixed by other hand)

Anterior subluxation of talus

Anterior talofibular ligament–torn

Talar-Tilt Sign
(Test for tear of calcaneofibular and anterior talofibular ligaments)

Examiner firmly rotates foot in varus. Tear of calcaneofibular ligament permits excessive mobility in this direction (leg firmly fixed by other hand)

Anterior talofibular ligament–torn

Calcaneofibular ligament–torn

Figure 8-36
Anterior drawer test.

Foot and Ankle

8

Detecting Tarsal Tunnel Syndrome

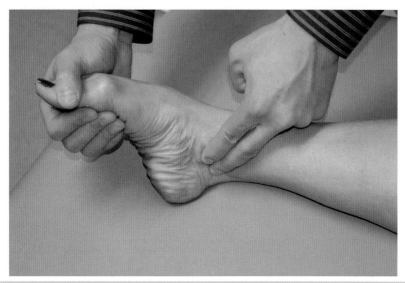

Figure 8-37
Triple compression test.

Test and Study Quality	Description	Positive Findings	Population	Reference Standard	Sens	Spec	+LR	−LR
Triple compression stress test[40] (see Video 8-4) ◆	Clinician positions patient's ankle in full plantarflexion and inversion while simultaneously applying direct digital pressure for 30 seconds over posterior tibial nerve behind the medial malleolus	Reproduction or intensified clinical symptoms and signs of tarsal tunnel syndrome	50 subjects with symptoms suggestive of tarsal tunnel syndrome and 40 healthy controls	Basic motor nerve conduction for tibial nerve	.86 (.76, .92)	1.00 (.93, 1.00)	Undefined	.14 (.08, .24)

Detecting Morton Neuroma

Test and Study Quality	Description	Positive Findings	Population	Reference Standard	Sens	Spec	+LR	−LR
Thumb index finger squeeze test[41]	The symptomatic intermetatarsal space is squeezed between the tips of the index finger (dorsal) and thumb (plantar). Splaying of the involved toes was used as a guide for correct positioning and pressure of the thumb and index finger	Positive if pain was produced			.96	1.00	Undefined*	.04*
Mulder's click[41]	The foot is clasped around the metatarsal heads with the fingers of 1 hand, and the thumb of the contralateral hand exerts firm pressure on the sole of the foot at the site of the MN. Firm lateral compression of the metatarsal heads is then applied with the fingers	Positive if a palpable click was felt	54 feet from 40 patients presenting with forefoot pain in a tertiary foot and ankle clinic	Ultrasonography	.62	1.00	Undefined*	0.38*
Foot squeeze test[41]	The foot is clasped with the fingers, and the metatarsal heads are squeezed together	Positive if localized pain was produced at the intermetatarsal space in question			.41	.00	.41*	Undefined*
Plantar and dorsal percussion tests[41]	The dorsal and plantar intermetatarsal spaces were percussed with a finger				.36	1.00	Undefined*	.64*
Light touch sensory test[41]	The toe tip is stroked with a finger	Positive if the subjective sensation was different from that on the adjacent toes			.25	1.00	Undefined*	.75*

*Values were calculated by the authors of this text.

8

Foot and Ankle

Outcome Measure		Scoring and Interpretation	Test-Retest Reliability and Study Quality	MCID
Lower Extremity Functional Scale (LEFS)		Users are asked to rate the difficulty of performing 20 functional tasks on a Likert-type scale ranging from 0 (extremely difficult or unable to perform activity) to 4 (no difficulty). A total score out of 80 is calculated by summing each score. The answers provide a score between 0 and 80, with lower scores representing more disability	ICC = .85–.99[42]	9[42]
Foot Function Index (FFI)		A self-administered questionnaire consisting of 23 items divided into pain, disability, and activity restriction subscales. A score between 0 and 100 is derived by dividing the visual analog scale into 10 segments. Higher scores indicate more impairment	ICC = .85[4]	Unknown
American Orthopaedic Foot and Ankle Society (AOFAS) scales	Ankle-Hindfoot	Each scale is administered by a clinician and has subjective and objective criteria, including range-of-motion, gait abnormalities, stability, alignment, and callus assessment. The answers provide a score between 0 and 100, with lower scores representing more disability	Unknown	9[43]
	Midfoot		Unknown	12[43]
	Hallux		ICC = .95[4]	25[43]
	MTP-IP joints		ICC = .80[4]	11[43]
Numeric Pain Rating Scale (NPRS)		Users rate their level of pain on an 11-point scale ranging from 0 to 10, with high scores representing more pain. Often asked as "current pain" and "least," "worst," and "average pain" in the past 24 hours	ICC = .72[44]	2[45,46]

ICC: Intraclass correlation coefficient; MCID: minimum clinically important difference.

1. Alonso A, Khoury L, Adams R. Clinical tests for ankle syndesmosis injury: reliability and prediction of return to function. *J Orthop Sports Phys Ther*. 1998;27:276–284.
2. Reischl SF, Noceti-DeWit LM. Foot and ankle. In: *Current Concepts of Orthopedic Physical Therapy*. La Crosse, Wisconsin: Orthopaedic Section, American Physical Therapy Association; 2001.
3. Bachmann LM, Kolb E, Koller MT, et al. Accuracy of Ottawa ankle rules to exclude fractures of the ankle and mid-foot: systematic review. *BMJ*. 2003;326:417.
4. Baumhauer JF, Nawoczenski DA, DiGiovanni BF, Wilding GE. Reliability and validity of the American Orthopaedic foot and ankle Society clinical Rating scale: a pilot study for the hallux and lesser toes. *Foot Ankle Int*. 2006;27:1014–1019.
5. Bennett JE, Reinking MF, Pluemer B, et al. Factors contributing to the development of medial tibial stress syndrome in high school runners. *J Orthop Sports Phys Ther*. 2001;31:504–510.
6. Binkley JM, Stratford PW, Lott SA, Riddle DL. The lower extremity functional scale (LEFS): scale development, measurement properties, and clinical application. North American Orthopaedic Rehabilitation Research Network. *Phys Ther*. 1999;79:371–383.
7. Cornwall MW, Fishco WD, McPoil TG, et al. Reliability and validity of clinically assessing first-ray mobility of the foot. *J Am Podiatr Med Assoc*. 2004,94.470–476.
8. Stiell IG, McKnight RD, Greenberg GH, et al. Interobserver agreement in the examination of acute ankle injury patients. *Am J Emerg Med*. 1992;10:14–17.
9. Großterlinden LG, Hartel M, Yamamura J, et al. Isolated syndesmotic injuries in acute ankle sprains: diagnostic significance of clinical examination and MRI. *Knee Surg Sports Traumatol Arthrosc*. 2016;24(4):1180–1186.
10. Barelds I, Krijnen WP, van de Leur JP, et al. Diagnostic accuracy of clinical decision rules to exclude fractures in acute ankle injuries: Systematic review and meta-analysis. *J Emerg Med*. 2017;53(3):353–368.
11. Beckenkamp PR, Lin C-WC, Macaskill P, et al. Diagnostic accuracy of the Ottawa Ankle and Midfoot Rules: A systematic review with meta-analysis. *Br J Sports Med*. 2017;51(6):504–510.
12. Dissmann PD, Han KH. The tuning fork test–a useful tool for improving specificity in "Ottawa positive" patients after ankle inversion injury. *Emerg Med J*. 2006;23:788–790.
13. Powden CJ, Hoch JM, Hoch MC. Reliability and minimal detectable change of the weight-bearing lunge test: A systematic review. *Man Ther*. 2015;20(4):524–532.
14. Menz HB, Tiedemann A, Kwan MM, et al. Reliability of clinical tests of foot and ankle characteristics in older people. *J Am Podiatr Med Assoc*. 2003;93:380–387.
15. Menadue C, Raymond J, Kilbreath SL, et al. Reliability of two goniometric methods of measuring active inversion and eversion range of motion at the ankle. *BMC Musculoskelet Disord*. 2006;7:60.
16. Croy T, Koppenhaver S, Saliba S, Hertel J. Anterior talocrural joint laxity: diagnostic accuracy of the anterior drawer test of the ankle. *J Orthop Sports Phys Ther*. 2013;43(12):911–919.
17. Elveru RA, Rothstein JM, Lamb RL. Goniometric reliability in a clinical setting. Subtalar and ankle joint measurements. *Phys Ther*. 1988;68:672–677.
18. Van Gheluwe B, Kirby KA, Roosen P, Phillips RD. Reliability and accuracy of biomechanical measurements of the lower extremities. *J Am Podiatr Med Assoc*. 2002;92:317–326.
19. Sell KE, Verity TM, Worrell TW, et al. Two measurement techniques for assessing subtalar joint position: a reliability study. *J Orthop Sports Phys Ther*. 1994;19:162–167.
20. Jonson SR, Gross MT. Intraexaminer reliability, interexaminer reliability, and mean values for nine lower extremity skeletal measures in healthy naval midshipmen. *J Orthop Sports Phys Ther*. 1997;25:253–263.
21. Sobel E, Levitz SJ, Caselli MA, et al. Reevaluation of the relaxed calcaneal stance position. Reliability and normal values in children and adults. *J Am Podiatr Med Assoc*. 1999;89:258–264.
22. Maurer C, Finley A, Martel J, et al. Ankle plantarflexor strength and endurance in 7-9 year old children as measured by the standing single leg heel-rise test. *Phys Occup Ther Pediatr*. 2007;27:37–54.
23. Menz HB, Zammit GV, Munteanu SE, Scott G. Plantarflexion strength of the toes: age and gender differences and evaluation of a clinical screening test. *Foot Ankle Int*. 2006;27:1103–1108.
24. Piva SR, Fitzgerald K, Irrgang JJ, et al. Reliability of measures of impairments associated with patellofemoral pain syndrome. *BMC Musculoskelet Disord*. 2006;7:33.
25. Saltzman CL, Nawoczenski DA, Talbot KD. Measurement of the medial longitudinal arch. *Arch Phys Med Rehabil*. 1995;76:45–49.
26. Root ML, Orien WP, Weed JH. *Biomechanical Examination of the Foot*. Los Angeles: Clinical Biomechanics Corp; 1971.
27. Sekir U, Yildiz Y, Hazneci B, et al. Reliability of a functional test battery evaluating functionality, proprioception, and strength in recreational athletes with functional ankle instability. *Eur J Phys Rehabil Med*. 2008;44:407–415.
28. Trojian TH, McKeag DB. Single leg balance test to identify risk of ankle sprains. *Br J Sports Med*. 2006;40:610–613. discussion 613.
29. Deshpande N, Connelly DM, Culham EG, Costigan PA. Reliability and validity of ankle proprioceptive measures. *Arch Phys Med Rehabil*. 2003;84:883–889.

8

Foot and Ankle

References

30. Keenan AM, Bach TM. Clinicians' assessment of the hindfoot: a study of reliability. *Foot Ankle Int.* 2006;27:451–460.

31. Payne C, Chuter V, Miller K. Sensitivity and specificity of the functional hallux limitus test to predict foot function. *J Am Podiatr Med Assoc.* 2002;92:269–271.

32. Rohner-Spengler M, Mannion AF, Babst R. Reliability and minimal detectable change for the figure-of-eight-20 method of, measurement of ankle edema. *J Orthop Sports Phys Ther.* 2007;37:199–205.

33. Petersen EJ, Irish SM, Lyons CL, et al. Reliability of water volumetry and the figure of eight method on subjects with ankle joint swelling. *J Orthop Sports Phys Ther.* 1999;29:609–615.

34. Maffulli N. The clinical diagnosis of subcutaneous tear of the Achilles tendon. A prospective study in 174 patients. *Am J Sports Med.* 1998;26(2):266–270.

35. De César PC, Avila EM, de Abreu MR. Comparison of magnetic resonance imaging to physical examination for syndesmotic injury after lateral ankle sprain. *Foot Ankle Int.* 2011;32(12):1110–1114.

36. Sman AD, Hiller CE, Rae K, et al. Diagnostic accuracy of clinical tests for ankle syndesmosis injury. *Br J Sports Med.* 2015;49(5):323–329.

37. Molloy S, Solan MC, Bendall SP. Synovial impingement in the ankle: a new physical sign. *J Bone Joint Surg B.* 2003;85:330–333.

38. Liu SH, Nuccion SL, Finerman G. Diagnosis of anterolateral ankle impingement. Comparison between magnetic resonance imaging and clinical examination. *Am J Sports Med.* 1997;25:389–393.

39. Hertel J, Denegar CR, Monroe MM, Stokes WL. Talocrural and subtalar joint instability after lateral ankle sprain. *Med Sci Sports Exerc.* 1999;31(11):1501–1508.

40. Abouelela AA, Zohiery AK. The triple compression stress test for diagnosis of tarsal tunnel syndrome. *Foot.* 2012;22(3):146–149.

41. Mahadevan D, Venkatesan M, Bhatt R, Bhatia M. Diagnostic accuracy of clinical tests for Morton's neuroma compared with ultrasonography. *J Foot Ankle Surg.* 2015;54(4):549–553.

42. Mehta SP, Fulton A, Quach C, et al. Measurement properties of the lower extremity functional scale: A systematic review. *J Orthop Sports Phys Ther.* 2016;46(3):200–216.

43. Dawson J, Doll H, Coffey J, Jenkinson C. Responsiveness and minimally important change for the Manchester-Oxford foot questionnaire (MOXFQ) compared with AOFAS and SF-36 assessments following surgery for hallux valgus. *Osteoarthritis Cartilage.* 2007;15:918–931.

44. Li L, Liu X, Herr K. Postoperative pain intensity assessment: a comparison of four scales in Chinese adults. *Pain Med.* 2007;8:223–234.

45. Farrar JT, Berlin JA, Strom BL. Clinically important changes in acute pain outcome measures: a validation study. *J Pain Symptom Manage.* 2003;25:406–411.

46. Farrar JT, Portenoy RK, Berlin JA, et al. Defining the clinically important difference in pain outcome measures. *Pain.* 2000;88:287–294.

Clinical Summary and Recommendations

Patient History	
Complaints	• Little is known about the utility of subjective complaints with shoulder pain. Although a report of trauma does not seem clinically useful, a history of popping, clicking, or catching may be minimally helpful in diagnosing a labral tear (+LRs [likelihood ratios] = 2.0).

Physical Examination	
Range-of-Motion, Strength, and Muscle Length Assessment	• Measuring shoulder range of motion has consistently been shown to be highly reliable but is of unknown diagnostic utility. Visual assessments and functional tests of range of motion are more variable and may be adequately reliable in some instances. • Assessing strength with manual muscle testing appears to be reliable. Weak abduction and/or external rotation may be fairly useful in identifying subacromial impingement and/or full-thickness rotator cuff tears. Weak internal rotation appears to be very helpful in identifying subscapularis tears (+LR = 7.5 to 20.0). • Assessments of shoulder muscle tightness are moderately reliable. However, the single study[1] done to test associated diagnostic utility found tight pectoralis minor muscles in all 90 participants regardless of whether they had shoulder problems or not (100% sensitivity, 0% specificity).
Special Tests	• Results of studies examining the diagnostic utility of tests to identify labral tears are highly variable. Even though most single tests do not appear very useful, a 2017 metaanalysis found the compression rotation and Yergason tests to be good at identifying labral tears (+LR of 3.9 and 2.5, respectively). • Although neither the Hawkins-Kennedy or Neer tests appear to be helpful for ruling in or ruling out subacromial impingement, a 2012 metaanalysis found the lift-off test to be very effective (+LR = 14), and the presence of a "painful arc" during elevation was also found to have some value in identifying the condition (+LR = 2.3). • In addition to rotator cuff muscle weakness (above), the external and internal rotation lag signs appear to be very helpful at identifying infraspinatus and subscapularis tears, respectively. Several other tests (the bear-hug, belly-press, and Napoleon tests) appear to be also very useful in diagnosing subscapularis tears. • Whereas several signs and symptoms are helpful in identifying brachial plexus nerve root avulsions, the shoulder protraction test appears to be the most useful (+LR = 4.8, −LR = .05). • Both the distension test in passive external rotation and the coracoid pain test appear to be moderately helpful in identifying adhesive capsulitis (+LR = 10.2 and 7.4, respectively).
Combinations of Findings	• Even though combinations of tests are generally better than single tests, combinations of tests are only moderately helpful in identifying labral tears. The most efficient pair seems to be the anterior apprehension and Jobe relocation tests (+LR = 5.4). • One study[2] showed that a combined history of popping, clicking, or catching in addition to a positive anterior slide test was moderately helpful in identifying a type II to IV SLAP lesion (+LR = 6.0). • Another study[3] reported even better diagnostic utility when specific combinations of three tests were used. By selecting two highly sensitive tests (compression rotation test, anterior apprehension test, and O'Brien test) and one highly specific test (Yergason test, biceps load II test, or Speed tests), users can be fairly confident in both ruling out and ruling in SLAP lesions.

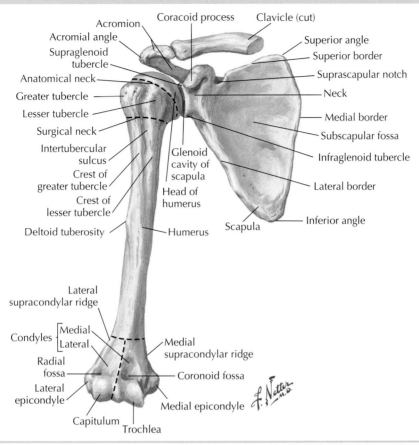

Figure 9-1
Anterior humerus and scapula.

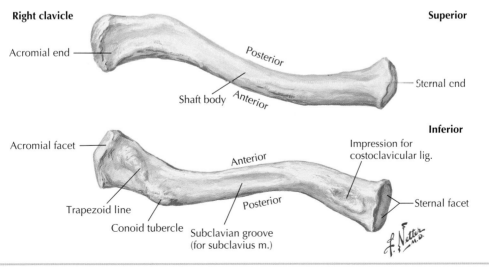

Figure 9-2
Superior and inferior surfaces of clavicle.

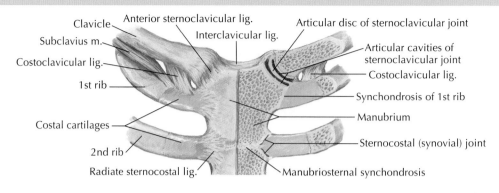

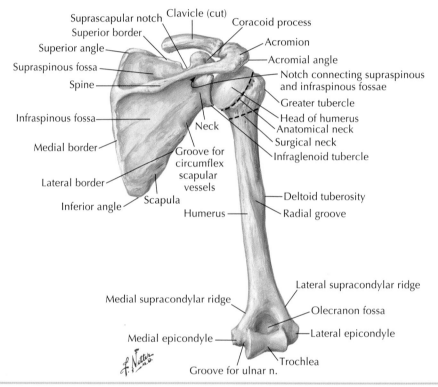

Figure 9-3
Sternoclavicular joint.

Joint	Type and Classification	Closed Packed Position	Capsular Pattern
Glenohumeral	Spheroidal	Full abduction and external rotation	External rotation limited more than abduction, limited more than internal rotation and flexion
Sternoclavicular	Saddle	Arm abducted to 90 degrees	Not reported
Acromioclavicular	Plane synovial	Arm abducted to 90 degrees	
Scapulothoracic	Not a true articulation	Not available	Not available

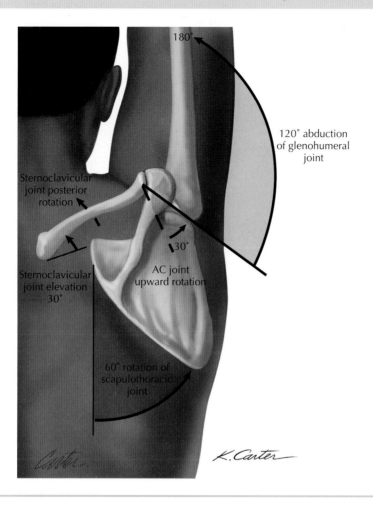

Figure 9-4
Scapulohumeral rhythm.

Scapulohumeral rhythm consists of integrated movements of the glenohumeral, scapulothoracic, acromioclavicular, and sternoclavicular joints occurring in sequential fashion to allow full functional motion of the shoulder complex. Scapulohumeral rhythm serves three functional purposes: It allows for greater overall shoulder range of motion; it maintains optimal contact between the humeral head and glenoid fossa; and it assists with maintaining an optimal length-tension relationship of the glenohumeral muscles.[4] To complete 180 degrees of abduction, the overall ratio of glenohumeral to scapulothoracic, acromioclavicular, and sternoclavicular motion is 2:1.

Inman and colleagues[5] were the first to explain scapulohumeral rhythm and described it as two phases that the shoulder complex completes to move through full abduction. During the first phase (0 degrees to 90 degrees), the scapula is set against the thorax to provide initial stability as the humerus abducts to 30 degrees.[4,5] From 30 degrees to 90 degrees of abduction, the glenohumeral joint contributes another 30 degrees of range of motion while the scapula rotates upward 30 degrees. The upward rotation results from clavicular elevation through the sternoclavicular and acromioclavicular joints. The second phase (90 degrees to –180 degrees) entails 60 degrees of glenohumeral abduction and 30 degrees of scapular upward rotation. The scapular rotation is associated with 5 degrees of elevation at the sternoclavicular joint and 25 degrees of rotation at the acromioclavicular joint.[5,6]

Shoulder 9

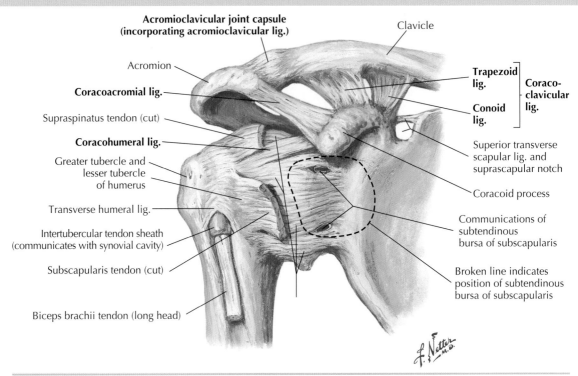

Figure 9-5
Shoulder ligaments: anterior view.

Ligaments	Attachments	Function
Glenohumeral	Glenoid labrum to neck of humerus	Reinforces anterior glenohumeral joint capsule
Coracohumeral	Coracoid process to greater tubercle of humerus	Strengthens superior glenohumeral joint capsule
Coracoclavicular *(trapezoid)*	Superior aspect of coracoid process to inferior aspect of clavicle	Anchors clavicle to coracoid process
Coracoclavicular *(conoid)*	Coracoid process to conoid tubercle on inferior clavicle	
Acromioclavicular	Acromion to clavicle	Strengthens acromioclavicular joint superiorly
Coracoacromial	Coracoid process to acromion	Prevents superior displacement of humeral head
Sternoclavicular	Clavicular notch of manubrium to medial base of clavicle anteriorly and posteriorly	Reinforces sternoclavicular joint anteriorly and posteriorly
Interclavicular	Medial end of one clavicle to medial end of other clavicle	Strengthens superior sternoclavicular joint capsule
Costoclavicular	Superior aspect of costal cartilage of first rib to inferior border of medial clavicle	Anchors medial end of clavicle to first rib

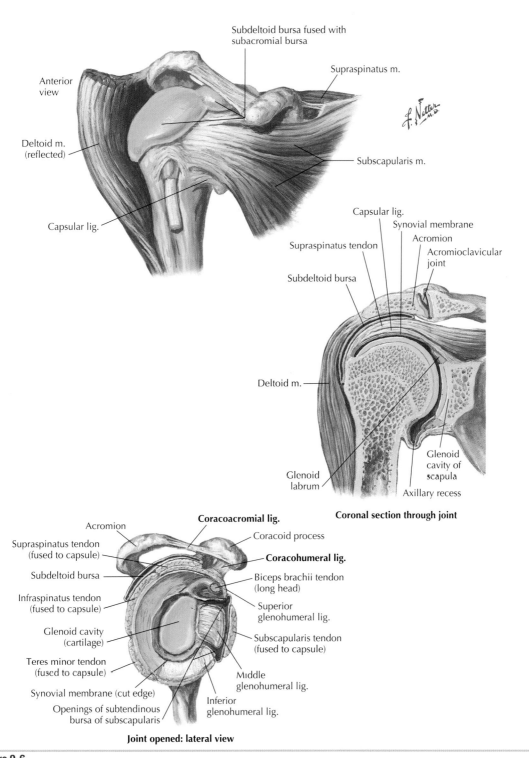

Subdeltoid bursa fused with
subacromial bursa

Supraspinatus m.

Anterior
view

Deltoid m.
(reflected)

Subscapularis m.

Capsular lig.

Capsular lig.

Synovial membrane

Supraspinatus tendon

Acromion

Acromioclavicular
joint

Subdeltoid bursa

Deltoid m.

Glenoid
cavity of
scapula

Glenoid
labrum

Axillary recess

Coronal section through joint

Coracoacromial lig.

Acromion

Coracoid process

Supraspinatus tendon
(fused to capsule)

Coracohumeral lig.

Subdeltoid bursa

Biceps brachii tendon
(long head)

Infraspinatus tendon
(fused to capsule)

Superior
glenohumeral lig.

Glenoid cavity
(cartilage)

Subscapularis tendon
(fused to capsule)

Teres minor tendon
(fused to capsule)

Middle
glenohumeral lig.

Synovial membrane (cut edge)

Inferior
glenohumeral lig.

Openings of subtendinous
bursa of subscapularis

Joint opened: lateral view

Figure 9-6
Shoulder (glenohumeral) joint.

Posterior Muscles of Shoulder

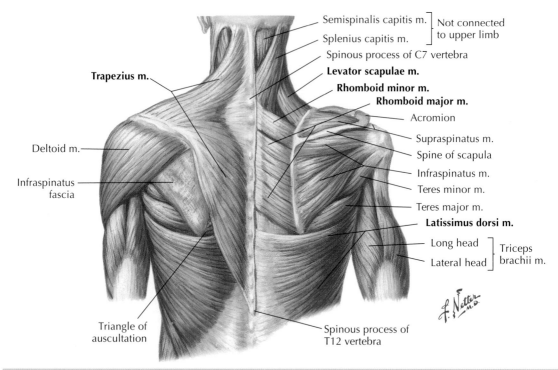

Figure 9-7
Muscles of the shoulder: posterior view.

Muscles	Origin	Insertion	Nerve and Segmental Level	Action
Upper trapezius	Occipital protuberance, nuchal line, ligamentum nuchae	Lateral clavicle and acromion	Cranial nerve XI; C2 to C4	Rotates glenoid fossa upwardly, elevates scapula
Middle trapezius	Spinous processes of T1 to T5	Acromion and spine of scapula	Cranial nerve XI; C2 to C4	Retracts scapula
Lower trapezius	Spinous processes of T6 to T12	Apex of spine of scapula	Cranial nerve XI; C2 to C4	Upward rotation of glenoid fossa, scapular depression
Levator scapulae	Transverse processes of C1 to C4	Superior medial scapula	Dorsal scapular nerve; C3 to C5	Elevates and adducts scapula
Rhomboids	Ligamentum nuchae and spinous processes of C7 to T5	Medial scapular border	Dorsal scapular nerve; C4 to C5	Retracts scapula
Latissimus dorsi	Inferior thoracic vertebrae, thoracolumbar fascia, iliac crest, and inferior ribs 3 and 4	Intertubercular groove of humerus	Thoracodorsal nerve; C6 to C8	Internally rotates, adducts, and extends humerus
Serratus anterior	Ribs 1 to 8	Anterior medial scapula	Long thoracic nerve; C5 to C8	Protracts and upwardly rotates scapula

Anterior Muscles of Shoulder

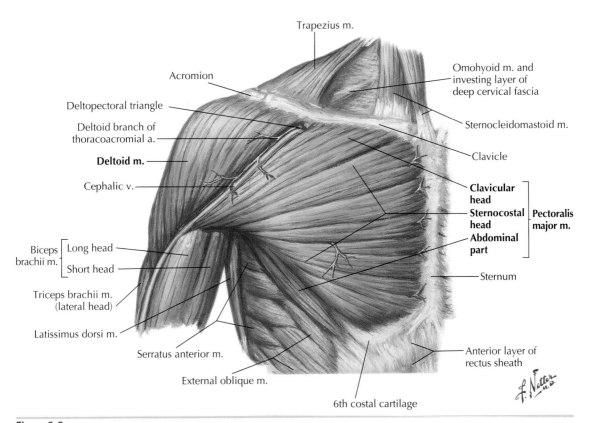

Figure 9-8
Muscles of the shoulder: anterior view.

Muscles	Origin	Insertion	Nerve and Segmental Level	Action
Deltoid	Clavicle, acromion, spine of scapula	Deltoid tuberosity of humerus	Axillary nerve; C5 to C6	Abducts arm
Pectoralis major (clavicular head)	Anterior medial clavicle	Intertubercular groove of humerus	Lateral and medial pectoral nerves; C5, C6, C7, C8, T1	Adducts and internally rotates humerus
Pectoralis major (sternocostal head)	Lateral border of sternum, superior six costal cartilages, and fascia of external oblique muscle			
Pectoralis minor	Just lateral to costal cartilage of ribs 3 to 5	Coracoid process	Medial pectoral nerve; C8, T1	Stabilizes scapula

Rotator Cuff Muscles

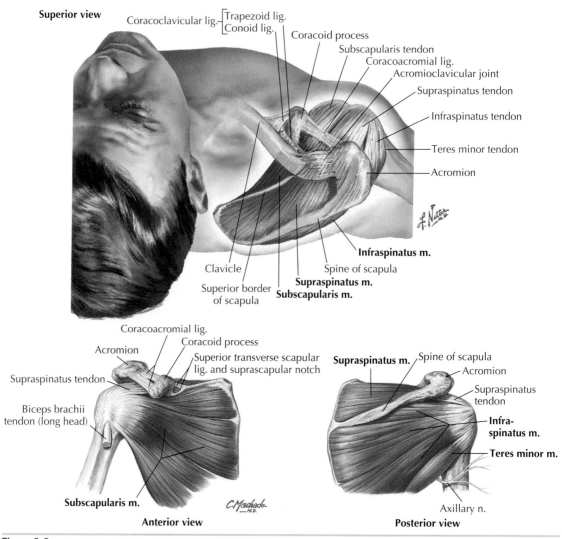

Figure 9-9
Muscles of the shoulder: rotator cuff.

Muscles	Origin	Insertion	Nerve and Segmental Level	Action
Supraspinatus	Supraspinous fossa of scapula	Greater tubercle of humerus	Suprascapular nerve; C4 to C6	Assists deltoid in abduction of humerus
Infraspinatus	Infraspinous fossa of scapula	Greater tubercle of humerus	Suprascapular nerve; C5 to C6	Externally rotates humerus
Teres minor	Lateral border of scapula	Greater tubercle of humerus	Axillary nerve; C5 to C6	Externally rotates humerus
Subscapularis	Subscapular fossa of scapula	Lesser tubercle of humerus	Upper and lower subscapular nerves; C5 to C6	Internally rotates humerus
Teres major	Inferior angle of scapula	Intertubercular groove of humerus	Lower subscapular nerve; C5 to C6	Internally rotates and adducts humerus

Nerves	Segmental Levels	Sensory	Motor
Radial	C5, C6, C7, C8, T1	Posterior aspect of forearm	Triceps brachii, anconeus, brachioradialis, extensor muscles of forearm
Ulnar	C7, C8, T1	Medial hand, including medial half of digit 4	Flexor carpi ulnaris, medial half of flexor digitorum profundus, most small muscles in hand
Musculocutaneous	C5, C6, C7	Becomes lateral antebrachial cutaneous nerve	Coracobrachialis, biceps brachii, brachialis
Axillary	C5, C6	Lateral shoulder	Teres minor, deltoid
Suprascapular	C4, C5, C6	No sensory	Supraspinatus, infraspinatus
Dorsal scapular	Ventral rami of C4, C5	No sensory	Rhomboids, levator scapulae
Lateral pectoral	C5, C6, C7	No sensory	Pectoralis major, pectoralis minor
Medial pectoral	C8, T1	No sensory	Pectoralis minor
Long thoracic	Ventral rami of C5, C6, C7	No sensory	Serratus anterior
Upper subscapular	C5, C6	No sensory	Subscapularis
Lower subscapular	C5, C6	No sensory	Teres major, subscapularis
Medial cutaneous of arm	C8, T1	Medial arm	No motor

9

Shoulder

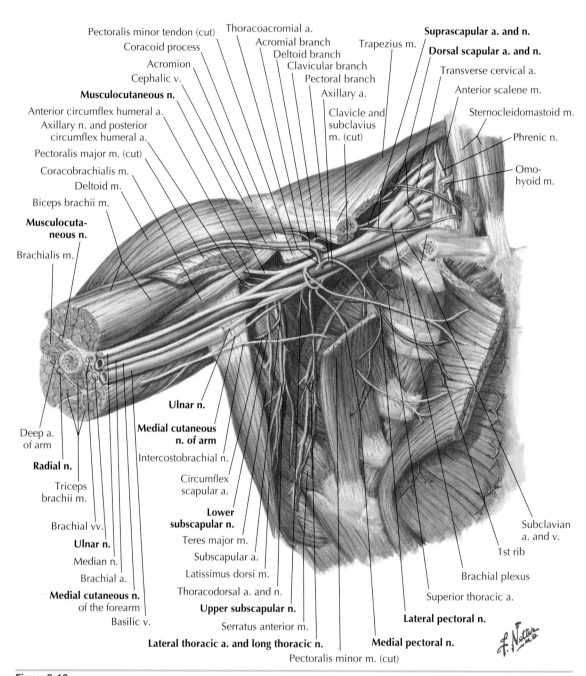

Pectoralis minor tendon (cut)
Coracoid process
Acromion
Cephalic v.
Musculocutaneous n.
Anterior circumflex humeral a.
Axillary n. and posterior
circumflex humeral a.
Pectoralis major m. (cut)
Coracobrachialis m.
Deltoid m.
Biceps brachii m.
**Musculocuta-
neous n.**
Brachialis m.

Thoracoacromial a.
Acromial branch
Deltoid branch
Clavicular branch
Pectoral branch
Axillary a.
Clavicle and
subclavius
m. (cut)

Trapezius m.

Suprascapular a. and n.
Dorsal scapular a. and n.
Transverse cervical a.
Anterior scalene m.
Sternocleidomastoid m.
Phrenic n.
Omo-
hyoid m.

Deep a.
of arm
Radial n.
Triceps
brachii m.
Brachial vv.
Ulnar n.
Median n.
Brachial a.
Medial cutaneous n.
of the forearm
Basilic v.

Ulnar n.
**Medial cutaneous
n. of arm**
Intercostobrachial n.
Circumflex
scapular a.
**Lower
subscapular n.**
Teres major m.
Subscapular a.
Latissimus dorsi m.
Thoracodorsal a. and n.
Upper subscapular n.
Serratus anterior m.
Lateral thoracic a. and long thoracic n.
Pectoralis minor m. (cut)

Subclavian
a. and v.
1st rib

Brachial plexus
Superior thoracic a.

Lateral pectoral n.
Medial pectoral n.

Figure 9-10
Anterior axilla.

Diagnostic Utility of the Patient History for Identifying the Need for Radiographs After Shoulder Dislocation

Patient Report and Study Quality	Population	Reference Standard	Sens	Spec	+LR	−LR
Quebec Decision Rule: "prereduction radiography" patients necessary if: (1) age < 40 and mechanism involves a motor vehicle collision, a fall from standing height, or sports injury, and (2) age ≥ 40 and first time dislocation or humeral ecchymosis[7] ◐	143 patients with shoulder dislocation presenting to emergency department	Radiographic evidence of fracture • age < 40 • age ≥ 40	.33 (.00, .91) 1.0 (.03, 1.0)	.60 (.50, .67) .50 (.28, .72)	0.8 (0.2, 4.2) 2.0 (1.3, 3.0)	1.1 (.50, 2.5) 0

Shoulder

9

Diagnostic Utility of the Patient History for Identifying Labrum and Rotator Cuff Tears

Patient Report and Study Quality	Population	Reference Standard	Sens	Spec	+LR	−LR
History of trauma[8] ◆	55 patients with shoulder pain scheduled for arthroscopy	Glenoid labral tear observed during arthroscopy	.50 (.35, .65)	.36 (.08, .65)	.79 (.46, 1.34)	1.38 (.60, 3.17)
History of popping, clicking, or catching[8] ◆			.55 (.40, .69)	.73 (.46, .99)	2.0 (.73, 5.45)	.63 (.38, 1.02)
Patient report of weakness[9] ◆	100 patients with shoulder pain	Rotator cuff tear observed via MRI arthrogram	.34	.54	0.8	1.2
Patient report of night pain[9] ◆			.89	.19	1.1	.58
History of trauma[10] ◆	448 patients with shoulder pain scheduled for arthroscopy	Rotator cuff tear observed during arthroscopy	.36	.73	1.33	.88
Reports of night pain[10] ◆			.88	.20	1.10	.60

Reliability of Range-of-Motion Measurements

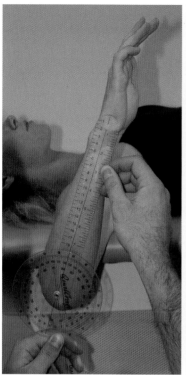

Measurement of internal rotation
in 90° of abduction

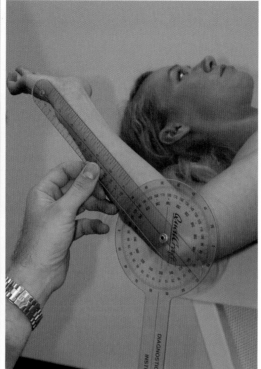

Measurement of external rotation
in 90° of abduction

Figure 9-11
Range-of-motion
measurements.

Test Procedure and Study Quality	Instrumentation	Population	Interexaminer Reliability
Passive flexion[11] ◆	Universal goniometer	21 patients with shoulder pain	ROM: ICC = .70 (.40, .87) Pain: κ = .70 (.39, .99)
Passive abduction[11] ◆			ROM: ICC = .76 (.5, .89) Pain: κ = .33 (.0, .72)
Passive external rotation[11] ◆			ROM: ICC = .74 (.44, .89) Pain: κ = .60 (.26, .95)
Passive internal rotation[11] ◆			ROM: ICC = .3 (.16, .65) Pain: κ = .49 (.19, .80)
Passive horizontal adduction[11] ◆			ROM: ICC = .46 (.03, .74) Pain: κ = −.22
Passive abduction[12] ◆	Inclinometer	50 patients with adhesive capsulitis	ICC = .83
Passive external rotation[12] ◆			ICC = .90
Passive internal rotation[12] ◆			ICC = .85
Passive external rotation[12] ◆			ICC = .90
Passive flexion[13] ◆	Universal goniometer	100 patients referred for physical therapy for shoulder impairments	Intraexaminer: ICC = .98 Interexaminer: ICC = .89
Passive extension[13] ◆			Intraexaminer: ICC = .94 Interexaminer: ICC = .27
Passive abduction[13] ◆			Intraexaminer: ICC = .98 Interexaminer: ICC = .87

9

Shoulder

Reliability of Range-of-Motion Measurements—cont'd

Test Procedure and Study Quality	Instrumentation	Population	Interexaminer Reliability
Active elevation[14] ◆	Visual estimation of range of motion	201 patients with shoulder pain	Affected side: ICC = .88 (.84, .91) Unaffected side: ICC = .76 (.67, .82)
Passive elevation[14] ◆			Affected side: ICC = .87 (.83, .90) Unaffected side: ICC = .73 (.66, .79)
Passive external rotation[14] ◆			Affected side: ICC = .73 (.22, .88) Unaffected side: ICC = .34 (.00, .65)
Passive horizontal adduction[14] ◆			Affected side: ICC = .36 (.22, .48) Unaffected side: ICC = .18 (.04, .32)
Active scaption (scapular plane shoulder elevation)[15] ◐	Goniometer	30 asymptomatic subjects	Intraexaminer: ICC = .87 (.74, .94) Interexaminer: ICC = .92 (.83, .96)
	Digital inclinometer		Intraexaminer: ICC = .88 (.75, .94) Interexaminer: ICC = .89 (.77, .95)

ICC, Intraclass correlation coefficient.

Reliability of Functional Range-of-Motion Tests

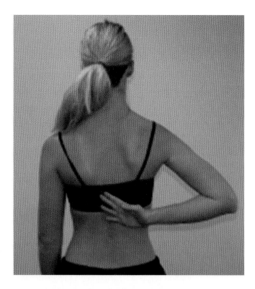

Figure 9-12
Hand behind back (functional internal rotation of shoulder test).

Test and Measure and Study Quality	Description	Population	Reliability
Hand behind back[12] ◆	Distance measured from PSIS to distal radius after reaching as high as possible behind back	50 patients with adhesive capsulitis	ICC = .91
Active abduction[17] ◆		91 patients with shoulder pain	Range of motion (ROM): ICC = .96 Pain: κ = .65
Passive abduction[17] ◆			ROM: ICC = .96 Pain: κ = .69
Painful arc with active abduction[17] ◆	Range of motion assessed visually to nearest 5 degrees. Pain assessed as "no pain," "little pain," "much pain," or "excruciating pain"		Presence of: κ = .46 Starting ROM: ICC = .72 Ending ROM: ICC = .57
Painful arc with passive abduction[17] ◆			Presence of: κ = .52 Starting ROM: ICC = .54 Ending ROM: ICC = .72
Passive external rotation[17] ◆			ROM: ICC = .70 Pain: κ = .50
Hand behind back[17] ◆	As above, except range of motion graded on a scale of 0 to 7		ROM: κ = .73 Pain: κ = .35
Hand on neck[17] ◆			ROM: κ = .52 Pain: κ = .52
Spring test for first rib[17] ◆	Examiner exerts force with the second metacarpophalangeal joint on the first rib of the patient, assessing range of motion (normal or restricted), pain (present or absent), and joint stiffness (present or absent)		ROM: κ = .26 Stiffness: κ = .09 Pain: κ = .66
Hand to neck[16] ●		46 patients with shoulder pain	Intraexaminer: ICC = .80 (.63, .93) Interexaminer: ICC = .90 (.69, .96)
Hand to scapula[16] ●	Visual estimation of range of motion graded on a scale of 0 to 3 or 4		Intraexaminer: ICC = .90 (.72, .92) Interexaminer: ICC = .90 (.69, .94)
Hand to opposite scapula[16] ●			Intraexaminer: ICC = .86 (.65, .90) Interexaminer: ICC = .83 (.75, .96)

9

Shoulder

Reliability of Assessing Muscular Strength and Endurance

Test and Measure and Study Quality	Description	Population	Reliability
Deltoid[11] ◆	Standard manual muscle test using grades 1–5	21 patients with shoulder pain. Estimates reported for right shoulder only	$\kappa = .47\ (.00, .93)$
Bicep[11] ◆			$\kappa = .45\ (.00, 1.0)$
Tricep[11] ◆			$\kappa = .77\ (.34, 1.0)$
External rotation[11] ◆			$\kappa = .30\ (.00, .68)$
Internal rotation[11] ◆			$\kappa = .32\ (.00, 1.0)$
Serratus anterior[11] ◆			$\kappa = .89\ (.64, 1.0)$

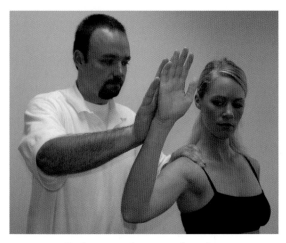

Resistance against external rotation

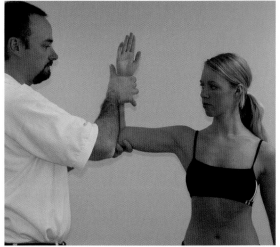

Resistance against internal rotation

Figure 9-13
Internal rotation resistance strength test.

Zaslav[18] investigated the usefulness of the internal rotation resistance strength (IRRS) test in distinguishing intraarticular pathologic conditions from impingement syndrome in a group of 115 patients who underwent arthroscopic shoulder surgery. The IRRS test is performed with the patient standing. The examiner positions the patient's arm in 90 degrees of abduction and 80 degrees of external rotation. The examiner applies resistance against external rotation and then internal rotation of the arm in this position. The test is considered positive for an intraarticular pathologic condition if the patient exhibits greater weakness in internal rotation than in external rotation. If the patient demonstrates greater weakness with external rotation, the test is considered positive for impingement syndrome. The IRRS test had a sensitivity of .88, a specificity of .96, a +LR of 22.0, and a –LR of .13.

Reliability of Assessing Passive Accessory Joint Motion

Test and Measure and Study Quality	Description	Population	Reliability
Inferior glenohumeral motion[11] ◆	Based on comparison to the opposite shoulder and based on the clinician's experience examining other patients with shoulder disorders, each motion was judged to be hypomobile, normal, or hypermobile	21 patients with shoulder pain. Estimates reported for right shoulder only	Mobility κ = .26 (0, .66) Pain κ = .61 (.01, 1.0)
Anterior glenohumeral motion[11] ◆			Mobility κ = .58 (.20, .95) Pain κ = .58 (.15, 1.0)
Posterior glenohumeral motion[11] ◆			Mobility κ = .83 (.50, 1.0) Pain κ = .39 (.00, .86)
Glenohumeral distraction[11] ◆			Mobility κ = .02 (.00, .50) Pain κ = .32 (.00, 1.0)
Anterior to posterior AC joint motion[11] ◆			Mobility κ = .02 (.00, .41) Pain κ = .77 (.46, 1.0)
Anterior to posterior SC joint motion[11] ◆			Mobility κ = .24 (.00, .75)

Reliability of Assessing Proprioception

Test and Measure and Study Quality	Description	Population	Test-Retest Reliability
Joint position sense[19] ●	With patient standing, examiner measures full external rotation and internal rotation of shoulder with inclinometer. Target angles are determined as 90% of internal rotation and 90% of external rotation. With patient blindfolded, examiner guides patient's arm into target angle position and holds it for 3 seconds. The patient's arm is returned to neutral. The patient is instructed to return the arm to the target angle. Examiner takes measurement with inclinometer	31 asymptomatic subjects	Internal rotation ICC = .98 External rotation ICC = .98

9

Shoulder

Reliability of Determining Muscle Length

Test and Measure and Study Quality	Description	Population	Test-Retest Reliability
Posterior shoulder tightness[20] ◆ **2019 Metaanalysis**	Seven different measurement techniques (low flexion, extension with internal rotation, horizonal adduction, internal rotation, diagnostic ultrasound, scapular-plane abduction, and myotonometer)	Pooled data from 12 studies on intrarater reliability and 6 studies on interrater reliability	Intrarater ICC = .93 (.90, .95) Interrater ICC = .89 (.80, .94)
Pectoralis minor muscle length[21] ◆	Patient is in supine position, with the elbows extended alongside the body and both palms placed on the examining table. The distance between the inferomedial aspect of the coracoid process and the caudal edge of the fourth rib at the sternum is measured with a vernier caliper during exhalation by the patient	25 patients with shoulder impingement symptoms and 25 controls	Patients: Intraexaminer ICC = .87 to .93 Interexaminer ICC = .65 to .72 Controls: Intraexaminer ICC = .76 to .87 Interexaminer ICC = .64 to .67
Pectoralis minor muscle length[11] ◆	Based on comparison to the opposite shoulder, and based on the clinician's experience examining other patients with shoulder disorders, each muscle was judged to be short or normal	21 patients with shoulder pain. Estimates reported for right shoulder only	$\kappa = .59$ (.16, 1.0)
Pectoralis major muscle length[11] ◆			$\kappa = .71$ (.41, 1.0)
Latissimus dorsi muscle length[11] ◆			$\kappa = .77$ (.46, 1.0)
Pectoralis minor muscle length[1] ◖	With the participant supine with hands resting on the abdomen, examiner measures the linear distance from the treatment table to the posterior aspect of the acromion using a plastic right angle	45 patients with shoulder pain and 45 asymptomatic persons	Single measure: ICC = .90 to .93 Mean of 3 measures: ICC = .92 to .97
Latissimus dorsi muscle length[22] ◖	With the subject supine with hips and knees flexed and feet flat on the treatment table in posterior pelvic tilt, the examiner passively flexes the subject's shoulder until a firm flexion end feel is noted or until the humerus begins to medially rotate. One arm of a goniometer is aligned with the humerus, the other arm of the goniometer is aligned parallel with the treatment table, and the axis of the goniometer is aligned with the center of the glenohumeral joint	30 asymptomatic subjects	Intraexaminer: ICC = .19

Diagnostic Utility of a Tight Pectoralis Minor Muscle in Identifying Shoulder Pain

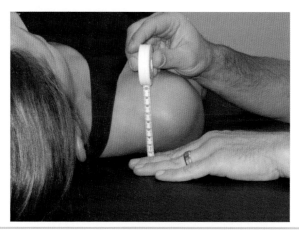

Figure 9-14
Measuring pectoralis minor muscle length.

Test and Study Quality	Description and Positive Findings	Population	Reference Standard	Sens	Spec	+LR	−LR
Tight pectoralis minor muscle[1]	As above, with a positive test being a measurement of less than 2.6 cm (1 inch)	45 patients with shoulder pain and 45 asymptomatic persons	Self-report of shoulder pain and/or restriction of shoulder movement	1.0*	0.0*	1.0	Undefined

*These results are due to the fact that all 90 symptomatic and asymptomatic participants were classified as "tight" using this definition.

Reliability of Palpating the Subacromial Space

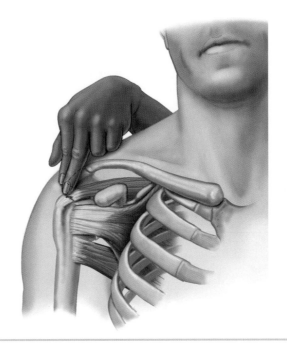

Figure 9-15
Palpation of subacromial space.

Test and Measure and Study Quality	Description	Population	Reliability
Palpation of subacromial space[24] ◐	Examiner palpates subacromial space and estimates distance as ¼, ½, ¾, or whole finger's breadth	36 patients with shoulder subluxation	Intraexaminer ICC = .90 to .94 Interexaminer ICC = .77 to .89

Reliability of Palpating the Myofascial Trigger Points and the Subacromial Space

Test and Measure and Study Quality	Description	Population	Reliability
Upper trapezius trigger point[23] ◆	Systematic palpation of each muscle of symptomatic side. Positive if at least 1 painful nodule	26 patients with symptoms of unilateral shoulder impingement syndrome	Intraexaminer κ = .65 Interexaminer κ = −.11
Lower trapezius trigger point[23] ◆			Intraexaminer κ = .29 Interexaminer κ = .26
Infraspinatus trigger point[23] ◆			Intraexaminer κ = .50 Interexaminer κ = .19
Supraspinatus trigger point[23] ◆			Intraexaminer κ = .48 Interexaminer κ = .37
Pectoralis minor trigger point[23] ◆			Intraexaminer κ = .30 Interexaminer κ = .44
Middle deltoid trigger point[23] ◆			Intraexaminer κ = .65 Interexaminer κ = .44
Palpation of subacromial space[24] ◉	Examiner palpates subacromial space and estimates distance as ¼, ½, ¾, or whole finger's breadth	36 patients with shoulder subluxation	Intraexaminer ICC = .90 to .94 Interexaminer ICC = .77 to .89

Diagnostic Utility of Palpation in Identifying Subacromial Impingement

Test and Study Quality	Description and Positive Findings	Population	Reference Standard	Sens	Spec	+LR	−LR
Supraspinatus palpation test[25] ◆	The examiner performs deep palpation of the tendon at the shoulder joint. Positive if tenderness is present with palpation	69 patients with shoulder pain	Evidence of subacromial impingement via sonographic examination	.92 (.78, .95)	.41 (.18, .64)	1.6	.20
Infraspinatus palpation test[25] ◆				.33 (.06, .79)	.66 (.54, .76)	.97	1.0
Subscapularis palpation test[25] ◆				.60 (.23, .88)	0 (0, .13)	.60	Undefined
Biceps palpation test[25] ◆				.85 (.67, .94)	.48 (.33, .62)	1.63	.31

Diagnostic Utility of Palpation in Identifying Labral Tears

Test and Study Quality	Description and Positive Findings	Population	Reference Standard	Sens	Spec	+LR	−LR
Bicipital groove tenderness[26] ◆ **2017 Meta-analysis**	Examiner gently presses the biceps groove with the patient's shoulder. Positive if pain occurs	Pooled estimates from 2 studies	Study dependent, but generally SLAP lesion visualized during arthroscopy	.26 (.17, .37)	.74 (.63, .82)	1.0	1.0

9

Shoulder

Reliability of Assessing Static Shoulder Posture

Test and Measure and Study Quality	Description and Positive Findings	Population	Reliability	
			Intraexaminer	Interexaminer
Position of posterior acromion[27] ◆	Measured from the posterior border of the acromion and the table surface with the patient supine	29 patients with shoulder pain	Not reported	ICC = .88 to .94
Position of medial scapular border[27] ◆	Measured from the medial scapular border to T4 spinous process		Not reported	ICC = .50 to .80
Position of posterior acromion[27] ◆	Measured from the posterior border of the acromion and the table surface with the patient supine		Not reported	ICC = .88 to .94
Position of medial scapular border[27] ◆	Measured from the medial scapular border to T4 spinous process		Not reported	ICC = .50 to .80
Clavicular tilt angle[28] ◆	With patient standing, the stationary arm of goniometer is aligned vertically between the jugular notch and xiphoid process, the movable arm of goniometer is aligned along long axis of the clavicle, and the axis of goniometer is placed at the intersection of the vertical line and the long axis of the clavicle	18 healthy subjects	Interexaminer ICC = .85 (.72, .92)	Intraexaminer ICC = .80 (.64, .89)
Thoracic kyphosis[29] ●	With patient standing, first inclinometer is placed over T1 to T2 spinal level and second inclinometer is placed over T12 to L1 spinal level. Thoracic kyphosis angle is calculated by the summation of the angles recorded by the two inclinometers	45 subjects with shoulder symptoms and 45 controls	Patients: ICC = .92 to .97 Controls: ICC = .94 to .97	

Reliability of Assessing Scapular Motion

Test and Measure and Study Quality		Description and Positive Findings	Population	Reliability	
				Intraexaminer	**Interexaminer**
Lateral scapular slide test[27] ◆	Position 1	With patient standing, examiner records measurement between inferior angle of scapula and spinous process of thoracic vertebra at same horizontal level in three positions. *Position 1:* With glenohumeral joint in neutral *Position 2:* At 45 degrees of shoulder abduction and internal rotation *Position 3:* With upper extremity in 90 degrees of abduction and full internal rotation A difference between sides of more than 1 cm is considered scapular asymmetry	29 patients with shoulder pain	Not reported	ICC = .82 (left) ICC = .96 (right)
	Position 2			Not reported	ICC = .85 (left) ICC = .95 (right)
	Position 3			Not reported	ICC = .70 (left) ICC = .85 (right)
Lateral scapular slide test[30] ◆	Position 1		46 subjects with shoulder dysfunction and 26 subjects without shoulder dysfunction	With dysfunction ICC = .52 (.10, .74) Without dysfunction ICC = .75 (.56, .85)	With dysfunction ICC = .79 (.46, .91) Without dysfunction ICC = .67 (.25, .85)
	Position 2			With dysfunction ICC = .66 (.36, .82) Without dysfunction ICC = .58 (.60, .86)	With dysfunction ICC = .45 (−.38, .78) Without dysfunction ICC = .43 (−.29, .75)
	Position 3			With dysfunction ICC = .62 (.27, .79) Without dysfunction ICC = .80 (.65, .88)	With dysfunction ICC = .57 (−.23, .85) Without dysfunction ICC = .74 (.41, .88)
Scapular dyskinesis test[31] ◆		The patient repeatedly performs active, weighted shoulder flexion and abduction while the clinician observes the scapulohumeral rhythm while standing behind the patient. The scapulohumeral rhythm was classified as either normal, subtle dyskinesis, or obvious dyskinesis	45 patients with shoulder impingement syndrome	κ = .86 (.72, .95)	κ = .59 (.32, .81)
Scapular motion during elevation[32] ◆		Examiners watched videos of scapular motion during elevation and indicated if symmetrical or not	6 patients with shoulder pain and 6 patients without shoulder pain	κ = .51	κ = .26
Movement evaluation during abduction[33] ◐		Examiner classifies scapular movement during shoulder abduction into categories 1 to 4: *Category 1:* Inferior angle tilts dorsally compared with contralateral side *Category 2:* Medial border tilts dorsally compared with contralateral side *Category 3:* Shoulder shrug initiates movement *Category 4:* Scapulae move symmetrically	20 subjects with shoulder impingement and 6 asymptomatic subjects	κ = .42	Not reported

*In addition to assessing reliability, Wassinger et al. (Wassinger et al., 2015) also evaluated the diagnostic ability of asymmetric scapular motion to identify patients seeking care for shoulder impingement. The report of asymmetric scapular motion had a sensitivity of .35 (.29, .41), specificity of .60 (.56, .64), and positive and negative likelihood ratios of 0.9 (0.7–1.1) and 1.1 (0.9–1.2), respectively.

9

Shoulder

Reliability of Assessing Scapular Motion—cont'd

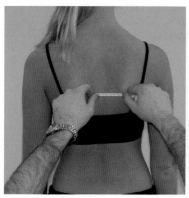
Lateral slide test position 1

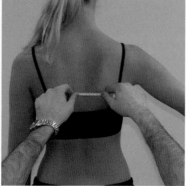
Lateral slide test position 2

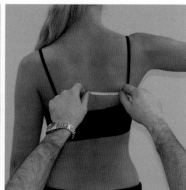
Lateral slide test position 3

Figure 9-16
Detecting scapular asymmetry.

Reliability of Classifying Shoulder Disorders

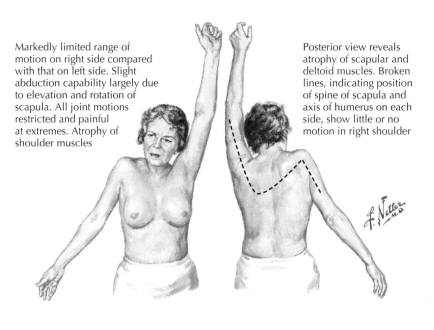

Markedly limited range of motion on right side compared with that on left side. Slight abduction capability largely due to elevation and rotation of scapula. All joint motions restricted and painful at extremes. Atrophy of shoulder muscles

Posterior view reveals atrophy of scapular and deltoid muscles. Broken lines, indicating position of spine of scapula and axis of humerus on each side, show little or no motion in right shoulder

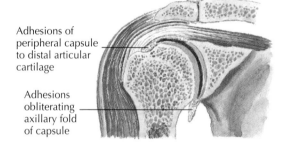

Adhesions of peripheral capsule to distal articular cartilage

Adhesions obliterating axillary fold of capsule

Coronal section of shoulder shows adhesions between capsule and periphery of humeral head

Figure 9-17
Adhesive capsulitis of the shoulder.

Classification and Study Quality	Description	Population	Interexaminer Reliability
Bursitis[34] ◆	Examiner uses patient history combined with "selective tissue tension" examination during active movements, passive movements, and isometric strength assessments	56 painful shoulders	κ = .35 to .58
Capsulitis[34] ◆			κ = .63 to .82
Rotator cuff lesion[34] ◆			κ − .71 to .79
Other diagnosis[34] ◆			κ = .69 to .78
Capsular syndrome[35] ◆	Examiner obtains patient history. Physical examination consists of active, passive, and resistive movements. The range of motion, presence of painful arc or capsular pattern, and degree of muscle weakness are identified	201 patients with shoulder pain	κ = .63 (.50, .76)
Acute bursitis[35] ◆			κ = .50 (−.10, 1.0)
Acromioclavicular syndrome[35] ◆			κ = .24 (−.06, .53)
Subacromial syndrome[35] ◆			κ = .56 (.45, .68)
Rest group (does not fit any category above)[35] ◆			κ = .39 (.24, .54)
Mixed group (patient presents with two or more of above classifications)[35] ◆			κ = .14 (−.03, .30)

9

Shoulder

Reliability of Tests to Identify Shoulder Instability

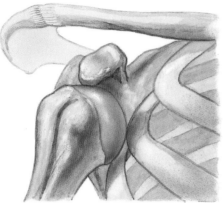

Subcoracoid dislocation (most common)

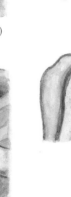

Subglenoid dislocation

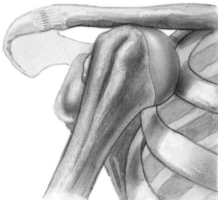

Subclavicular dislocation (uncommon).
Very rarely, humeral head penetrates
between ribs, producing intrathoracic
dislocation

Figure 9-18
Shoulder instability.

Reliability of Tests to Identify Shoulder Instability—cont'd

Test and Measure and Study Quality	Description and Positive Findings	Population	Interexaminer Reliability
Apprehension[36] ◆	With patient supine, examiner passively abducts and externally rotates humerus. Positive if patient complains of pain or instability	13 patients with shoulder instability and 27 asymptomatic participants	$\kappa = .65\ (.38, .85)$
Relocation[36] ◆	From the end position of the apprehension test the humeral head is gently forced posteriorly. Positive if relief of pain or instability		$\kappa = .39\ (.07, .68)$
Surprise[36] ◆	From end position of the relocation test the posteriorly directed force at the humeral head is quickly removed. Positive if patient complains of pain or instability		$\kappa = .65\ (.38, 85)$
Load and shift[36] ◆	From supine, the humeral head is loaded gently into the glenoid through axial pressure at the elbow and humeral head movement is then evaluated using a four-level laxity scale		$\kappa = .48\ (.00, 1.0)$
Gagey[36] ◆	From sitting, the shoulder girdle is stabilized while the individual's arm is passively moved into end range in horizontal abduction. A mirror in front of the individual is used to evaluate the shoulder abduction angle. Rated as positive with abduction exceeding 105°		$\kappa = .73\ (.46, .94)$
Sulcus sign[36] ◆			$\kappa = .43\ (.17, .72)$
Sulcus sign[37] ◉	With patient supine, examiner applies inferior distraction to shoulder. Amount of laxity is graded on a 0 to 3+ scale. 0 represents no laxity; 3+ represents maximum laxity	43 healthy college athletes	Interexaminer κ = .03 to .06 Intraexaminer κ = .01 to .20
Sulcus sign test[38] ◉		113 patients with shoulder pain	Interexaminer κ = .36 (.09, .64)
Apprehension test[38] ◉	With patient standing, examiner places both patient's arms in 90 degrees of abduction and 90 degrees of external rotation	113 patients with shoulder pain	Interexaminer κ = .32 (.14, .50)
Relocation test[30] ◉	With patient supine with glenohumeral joint at edge of table, examiner places arm in 90 degrees of abduction, full external rotation, and 90 degrees of elbow flexion. Examiner then applies a posterior force on head of humerus. Positive if patient's pain or apprehension diminishes with applied force	113 patients with shoulder pain	Interexaminer κ = .27 (.00, .58)

9

Shoulder

Diagnostic Utility of the Apprehension Test in Identifying Shoulder Instability

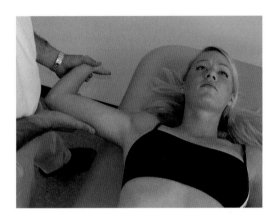

Figure 9-19
Apprehension test.

Test and Study Quality	Description and Positive Findings	Population	Reference Standard	Sens	Spec	+LR	−LR
Anterior apprehension test[26] ◆ **2017 Meta-analysis**	With patient supine, examiner passively abducts and externally rotates humerus. Positive if patient complains of pain or instability	Pooled estimates from 2 studies	Study dependent, but generally visualized arthroscopy	.74 (.61, .84)	.45 (.35, .55)	1.4	.58

Diagnostic Utility of the Apprehension and Relocation Tests in Identifying Shoulder Instability

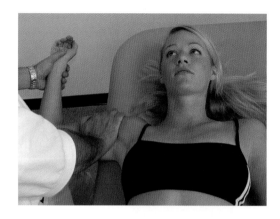

Figure 9-20
Relocation test.

Test and Study Quality	Description and Positive Findings	Population	Reference Standard	Sens	Spec	+LR	−LR
Relocation test[26] ◆ **2017 Meta-analysis**	With patient supine with glenohumeral joint at edge of table, examiner places arm in 90 degrees of abduction, full external rotation, and 90 degrees of elbow flexion. Examiner then applies a posterior force on head of humerus. Positive if patient's pain or apprehension diminishes with applied force	Pooled estimates from 2 studies	Study dependent, but generally visualized arthroscopy	.61 (.48, .72)	.47 (.37, .57)	1.2	.83

9

Shoulder

Diagnostic Utility of the Anterior Drawer Test in Identifying Shoulder Instability

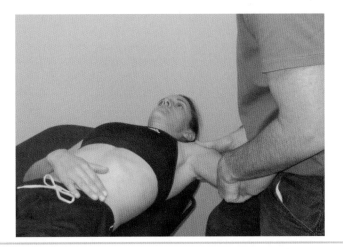

Figure 9-21
Anterior drawer test.

Test and Study Quality	Description and Positive Findings	Population	Reference Standard	Sens	Spec	+LR	−LR
Anterior drawer test (pain)[39]	With patient supine with glenohumeral joint at edge of table, examiner places arm in 60 degrees to 80 degrees of abduction and neutral rotation and then translates the humeral head anteriorly. Positive if patient reports pain or reproduction of instability symptoms	363 patients scheduled to undergo shoulder surgery	Either radiographic documentation of an anterior shoulder dislocation after trauma or demonstration of a Hill-Sachs lesion, a Bankart lesion, or a humeral avulsion of the glenohumeral ligament at the time of arthroscopy	.28	.71	1.0	1.01
Anterior drawer test (instability symptoms)[39]				.53	.85	3.6	.56

Reliability of the Crank Test

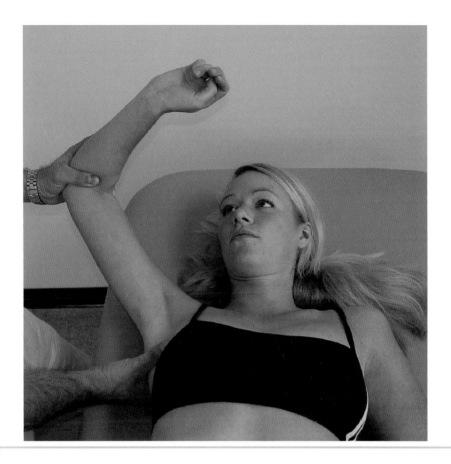

Figure 9-22
Crank test.

Test and Study Quality	Description and Positive Findings	Population	Interexaminer Reliability
Crank test[40] ◆	Patient is supine with shoulder in 160 degrees of abduction and elbow in 90 degrees of flexion. The examiner applies a compressive force to the humerus while repeatedly rotating it into internal and external rotation. Positive if click is produced during the test	40 subjects with shoulder pain	$\kappa = .36$ $(-.07, .59)$
Crank test[8] ◆	As above	55 patients with shoulder pain scheduled for arthroscopic surgery	$\kappa = .20$ $(-.05, .46)$

9

Shoulder

Diagnostic Utility of the Crank Test in Identifying Labral Tears

Test and Study Quality	Description and Positive Findings	Population	Reference Standard	Sens	Spec	+LR	−LR
Crank test[26] ◆ **2017 Meta-analysis**	Patient is supine while examiner elevates humerus 160 degrees in scapular plane. Axial load is applied to humerus while shoulder is internally and externally rotated. Positive if pain is elicited	Pooled esti-mates from 2 studies	Study de-pendent, but generally labral tear diagnosed arthroscopically	.46 (.33, .60)	.72 (.54, .85)	1.6	.75
Crank test[41] ◆ **2012 Meta-analysis**		Pooled esti-mates from 4 studies (n = 282)	Labral tear diagnosed by arthroscopy	.34 (.19, .53)	.75 (.65, .83)	1.4 (.84, 2.2)	.88 (.69, 1.1)

Diagnostic Utility of the Compression Rotation Test in Identifying Labral Tears

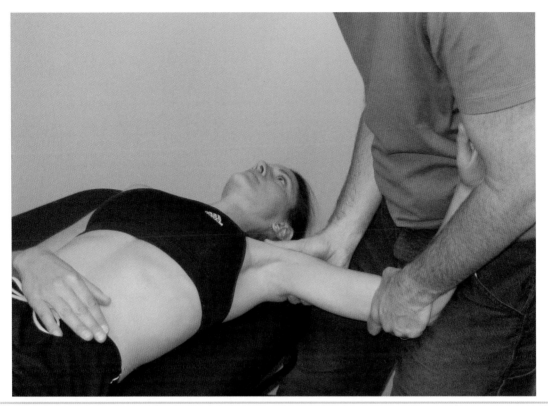

Figure 9-23
Compression rotation test.

Test and Study Quality	Description and Positive Findings	Population	Reference Standard	Sens	Spec	+LR	−LR
Compression rotation test[26] ◆ **2017 Meta-analysis**	With patient supine with arm abducted to 90 degrees and elbow flexed to 90 degrees, examiner applies axial force to humerus. Humerus is circumducted and rotated. Positive if pain or clicking is elicited	Pooled estimates from 2 studies	Study dependent, but generally labral tear diagnosed arthroscopically	.43 (.31, .56)	.89 (.67, .97)	3.9	.64
Compression rotation test[42] ◆		93 patients suspected of having SLAP lesions	SLAP lesion visualized during arthroscopy or MRI arthrogram	.14 (.06, .31)	.93 (.83, .97)	1.8	.93

Shoulder 9

Diagnostic Utility of the Speed Test in Identifying Superior Labrum Anterior and Posterior and/ or Long Head of the Bicep Lesions

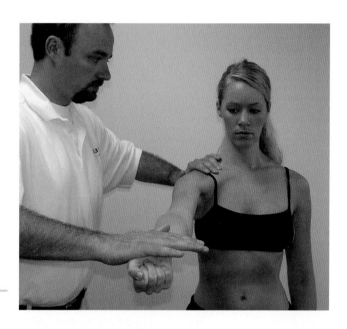

Figure 9-24
Speed test.

Test and Study Quality	Description and Positive Findings	Population	Reference Standard	Sens	Spec	+LR	−LR
Speed test[26] ◆ **2017 Meta-analysis**		Pooled estimates from 3 studies	Study dependent, but generally SLAP lesion diagnosed arthroscopically	.20 (.11, .32)	.88 (.73, .95)	1.7	.91
Speed test[41] ◆ **2012 Meta-analysis**	Patient elevates humerus to 90 degrees with elbow extended and forearm in supination. Patient holds this position while examiner applies resistance against elevation. Positive if pain is elicited in the bicipital groove area	Pooled estimates from 4 studies (n = 327)	SLAP lesion diagnosed by arthroscopy	.20 (.05, .53)	.78 (.58, .90)	.90 (.43, 1.9)	1.0 (.86, 1.2)
Speed test[45] ◆ **2008 Meta-analysis**		Pooled estimates from 4 high-quality studies	SLAP lesion visualized during arthroscopy	.32 (.24, .42)	.61 (.54, .68)	.80	1.11
Speed test[46] ◆		65 patients scheduled to undergo arthroscopic shoulder surgery		.61	.71	2.1	.55
Speed test[47] ◆		143 patients with chronic shoulder pain. Patients with SLAP lesions were excluded	Inflammation, partial tear, complete rupture of the tendon, and instability of the long head of the biceps visualized during arthroscopy	.49	.67	1.48	.76
Speed test[42] ◆		93 patients suspected of having SLAP lesions	SLAP lesion visualized during arthroscopy or MRI arthrogram	.28 (.15, .48)	.71 (.59, .81)	1.0	1.0

Reliability of the Active Compression/O'Brien Test

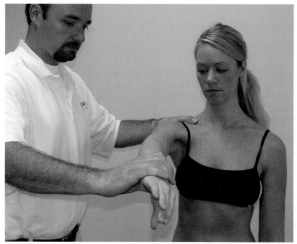

Active compression test with internal rotation

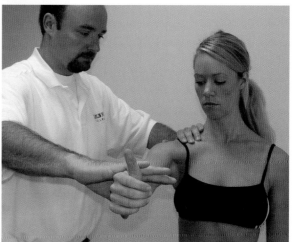

Active compression test with external rotation

Figure 9-25
Active compression test.

Test and Study Quality	Description and Positive Findings	Population	Interexaminer Reliability
Active compression test[40] ◆	Patient is standing with involved shoulder flexed 90 degrees, horizontally adducted 10 degrees, and in maximum internal rotation and the elbow in full extension. Patient resists a downward force applied to the wrist of the involved extremity. The same procedure is repeated with the shoulder in maximum external rotation. Positive with shoulder pain that is worse in the position of internal rotation and relieved in the position of external rotation	40 subjects with shoulder pain	Acromioclavicular joint: $\kappa = .22$ (−.24, .68) Labral pathologic condition: $\kappa = .38$ (.10, .65)
Active compression test[8] ◆		55 patients with shoulder pain scheduled for arthroscopic surgery	$\kappa = .24$ (−.02, .50)
Active compression test[38] ◐		113 patients with shoulder pain	Interexaminer $\kappa = .46$ (.29, .63)

9

Shoulder

Diagnostic Utility of the Active Compression/O'Brien Test

Test and Study Quality	Description and Positive Findings	Population	Reference Standard	Sens	Spec	+LR	−LR
O'Brien test[26] ◆ **2017 Meta-analysis**	Patient stands and flexes arm to 90 degrees with elbow in full extension. Patient then adducts arm 10 degrees internally and rotates humerus. Examiner applies downward force to arm as patient resists. Patient then fully supinates arm and repeats procedure. Positive if pain is elicited with first maneuver and reduced with second maneuver	Pooled estimates from 3 studies	Study dependent, but generally SLAP lesion diagnosed arthroscopically	.66 (.55, .75)	.36 (.21, .55)	1.0	.94
Active compression test[41] ◆ **2012 Meta-analysis**		Pooled estimates from 6 studies (n = 782)		.67 (.51, .80)	.37 (.22, .54)	1.1 (.90, 1.3)	.89 (.67, 1.2)
Active compression test[42] ◆		93 patients suspected of having SLAP lesions	SLAP lesion visualized during arthroscopy or MRI arthrogram	.33 (.19, .51)	.61 (.49, .72)	0.9	1.1

Diagnostic Utility of the Yergason Test in Identifying Labral and/or Long Head of the Bicep Lesions

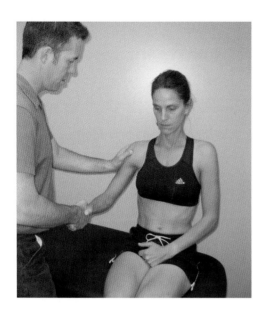

Figure 9-26
Yergason test.

Test and Study Quality	Description and Positive Findings	Population	Reference Standard	Sens	Spec	+LR	−LR
Yergason test[26] ◆ **2017 Meta-analysis**		Pooled estimates from 3 studies	Study de-pendent, but generally labral tear diagnosed by arthroscopy	.20 (13, .30)	.92 (.81, .97)	2.5	.87
Yergason test[41] ◆ **2012 Meta-analysis**	With patient stand-ing or sitting with elbow at 90 degrees of flexion, patient supinates forearm against examiner's resistance. During procedure, examiner palpates long head of biceps tendon. Positive if pain at biceps tendon	Pooled estimates from 4 studies (n = 246)		.12	.95	2.5	.91
Yergason test[46] ◆		65 patients scheduled to un-dergo arthroscop-ic shoulder surgery	Lesion of long head of biceps tendon visual-ized during arthroscopy	.37	.83	2.2	.76
Yergason test[47] ◆		143 patients with chronic shoulder pain. Patients with SLAP lesions were excluded	Inflamma-tion, partial tear, complete rupture of the tendon, and instability of the long head of the biceps vi-sualized during arthroscopy	.45	.62	1.2	.89

9

Shoulder

Reliability of the Anterior Slide Test/Kibler Test

Test and Study Quality	Description	Population	Interexaminer Reliability
Anterior slide test[8] ◆	See next table	55 patients with shoulder pain scheduled for arthroscopic surgery	κ = .21 (−.05, .46)

Diagnostic Utility of the Anterior Slide Test/Kibler Test in Identifying Labral Tears

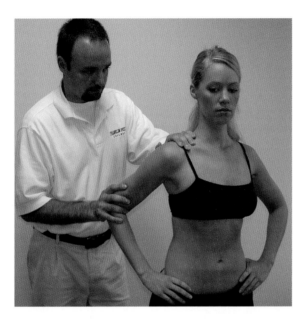

Figure 9-27
Anterior slide test/Kibler test.

Test and Study Quality	Description and Positive Findings	Population	Reference Standard	Sens	Spec	+LR	−LR
Anterior slide (Kibler) test[26] ◆ **2017 Meta-analysis**	With patient standing or sitting with hands on hips and thumbs facing posteriorly, examiner stabilizes scapula with one hand and, with other hand on elbow, applies anteriorly and superiorly directed force through humerus. Patient pushes back against force. Positive if pain or click is elicited in anterior shoulder	Pooled estimates from 3 studies	Study dependent, but generally labral tear diagnosed by arthroscopy	.10 (.04, .23)	.85 (.73, .93)	.67	1.1
Anterior slide test[41] ◆ **2012 Meta-analysis**		Pooled estimates from 4 studies (n = 831)		.17 (.03, .55)	.86 (.81, .89)	1.2 (.22, 6.5)	.97 (.96, 1.4)
Anterior slide test[42] ◆		93 patients suspected of having SLAP lesions	SLAP lesion visualized during arthroscopy or MRI arthrogram	.20 (.10, .37)	.74 (.62, .83)	0.8	1.1

Reliability of Various Tests in Identifying Labral Tears

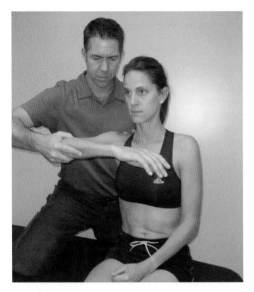

Figure 9-28
Jerk test.

Test and Study Quality	Description and Positive Findings	Population	Reliability
Passive compression test[48] ◆	Patient is side-lying with the affected shoulder up and the examiner standing behind the patient. The examiner stabilizes the patient's affected shoulder by holding the acromioclavicular joint with one hand and the patient's elbow with the other hand. The examiner rotates the patient's shoulder externally with 30 degrees of abduction and then pushes the arm proximally while extending the arm. The test is positive if pain or a painful click is elicited in the glenohumeral joint.	61 patients undergoing arthroscopy for shoulder pain	Interexaminer κ = .77
Kim test[40] ◆	With patient sitting with arm abducted 90 degrees, examiner holds the elbow and lateral aspect of the proximal arm and applies a strong axial loading force. Examiner then elevates the arm to 135 degrees and adds a posterior/inferior force. Positive if sudden onset of posterior shoulder pain	40 subjects with shoulder pain	Interexaminer κ = −.04 (−.12, .03)
Kim test[49] ◐		172 painful shoulders	Interexaminer κ = .91
Kim test[38] ◐		113 patients with shoulder pain	Interexaminer κ = .34 (.14, .53)
Biceps load II test[38] ◐	With patient supine, examiner grasps patient's wrist and elbow. Arm is elevated 120 degrees and fully externally rotated, with elbow held in 90 degrees of flexion and forearm supinated. Examiner then resists elbow flexion by patient. Positive if resisted elbow flexion causes pain		Interexaminer κ = .31 (.01, .60)

9

Shoulder

Diagnostic Utility of Other Tests in Identifying Labral and/or Long Head of the Bicep Lesions

Test and Study Quality	Description and Positive Findings	Population	Reference Standard	Sens	Spec	+LR	−LR
Upper cut test[46] ◆	With shoulder in a neutral position, the elbow flexed to 90 degrees, the forearm supinated, and the patient making a fist, the patient was asked to rapidly bring the hand up and toward the chin, as the examiner resists the motion. A positive test result is pain over the anterior portion of the shoulder	65 patients scheduled to undergo arthroscopic shoulder surgery	Lesion of long head of biceps tendon visualized during arthroscopy	.61	.63	1.63	.07
Backward traction[47] test ◆	With the patient standing and the involved shoulder relaxed and hanging down naturally, the examiner fixes the shoulder with one hand and holds the wrist with the other hand. The examiner then pulls the involved arm backward in the extreme internally rotated position. A positive test result is denoted by pain or a painful click in the anterior shoulder in the extreme externally rotated or internally rotated position	143 patients with chronic shoulder pain. Patients with SLAP lesions were excluded	Inflammation, partial tear, complete rupture of the tendon, and instability of the long head of the biceps visualized during arthroscopy	.49	.67	1.48	.76
Kim test[49] ⬤	With patient sitting with arm abducted 90 degrees, examiner holds the elbow and lateral aspect of the proximal arm and applies a strong axial loading force. Examiner then elevates the arm to 135 degrees and adds a posterior/inferior force. Positive if sudden onset of posterior shoulder pain	172 painful shoulders	Labral tear visualized during arthroscopy	.80	.94	13.3	.21

Diagnostic Utility of the Biceps Load Test in Identifying Labral Tears

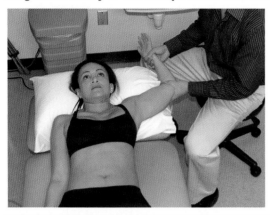

Figure 9-29
Biceps load test II.

Test and Study Quality	Description and Positive Findings	Population	Reference Standard	Sens	Spec	+LR	−LR
Biceps load II test[42] ◆	With patient supine, examiner grasps patient's wrist and elbow. Arm is elevated 120 degrees and fully externally rotated, with elbow held in 90 degrees of flexion and forearm supinated. Examiner then resists elbow flexion by patient. Positive if resisted elbow flexion causes pain	93 patients suspected of having SLAP lesions	SLAP lesion visualized during arthroscopy or MRI arthrogram	.28 (.15, .46)	.78 (.65, .87)	1.2	.93
Biceps load test II[54] ◆	With patient supine, the examiner places the patient's shoulder in 120 degrees of abduction, the elbow in 90 degrees of flexion, and the forearm in supination. The examiner moves the patient's shoulder to end-range external rotation and asks the patient to flex his or her elbow while the examiner resists this movement. A positive test is indicated as reproduction of pain during resisted elbow flexion	87 individuals with variable shoulder pathologic conditions	SLAP lesion diagnosed by arthroscopy	.55 (.46, .64)	.53 (.38, .68)	1.2 (.73, 2.0)	.85 (.53, 1.4)
Biceps load test II[3] ◆	With patient supine, examiner grasps patient's wrist and elbow. Arm is elevated 120 degrees and fully externally rotated, with elbow held in 90 degrees of flexion and forearm supinated. Examiner then resists elbow flexion by patient. Positive if resisted elbow flexion causes pain	68 patients with type II SLAP lesions and 78 age-matched controls who underwent shoulder arthroscopy	Type II SLAP lesion visualized during arthroscopy	.30	.78	1.4	.90
Biceps load test II[50] ◉		127 patients experiencing shoulder pain scheduled to undergo arthroscopy		.90	.97	30	.10
Biceps load test[51] ◉	With patient supine, examiner grasps wrist and elbow. Arm is abducted to 90 degrees, with elbow flexed to 90 degrees and forearm supinated. Examiner externally rotates arm until patient becomes apprehensive, at which time external rotation is stopped. Patient flexes elbow against examiner's resistance. Positive if patient's apprehension remains or pain is produced	75 patients with unilateral recurrent anterior shoulder dislocations	SLAP lesion diagnosed by arthroscopy	.90	.97	30	.10

9

Shoulder

Diagnostic Utility of Various Tests in Identifying Labral Tears

Test and Study Quality	Description and Positive Findings	Population	Reference Standard	Sens	Spec	+LR	−LR
Passive compression test[48] ◆	With patient side-lying with affected side up, examiner places one hand over the acromioclavicular joint to stabilize the shoulder and places the other hand on the elbow. Examiner then externally rotates the shoulder in 30 degrees of abduction and gives axial compression while extending the arm. Positive if pain occurs	61 patients undergoing arthroscopy for shoulder pain	SLAP lesion visualized during arthroscopy	.82	.86	5.90	.21
Supine flexion resistance test[52] ◆	With patient supine with arm resting in full flexion and palm up, examiner grasps patient's arm just distal to the elbow and asks the patient to lift the arm as if throwing. Positive if pain is felt deep inside the shoulder joint	133 patients who underwent diagnostic arthroscopy of the shoulder	SLAP lesion visualized during arthroscopy	.80	.69	2.6	.29
Resisted supination external rotation test[53] ◆	With patient supine with arm abducted 90 degrees and elbow flexed 70 degrees, examiner supports the arm by the elbow. Examiner resists supination and gently maximally externally rotates the shoulder. Positive if shoulder pain, clicking, or catching is elicited	40 athletes with shoulder pain		.83	.82	4.6	.21
Dynamic labral shear test (O'Driscoll test)[54] ◆	Patient is sitting with the arm at the side and the elbow flexed 90 degrees. Examiner externally rotates patient's arm 90 degrees and brings the arm into 90 degrees of abduction. With the elbow flexed, the arm is abducted from 90 degrees to 120 degrees. Test is positive if pain is reproduced in the abduction range of 90 to 120 degrees	87 individuals with variable shoulder pathologic conditions	SLAP lesion diagnosed by arthroscopy	.89 (.81, .95)	.30 (.17, .41)	1.3 (.98, 1.6)	.40 (.10, 1.1)
Labral tension test[54] ◆	Patient is supine with arm placed in 120 degrees of abduction and neutral forearm rotation. The shoulder is then taken to end-range external rotation. At end-range rotation, the examiner grasps the patient's hand and asks him or her to supinate the forearm, against resistance, from the neutral position. Positive if patient reports increased pain with resisted supination			.28 (.20, .36)	.76 (.61, .88)	1.2 (.50, 2.9)	.94 (.73, 1.3)

Diagnostic Utility of Various Tests in Identifying Labral Tears—cont'd

Test and Study Quality	Description and Positive Findings	Population	Reference Standard	Sens	Spec	+LR	−LR
Whipple test[3] ◆	The arm is flexed 90 degrees and adducted until the hand is opposite the other shoulder. The patient resists while examiner pushes downward on the arm. Positive if pain occurs	68 patients with type II SLAP lesions and 78 age-matched controls who underwent shoulder arthroscopy	Type II SLAP lesion visualized during arthroscopy	.65	.42	1.1	.83
Posterior jerk test[44]	Not described	54 throwing athletes with shoulder pain		.25	.80	1.3	.72
Jerk test[49]	With patient sitting, examiner holds scapula with one hand and internally rotates and abducts the patient's arm to 90 degrees with the other hand. Examiner then horizontally adducts the arm while applying an axial loading force. Sharp pain indicates a positive test	172 painful shoulders	Labral tear visualized during arthroscopy	.73	.98	36.5	.28

9

Shoulder

Reliability of the Hawkins-Kennedy Test

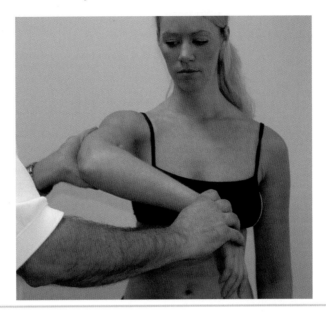

Figure 9-30
Hawkins-Kennedy test.

Test and Study Quality	Description and Positive Findings	Population	Reliability
Hawkins-Kennedy test[55] ◆ **2017 Metaanalysis**	Examiner flexes the humerus and elbow to 90 degrees and then maximally internally rotates the shoulder and applies overpressure. Positive with reproduction of pain of the superior shoulder	Pooled estimates from 7 studies (n = 437)	Interexaminer κ = .47 (.28, .67)
Hawkins-Kennedy test[38] ◐		113 patients with shoulder pain	Interexaminer κ = .33 (.15, .51)

Diagnostic Utility of the Hawkins-Kennedy Test in Identifying Subacromial Impingement

Test and Study Quality	Description and Positive Findings	Population	Reference Standard	Sens	Spec	+LR	−LR
Hawkins-Kennedy test[26] ◆ 2017 Metaanalysis	The examiner places the patient's arm in 90 degrees of forward flexion and then gently internally rotates the arm. The end point for internal rotation is either when the patient feels pain or when the rotation of the scapula is felt or observed by the examiner. The test is positive when the patient experiences pain during the maneuver	Pooled estimates from 2 studies	Study dependent, but generally impingement syndrome diagnosed by arthroscopy	.58 (.50, .66)	.67 (.47, .83)	1.8	.63
Hawkins-Kennedy test[56] ◆ 2012 Meta-analysis		Pooled estimates from 6 studies (n = 1029)		.74 (.57, .85)	.57 (.46, .67)	1.7	.46
Hawkins-Kennedy test[41] ◆ 2012 Meta-analysis		Pooled estimates from 7 studies (n = 944)		.80 (.72, 086)	.56 (.45, .67)	1.8 (1.5, 2.3)	0.35 (0.27, 0.46)
Hawkins-Kennedy test[5] ◆ 2008 Meta-analysis		Pooled estimates from 4 high-quality studies		.79 (.75, .82)	.59 (.53, .64)	1.9	.36

9

Shoulder

Reliability of the Neer Test

Test and Study Quality	Description and Positive Findings	Population	Reliability
Neer test[55] ◆ **2017 Metaanalysis**	Examiner stabilizes the scapula with a downward force while fully flexing the humerus overhead while applying overpressure. Positive with reproduction of pain of the superior shoulder	Pooled estimates from 7 studies (n = 534)	Interexaminer κ = .54 (.33, .74)
Neer test[38] ◐		113 patients with shoulder pain	Interexaminer κ = .43 (.23, .62)

Diagnostic Utility of the Neer Test in Identifying Subacromial Impingement

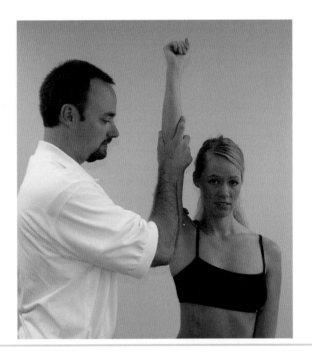

Figure 9-31
Neer test.

Diagnostic Utility of the Neer Test in Identifying Subacromial Impingement—cont'd

Test and Study Quality	Description and Positive Findings	Population	Reference Standard	Sens	Spec	+LR	−LR
Neer test[26] ◆ 2017 Meta-analysis	The examiner stabilizes the scapula and has the patient passively or actively forward flex the arm until he or she reports pain or until full elevation is reached. Positive if pain is produced	Pooled estimates from 2 studies	Study dependent, but generally impingement syndrome diagnosed by arthroscopy	.59 (.52, .67)	.60 (.40, .77)	1.5	.68
Neer test[56] ◆ 2012 Metaanaly-sis		Pooled estimates from 5 studies (n = 1127)		.78 (.68, .87)	.58 (.47, .68)	1.9	.38
Neer test[41] ◆ 2012 Metaanaly-sis		Pooled estimates from 7 studies (n = 946)		.72 (.60, .81)	.60 (.40, .77)	1.8 (1.2, 2.6)	.47 (.39, .56)
Neer test[45] ◆ 2008 Metaanaly-sis		Pooled estimates from 4 high-quality studies		.79 (.75, .82)	.53 (.48, .58)	1.7	.40

9

Shoulder

Reliability of the Painful Arc Test in Identifying Subacromial Impingement

Test and Study Quality	Description and Positive Findings	Population	Reliability
Painful arc test[55] ◆ **2017 Metaanalysis**	Patient asked to actively abduct shoulder and report any pain during abduction. If pain of the superior shoulder is noted between 60 degrees and 120 degrees of abduction, the test is considered positive	Pooled estimates from 5 studies (n = 489)	Interexaminer κ = .57 (.37, .78)

Diagnostic Utility of the Painful Arc Test in Identifying Subacromial Impingement

Test and Study Quality	Description and Positive Findings	Population	Reference Standard	Sens	Spec	+LR	−LR
Painful arc test[41] ◆ **2012 Meta-analysis**	Not described	Pooled estimates from 4 studies (n = 756)	Impingement syndrome diagnosed by arthroscopy and ultrasound	.53 (.31, .74)	.76 (.68, .84)	2.3 (1.2, 4.1)	.62 (.37, 1.0)
Painful arc sign[57] ◆	Patient actively elevates arm in scapular plane to full elevation. Positive if patient experiences pain between 60 degrees and 120 degrees	552 patients with shoulder pain	Arthroscopic visualization				
			• All impingement	.74	.81	3.9	.32
			• Bursitis	.71	.47	1.3	.62
			• Partial thickness rotator cuff tear	.67	.47	1.3	.70
			• Full-thickness rotator cuff tear	.76	.72	2.7	.33
Painful arc test[59] ◆	Patient is asked to actively abduct shoulder and report any pain during abduction. If pain of the superior shoulder is noted between 60 degrees and 120 degrees of abduction, the test is considered positive	55 patients with shoulder pain	Impingement diagnosed via arthroscopy	.75 (.54, .96)	.67 (.52, .81)	2.3 (1.3, 3.8)	.38 (.16, .90)
Painful arc test[58] ◑	Patient is instructed to perform straight plane abduction throughout full range of motion. Positive if pain occurs between 60 degrees and 100 degrees of abduction	125 painful shoulders	Subacromial impingement diagnosed via subacromial injection	.33	.33	1.74	.83

Reliability of the Drop-Arm Test in Identifying Subacromial Impingement

Test and Study Quality	Description and Positive Findings	Population	Reliability
Drop-arm test[40] ◆	The examiner passively abducts the patient's arm to 90 degrees. The examiner releases the patient's arm with instructions to hold the arm in the same position. Positive with inability to hold the arm at 90 degrees of abduction or with a sudden drop of the arm	40 subjects with shoulder pain	κ = .57 (−.14, .57)

Diagnostic Utility of the Drop-Arm Test in Identifying Subacromial Impingement

Test and Study Quality	Description and Positive Findings	Population	Reference Standard	Sens	Spec	+LR	−LR
Drop-arm test[56] ◆ 2012 Meta-analysis	The patient fully elevates the arm and then slowly reverses the motion in the same arc. If the arm is dropped suddenly or the patient has severe pain, the test is considered to be positive	Pooled estimates from 5 studies (n = 1213)	Impingement syndrome diagnosed by arthroscopy	.21 (.14, .30)	.92 (.86, .96)	2.6	.86
Drop-arm test[58] ◕	Patient is instructed to abduct shoulder to 90 degrees and then lower it slowly to neutral position. Positive if patient is unable to do this because of pain	125 painful shoulders	Subacromial impingement diagnosed via subacromial injection	.08	.97	2.67	.95

Reliability of the Empty Can Test in Identifying Subacromial Impingement

Test and Study Quality	Description and Positive Findings	Population	Reliability
Empty can/Supraspinatus test[55] ◆ 2017 Metaanalysis	Examiner elevates patient's shoulder to 90 degrees in the scapular plane and places the humerus in internal rotation by asking the patient to rotate the shoulder so that his or her thumb is pointing toward the floor. The examiner then applies a downward directed force at the wrist while the patient attempts to resist. Test is considered positive if weakness is detected of the involved shoulder	Pooled estimates from 4 studies (n = 195)	Interexaminer κ = .71 (.45, .97)

9

Shoulder

Diagnostic Utility of the Empty Can Test in Identifying Subacromial Impingement

Test and Study Quality	Description and Positive Findings	Population	Reference Standard	Sens	Spec	+LR	−LR
Empty can test[56] ◆ **2012 Meta-analysis**	The examiner asks the patient to elevate and internally rotate the arm with thumbs pointing downward in the scapular plane. The elbow should be fully extended. In this position the examiner applies downward pressure on the upper surface of the arm. Test is positive with weakness	Pooled estimates from 6 studies (n = 695)	Impingement syndrome diagnosed by arthroscopy	.69 (.54, .81)	.62 (.38, .81)	1.8	.50
Empty can test (Jobe test)[59] ◆	Examiner elevates patient's shoulder to 90 degrees in the scapular plane and then places the shoulder in internal rotation by asking the patient to rotate the shoulder so that his or her thumb is pointing toward the floor. The examiner then applies a downward directed force at the wrist while the patient attempts to resist. Test is considered positive if weakness is detected of the involved shoulder as compared bilaterally	55 patients with shoulder pain	Impingement diagnosed via arthroscopy	.50 (.26, .75)	.87 (.77, .98)	3.9 (1.5, 10.1)	.57 (.35, .95)
Weakness with elevation (empty can test)[60] ◆	With patient standing with arms elevated to shoulder level in scapular plane and thumbs pointing down, examiner applies downward force and patient resists. Positive if weakness is present	30 patients with new onset of shoulder pain	MRI has confirmed • Subacromial impingement • Subacromial bursitis	.74 .73	.30 .29	1.1 1.0	.87 .93
Supraspinatus muscle test[60] ◆	Examiner resists abduction of the arm at 90 degrees with patient's arm neutral or internally rotated. Positive if patient gives way	30 patients with new onset of shoulder pain	MRI has confirmed • Subacromial impingement • Subacromial bursitis	.58 .73	.20 .43	.70 1.3	2.10 .63

Diagnostic Utility of the Lift-Off Test in Identifying Subacromial Impingement

Test and Study Quality	Description and Positive Findings	Population	Reference Standard	Sens	Spec	+LR	−LR
Lift-off test[56] ◆ 2012 Meta-analysis	The patient internally rotates the shoulder, placing the hand on the ipsilateral buttock. Patient is then asked to lift the hand off the buttock against resistance. Test is positive with weakness of this action	Pooled estimates from 4 studies (n = 267)	Impingement syndrome diagnosed by arthroscopy	.42 (.19, .69)	.97 (.79, 1.0)	14	.60
Lift-off test (Gerber test)[60] ◆	Patient attempts to lift the affected arm off the back. Positive if unable to lift off back	30 patients with new onset of shoulder pain	Subacromial impingement confirmed by MRI	.68	.50	1.4 (.70, 2.7)	.64
			Subacromial bursitis confirmed by MRI	.93	.71	3.3 (1.4, 7.6)	.10
Lift-off test (Gerber test)[62] ◆		847 patients who underwent diagnostic arthroscopy of the shoulder	Partial biceps tendon tear visualized during arthroscopy	.28	.89	2.5	.81

Reliability of Various Tests in Identifying Subacromial Impingement

Test and Study Quality	Description and Positive Findings	Population	Reliability
External rotation resistance test[38] ◉	With patient's arm at the side and elbow flexed to 90 degrees, a medially directed force is exerted on the distal forearm to resist shoulder external rotation. Test is considered positive if weakness is detected on the involved shoulder as compared bilaterally	113 patients with shoulder pain	Interexaminer κ = .50 (.34, .66)
External rotation resistance test[59] ◉	With patient's arm at the side and elbow flexed to 90 degrees, a medially directed force is exerted on the distal forearm to resist shoulder external rotation. Test is considered positive if weakness is detected on the involved shoulder as compared bilaterally	55 patients with shoulder pain	Interexaminer κ = .67 (.40, .94)

9

Shoulder

Diagnostic Utility of Various Tests in Identifying Subacromial Impingement

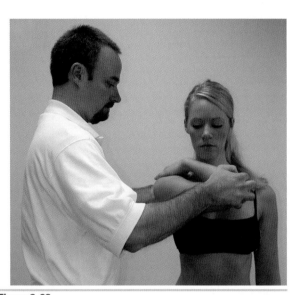

Figure 9-32
Horizontal adduction test.

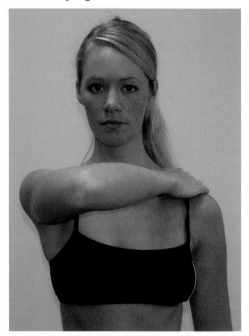

Figure 9-33
Yocum test.

Test and Study Quality	Description and Positive Findings	Population	Reference Standard	Sens	Spec	+LR	−LR
Cross-body adduction test[57] ◆	With patient's arm at 90 degrees of flexion, examiner adducts arm across the patient's body. Positive if shoulder pain is produced	552 patients with shoulder pain	Arthroscopic visualization				
			• All impingement	.23	.82	1.3	.94
			• Bursitis	.25	.80	1.3	.94
			• Partial thickness RCT	.17	.79	.80	1.05
			• Full-thickness RCT	.23	.81	1.2	.95
Yocum test[60] ◆	With patient seated or standing, patient places hand of involved shoulder on contralateral shoulder and raises elbow. Positive if pain is elicited	30 patients with new onset of shoulder pain	Subacromial impingement confirmed by MRI	.79	.40	1.3 (.80, 2.3)	.53
			Subacromial bursitis confirmed by MRI	.80	.36	1.2 (.08, 2.0)	.56
External rotation resistance test[59] ◆	With patient's arm at the side and elbow flexed to 90 degrees, a medially directed force is exerted on the distal forearm to resist shoulder external rotation. Test is considered positive if weakness of the involved shoulder is detected as compared bilaterally	55 patients with shoulder pain	Impingement diagnosed via arthroscopy	.56 (.32, .81)	.87 (.77, .98)	4.4 (1.7, 11.1)	.50 (.28, .89)
Horizontal adduction test[58] ◉	Examiner forces patient's arm into horizontal adduction while elbow is flexed. Positive if pain is elicited	125 painful shoulders	Subacromial impingement via subacromial injection	.82	.28	1.14	.64

Reliability of Special Tests for Identifying Supraspinatus and/or Infraspinatus Tears

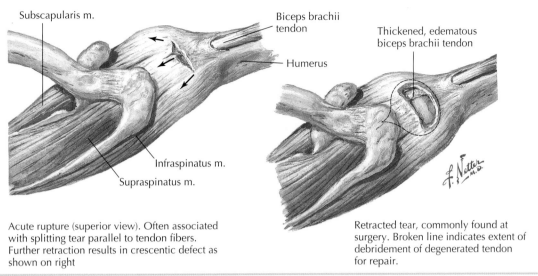

Acute rupture (superior view). Often associated with splitting tear parallel to tendon fibers. Further retraction results in crescentic defect as shown on right

Retracted tear, commonly found at surgery. Broken line indicates extent of debridement of degenerated tendon for repair.

Figure 9-34
Superior rotator cuff tear.

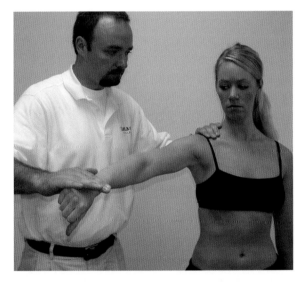

Figure 9-35
Supraspinatus muscle test (empty can test).

Test and Study Quality	Description and Positive Findings	Population	Reliability
Supraspinatus muscle test (empty can test)[61] ◆	Patient's arm is elevated to shoulder level in scapular plane and thumbs pointing down, examiner applies downward force and patient resists. Positive if weakness is present	33 patients with shoulder pain	Test-retest κ = 1.0 Interexaminer κ = .94
Patte maneuver[61] ◆	Shoulder and elbow at 90 degrees with arm internally rotated. Examiner then resists internal rotation force. Positive if patient gives way		Test-retest κ = 1.0 Interexaminer κ = 1.0
Empty can test[38] ◐	Patient's arm is elevated to shoulder level in scapular plane and thumbs pointing down, examiner applies downward force and patient resists. Positive if weakness is present	113 patients with shoulder pain	Interexaminer κ = .51 (.34, .66)
Full can test[38] ◐	Same as empty can, but with thumb up	113 patients with shoulder pain	Interexaminer κ = .62 (.47, .78)

9 | Shoulder

Diagnostic Utility of Special Tests for Identifying Supraspinatus and/or Infraspinatus Tears

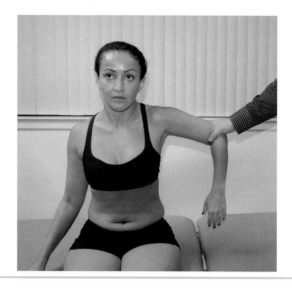

Figure 9-36
Lateral Jobe test.

Test and Study Quality	Description and Positive Findings	Population	Reference Standard	Sens	Spec	+LR	−LR
Supraspinatus/Empty can test[26] ◆ **2017 Meta-analysis**	Patient's arm elevated to shoulder level in scapular plane and thumbs pointing down, examiner applies downward force and patient resists. Positive if weakness is present	Pooled estimates from 3 studies	Arthroscopic evidence of: • Any rotator cuff tear • Full thickness rotator cuff tear • Full thickness supraspinatus tear	.60 (.52, .68) .74 (.39, .92) .60 (.46, .72)	.63 (.55, .71) .77 (.69, .83) .70 (.61, .78)	1.6 3.2 2.0	.63 .63 .57
Empty can test[63] ◆		91 patients undergoing arthrography	Arthroscopic evidence of: • Partial thickness supraspinatus tear • Full thickness supraspinatus tear	.88 .91	.46 .46	1.7 1.7	.25 .20
Full can test[63] ◆	As above for empty can test, but with thumb pointing up		Arthroscopic evidence of: • Partial thickness supraspinatus tear • Full thickness supraspinatus tear	.79 .79	.69 .70	2.6 2.6	.30 .30

Diagnostic Utility of Special Tests for Identifying Supraspinatus and/or Infraspinatus Tears—cont'd

Test and Study Quality	Description and Positive Findings	Population	Reference Standard	Sens	Spec	+LR	−LR
Lateral Jobe test[64] ◆ (see Video 9-1)	Patient's shoulder is abducted 90 degrees in the coronal plane and internally rotated so that with the elbow flexed 90 degrees the fingers point inferiorly and thumb medially. Test is positive with pain or weakness on resisting an inferiorly directed force applied to the distal arm or an inability to perform the test	175 patients undergoing arthrography	Arthrographic confirmation of complete or partial rotator cuff tear	.81	.89	7.36	.21
Drop-arm test[63] ◆	Patient elevates arm fully and then slowly lowers arm. Positive if the arm suddenly drops or patient has severe pain	91 patients undergoing arthrography	Arthroscopic evidence of:				
			• Partial thickness supraspinatus tear	.23	.77	1.0	.99
			• Full thickness supraspinatus tear	.25	.77	1.1	.98
Drop-arm test[57] ◆	Patient elevates arm fully and then slowly lowers arm. Positive if the arm suddenly drops or patient has severe pain	552 patients with shoulder pain	Arthroscopic visualization of				
			• All impingement	.27	.88	2.3	.83
			• Bursitis	.14	.77	.60	1.12
			• Partial thickness RCT	.14	.78	.60	1.10
			• Full-thickness RCT	.35	.88	2.9	.74
Infraspinatus muscle test (Patte test)[60] ◆	Elbow at 90 degrees with arm neutrally rotated and adducted to the trunk. Examiner then resists internal rotation force. Positive if patient gives way	30 patients with new onset of shoulder pain	MRI has confirmed				
			• Subacromial impingement	.58	.60	1.5	.70
			• Subacromial bursitis	.73	.71	2.5	.38
Infraspinatus muscle test[57] ◆		552 patients with shoulder pain	Arthroscopic visualization of				
			• All impingement	.42	.90	4.2	.64
			• Bursitis	.25	.69	.80	1.09
			• Partial thickness RCT	.19	.69	.60	1.17
			• Full-thickness RCT	.51	.84	3.2	.58

Continued

9

Shoulder

Diagnostic Utility of Special Tests for Identifying Supraspinatus and/or Infraspinatus Tears—cont'd

Test and Study Quality	Description and Positive Findings	Population	Reference Standard	Sens	Spec	+LR	−LR
External rotation lag sign[65] ◆	With patient sitting, examiner holds the patient's arm in 20 degrees of shoulder elevation (in the scapular plane), 5 degrees from full external rotation, and 90 degrees of elbow extension. Patient maintains the position when examiner releases arm. Positive if unable to hold position	37 patients with shoulder pain	Supraspinatus or infraspinatus tear diagnosed via ultrasound	.46	.94	7.2 (1.7, 31.0)	.60 (.40, .90)
Drop sign[65] ◆	With patient sitting, examiner holds the arm in 90 degrees of abduction and full external rotation. Patient is asked to maintain the position when examiner releases arm. Positive if unable to hold position			.73	.77	3.2 (1.5, 6.7)	.30 (.20, .80)
Scapular retraction[63] test ◆	After performing a resisted empty can test, the test is then repeated with additional manual stabilization of the patient's medial scapular border and anterior shoulder at the clavicle. Positive when weakness during the empty can test is normalized with stabilization	91 patients undergoing arthrography	Arthroscopic evidence of: • Partial thickness supraspinatus tear • Full thickness supraspinatus tear	.38 .45	.38 .38	0.6 0.7	1.6 1.4
Scapular retraction test[66] ◉		331 patients with shoulder pain	Full-thickness rotator cuff tear visualized on MRI	.82 (.77, .85)	.81 (.76, .85)	4.3 (3.1, 5.8)	.23 (.17, .30)
Subacromial grind test[67] ◉	With patient standing, examiner passively abducts the arm in the scapular plane, then internally and externally rotates the shoulder. The other hand is placed over the anterior and lateral acromion. A positive test is palpable crepitus	50 patients undergoing shoulder arthroscopy	Arthroscopic visualization of supraspinatus tear: • Any tear • Full thickness tear	.63 (.42, .81) .82 (.57, .96)	.95 (.75, 1.0) .87 (.69, .96)	12.6 (1.8, 86.9) 6.2 (2.4, 15.8)	.39 (.24, .64) .20 (.07, .57)

Diagnostic Utility of Special Tests for Identifying Supraspinatus and/or Infraspinatus Tears—cont'd

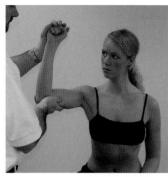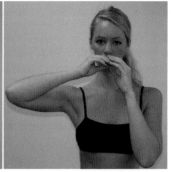

Patients with a positive Hornblower sign often have difficulty raising their hand to their mouth without abducting the shoulder

Figure 9-37
Hornblower sign.

Test and Study Quality	Description and Positive Findings	Population	Reference Standard	Sens	Spec	+LR	−LR
Passive elevation of less than 170 degrees[10] ◆	With patient supine, examiner maximally elevates shoulder			.30	.78	1.36	.90
Passive external rotation of less than 70 degrees[10] ◆	With patient supine with arm at side, examiner externally rotates arm			.19	.84	1.19	.96
Arc of pain sign[10] ◆	With patient standing, examiner passively abducts arm to 170 degrees. Patient then slowly lowers arm to side. Positive if patient reports pain at 120 degrees to 70 degrees of abduction	448 patients undergoing arthrography	Arthrographic confirmation of complete or partial rotator cuff tear	.98	.10	1.09	.20
Atrophy of the supraspinatus muscle[10] ◆	Examiner determines atrophy through visual inspection			.56	.73	2.07	.60
Atrophy of the infraspinatus muscle[10] ◆				.56	.73	2.07	.60

9

Shoulder

Reliability of Special Tests for Identifying Subscapularis Tears

Test and Study Quality	Description and Positive Findings	Population	Reliability
Belly-press test[40] ◆	With elbow at 90 degrees and hand on belly, patient forcefully presses into a tensiometer on the belly. Positive if weak compared with other side or if patient uses elbow or shoulder extension to push. Positive with weakness of 30% or more compared with the opposite shoulder measured with a handheld dynamometer	40 subjects with shoulder pain	κ = .65 (.33, .96)

Diagnostic Utility of Special Tests for Identifying Subscapularis Tears

Test and Study Quality	Description and Positive Findings	Population	Reference Standard	Sens	Spec	+LR	−LR
Internal rotation lag sign[65] ◆	With patient sitting, examiner holds patient's hand behind the lumbar region in full internal rotation. Patient maintains the position when examiner releases arm. Positive if patient is unable to hold position	37 patients with shoulder pain	Subscapularis tear diagnosed via ultrasound	1.0	.84	6.2 (1.9, 12.0)	.00 (.00, 2.50)
Internal rotation lag sign[69] ◆	Examiner places the hand of the patient's affected arm on the back at the midlumbar region; it is held by the examiner at almost maximum internal rotation. The back of the hand is passively lifted away from the body until almost full internal rotation is reached. The patient is then asked to actively maintain this position. The test is considered positive if the patient is unable to maintain this position and the hand has dropped back to the lumbar region	55 patients suffering from subacromial and/or glenohumeral impingement syndrome scheduled for an arthroscopic procedure	Subscapularis tear diagnosed via arthroscopic visualization	.71	.60	1.8	.48
Internal rotation lag sign[70] ◆	The patient's affected arm is placed on the back in the middle lumbar region. The dorsum of the hand is then passively lifted away from the body until almost full internal rotation is reached, and the patient is asked to actively maintain this position. The sign is considered positive if lag occurs	312 patients scheduled to undergo arthroscopic shoulder surgery	Subscapularis tear diagnosed via arthroscopic visualization	.20	.97	6.7	.83
Internal rotation lag sign[71] ●	The patient's affected arm is placed on the back in the middle lumbar region. The dorsum of the hand is then passively lifted away from the body until almost full internal rotation is reached, and the patient is asked to actively maintain this position. The sign is considered positive if lag occurs	106 patients undergoing shoulder arthroscopy	Subscapularis tear diagnosed via arthroscopic visualization	.41	.91	4.6	.60

Diagnostic Utility of Special Tests for Identifying Subscapularis Tears—cont'd

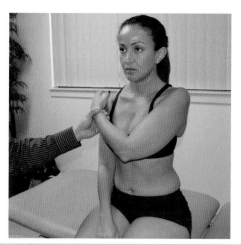

Figure 9-38
Bear-hug test.

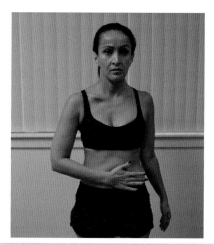

Figure 9-39
Belly-press test.

Test and Study Quality	Description and Positive Findings	Population	Reference Standard	Sens	Spec	+LR	−LR
Bear-hug test[70] ◆ (see Video 9-2)	The palm of the hand on the patient's involved side is placed on the opposite shoulder with fingers extended, and the elbow is positioned anterior to the body. The patient is then asked to hold that position as the examiner tries to pull the patient's hand from the shoulder with an external rotation force applied perpendicular to the forearm. The test is considered positive if the patient is unable to resist the examiner's external rotation power and if the affected arm exhibits weakness compared with the contralateral side	165 patients scheduled to undergo arthroscopic shoulder surgery	Subscapularis tear diagnosed via arthroscopic visualization	.19	.99	19	.82
Bear-hug test[72] ◆		130 patients scheduled to undergo arthroscopic shoulder surgery	Subscapularis tear diagnosed via arthroscopic visualization	.74 (.57, .86)	.97 (.90, 1.0)	28.4 (7.1, 112.9)	.27 (.16, .46)
Bear-hug test[71] ◉		106 patients undergoing shoulder arthroscopy	Subscapularis tear diagnosed via arthroscopic visualization	.52	.85	3.5	.60

9

Shoulder

Diagnostic Utility of Special Tests for Identifying Subscapularis Tears—cont'd

Test and Study Quality	Description and Positive Findings	Population	Reference Standard	Sens	Spec	+LR	−LR
Bear-hug test[73] ●	Patient places palm of hand on involved side on the opposite shoulder, and fingers are extended. Examiner attempts to pull the hand off the shoulder into external rotation while the patient resists. Positive if patient is unable to maintain hand on shoulder or there is weakness at more than 20 degrees compared with the other side	68 shoulders scheduled to undergo arthroscopic shoulder surgery	Subscapularis tear diagnosed via arthroscopic visualization	.60	.92	7.5	.43
Belly-press test[73] ●	With elbow at 90 degrees and hand on belly, patient forcefully presses into a tensiometer on the belly. Positive if weak compared with other side or if patient uses elbow or shoulder extension to push			.40	.98	20.0	.61

Diagnostic Utility of Special Tests for Identifying Subscapularis Tears—cont'd

Test and Study Quality	Description and Positive Findings	Population	Reference Standard	Sens	Spec	+LR	−LR
Belly-press test[70] ◆ (see Video 9-3)	The patient's arm is at the side and the elbow is flexed. The patient is asked to press the palm into his or her abdomen by internally rotating the shoulder. The test is considered positive if the patient pushes the hand against the belly by wrist flexion, despite instruction to the contrary	312 patients scheduled to undergo arthroscopic shoulder surgery	Subscapularis tear diagnosed via arthroscopic visualization	.28	.99	28	.73
Belly-press test[74] ◆		134 patients with suspected rotator cuff pathology	Subscapularis tear diagnosed via arthroscopic visualization or MRI arthrogram	.30 (.15, .52)	.97 (.92 (.99)	11.0	.72
Belly-press test[71] ●		106 patients undergoing shoulder arthroscopy	Subscapularis tear diagnosed via arthroscopic visualization	.34	.96	8.5	.70
Belly-off sign[71] ●	The arm of the patient is passively brought into flexion and maximum internal rotation with the elbow flexed at 90 degrees. The elbow is supported by one hand of the examiner while the examiner's other hand brings the arm into maximum internal rotation, placing the palm of the patient's hand on the abdomen. The patient is asked to keep the wrist straight and actively maintain the position of internal rotation as the examiner releases the wrist. Test is positive if the patient cannot maintain that position, if the wrist is flexed or lag occurs, and if the hand is lifted off the abdomen	106 patients undergoing shoulder arthroscopy	Subscapularis tear diagnosed via arthroscopic visualization	.31	.97	10.3	.70

9

Shoulder

Diagnostic Utility of Special Tests for Identifying Subscapularis Tears—cont'd

Test and Study Quality	Description and Positive Findings	Population	Reference Standard	Sens	Spec	+LR	−LR
Modified belly-press test[69] ◆	With the hand flat on the abdomen and the elbow close to the body, the patient is asked to bring the elbow forward and straighten the wrist. The final wrist flexion position or belly-press angle of the wrist is then measured by a goniometer. The test is considered positive if the measured belly-press angle at the wrist shows a side-to-side difference of at least 10 degrees	55 patients suffering from subacromial and/or glenohumeral impingement syndrome scheduled for an arthroscopic procedure	Subscapularis tear diagnosed via arthroscopic visualization	.80	.88	6.7	.23
Belly-off sign[69] ◆	The arm of the patient is passively brought into flexion and maximum internal rotation with the elbow flexed at 90 degrees. The elbow is supported by one hand of the examiner while the examiner's other hand brings the arm into maximum internal rotation, placing the palm of the patient's hand on the abdomen. The patient is asked to keep the wrist straight and actively maintain the position of internal rotation as the examiner releases the wrist. Test is positive if the patient cannot maintain that position, if the wrist is flexed or lag occurs, and if the hand is lifted off the abdomen			.86	.91	9.6	.15
Lift-off test[69] ◆	Examiner places the hand of the patient's affected arm on the back at the midlumbar region and asks the patient to rotate the arm internally and lift the hand posteriorly off the back. The test is considered positive if the patient is unable to do so			.40	.79	1.9	.76
Lift-off test[72] ◆		130 patients scheduled to undergo arthroscopic shoulder surgery	Subscapularis tear diagnosed via arthroscopic visualization	.65 (.50, .78)	.95 (.86, .98)	11.9 (4.5, 31.6)	.37 (.25, .55)

Diagnostic Utility of Special Tests for Identifying Subscapularis Tears—cont'd

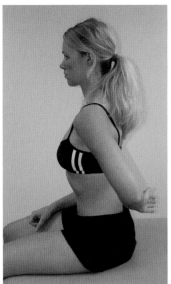
Negative test

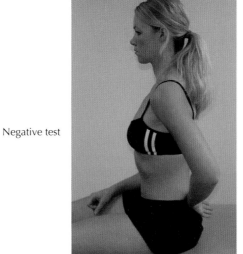
Positive test

Figure 9-40
Lift-off test.

Test and Study Quality	Description and Positive Findings	Population	Reference Standard	Sens	Spec	+LR	−LR
Lift-off test[70] ◆	Hand of the affected arm is placed on the back and patient is asked to internally rotate the arm so as to lift the hand off the back. The test is considered positive if the patient is unable to lift the hand off or if the patient performs the lifting maneuver by extending the elbow or shoulder	312 patients scheduled to undergo arthroscopic shoulder surgery	Subscapularis tear diagnosed via arthroscopic visualization	.12	1.0	Undefined	.88
Lift-off test[74] ◆		134 patients with suspected rotator cuff pathology	Subscapularis tear diagnosed via arthroscopic visualization or MRI arthrogram	.21 (.07, .59)	.96 (.91, .99)	5.7	.82
Lift-off test[71] ◉		106 patients undergoing shoulder arthroscopy	Subscapularis tear diagnosed via arthroscopic visualization	.35	.98	17.5	.70

9

Shoulder

Diagnostic Utility of Special Tests for Identifying Subscapularis Tears—cont'd

Test and Study Quality	Description and Positive Findings	Population	Reference Standard	Sens	Spec	+LR	−LR
Lift-off test[73] ◐	Patient places the hand of the affected arm on the back (at the position of the midlumbar spine) and then attempts to internally rotate the arm to lift the hand posteriorly off the back. Test is positive if patient is unable to lift the arm off the back or if patient performs the lifting maneuver by extending the elbow or the shoulder	68 shoulders scheduled to undergo arthroscopic surgery	Subscapularis tear diagnosed via arthroscopic visualization	18	1.0	Undefined	.82
Napoleon test[73] ◐	Patient sitting or supine. The examiner places the patient's hand on his or her belly and asks the patient to lift his or her elbow. Positive if patient is unable to lift the elbow			.25	.98	12.5	.77
Napoleon test[72] ◆		130 patients scheduled to undergo arthroscopic shoulder surgery	Subscapularis tear diagnosed via arthroscopic visualization	.84 (.71, .92)	.96 (.88, .99)	21.9 (7.2–66.9)	.16 (.09, .31)

Diagnostic Utility of Special Tests for Identifying Teres Minor and/or Infraspinatus Tears

Test and Study Quality	Description and Positive Findings	Population	Reference Standard	Sens	Spec	+LR	−LR
External rotation lag sign > 10°[75] ◆	With the patient seated, the elbow flexed to 90° and the shoulder elevated 20° in the scapular plane, the arm is passively taken to maximal external rotation. The patient was asked to maintain that position as the clinician released the wrist. A positive test is defined as any internal rotation greater than 10°	100 patients with massive rotator cuff tears	Teres minor tear diagnosed via CT arthro-gram	1.0 (.80, 1.0)	.51 (.40, .61)	2.0	.00
External rotation lag sign > 40°[75] ◆	As above, but a positive test is defined as internal rotation greater than 40°			1.0 (.80, 1.0)	.92 (.84, .96)	12.5	.00
Patte sign[75] ◆	With the patient seated, arm at 90° abduction in the scapular plane and elbow flexed to 90°, the patient is asked to perform external ro-tation of the shoulder against resistance. A positive test is external rotation strength less than 4/5			.93 (.70, .99)	.72 (.23, .80)	3.3	.10
Patte sign[76] ◆		91 patients undergoing arthrography	Arthroscopic evidence of: • Partial thickness infraspina-tus tear	.66	.30	1.0	1.1
			• Full thickness infraspina-tus tear	.89	.36	1.4	.29
Drop sign[75] ◆	With the patient seated, arm at 90° abduction in the scapular plane, elbow flexed to 90°, and shoulder externally rotated to 90°, the patient is asked to maintain the position against gravity. Failure to resist gravity and internal rotation of the arm is considered a positive test	100 patients with massive rotator cuff tears	Teres minor tear diagnosed via CT arthro-gram	.87 (.62, .96)	.88 (.80, .93)	7.3	.15
Hornblower sign[76] ◆	With patient seated, examiner places patient's arm in 90 degrees of scaption and patient attempts to externally rotate arm against resistance. Positive if patient is unable to externally rotate shoulder	91 patients undergoing arthrography	Arthroscopic evidence of: • Partial thickness infraspina-tus tear	.33	.95	6.8	.70
			• Full thickness infraspina-tus tear	.05	.91	0.6	1.0

9

Shoulder

Diagnostic Utility of Special Tests for Identifying Teres Minor and/or Infraspinatus Tears—cont'd

Test and Study Quality	Description and Positive Findings	Population	Reference Standard	Sens	Spec	+LR	−LR
External rotation lag[76] sign ◆	With patient seated, examiner places patient's shoulder in 0 degrees of abduction and 45 degrees of external rotation, with elbow flexed to 90 degrees. Patient holds position when examiner releases forearm. Positive if patient is unable to hold position and arm returns to 0 degrees of external rotation	91 patients undergoing arthrography	Arthroscopic evidence of: • Partial thickness infraspinatus tear • Full thickness infraspinatus tear	.22 .21	.91 .93	2.6 3.0	.85 .85
Drop sign[76] ◆	With patient seated, examiner places patient's shoulder in 0 degrees of abduction and 45 degrees of external rotation, with elbow flexed to 90 degrees. Patient holds position when examiner releases forearm. Positive if patient is unable to hold position and arm returns to 0 degrees of external rotation	91 patients undergoing arthrography	Arthroscopic evidence of: • Partial thickness infraspinatus tear • Full thickness infraspinatus tear	.33 .47	.74 .79	1.3 2.2	.90 .66

Diagnostic Utility of Special Tests for Identifying Nerve Root Avulsion in People with Brachial Plexus Palsy

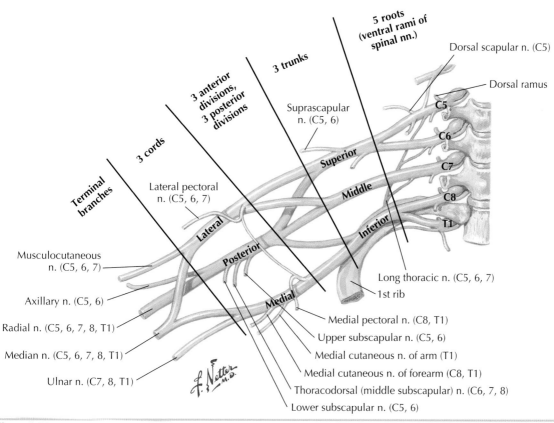

Figure 9-41
Brachial plexus: schema.

Test and Study Quality	Description and Positive Findings	Population	Reference Standard	Sens	Spec	+LR	−LR
Tinel sign C5[78] ◉	Gentle percussion on the supraclavicular region. Positive if painful paresthesias radiate into forearm	32 patients with complete brachial plexus palsy	CT myelography agreement with surgical findings	.85	.67	2.6	.22
Tinel sign C6[78] ◉	As above, except painful paresthesias radiate into hand			.50	.81	2.6	.62
Shoulder protraction test[78] ◉	From supine position, patient protracts the shoulder against resistance of the examiner's hand placed on the patient's anterior shoulder. Test is positive if the shoulder is weaker than the opposite shoulder			.96	.80	4.8	.05
Hand pain[78] ◉	Positive if reported as severe burning or crushing sensation			.86	.75	3.4	.19

9

Shoulder

Diagnostic Utility of Special Tests for Identifying Acromioclavicular Lesions

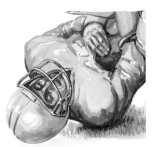 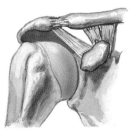 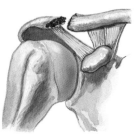 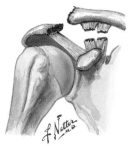

Injury to acromioclavicular joint. Usually caused by fall on tip of shoulder, depressing acromion (shoulder separation)

Grade I. Acromioclavicular ligaments stretched but not torn; coracoclavicular ligaments intact

Grade II. Acromioclavicular ligaments ruptured and joint separated; coracoclavicular ligaments intact

Grade III. Coracoclavicular and acromioclavicular ligaments rupture with wide separation of joint

Figure 9-42
Common mechanism of injury for acromioclavicular tears.

Test and Study Quality	Description and Positive Findings	Population	Reference Standard	Sens	Spec	+LR	−LR
O'Brien sign[79] ◆	Patient is standing. Examiner asks patient to flex arm to 90 degrees with elbow in full extension. Patient then adducts arm 10 degrees and internally rotates humerus. Examiner applies downward force to arm as patient resists. Patient fully supinates arm and repeats procedure. Positive if pain is localized to acromioclavicular joint	1013 patients with pain between midclavicle and deltoid	Acromioclavicular joint infiltration test: Acromioclavicular joint was injected with lidocaine. Patients who experienced a reduction in symptoms of at least 50% within 10 minutes were considered to have an acromioclavicular pathologic condition	.16	.90	1.6	.93
Paxinos sign[79] ◆	Patient sits with arm by side. With one hand, examiner places thumb over posterolateral aspect of acromion and index finger superior to midportion of clavicle. Examiner then applies compressive force. Positive if pain is reported in area of acromioclavicular joint			.79	.50	1.58	.42
Palpation of acromioclavicular joint[79] ◆	Not reported			.96	.10	1.07	.40

Diagnostic Utility of Special Tests for Identifying Adhesive Capsulitis

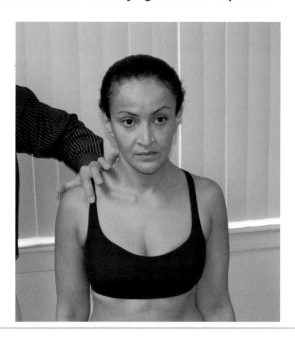

Figure 9-43
Coracoid pain test.

Test and Study Quality	Description and Positive Findings	Population	Reference Standard	Sens	Spec	+LR	−LR
Distension test in passive external rotation[80] ◐	With patients standing, arm down and elbow at 90 degrees, the examiner slowly and passively externally rotates the shoulder until reaching maximum painless external rotation. The examiner then quickly attempts to induce more external rotation, which causes intense pain in a positive test	135 patients with shoulder pain	Clear limitation of passive external rotation during motion under anesthesia	1.0 (.92, 1.0)	.90 (.82, .95)	10.2 (5.5, 19.0)	.00
Coracoid pain test[81] ◐	Digital pressure is applied on the area of the coracoid process, the acromioclavicular joint, and the anterolateral subacromial area. The test is positive if the severity of pain in the coracoid area is 3 points or higher on the visual analog scale (VAS) and pain in the coracoid area is more severe than pain in the other two areas	830 patients (85 with adhesive capsulitis, 595 with other shoulder pain, 150 asymptomatic)	Codman criteria, shoulder stiffness, MRI, and x-ray	.96 (.90, .99)	.87 (.76, .96)	7.4	.05

9

Shoulder

Diagnostic Utility of Combinations of Tests for Identifying Glenoid Labral Tears

Test* and Study Quality	Patient Population	Reference Standard	Sens	Spec	+LR	−LR
Popping + Crank test[8] ◆	55 patients with shoulder pain scheduled for arthroscopic surgery	Glenoid labral tear observed during arthroscopy	.27 (.14, .40)	.91 (.74, 1.08)	3.0 (.44, 20.67)	.80 (.62, 1.04)
Popping + Anterior slide test[8] ◆			.16 (.05, .27)	1.0 (1.0, 1.0)	Undefined	.84 (.74, .96)
Active compression test + Anterior slide test[8] ◆			.25 (.12, .38)	.91 (.74, 1.08)	2.75 (.40, 19.09)	.83 (.64, 1.06)
Anterior slide test + Crank test[8] ◆			.34 (.20, .48)	.91 (.74, 1.08)	3.75 (.55, 25.41)	.73 (.55, .96)
Crank test + Apprehension test + Relocation test + Load and shift test + Inferior sulcus sign[82] ◉	54 patients with shoulder pain	Arthroscopic visualization	.90	.85	6.0	.12
Jobe relocation test + O'Brien test[83] ◉	62 shoulders scheduled to undergo arthroscopy	As above	.41	.91	4.56	.65
Jobe relocation test + Anterior apprehension test[83] ◉			.38	.93	5.43	.67
O'Brien test + Anterior apprehension test[83] ◉			.38	.82	2.11	.76
Jobe test + O'Brien test + Apprehension test[83] ◉			.34	.91	3.78	.73

*See test descriptions under single tests.

Diagnostic Utility of Combinations of Tests for Identifying SLAP Lesions

Oh and colleagues[3] studied the usefulness of combinations of two and three special tests in identifying type II SLAP lesions. Although combinations of two tests were not useful in substantially increasing the overall diagnostic utility, several combinations of three tests were. When two tests were chosen from the group with relatively high sensitivities and one from the group with relatively high specificities, the sensitivities of the three "or" combinations were approximately 75% and the specificities of the three "and" combinations were approximately 90%.

High Sensitivity (choose 2)	High Specificity (choose 1)
Compression rotation test + Anterior apprehension test + O'Brien test	Yergason test + Biceps load test II + Speed test

Diagnostic Utility of Combinations of Tests for Identifying Type II to IV SLAP Lesions

Test and Study Quality	Test Combination	Population	Reference Standard	Sens	Spec	+LR	−LR
History of popping, clicking, or catching + Anterior slide test[2] ◆	History and test positive	55 patients with shoulder pain	Arthroscopic visualization	.40 (.10, .70)	.93 (.86, 1.0)	6.0 (1.6, 22.7)	.64 (.39, 1.1)

Diagnostic Utility of Combinations of Tests for Identifying Subacromial Impingement

Test* and Study Quality	Test Combination	Population	Reference Standard	Sens	Spec	+LR	−LR
Hawkins-Kennedy impinge-ment test + Painful arc sign + Infraspina-tus muscle test[57] ◆	All three tests positive	552 patients with shoulder pain	Arthroscopic visualiza-tion of • Any impingement • Full-thickness RCT	.26 .33	.98 .98	10.6 15.9	.75 .69
	Two of three tests positive		Arthroscopic visualiza-tion of • Any impingement • Full-thickness RCT	.26 .35	.98 .90	10.6 3.6	.75 .72
Hawkins test + Jobe test + Patte test + Gerber test + Speed test[84] ◆	A scale of elicited pain ranging from 0 to 2 (0 = none, 1 = moderate, 2 = severe) is scored for each clinical test. Positive if total score is more than 4	203 patients with shoulder pain	Impingement diag-nosed via ultrasonog-raphy assessment	.37 (.29, .44)	.98 (.87, 1.0)	11	.70
Neer test + Hawkins test + Horizontal adduction test + Painful arc test + Drop-arm test + Yergason test + Speed test[58] ◉	All seven tests positive	125 painful shoulders	Impingement diag-nosed via subacromial injection test	.04	.97	1.33	.99
	At least six tests positive			.30	.89	2.73	.79
	At least five tests positive			.38	.86	2.71	.72
	At least four tests positive			.70	.67	2.12	.45
	At least three tests positive			.84	.44	1.95	.28

*See test descriptions under single tests.

Outcome Measure	Scoring and Interpretation	Test-Retest Reliability	MCID
Upper Extremity Functional Index	Users are asked to rate the difficulty of performing 20 functional tasks on a Likert-type scale ranging from 0 (extremely difficult or unable to perform activity) to 4 (no difficulty). A total score out of 80 is calculated by summing each score. The answers provide a score between 0 and 80, with lower scores representing more disability	ICC = .95[85]	Unknown (MDC = 9.1)[85]
Disabilities of the Arm, Shoulder, and Hand (DASH)	Users are asked to rate the difficulty of performing 30 functional tasks on a Likert-type scale. Twenty-one items relate to physical function, 5 items relate to pain symptoms, and 4 items relate to emotional and social functioning. A total score out of 100 is calculated, with higher scores representing more disability	ICC = .90[86] ◆	10.2[86]
Shortened Version of Disabilities of the Arm, Shoulder, and Hand Questionnaire (QuickDASH)	Users are asked to rate questions on an 11-item questionnaire that addresses symptoms and physical function. A total score out of 100 is calculated, with higher scores representing more disability	ICC = .90[87]	8.0[87]
Shoulder Pain and Disability Index (SPADI)	Users are asked to rate their shoulder pain and disability on 13 items, each on a VAS from 0 (no pain/difficulty) to 100 (worst pain imaginable/so difficult requires help). Eight items relate to physical function, and 5 items relate to pain symptoms. A total score out of 100 is calculated, with higher scores representing more disability	ICC = .89[86] ◆	13.1[86]
Penn Shoulder Score (PSS)	Users are asked to rate their level of pain, satisfaction, and function on three subscales. The pain subscale is based on a 10-point numeric rating scale with "no pain" and "worst pain possible" as end points. The satisfaction subscale is also based on a 10-point numeric rating scale with "not satisfied" and "very satisfied" as end points. The function subscale is based on a 4-point Likert scale with "can't do at all," "much difficulty," "with some difficulty," and "no difficulty" as response options. A maximum score of 100 indicates low pain, high satisfaction, and high function	ICC = .94[88]	11.4[88]
American Shoulder and Elbow Surgeons (ASES) score	Users are asked to rate their shoulder pain on a 1-item scale and VAS and functional ability on 10 items on a Likert-type scale ranging from 0 to 4. Pain and function are equally weighted to create a total score out of 100. Lower scores represent more pain and disability	ICC = .91[86] ◆	6.4[86]
Numeric Pain Rating Scale (NPRS)	Users rate their level of pain on an 11-point scale ranging from 0 to 10, with high scores representing more pain. Often asked as "current pain" and "least," "worst," and "average" pain in the past 24 hours	ICC = .72[89]	2[90,91]

ICC, Intraclass correlation coefficient; MDC, minimal detectable change; MCID, minimum clinically important difference.

9

Shoulder

1. Lewis JS, Valentine RE. The pectoralis minor length test: a study of the intra-rater reliability and diagnostic accuracy in subjects with and without shoulder symptoms. *BMC Musculoskelet Disord.* 2007;8:64.

2. Michener LA, Doukas WC, Murphy KP, Walsworth MK. Diagnostic accuracy of history and physical examination of superior labrum anterior-posterior lesions. *J Athl Train.* 2011;46(4):343–348.

3. Oh JH, Kim JY, Kim WS, et al. The evaluation of various physical examinations for the diagnosis of type II superior labrum anterior and posterior lesion. *Am J Sports Med.* 2008;36:353–359.

4. Norkin CC, Levangie PK. The shoulder complex. In: *Joint Structure and Function: A Comprehensive Analysis.* 2nd ed. Philadelphia: FA Davis; 1992:240–261.

5. Inman VT, Saunders SJB, Abbott LC. Observations on the function of the shoulder joint. 1944. *Clin Orthop.* 1996;330:3–12.

6. Neumann DA. Shoulder complex. In: *Kinesiology of Musculoskeletal System: Foundations for Physical Rehabilitation.* St. Louis: Mosby; 2002:189–248.

7. Bolvardi E, Alizadeh B, Foroughian M, et al. Quebec decision rule in determining the need for radiography in reduction of shoulder dislocation; a diagnostic accuracy study. *Arch Acad Emerg Med.* 2019;7(1):e21.

8. Walsworth MK, Doukas WC, Murphy KP, et al. Reliability and diagnostic accuracy of history and physical examination for diagnosing glenoid labral tears. *Am J Sports Med.* 2008;36:162–168.

9. van Kampen DA, van den Berg T, van der Woude HJ, et al. The diagnostic value of the combination of patient characteristics, history, and clinical shoulder tests for the diagnosis of rotator cuff tear. *J Orthop Surg Res.* 2014;9:70.

10. Litaker D, Pioro M, El Bilbeisi H, et al. Returning to the bedside: using the history and physical examination to identify rotator cuff tears. *J Am Geriatr Soc.* 2000;48:1633–1637.

11. Burns SA, Cleland JA, Carpenter K, Mintken PE. Interrater reliability of the cervicothoracic and shoulder physical examination in patients with a primary complaint of shoulder pain. *Phys Ther Sport.* 2016;18:46–55.

12. Sharma S, Bærheim A, Kvåle A. Passive range of motion in patients with adhesive shoulder capsulitis, an intertester reliability study over eight weeks. *BMC Musculoskelet Disord.* 2015;16(1):37.

13. Riddle DL, Rothstein JM, Lamb RL. Goniometric reliability in a clinical setting. Shoulder measurements. *Phys Ther.* 1987;67:668–673.

14. Terwee CB, de Winter AF, Scholten RJ, et al. Interobserver reproducibility of the visual estimation of range of motion of the shoulder. *Arch Phys Med Rehabil.* 2005;86:1356–1361.

15. Kolber MJ, Fuller C, Marshall J, et al. The reliability and concurrent validity of scapular plane shoulder elevation measurements using a digital inclinometer and goniometer. *Physiother Theory Pract.* 2012;28(2):161–168.

16. Yang JL, Lin JJ. Reliability of function-related tests in patients with shoulder pathologies. *J Orthop Sports Phys Ther.* 2006;36:572–576.

17. Nomden JG, Slagers AJ, Bergman GJ, et al. Interobserver reliability of physical examination of shoulder girdle. *Man Ther.* 2009;14:152–159.

18. Zaslav KR. Internal rotation resistance strength test: a new diagnostic test to differentiate intraarticular pathology from outlet (Neer) impingement syndrome in the shoulder. *J Shoulder Elbow Surg.* 2001;10:23–27.

19. Dover G, Powers ME. Reliability of joint position sense and force-reproduction measures during internal and external rotation of the shoulder. *J Athl Train.* 2003;38:304–310.

20. Salamh PA, Liu X, Kolber MJ, et al. The reliability, validity, and methodologic quality of measurements used to quantify posterior shoulder tightness: A systematic review of the literature with meta-analysis. *J Shoulder Elbow Surg.* 2019;28(1):178–185.

21. Struyf F, Meeus M, Fransen E, et al. Interrater and intrarater reliability of the pectoralis minor muscle length measurement in subjects with and without shoulder impingement symptoms. *Man Ther.* 2014;19(4):294–298.

22. Borstad JD, Briggs MS. Reproducibility of a measurement for latissimus dorsi muscle length. *Physiother Theory Pract.* 2010;26(3):195–203.

23. do Nascimento JDS, Alburquerque-Sendín F, Vigolvino LP, et al. Inter- and intraexaminer reliability in identifying and classifying myofascial trigger points in shoulder muscles. *Arch Phys Med Rehabil.* 2018;99(1):49–56.

24. Boyd EA, Torrance GM. Clinical measures of shoulder subluxation: their reliability. *Can J Public Health.* 1992;83(suppl 2):S24–S28.

25. Toprak U, Ustuner E, Ozer D, et al. Palpation tests versus impingement tests in Neer stage I and II subacromial impingement syndrome. *Knee Surg Sports Traumatol Arthrosc.* 2013;21(2):424–429.

26. Gismervik SØ, Drogset JO, Granviken F, et al. Physical examination tests of the shoulder: a systematic review and meta-analysis of diagnostic test performance. *BMC Musculoskelet Disord.* 2017;18:41.

27. Nijs J, Roussel N, Vermeulen K, et al. Scapular positioning in patients with shoulder pain: a study examining the reliability and clinical importance of 3 clinical tests. *Arch Phys Med Rehabil.* 2005;86:1349–1355.

28. Ha S, Kwon O, Weon J, et al. Reliability and validity of goniometric and photographic measurements of clavicular tilt angle. *Man Ther.* 2013;18(5):367–371.

29. Lewis JS, Valentine RE. Clinical measurement of the thoracic kyphosis. A study of the intra-rater reliability in subjects with and without shoulder pain. *BMC Musculoskelet Disord.* 2010;11:39.

30. Odom CJ, Taylor AB, Hurd CE, et al. Measurement of scapular asymmetry and assessment of shoulder dysfunction using the Lateral Scapular Slide Test: a reli-

ability and validity study. *Phys Ther*. 2001;81:799–809.

31. Christiansen DH, Møller AD, Vestergaard JM, et al. The scapular dyskinesis test: reliability, agreement, and predictive value in patients with subacromial impingement syndrome. *J Hand Ther*. 2017;30(2):208–213.

32. Wassinger CA, Williams DA, Milosavljevic S, Hegedus EJ. Clinical reliability and diagnostic accuracy of visual scapulohumeral movement evaluation in detecting patients with shoulder impairment. *Int J Sports Phys Ther*. 2015;10(4):456–463.

33. Kibler WB, Uhl TL, Maddux JW, et al. Qualitative clinical evaluation of scapular dysfunction: a reliability study. *J Shoulder Elbow Surg*. 2002;11:550–556.

34. Hanchard NC, Howe TE, Gilbert MM. Diagnosis of shoulder pain by history and selective tissue tension: agreement between assessors. *J Orthop Sports Phys Ther*. 2005;35:147–153.

35. de Winter AF, Jans MP, Scholten RJ, et al. Diagnostic classification of shoulder disorders: interobserver agreement and determinants of disagreement. *Ann Rheum Dis*. 1999;58:272–277.

36. Eshoj H, Ingwersen KG, Larsen CM, et al. Intertester reliability of clinical shoulder instability and laxity tests in subjects with and without self-reported shoulder problems. *BMJ Open*. 2018;8(3). e018472.

37. Levy AS, Lintner S, Kenter K, et al. Intra- and interobserver reproducibility of the shoulder laxity examination. *Am J Sports Med*. 1999;27:460–463.

38. Apeldoorn AT, Den Arend MC, Schuitemaker R, et al. Interrater agreement and reliability of clinical tests for assessment of patients with shoulder pain in primary care. *Physiother Theory Pract*. 2019:1–20.

39. Farber AJ, Castillo R, Clough M, et al. Clinical assessment of three common tests for traumatic anterior shoulder instability. *J Bone Joint Surg Am*. 2006;88:1467–1474.

40. Cadogan A, Laslett M, Hing W, et al. Interexaminer reliability of orthopaedic special tests used in the assessment of shoulder pain. *Man Ther*. 2011;16(2):131–135.

41. Hegedus EJ, Goode AP, Cook CE, et al. Which physical examination tests provide clinicians with the most value when examining the shoulder? Update of a systematic review with meta-analysis of individual tests. *Br J Sports Med*. 2012;46(14):964–978.

42. Somerville LE, Willits K, Johnson AM, et al. Clinical assessment of physical examination maneuvers for superior labral anterior to posterior lesions. *Surg J (N Y)*. 2017;3(4):e154–e162.

43. McFarland EG, Kim TK, Savino RM. Clinical assessment of three common tests for superior labral anterior-posterior lesions. *Am J Sports Med*. 2002;30:810–815.

44. Nakagawa S, Yoneda M, Hayashida K, et al. Forced shoulder abduction and elbow flexion test: a new simple clinical test to detect superior labral injury in the throwing shoulder. *Arthroscopy*. 2005;21:1290–1295A.

45. Hegedus EJ, Goode A, Campbell S, et al. Physical examination tests of the shoulder: a systematic review with meta-analysis of individual tests. *Br J Sports Med*. 2008;42:80–92, discussion 92.

46. Cardoso A, Amaro P, Barbosa L, et al. Diagnostic accuracy of clinical tests directed to the long head of biceps tendon in a surgical population: a combination of old and new tests. *J Shoulder Elbow Surg*. 2019;28(12):2272–2278.

47. Li D, Wang W, Liu Y, et al. The backward traction test: a new and effective test for diagnosis of biceps and pulley lesions. *J Shoulder Elbow Surg*. 2020;29:e37–e44.

48. Kim YS, Kim JM, Ha KY, et al. The passive compression test: a new clinical test for superior labral tears of the shoulder. *Am J Sports Med*. 2007;35:1489–1494.

49. Kim SH, Park JS, Jeong WK, et al. The Kim test: a novel test for posteroinferior labral lesion of the shoulder—a comparison to the jerk test. *Am J Sports Med*. 2005;33:1188–1192.

50. Kim SH, Ha KI, Ahn JH, et al. Biceps load test II: a clinical test for SLAP lesions of the shoulder. *Arthroscopy*. 2001;17:160–164.

51. Kim SH, Ha KI, Han KY. Biceps load test: a clinical test for superior labrum anterior and posterior lesions in shoulders with recurrent anterior dislocations. *Am J Sports Med*. 1999;27:300–303.

52. Ebinger N, Magosch P, Lichtenberg S, Habermeyer P. A new SLAP test: the supine flexion resistance test. *Arthroscopy*. 2008;24:500 505.

53. Myers TH, Zemanovic JR, Andrews JR. The resisted supination external rotation test: a new test for the diagnosis of superior labral anterior posterior lesions. *Am J Sports Med*. 2005;33:1315–1320.

54. Cook C, Beaty S, Kissenberth MJ, et al. Diagnostic accuracy of five orthopedic clinical tests for diagnosis of superior labrum anterior posterior (SLAP) lesions. *J Shoulder Elbow Surg*. 2012;21(1):13–22.

55. Lange T, Matthijs O, Jain NB, et al. Reliability of specific physical examination tests for the diagnosis of shoulder pathologies: a systematic review and meta-analysis. *Br J Sports Med*. 2017;51(6):511–518.

56. Alqunaee M, Galvin R, Fahey T. Diagnostic accuracy of clinical tests for subacromial impingement syndrome: a systematic review and meta-analysis. *Arch Phys Med Rehabil*. 2012;93(2):229–236.

57. Park HB, Yokota A, Gill HS, et al. Diagnostic accuracy of clinical tests for the different degrees of subacromial impingement syndrome. *J Bone Joint Surg Am*. 2005;87:1446–1455.

58. Calis M, Akgun K, Birtane M, et al. Diagnostic values of clinical diagnostic tests in subacromial impingement syndrome. *Ann Rheum Dis*. 2000;59:44–47.

59. Michener LA, Walsworth MK, Doukas WC, Murphy KP. Reliability and diagnostic accuracy of 5 physical examination tests and combination of tests for

9

Shoulder

References

subacromial impingement. *Arch Phys Med Rehabil.* 2009;90(11):1898–1903.

60. Silva L, Andreu JL, Munoz P, et al. Accuracy of physical examination in subacromial impingement syndrome. *Rheumatology (Oxford).* 2008;47:679–683.

61. Johansson K, Ivarson S. Intra- and interexaminer reliability of four manual shoulder maneuvers used to identify subacromial pain. *Man Ther.* 2009;14:231–239.

62. Gill HS, El Rassi G, Bahk MS, et al. Physical examination for partial tears of the biceps tendon. *Am J Sports Med.* 2007;35:1334–1340.

63. Sgroi M, Loitsch T, Reichel H, Kappe T. Diagnostic value of clinical tests for supraspinatus tendon tears. *Arthroscopy.* 2018;34(8):2326–2333.

64. Gillooly JJ, Chidambaram R, Mok D. The lateral Jobe test: a more reliable method of diagnosing rotator cuff tears. *Int J Shoulder Surg.* 2010;4(2):41–43.

65. Miller CA, Forrester GA, Lewis JS. The validity of the lag signs in diagnosing full-thickness tears of the rotator cuff: a preliminary investigation. *Arch Phys Med Rehabil.* 2008;89:1162–1168.

66. Khazzam M, Gates ST, Tisano BK, Kukowski N. Diagnostic accuracy of the scapular retraction test in assessing the status of the rotator cuff. *Orthop J Sports Med.* 2018;6(10). 2325967118799308.

67. Sawalha S, Fischer J. The accuracy of "subacromial grind test" in diagnosis of supraspinatus rotator cuff tears. *Int J Shoulder Surg.* 2015;9(2):43–46.

68. Holtby R, Razmjou H. Validity of the supraspinatus test as a single clinical test in diagnosing patients with rotator cuff pathology. *J Orthop Sports Phys Ther.* 2004;34:194–200.

69. Bartsch M, Greiner S, Haas NP, Scheibel M. Diagnostic values of clinical tests for subscapularis lesions. *Knee Surg Sports Traumatol Arthrosc.* 2010;18(12):1712–1717.

70. Yoon JP, Chung SW, Kim SH, Oh JH. Diagnostic value of four clinical tests for the evaluation of subscapularis integrity. *J Shoulder Elbow Surg.* 2013;22(9):1186–1192.

71. Kappe T, Sgroi M, Reichel H, Daexle M. Diagnostic performance of clinical tests for subscapularis tendon tears. *Knee Surg Sports Traumatol Arthrosc.* 2018;26(1):176–181.

72. Takeda Y, Fujii K, Miyatake K, et al. Diagnostic value of the supine Napoleon test for subscapularis tendon lesions. *Arthroscopy.* 2016;32(12):2459–2465.

73. Barth JR, Burkhart SS, De Beer JF. The bear-hug test: a new and sensitive test for diagnosing a subscapularis tear. *Arthroscopy.* 2006;22:1076–1084.

74. Somerville LE, Willits K, Johnson AM, et al. Clinical assessment of physical examination maneuvers for rotator cuff lesions. *Am J Sports Med.* 2014;42(8):1911–1919.

75. Collin P, Treseder T, Denard PJ, et al. What is the best clinical test for assessment of the teres minor in massive rotator cuff tears? *Clin Orthop Relat Res.* 2015;473(9):2959–2966.

76. Sgroi M, Loitsch T, Reichel H, Kappe T. Diagnostic value of clinical tests for infraspinatus tendon tears. *Arthroscopy.* 2019;35(5):1339–1347.

77. Deleted in review.

78. Bertelli JA, Ghizoni MF. Use of clinical signs and computed tomography myelography findings in detecting and excluding nerve root avulsion in complete brachial plexus palsy. *J Neurosurg.* 2006;105:835–842.

79. Walton J, Mahajan S, Paxinos A, et al. Diagnostic values of tests for acromioclavicular joint pain. *J Bone Joint Surg Am.* 2004;86A:807–812.

80. Noboa E, López-Graña G, Barco R, Antuña S. Distension test in passive external rotation: validation of a new clinical test for the early diagnosis of shoulder adhesive capsulitis. *Rev Esp Cir Ortop Traumatol (English Edition).* 2015;59(5):354–359.

81. Carbone S, Gumina S, Vestri AR, Postacchini R. Coracoid pain test: a new clinical sign of shoulder adhesive capsulitis. *Int Orthop.* 2010;34(3):385–388.

82. Liu SH, Henry MH, Nuccion SL. A prospective evaluation of a new physical examination in predicting glenoid labral tears. *Am J Sports Med.* 1996;24:721–725.

83. Guanche CA, Jones DC. Clinical testing for tears of the glenoid labrum. *Arthroscopy.* 2003;19:517–523.

84. Salaffi F, Ciapetti A, Carotti M, et al. Clinical value of single versus composite provocative clinical tests in the assessment of painful shoulder. *J Clin Rheumatol.* 2010;16(3):105–108.

85. Stratford PW, Binkley JM, Stratford DM. Development and initial validation of the upper extremity functional index. *Physiotherapy Canada.* 2001;53:259–263.

86. Roy JS, MacDermid JC, Woodhouse LJ. Measuring shoulder function: a systematic review of four questionnaires. *Arthritis Rheum.* 2009;61:623–632.

87. Mintken PE, Glynn P, Cleland JA. Psychometric properties of the shortened Disabilities of the Arm, Shoulder, and Hand Questionnaire (QuickDASH) and Numeric Pain Rating Scale in patients with shoulder pain. *J Shoulder Elbow Surg.* 2009;18(6):920–926.

88. Leggin BG, Michener LA, Shaffer MA, et al. The Penn shoulder score: reliability and validity. *J Orthop Sports Phys Ther.* 2006;36(3):138–151.

89. Li L, Liu X, Herr K. Postoperative pain intensity assessment: a comparison of four scales in Chinese adults. *Pain Med.* 2007;8:223–234.

90. Farrar JT, Berlin JA, Strom BL. Clinically important changes in acute pain outcome measures: a validation study. *J Pain Symptom Manage.* 2003;25:406–411.

91. Farrar JT, Portenoy RK, Berlin JA, et al. Defining the clinically important difference in pain outcome measures. *Pain.* 2000;88:287–294.

Clinical Summary and Recommendations

Patient History	
Complaints	• Little is known about the utility of subjective complaints with elbow pain.
Physical Examination	
Range-of-Motion Measurements	• Measuring elbow range of motion has consistently exhibited good to high reliability for assessing flexion, extension, supination, and pronation.
Strength Assessment	• Grip strength testing in patients with lateral epicondylalgia exhibits high interrater reliability.
Special Tests	• In general, few studies have examined the diagnostic utility of special tests of the elbow. • The elbow extension test has consistently been shown to be an excellent test for ruling out the presence of bony or joint injury (sensitivity values between .91 and .97 and −LR values between .04 and .13). • The pressure provocation test, the flexion test, the shoulder internal rotation test, and the Tinel sign at the elbow have been found to be useful tests for identifying the presence of cubital tunnel syndrome. • The moving valgus stress test has been shown to exhibit superior diagnostic accuracy when compared with the valgus stress test for identifying a medial collateral tear. • No studies to date have examined the utility of the varus stress test for identifying the presence of a lateral collateral tear. • The hook test, the passive forearm pronation test, and the biceps crease interval test have been shown to have 100% sensitivity and specificity for identifying distal biceps tendon rupture when the outcomes on all three tests are positive.

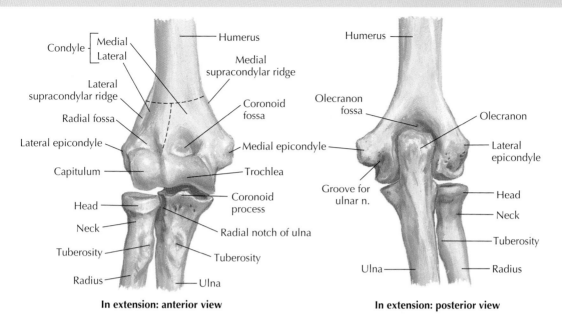

Condyle [Medial
Lateral]

Lateral
supracondylar ridge

Radial fossa

Lateral epicondyle

Capitulum

Head

Neck

Tuberosity

Radius

Humerus

Medial
supracondylar ridge

Coronoid
fossa

Medial epicondyle

Trochlea

Coronoid
process

Radial notch of ulna

Tuberosity

Ulna

In extension: anterior view

Humerus

Olecranon
fossa

Groove for
ulnar n.

Ulna

Humerus

Olecranon

Lateral
epicondyle

Head

Neck

Tuberosity

Radius

In extension: posterior view

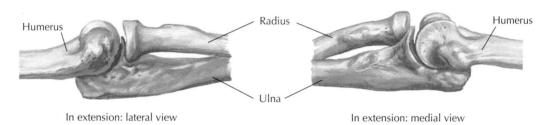

Humerus

Radius

Ulna

In extension: lateral view

Humerus

Radius

Ulna

In extension: medial view

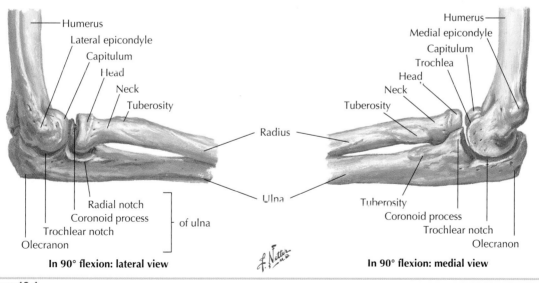

Humerus

Lateral epicondyle

Capitulum

Head

Neck

Tuberosity

Radius

Ulna

Radial notch
Coronoid process of ulna
Trochlear notch

Olecranon

In 90° flexion: lateral view

Humerus

Medial epicondyle

Capitulum

Trochlea

Head

Neck

Tuberosity

Radius

Ulna

Tuberosity

Coronoid process

Trochlear notch

Olecranon

In 90° flexion: medial view

Figure 10-1
Bones of elbow.

10

Elbow and Forearm

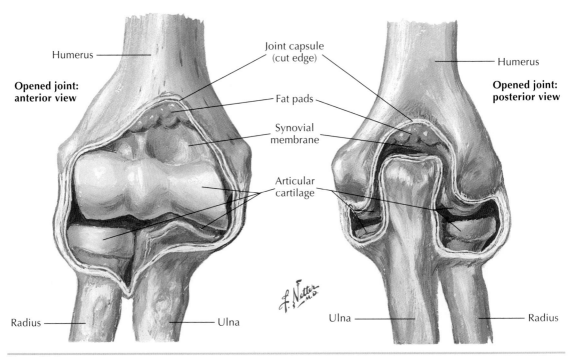

Figure 10-2
Anterior and posterior opened elbow joint.

Joint	Type and Classification	Closed Packed Position	Capsular Pattern
Humeroulnar	Synovial: hinge	Elbow extension	Flexion is limited more than extension
Humeroradial	Synovial: condyloid	0 degrees of flexion, 5 degrees of supination	Flexion is limited more than extension
Proximal radioulnar	Synovial: trochoid	5 degrees of supination	Pronation = supination
Distal radioulnar	Synovial: trochoid	5 degrees of supination	Pronation = supination

Elbow

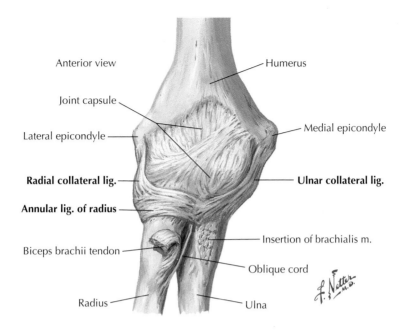

Anterior view

Humerus

Joint capsule

Lateral epicondyle

Medial epicondyle

Radial collateral lig.

Ulnar collateral lig.

Annular lig. of radius

Insertion of brachialis m.

Biceps brachii tendon

Oblique cord

Radius

Ulna

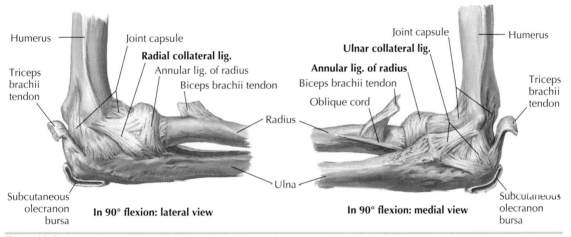

Humerus — Joint capsule

Radial collateral lig.

Annular lig. of radius

Triceps brachii tendon

Biceps brachii tendon

Radius

Ulna

Subcutaneous olecranon bursa

In 90° flexion: lateral view

Joint capsule — Humerus

Ulnar collateral lig.

Annular lig. of radius

Biceps brachii tendon

Triceps brachii tendon

Oblique cord

Subcutaneous olecranon bursa

In 90° flexion: medial view

Figure 10-3
Ligaments of the elbow.

Ligaments	Attachments	Function
Radial collateral	Lateral epicondyle of humerus to annular ligament of radius	Resists varus stress
Annular ligament of radius	Coronoid process of ulna, around radial head to lateral border of radial notch of ulna	Holds head of radius in radial notch of ulna and allows forearm supination and pronation
Ulnar collateral	Medial epicondyle of humerus to coronoid process and olecranon of ulna	Resists valgus stress

10

Elbow and Forearm

Forearm

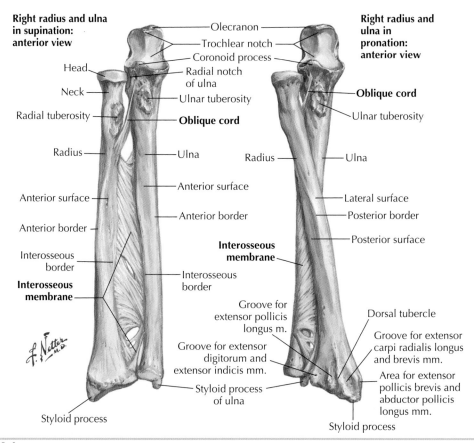

Right radius and ulna in supination: anterior view

Olecranon
Trochlear notch
Coronoid process
Radial notch of ulna
Ulnar tuberosity
Oblique cord

Head
Neck
Radial tuberosity
Radius
Ulna
Anterior surface
Anterior border
Anterior surface
Anterior border
Interosseous border
Interosseous membrane

Interosseous border

Groove for extensor pollicis longus m.
Groove for extensor digitorum and extensor indicis mm.
Styloid process of ulna

Styloid process

Right radius and ulna in pronation: anterior view

Oblique cord
Ulnar tuberosity
Radius
Ulna
Lateral surface
Posterior border
Posterior surface
Interosseous membrane

Dorsal tubercle
Groove for extensor carpi radialis longus and brevis mm.
Area for extensor pollicis brevis and abductor pollicis longus mm.
Styloid process

Figure 10-4
Ligaments of the forearm.

Ligaments	Attachments	Function
Oblique cord	Tuberosity of ulna to just distal to tuberosity of radius	Transfers forces from radius to ulna and reinforces proximity of ulna to radius
Interosseous membrane	Lateral border of ulna to medial border of radius	Transfers force from radius to ulna and reinforces proximity of ulna to radius

Anterior and Posterior Muscles of Arm

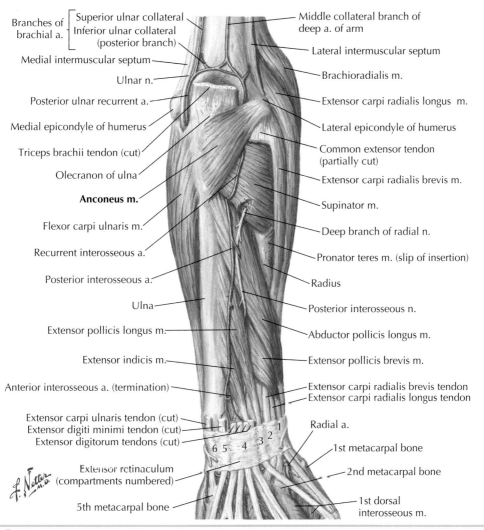

Branches of brachial a. — Superior ulnar collateral
Inferior ulnar collateral (posterior branch)

Medial intermuscular septum

Ulnar n.

Posterior ulnar recurrent a.

Medial epicondyle of humerus

Triceps brachii tendon (cut)

Olecranon of ulna

Anconeus m.

Flexor carpi ulnaris m.

Recurrent interosseous a.

Posterior interosseous a.

Ulna

Extensor pollicis longus m.

Extensor indicis m.

Anterior interosseous a. (termination)

Extensor carpi ulnaris tendon (cut)
Extensor digiti minimi tendon (cut)
Extensor digitorum tendons (cut)

Extensor retinaculum (compartments numbered)

5th metacarpal bone

Middle collateral branch of deep a. of arm

Lateral intermuscular septum

Brachioradialis m.

Extensor carpi radialis longus m.

Lateral epicondyle of humerus

Common extensor tendon (partially cut)

Extensor carpi radialis brevis m.

Supinator m.

Deep branch of radial n.

Pronator teres m. (slip of insertion)

Radius

Posterior interosseous n.

Abductor pollicis longus m.

Extensor pollicis brevis m.

Extensor carpi radialis brevis tendon
Extensor carpi radialis longus tendon

Radial a.

1st metacarpal bone

2nd metacarpal bone

1st dorsal interosseous m.

Figure 10-5
Muscles of forearm: posterior view.

Muscle	Proximal Attachment	Distal Attachment	Nerve and Segmental Level	Action
Triceps brachii (long head)	Infraglenoid tubercle of scapula	Olecranon process of ulna	Radial nerve (C6, C7, C8)	Extends elbow
Triceps brachii (lateral head)	Superior to radial groove of humerus			
Triceps brachii (medial head)	Inferior to radial groove of humerus			
Anconeus	Lateral epicondyle of humerus	Superoposterior aspect of ulna	Radial nerve (C7, C8, T1)	Assists in elbow extension, stabilizes elbow joint

10

Elbow and Forearm

Anterior and Posterior Muscles of Arm—cont'd

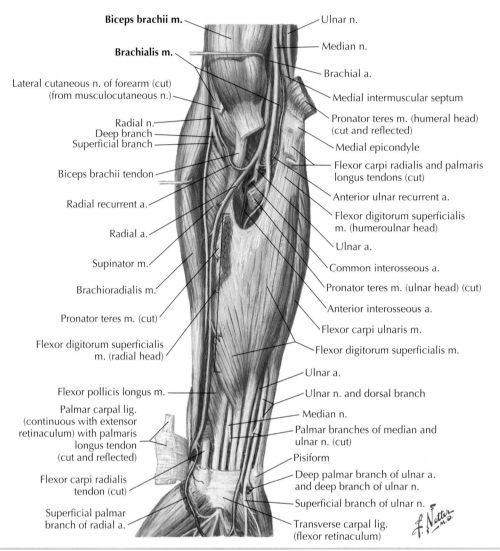

Biceps brachii m.

Brachialis m.

Lateral cutaneous n. of forearm (cut)
(from musculocutaneous n.)

Radial n.
Deep branch
Superficial branch

Biceps brachii tendon

Radial recurrent a.

Radial a.

Supinator m.

Brachioradialis m.

Pronator teres m. (cut)

Flexor digitorum superficialis
m. (radial head)

Flexor pollicis longus m.

Palmar carpal lig.
(continuous with extensor
retinaculum) with palmaris
longus tendon
(cut and reflected)

Flexor carpi radialis
tendon (cut)

Superficial palmar
branch of radial a.

Ulnar n.

Median n.

Brachial a.

Medial intermuscular septum

Pronator teres m. (humeral head)
(cut and reflected)

Medial epicondyle

Flexor carpi radialis and palmaris
longus tendons (cut)

Anterior ulnar recurrent a.

Flexor digitorum superficialis
m. (humeroulnar head)

Ulnar a.

Common interosseous a.

Pronator teres m. (ulnar head) (cut)

Anterior interosseous a.

Flexor carpi ulnaris m.

Flexor digitorum superficialis m.

Ulnar a.

Ulnar n. and dorsal branch

Median n.

Palmar branches of median and
ulnar n. (cut)

Pisiform

Deep palmar branch of ulnar a.
and deep branch of ulnar n.

Superficial branch of ulnar n.

Transverse carpal lig.
(flexor retinaculum)

Figure 10-6
Muscles of forearm: anterior view.

Muscle	Proximal Attachment	Distal Attachment	Nerve and Segmental Level	Action
Biceps brachii (short head)	Coronoid process of scapula	Radial tuberosity and fascia of forearm	Musculocutaneous nerve (C5, C6)	Supinates forearm and flexes elbow
Biceps brachii (long head)	Supraglenoid tubercle of scapula			Flexes and abducts shoulder, supinates forearm, and flexes elbow
Brachialis	Distal aspect of humerus	Coronoid process and tuberosity of ulna	Musculocutaneous nerve (C5, C6)	Flexes elbow

Supinators and Pronators of the Forearm

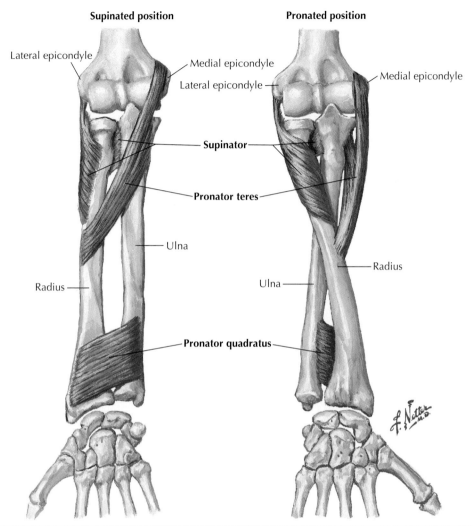

Figure 10-7
Individual muscles of forearm: rotators of radius.

Muscle	Proximal Attachment	Distal Attachment	Nerve and Segmental Level	Action
Supinator	Lateral epicondyle of humerus, supinator fossa, and crest of ulna	Proximal aspect of radius	Deep branch of radial nerve (C5, C6)	Supinates forearm
Pronator teres	Medial epicondyle of humerus and coronoid process of ulna	Lateral aspect of radius	Median nerve (C6, C7)	Pronates forearm and flexes elbow
Pronator quadratus	Distal anterior aspect of ulna	Distal anterior aspect of radius	Anterior interosseous nerve (C8, T1)	Pronates forearm

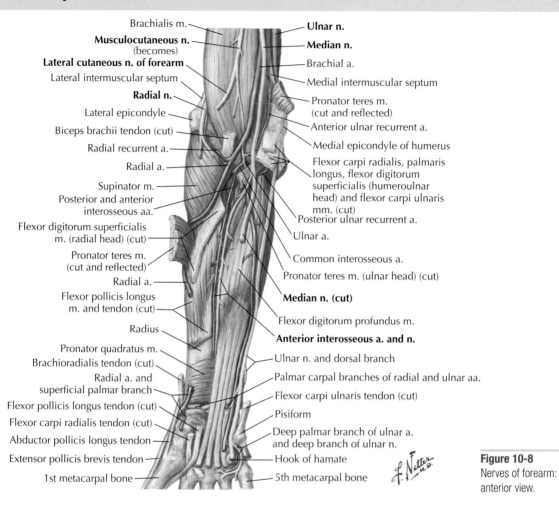

Brachialis m.
Musculocutaneous n. (becomes)
Lateral cutaneous n. of forearm
Lateral intermuscular septum
Radial n.
Lateral epicondyle
Biceps brachii tendon (cut)
Radial recurrent a.
Radial a.
Supinator m.
Posterior and anterior interosseous aa.
Flexor digitorum superficialis m. (radial head) (cut)
Pronator teres m. (cut and reflected)
Radial a.
Flexor pollicis longus m. and tendon (cut)
Radius
Pronator quadratus m.
Brachioradialis tendon (cut)
Radial a. and superficial palmar branch
Flexor pollicis longus tendon (cut)
Flexor carpi radialis tendon (cut)
Abductor pollicis longus tendon
Extensor pollicis brevis tendon
1st metacarpal bone

Ulnar n.
Median n.
Brachial a.
Medial intermuscular septum
Pronator teres m. (cut and reflected)
Anterior ulnar recurrent a.
Medial epicondyle of humerus
Flexor carpi radialis, palmaris longus, flexor digitorum superficialis (humeroulnar head) and flexor carpi ulnaris mm. (cut)
Posterior ulnar recurrent a.
Ulnar a.
Common interosseous a.
Pronator teres m. (ulnar head) (cut)
Median n. (cut)
Flexor digitorum profundus m.
Anterior interosseous a. and n.
Ulnar n. and dorsal branch
Palmar carpal branches of radial and ulnar aa.
Flexor carpi ulnaris tendon (cut)
Pisiform
Deep palmar branch of ulnar a. and deep branch of ulnar n.
Hook of hamate
5th metacarpal bone

Figure 10-8
Nerves of forearm: anterior view.

Nerves	Segmental Levels	Sensory	Motor
Musculocutaneous	C5, C6, C7	Lateral antebrachial cutaneous nerve	Coracobrachialis, biceps brachii, brachialis
Lateral cutaneous of forearm	C5, C6, C7	Lateral forearm	No motor
Median	C6, C7, C8, T1	Palmar and distal dorsal aspects of lateral 3½ digits and lateral palm	Flexor carpi radialis, flexor digitorum superficialis, lateral ½ of flexor digitorum profundus, flexor pollicis longus, pronator quadratus, pronator teres, most thenar muscles, and lateral lumbricales
Anterior interosseous	C6, C7, C8, T1	No sensory	Flexor digitorum profundus, flexor pollicis longus, pronator quadratus
Ulnar	C7, C8, T1	Medial hand, including medial ½ of digit 4	Flexor carpi ulnaris, medial ½ of flexor digitorum profundus, and most small muscles in hand
Radial	C5, C6, C7, C8, T1	Posterior aspect of forearm	Triceps brachii, anconeus, brachioradialis, extensor muscles of forearm
Posterior interosseous	C5, C6, C7, C8, T1	None	Abductor pollicis longus, extensor pollicis brevis and longus, extensor digitorum communis, extensor indicis, extensor digiti minimi

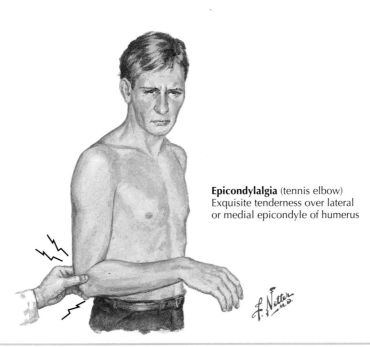

Epicondylalgia (tennis elbow)
Exquisite tenderness over lateral
or medial epicondyle of humerus

Figure 10-9
Palpation of lateral epicondyle.

History	Initial Hypothesis
Pain over lateral elbow during gripping activities	Possible lateral opicondylitis[1-4] Possible radial tunnel syndrome[5-7]
Pain over medial elbow during wrist flexion and pronation	Possible medial epicondylitis[8,9]
Reports of numbness and tingling in ulnar nerve distribution distal to elbow	Possible cubital tunnel syndrome[9,10]
Pain in anterior aspect of elbow and forearm that is exacerbated by wrist flexion combined with elbow flexion and forearm pronation	Possible pronator syndrome[11]
Reports of pain during movement with sensations of catching or instability	Possible rotatory instability[11]
Reports of posterior elbow pain during elbow hyperextension	Possible valgus extension overload syndrome[11]

10

Elbow and Forearm

Reliability of Elbow Flexion and Extension Measurements

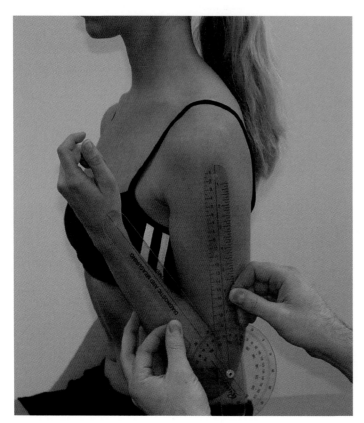

Figure 10-10
Measurement of elbow flexion.

Test and Measure and Study Quality	Instrumentation	Population	Reliability ICC	
			Intraexaminer	Interexaminer
Active range of motion (AROM) elbow flexion[12] ◆	12-inch metal goniometer	24 patients referred to physical therapy in whom range-of-motion measurements of elbow were appropriate	.94	.89
	10-inch plastic goniometer		.97	.96
	6-inch plastic goniometer		.96	.90
AROM elbow extension[12] ◆	12-inch metal goniometer		.86	.96
	10-inch plastic goniometer		.96	.94
	6-inch plastic goniometer		.99	.93
AROM elbow flexion[14] ◆	Universal plastic goniometer	30 healthy subjects	Not reported	.53
	Fluid-filled bubble inclinometer		Not reported	.92
AROM elbow flexion[13] ●	Universal standard goniometer	38 patients who had undergone a surgical procedure for injury at elbow, forearm, or wrist	.55 to .98	.58 to .62
AROM elbow extension[13] ●			.45 to .98	.58 to .87

Reliability of Forearm Supination and Pronation Measurements

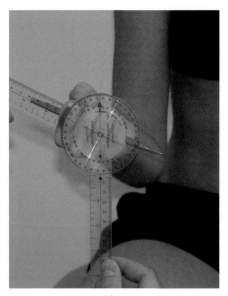

Measurement of forearm supination

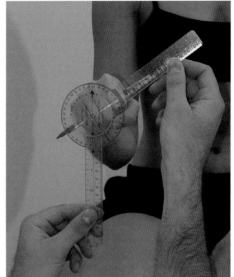

Measurement of forearm pronation

Figure 10-11
Forearm supination and pronation measurements.

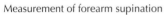

Test and Measure and Study Quality		Instrumentation	Population		Reliability ICC	
					Intraexaminer	Interexaminer
Passive range of motion (PROM) [17] ◆	Supination	Plumb line goniometer	30 hand therapy patients		.95	Not reported
	Pronation				.87	Not reported
	Supination	Standard goniometer			.95	Not reported
	Pronation				.79	Not reported
Active range of motion (AROM) [13]	Supination	Universal standard goniometer	38 patients who had undergone a surgical procedure for elbow, forearm, or wrist injury		.96 to .99	.90 to .93
	Pronation				.96 to .99	.83 to .86
AROM [15]	Supination	14.5-cm plastic goniometer	40 subjects, 20 injured and 20 not injured	Injured	.98	.96
				Not injured	.96	.94
	Pronation			Injured	.95 to .97	.95
				Not injured	.86 to .98	.92
	Supination	Plumb line goniometer: a 14.5-cm single-arm plastic goniometer with a plumb line attached to the center of its 360 degrees. The plumb line is used as the second arm to take measurement.		Injured	.98	.96
				Not injured	.94 to .98	.96
	Pronation			Injured	.96 to .98	.92
				Not injured	.95 to .97	.91
AROM supination/ pronation [16]		8-inch steel goniometer	31 asymptomatic subjects		.81 to .97	Not reported

ICC, Intraclass correlation coefficient.

10

Elbow and Forearm

Reliability of Classification According to End Feel for Elbow Flexion and Extension

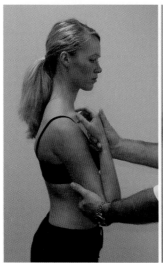

Assessment of flexion end-feel

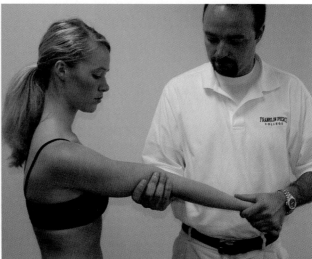

Assessment of extension end-feel

Figure 10-12
End feel for elbow flexion and extension assessment.

Test and Measure and Study Quality	Description and Positive Findings	Population	Interexaminer Reliability
Flexion/extension[18] ◆	With patient standing, examiner stabilizes humerus with one hand and maintains forearm in neutral with the other hand. Examiner extends or flexes elbow and assesses end feel. End feel is graded as "soft tissue approximation," "muscular," "cartilage," "capsule," or "ligament"	20 asymptomatic subjects	Flexion $\kappa = .40$ Extension $\kappa = .73$

Assessing Strength

Reliability of Grip Strength Testing in Patients with Lateral Epicondylalgia

Test and Study Quality	Description	Population	Interexaminer Reliability
Pain-free grip strength test[19] ●	With patient standing with elbow extended and forearm in neutral, patient squeezes dynamometer until discomfort is felt	50 patients diagnosed with lateral epicondylalgia on clinical examination	ICC = .97
Maximum grip strength test[19] ●	As above, except patient is instructed to squeeze dynamometer as hard as possible		ICC = .98

Indication of Bony or Joint Injury

Test and Study Quality	Description	Positive Findings	Population	Reference Standard	Sens (95% CI)	Spec (95% CI)	+LR	−LR
4-way range of motion test after blunt elbow trauma[20] ◆	Patient is seated or standing with the injured arm at the patient's side in the anatomical position, extended at the elbow with the palm forward. Patient tested on ability to actively extend to a full locked position, flex to at least 90°, and actively pronate and supinate to full range of motion while flexed as close to 90° as possible	Positive if any limitation of range of motion, in any of the 4 maneuvers	251 patients 5 years and older with an acute (<24 hours) nonpenetrating elbow injury presenting to a medical center	Radiographic evaluation	.99 (.94–1.00)	.60 (.52–.68)	2.47 (2.03–3.00)	0.02 (.00–.12)
Elbow extension test[21] ◆	With patient seated with arms supinated, patient flexes shoulders to 90 degrees and then extends both elbows	Positive if the involved elbow has less extension than the contralateral side	2127 adults and children presenting to the emergency department	Radiographic evaluation and/or a 7- to 10-day phone call follow-up	96.8 (95.0, 98.2)	48.5 (45.6, 51.4)	1.88 (1.78, 1.99)	.06 (.04, .10)
Elbow extension test[22] ◆	Supine patient fully extends elbow	Positive if patient is unable to fully extend elbow	114 patients with acute elbow injuries	Radiographic evaluation	.97	.69	3.13	.04
Elbow extension test[23] ◐	As above, except patient is standing	As above	100 patients presenting to an emergency department with elbow injury	As above	.91 (.81, 1.0)	.70 (.61, .78)	3.03	.13

10

Elbow and Forearm

Indication of Bony or Joint Injury—cont'd

Test and Study Quality	Description	Positive Findings	Population	Reference Standard	Sens (95% CI)	Spec (95% CI)	+LR	−LR
Elbow extension test[24] ◆	Active elbow extension to fully locked position with patient in supine or sitting position	Positive if patient is unable to fully extend elbow	113 patients presenting to an emergency department with elbow injury	Radiographic evaluation	1.0 (.93, 1.0)	1.0 (.94, 1.0)	Undefined	0.0
Elbow flexion test[24] ◆	Active elbow flexion to at least 90 degrees with patient in supine or sitting position				.64 (.50, .69)	1.0 (.94, 1.0)	Undefined	.36
Elbow pronation test[24] ◆	Full active elbow pronation from anatomic position with patient in supine or sitting position				.34 (.22, .48)	1.0 (.94, 1.0)	Undefined	.66
Elbow supination test[24] ◆	Full active elbow supination from anatomic position with patient in supine or sitting position				.43 (.30, .58)	.97 (.89, 1.0)	14.3	.59

CI, Confidence interval.

Detecting Cubital Tunnel Syndrome

Test and Measure and Study Quality	Description	Positive Findings	Population	Reference Standard	Sens	Spec	+LR	−LR
Shoulder internal rotation test[25] ⬤ (see Video 10-1)	Patient holds shoulder at 90 degrees of abduction, maximal internal rotation, and 10 degrees of flexion; elbow at 90 degrees of flexion; forearm and wrist in neutral position; and fingers fully extended. Position is held for 10 seconds	Positive if patient reports symptoms in distribution of ulnar nerve	93 subjects, 25 with cubital tunnel syndrome, 14 with cervical or upper extremity neuropathy other than cubital tunnel syndrome, and 54 asymptomatic subjects	Electrodiag-nostically proven cubital tunnel syndrome	.80	1.00	Undefined	.20
Flexion test[26] ⬤	Patient's shoulder is in anatomic position; elbow is placed in maximum flexion; forearm is in full supination; and wrist is in extension. Position is held for 10 seconds				.60	1.00	Undefined	.40
Flexion test[27] ⬤	Patient's elbow is placed in maximum flexion with full supination of forearm and wrist in neutral. Position is held for 60 seconds	Positive if patient reports symptoms in distribution of ulnar nerve			.75	.99	75	.25
Pressure provocative test[27] ⬤	With patient's elbow in 20 degrees of flexion and forearm supination, examiner applies pressure to ulnar nerve just proximal to cubital tunnel for 60 seconds	As above	55 subjects, 32 with cubital tunnel syndrome and 33 asymptomatic subjects	Electrodiag-nostically proven cubital tunnel syndrome	.89	.98	44.5	.11
Combined pressure and flexion provocative test[27] ⬤	Patient's arm is in maximum elbow flexion and forearm supination. Examiner applies pressure on ulnar nerve just proximal to cubital tunnel. Pressure is held for 60 seconds	As above			.98	.95	19.6	.02
Tinel sign[27] ⬤	Examiner applies four to six taps to patient's ulnar nerve just proximal to cubital tunnel	Positive if tingling sensation in distribution of ulnar nerve			.70	.98	35	.31

10

Elbow and Forearm

Detecting Cubital Tunnel Syndrome—cont'd

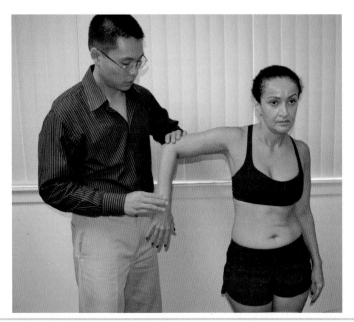

Figure 10-13
Shoulder internal rotation test.

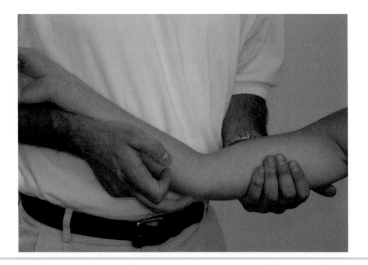

Figure 10-14
Tinel sign.

Detecting Medial Collateral Tears

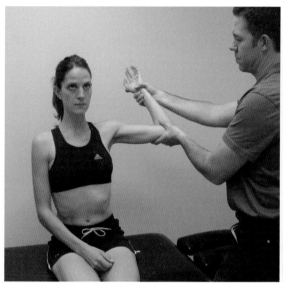

With the shoulder at 90 degrees of abduction and full external rotation, the clinician maximally flexes the patient's elbow while simultaneously applying a valgus force.

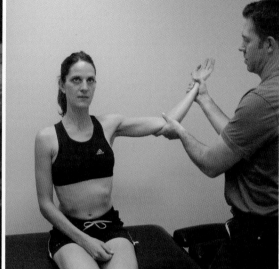

The clinician quickly extends the patient's elbow.

Figure 10-15
Moving valgus stress test.

Test and Measure and Study Quality	Description	Positive Findings	Patient Population	Reference Standard	Sens	Spec	+LR	−LR
Moving valgus stress test[28] ◆ (see Video 10-2)	Patient's shoulder is abducted to 90 degrees with maximal external rotation. Clinician maximally flexes the elbow and applies a valgus stress. The clinician quickly extends the elbow to 30 degrees	If patient experiences maximal medial elbow pain between 120 and 70 degrees of elbow flexion, test is considered positive	21 patients referred with chronic medial collateral ligament injuries	Surgical visualization	1.0 (.81, 1.0)	.75 (.19, .99)	4.0 (.73, 21.8)	.04 (.00, .72)
Valgus stress test at 30, 60, 70, or 90 degrees of elbow flexion[28] ◆	Valgus stress is applied to the elbow at 30, 60, 70, and 90 degrees of elbow flexion	If the clinician identifies laxity or the patient reports pain, the test is considered positive	21 patients referred with chronic medial collateral ligament injuries	Surgical visualization	Pain: .65 (.38, .86) Laxity: .19 (.04, .46)	Pain: .50 (.70, .93) Laxity: 1.0 (.40, 1.0)	Pain: 1.3 Laxity: Unde-fined	Pain: .70 Laxity: .81

Detecting Complete Distal Biceps Tendon Rupture

Test and Measure and Study Quality	Description	Positive Findings	Patient Population	Reference Standard	Sens	Spec	+LR	−LR
Biceps squeeze test[29] ◆	Patient seated with forearm resting in patient's lap, elbow flexed 60 to 80 degrees, and forearm in slight pronation. Examiner squeezes the biceps firmly with both hands (one hand around the muscle belly and one hand at the distal myotendinous junction)	Lack of forearm supination as the biceps is squeezed	25 patients with suspected distal biceps tendon injuries	Surgical visualization or magnetic resonance imaging (MRI) studies	.96	1.0	Undefined	.04
Bicipital aponeurosis flex test[26] ◆	Patient is asked to make a fist and actively flex the wrist with a supinated forearm. While maintaining the flexed wrist and hand, the patient is asked to flex the elbow and maintain it in 75 degrees of flexion. The examiner palpates the medial part of the antecubital fossa for the sharp, thin edge of the aponeurosis	Absence of palpable sharp, thin edge of the aponeurosis on the medial part of the antecubital fossa	17 patients with suspected distal biceps tendon injuries	Surgical visualization	1.0	.90	10	.00

Detecting Complete Distal Biceps Tendon Rupture—cont'd

Test and Measure and Study Quality	Description	Positive Findings	Patient Population	Reference Standard	Sens	Spec	+LR	−LR
Hook test[30] ⬤	Examiner uses index finger to palpate patient's flexed elbow from the lateral side of the antecubital fossa in an attempt to "hook" the distal biceps tendon	No cord-like structure under which the examiner can hook the finger	48 patients with suspected distal biceps tendon injuries	Surgical visualization and/or MRI studies	.81	1.0	Undefined	.19
Passive forearm pronation test[30] ⬤	Examiner passively moves the patient's forearm from a supinated position to pronation	Loss of visible and palpable proximal-to-distal movement of the biceps muscle belly			.09	1.0	Undefined	.91
Biceps crease interval test[30] ⬤	The distance is measured between the antecubital crease and the cusp of the distal descent of the biceps muscle	Biceps crease interval greater than 6 cm			.88	.50	1.76	.24
Hook test + Passive forearm pronation test + Biceps crease interval test[30] ⬤	As described for each test above	As described for each test above			1.0	1.0	Undefined	0.0

Detecting Complete Distal Biceps Tendon Rupture—cont'd

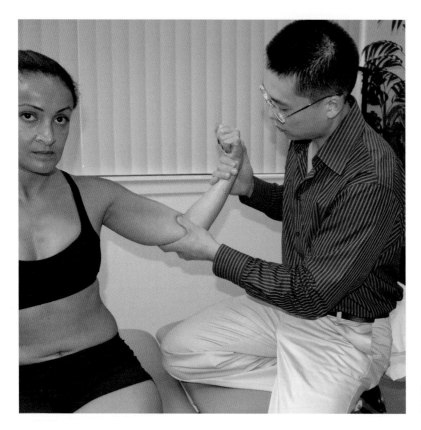

Figure 10-16
Bicipital aponeurosis flex test.

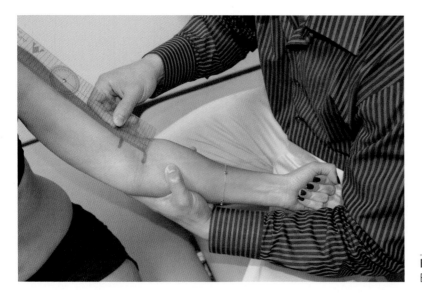

Figure 10-17
Biceps crease interval test.

Diagnostic Utility of History and Physical Examination Findings for Predicting a Favorable Short-Term Response to Mobilization with Movement and Exercise in Patients with Lateral Epicondylalgia

Vicenzino and colleagues[31] have developed a preliminary clinical prediction rule to identify individuals with lateral epicondylalgia who are likely to benefit from mobilization with movement and exercise. The study identified a number of predictor variables.

Test and Study Quality	Population	Reference Standard	Sens	Spec	+LR
Age less than 49 years[31] ●			.61 (.46, .74)	.77 (.46, .94)	2.6 (.96, 7.3)
Affected pain-free grip more than 112 newtons (N)[31] ●	62 patients with lateral epicondylalgia	A global perceived effect of improved, much improved, or completely recovered	.53 (.38, .67)	.77 (.46, .93)	2.3 (.82, 6.4)
Unaffected pain-free grip less than 336 N[31] ●			.49 (.35, .63)	.77 (.46, .94)	2.1 (.76, 6.0)
Change in pain-free grip following the mobilization with movement of more than 25%[31] ●			.75 (.58, .87)	.5 (.78, 2.9)	1.5 (.78, 2.9)

The following three variables formed the clinical prediction rule:
1. Age younger than 49 years
2. Affected pain-free grip more than 112 N
3. Unaffected pain-free grip less than 336 N

Diagnostic Accuracy for the Clinical Prediction Rule			
Number of Variables Present	Sens	Spec	+LR
3	.01 (.03, .20)	1.0 (.70, 1.0)	Undefined
2	.57 (.42, .71)	.85 (.54, .97)	3.7 (1.0, 13.6)
1	.98 (.88, .99)	.46 (.20, .74)	1.8 (1.1, 3.0)

10

Elbow and Forearm

Outcome Measure	Scoring and Interpretation	Test-Retest Reliability and Study Quality	MCID
20-item Upper Extremity Functional Index (UEFI-20)	Users are asked to rate the difficulty of performing 20 functional tasks on a Likert-type scale ranging from 0 (extremely difficult or unable to perform activity) to 4 (no difficulty). A total score out of 80 is calculated by summing each score. The answers provide a score between 0 and 80, with lower scores representing more disability	ICC = .94[32]	9.4
15-item Upper Extremity Functional Index (UEFI-15)	Users are asked to rate the difficulty of performing 15 functional tasks on a Likert-type scale ranging from 0 (extremely difficult or unable to perform activity) to 4 (no difficulty) for most questions. A total score out of 100 is calculated by summing each score. The answers provide a score between 0 and 100, with lower scores representing more disability	ICC = .94[32]	8.8
Numeric Pain Rating Scale (NPRS)	Users rate their level of pain on an 11-point scale ranging from 0 to 10, with high scores representing more pain. Often asked as "current pain" and, "least," "worst," and "average" pain in the past 24 hours	ICC = .72[33] ⬤	2[34,35]

ICC, Intraclass correlation coefficient; MCID, minimum clinically important difference; MDC, minimal detectable change.

1. Baquie P. Tennis elbow. Principles of ongoing management. *Aust Fam Physician.* 1999;28:724–725.

2. Borkholder CD, Hill VA, Fess EE. The efficacy of splinting for lateral epicondylitis: a systematic review. *J Hand Ther.* 2004;17:181–199.

3. Vicenzino B. Lateral epicondylalgia: a musculoskeletal physiotherapy perspective. *Man Ther.* 2003;8:66–79.

4. Vicenzino B, Wright A. Lateral epicondylalgia I: epidemiology, pathophysiology, aetiology and natural history. *Phys Ther Rev.* 1996;1:23–34.

5. Pecina MM, Bojanic I. *Overuse Injuries of the Musculoskeletal System.* Boca Raton, Florida: CRC Press; 1993.

6. Ellenbecker TS, Mattalino AJ. *The Elbow in Sport.* Champaign, Illinois: Human Kinetics; 1997.

7. Ekstrom R, Holden K. Examination of and intervention for a patient with chronic lateral elbow pain with signs of nerve entrapment. *Phys Ther.* 2002;82:1077–1086.

8. Pienimäki TT, Siira PT, Vanharanta H. Chronic medial and lateral epicondylitis: a comparison of pain, disability, and function. *Arch Phys Med Rehabil.* 2002;83:317–321.

9. Hertling D, Kessler RM. The elbow and forearm. In: *Management of Common Musculoskeletal Disorders: Physical Therapy Principles and Methods.* 3rd ed. Lippincott; 1990:217–242.

10. Kingery WS, Park KS, Wu PB, Date ES. Electromyographic motor Tinel's sign in ulnar mononeuropathies at the elbow. *Am J Phys Med Rehabil.* 1995;74:419–426.

11. Elbow Ryan J. *In: Current Concepts of Orthopaedic Physical Therapy, Orthopaedic Section.* American Physical Therapy Association; 2001.

12. Rothstein JM, Miller PJ, Roettger RF. Goniometric reliability in a clinical setting. Elbow and knee measurements. *Phys Ther.* 1983;63:1611–1615.

13. Armstrong AD, MacDermid JC, Chinchalkar S, et al. Reliability of range-of-motion measurement in the elbow. *J Elbow Shoulder Surg.* 1998;7:573–580.

14. Petherick M, Rheault W, Kimble S, et al. Concurrent validity and intertester reliability of universal and fluid-based goniometers for active elbow range of motion. *Phys Ther.* 1988;68:966–969.

15. Karagiannopoulos C, Sitler M, Michlovitz S. Reliability of 2 functional goniometric methods for measuring forearm pronation and supination active range of motion. *J Orthop Sports Phys Ther.* 2003;33:523–531.

16. Gajdosik RL. Comparison and reliability of three goniometric methods for measuring forearm supination and pronation. *Percept Mot Skills.* 2001;93:353–355.

17. Flowers KR, Stephens-Chisar J, LaStayo P, Galante BL. Intrarater reliability of a new method and instrumentation for measuring passive supination and pronation. *J Hand Ther.* 2001;14:30–35.

18. Patla C, Paris S. Reliability of interpretation of the Paris classification of normal end feel for elbow flexion and extension. *J Man Manipulative Ther.* 1993;1:60–66.

19. Smidt N, van der Windt DA, Assendelft WJ, et al. Interobserver reproducibility of the assessment of severity of complaints, grip strength, and pain pressure threshold in patients with lateral epicondylitis. *Arch Phys Med Rehabil.* 2002;83:1145–1150.

20. Vinson DR, Kann GS, Gaona SD, Panacek EA. Performance of the 4-way range of motion test for radiographic injuries after blunt elbow trauma. *Am J Emerg Med.* 2016;34(2):235–239.

21. Appelboam A, Reuben AD, Benger JR, et al. Elbow extension test to rule out elbow fracture: multicentre, prospective validation and observational study of diagnostic accuracy in adults and children. *Br Med J.* 2008;337:a2428.

22. Docherty MA, Schwab RA, Ma OJ. Can elbow extension be used as a test of clinically significant injury? *South Med J.* 2002;95:539–541.

23. Hawksworth CR, Freeland P. Inability to fully extend the injured elbow: an indicator of significant injury. *Arch Emerg Med.* 1991;8:253–256.

24. Darracq MA, Vinson DR, Panacek EA. Preservation of active range of motion after acute elbow trauma predicts absence of elbow fracture. *Am J Emerg Med.* 2008;26(7):779–782.

25. Ochi K, Horiuchi Y, Tanabe A, et al. Comparison of shoulder internal rotation test with the elbow flexion test in the diagnosis of cubital tunnel syndrome. *J Hand Surg [Am].* 2011;36(5):782–787.

26. El Maraghy A, Devereaux M. The "bicipital aponeurosis flex test": evaluating the integrity of the bicipital aponeurosis and its implications for treatment of distal biceps tendon ruptures. *J Shoulder Elbow Surg.* 2013;22(7):908–914.

27. Novak CB, Lee GW, Mackinnon SE, Lay L. Provocative testing for cubital tunnel syndrome. *J Hand Surg [Am].* 1994;19:817–820.

28. O'Driscoll SW, Lawton RL, Smith AM. The "moving valgus stress test" for medial collateral ligament tears of the elbow. *Am J Sports Med.* 2005;33:231–239.

29. Ruland RT, Dunbar RP, Bowen JD. The biceps squeeze test for diagnosis of distal biceps tendon ruptures. *Clin Orthop Relat Res.* 2005;437:128–131.

30. Devereaux MW, El Maraghy AW. Improving the rapid and reliable diagnosis of complete distal biceps tendon rupture: a nuanced approach to the clinical examination. *Am J Sports Med.* 2013;41(9):1998–2004.

31. Vicenzino B, Smith D, Cleland J, Bisset L. Development of a clinical prediction rule to identify initial responders to mobilisation with movement and exercise for lateral epicondylalgia. *Man Ther.* 2009;14:550–554.

10

Elbow and Forearm

32. Chesworth BM, Hamilton CB, Walton DM, et al. Reliability and validity of two versions of the upper extremity functional index. *Physiother Can.* 2014;66(3):243–253.

33. Li L, Liu X, Herr K, et al. Postoperative pain intensity assessment: a comparison of four scales in Chinese adults. *Pain Med.* 2007;8:223–234.

34. Farrar JT, Young Jr JP, LaMoreaux L, et al. Clinical importance of changes in chronic pain intensity measured on an 11-point numerical pain rating scale. *Pain.* 2001;94:149–158.

35. Farrar JT, Portenoy RK, Berlin JA, et al. Defining the clinically important difference in pain outcome measures. *Pain.* 2000;88:287–294.

Wrist and Hand **11**

Clinical Summary and Recommendations

Patient History	
Complaints	• Overall subjective complaints do not appear useful in identifying carpal tunnel syndrome. Only reports of "dropping objects" and "shaking hand improves symptoms" statistically altered the probability of the diagnosis and then only minimally (+LR [likelihood ratio] = 1.7 to 1.9, −LR = .34 to .47).

Physical Examination	
Screening	• Physical examination cannot accurately rule in scaphoid fracture, but the absence of snuffbox tenderness can substantially reduce the probability of scaphoid fracture (+LR = 1.5, −LR = 0.15). • Clinical prediction rules for identifying wrist fractures in adults and children based on eight variables (age, sex, swelling of the wrist, swelling of the anatomical snuffbox, visible deformation, distal radius tender to palpation, pain on radial deviation, and painful axial compression of the thumb) can be useful to screen patients with acute wrist trauma (app and calculator available at http://www.amsterdamwristrules.nl/).
Range-of-Motion, Strength, and Sensation Assessments	• Measuring wrist range of motion appears to be highly reliable but is of unknown diagnostic utility. Measuring finger and thumb range of motion is less reliable, even when it is performed by the same examiner. • Assessing strength with dynamometry has consistently been shown to be highly reliable but, again, is of unknown diagnostic utility. Manual muscle testing of the abductor pollicis brevis muscle does not appear to be very helpful in identifying carpal tunnel syndrome. • Sensory testing of the hand is of poor to moderate reliability. Only *sensory loss at the pad of the thumb* appears helpful in identifying carpal tunnel syndrome, and then only minimally (+LR = 2.2, −LR = .49).
Special Tests	• Evidence for the diagnostic utility of the Tinel sign, Phalen test, and carpal tunnel compression test is highly variable. The highest-quality studies of each suggest that none of the three tests is particularly helpful in identifying carpal tunnel syndrome. Additionally, one study[1] found all three tests to be both more sensitive and more specific in identifying tenosynovitis than carpal tunnel syndrome. • The ulnar fovea sign appears to be very useful at ruling in or ruling out foveal disruption of the distal radioulnar ligaments and ulnotriquetral ligament injuries (+LR = 7.1, −LR =.06). • The metacarpal adduction (+LR = 13.4, −LR = .06) and extension provocation maneuvers (+LR = 18.8, −LR = .06) appear to be useful at ruling in or ruling out trapeziometacarpal arthritis.
Combinations of Findings	• Although not yet validated, a clinical prediction rule appears to be very effective at identifying carpal tunnel syndrome. The presence of five variables (a Hand Severity Scale score of more than 1.9, a wrist ratio index higher than .67, a patient report of shaking the hand for symptom relief, diminished sensation on the thumb pad, and age over 45 years) was found to be associated with a +LR of 18.3.

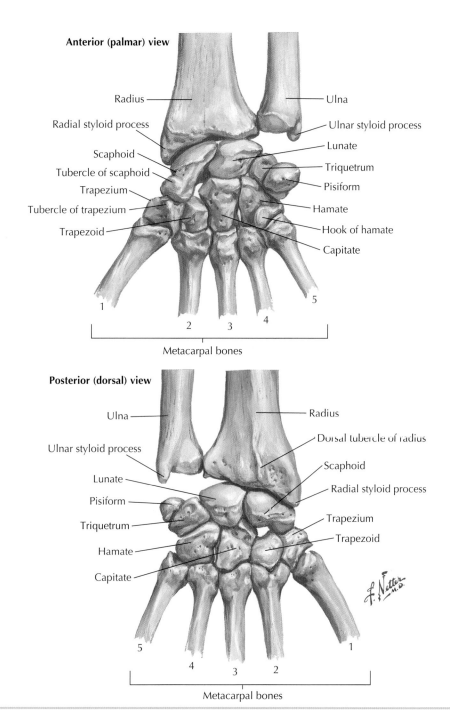

Figure 11-1
Carpal bones.

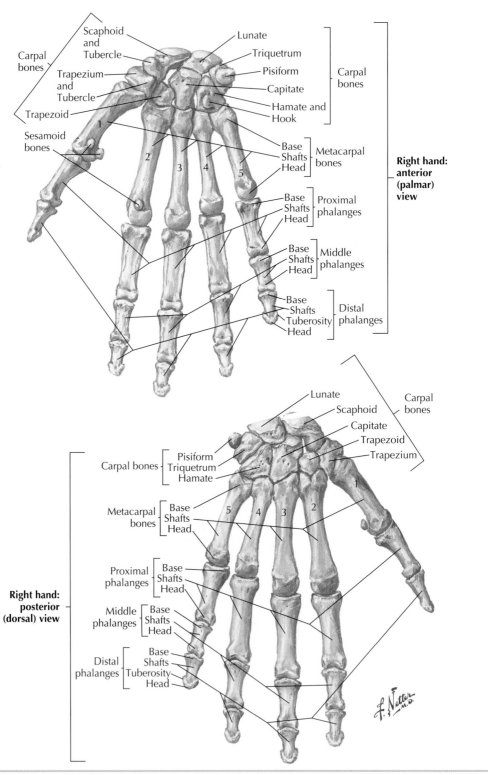

Figure 11-2
Bones of wrist and hand.

Coronal section: dorsal view

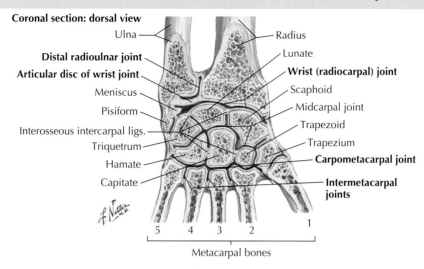

Ulna
Radius
Distal radioulnar joint
Lunate
Articular disc of wrist joint
Wrist (radiocarpal) joint
Meniscus
Scaphoid
Pisiform
Midcarpal joint
Interosseous intercarpal ligs.
Trapezoid
Triquetrum
Trapezium
Hamate
Carpometacarpal joint
Capitate
Intermetacarpal joints

5   4   3   2   1

Metacarpal bones

Sagittal sections through wrist and first finger

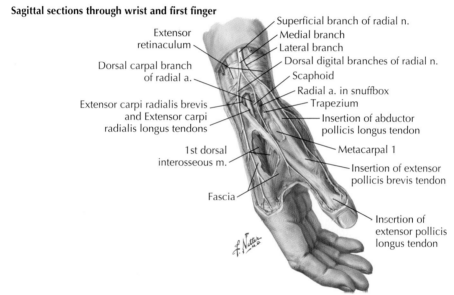

Superficial branch of radial n.
Extensor retinaculum
Medial branch
Lateral branch
Dorsal carpal branch of radial a.
Dorsal digital branches of radial n.
Scaphoid
Extensor carpi radialis brevis and Extensor carpi radialis longus tendons
Radial a. in snuffbox
Trapezium
Insertion of abductor pollicis longus tendon
1st dorsal interosseous m.
Metacarpal 1
Insertion of extensor pollicis brevis tendon
Fascia
Insertion of extensor pollicis longus tendon

Figure 11-3
Wrist joint.

Joints	Type and Classification	Closed Packed Position	Capsular Pattern
Radiocarpal	Synovial: condyloid	Full extension	Limitation equal in all directions
Intercarpal	Synovial: plane	Extension	Limitation equal in all directions
Carpometacarpal (CMC)	Synovial: plane, except for first CMC, which is sellar	Full opposition	Limitation equal in all directions
Metacarpophalangeal (MCP)	Synovial: condyloid	Extension except for first digit	Limitation equal in all directions
Interphalangeal (IP)	Synovial: hinge	Extension	Flexion greater than extension

11

Wrist and Hand

Palmar Ligaments of the Wrist

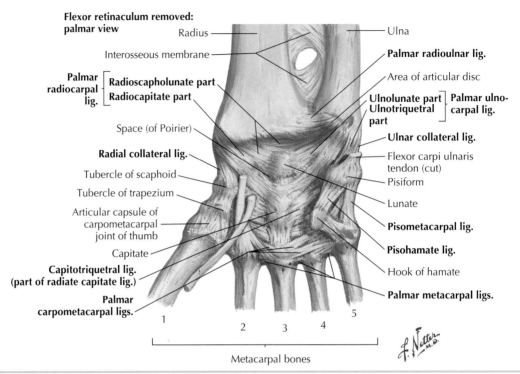

Figure 11-4
Palmar ligaments of wrist.

Ligaments	Attachments	Function
Transverse carpal	Hamate and pisiform medially, and scaphoid and trapezium laterally	Prevents bowstringing of finger flexor tendons
Palmar radiocarpal (radioscapholunate and radiocapitate portions)	Distal radius to both rows of carpal bones	Reinforces fibrous capsule of wrist volarly
Palmar ulnocarpal (ulnolunate and ulnotriquetral portions)	Distal ulna to both rows of carpal bones	Reinforces fibrous capsule of wrist volarly
Palmar radioulnar	Distal radius to distal ulna	Reinforces volar aspect of distal radioulnar joint
Radial collateral	Radial styloid process to scaphoid	Reinforces fibrous capsule of wrist laterally
Ulnar collateral	Ulnar styloid process to triquetrum	Reinforces fibrous capsule of wrist medially
Pisometacarpal	Pisiform to base of fifth metacarpal	Reinforces fifth CMC joint
Pisohamate	Pisiform to hook of hamate	Maintains proximity of pisiform and hamate
Capitotriquetral	Capitate to triquetrum	Maintains proximity of capitates and triquetrum
Palmar CMC	Palmar aspect of carpals to bases of metacarpals 2 to 5	Reinforces volar aspect of CMC joints 2 to 5
Palmar metacarpal	Attaches bases of metacarpals 2 to 5	Maintains proximity between metacarpals

Posterior Ligaments of the Wrist

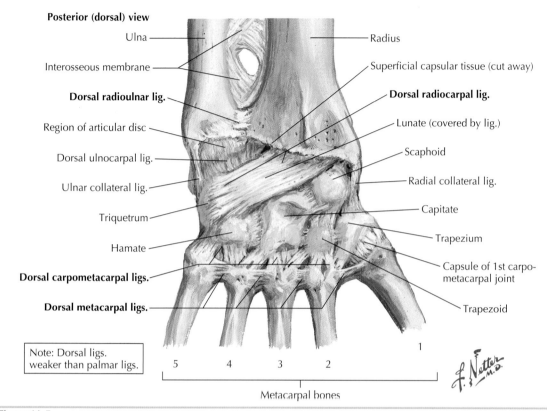

Posterior (dorsal) view

Ulna

Interosseous membrane

Dorsal radioulnar lig.

Region of articular disc

Dorsal ulnocarpal lig.

Ulnar collateral lig.

Triquetrum

Hamate

Dorsal carpometacarpal ligs.

Dorsal metacarpal ligs.

Note: Dorsal ligs. weaker than palmar ligs.

Radius

Superficial capsular tissue (cut away)

Dorsal radiocarpal lig.

Lunate (covered by lig.)

Scaphoid

Radial collateral lig.

Capitate

Trapezium

Capsule of 1st carpo-metacarpal joint

Trapezoid

5   4   3   2   1

Metacarpal bones

Figure 11-5
Posterior ligaments of wrist.

Ligaments	Attachments	Function
Dorsal radioulnar	Distal radius to distal ulnar	Reinforces dorsal aspect of distal radioulnar joint
Dorsal radiocarpal	Distal radius to both rows of carpal bones	Reinforces fibrous capsule of wrist dorsally
Dorsal CMC	Dorsal aspect of carpals to bases of meta carpals 2 to 5	Reinforces dorsal aspect of CMC joints 2 to 5
Dorsal metacarpal	Attaches bases of metacarpals 2 to 5	Maintains proximity between metacarpals

Metacarpophalangeal and Interphalangeal Ligaments

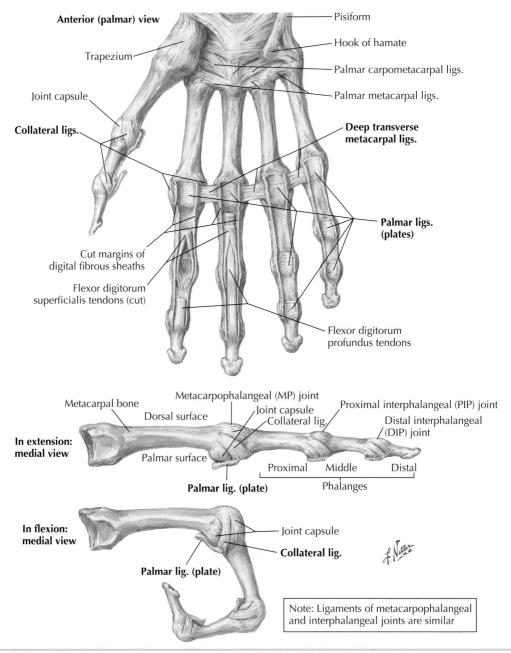

Figure 11-6
Metacarpophalangeal and interphalangeal ligaments.

Ligaments	Attachments	Function
Collateral ligaments of IP joints	Sides of distal aspect of proximal phalanx to proximal aspect of distal phalanx	Reinforces medial and lateral capsules of IP joints
Deep transverse metacarpal ligaments	Connects adjacent MCP joints	Reinforces MCP joints
Palmar ligament (volar plate)	Individual plates attach to palmar aspect of MCP and IP joints	Reinforces palmar aspect of MCP and IP joints

Extensor Muscles of the Wrist and Digits

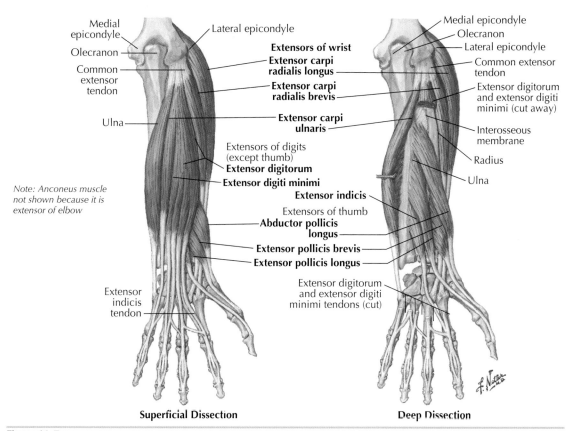

Figure 11-7
Extensors of wrist and digits.

Muscles	Proximal Attachments	Distal Attachments	Nerve and Segmental Level	Action
Extensor carpi radialis longus	Lateral supracondylar ridge of humerus	Base of second metacarpal	Radial nerve (C6, C7)	Extends and radially deviates wrist
Extensor carpi radialis brevis	Lateral epicondyle of humerus	Base of third metacarpal	Deep branch of radial nerve (C7, C8)	Extends and radially deviates wrist
Extensor carpi ulnaris	Lateral epicondyle of humerus	Base of fifth metacarpal	Radial nerve (C6, C7, C8)	Extends and ulnarly deviates wrist
Extensor digitorum	Lateral epicondyle of humerus	Extensor expansions of digits 2 to 5	Posterior interosseous nerve (C7, C8)	Extends digits 2 to 5 at MCP and IP joints
Extensor digiti minimi	Lateral epicondyle of humerus	Extensor expansion of fifth digit	Posterior interosseous nerve (C7, C8)	Extends fifth digit at MCP and IP joints

Continued

11

Wrist and Hand

Extensor Muscles of the Wrist and Digits—cont'd

Muscles	Proximal Attachments	Distal Attachments	Nerve and Segmental Level	Action
Extensor indicis	Posterior aspect of ulna and interosseous membrane	Extensor expansion of second digit	Posterior interosseous nerve (C7, C8)	Extends second digit and assists with wrist extension
Abductor pollicis longus	Posterior aspect of ulnar, radius, and interosseous membrane	Base of first metacarpal	Posterior interosseous nerve (C7, C8)	Abducts and extends thumb
Extensor pollicis brevis	Posterior aspect of radius and interosseous membrane	Base of proximal phalanx of thumb	Posterior interosseous nerve (C7, C8)	Extends thumb
Extensor pollicis longus	Posterior aspect of ulnar and interosseous membrane	Base of distal phalanx of thumb	Posterior interosseous nerve (C7, C8)	Extends distal phalanx of thumb at MCP and IP joints

Flexor Muscles of the Wrist and Digits

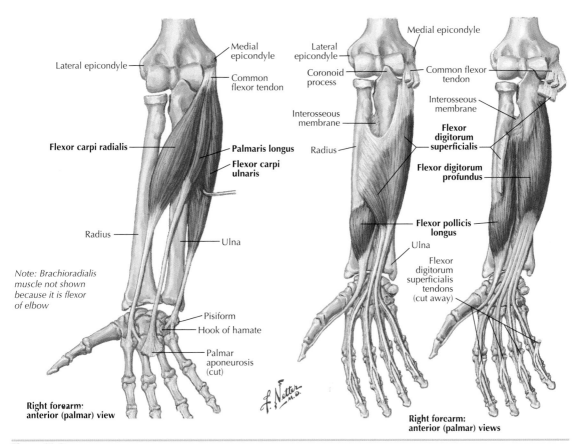

Figure 11-8
Flexors of wrist and digits.

Muscles	Proximal Attachments	Distal Attachments	Nerve and Segmental Level	Action
Flexor carpi radialis	Medial epicondyle of humerus	Base of second meta-carpal bone	Median nerve (C6, C7)	Flexes and radially deviates hand
Flexor carpi ulnaris	Medial epicondyle of humerus and olecranon and posterior border of ulna	Pisiform, hook of hamate, and fifth metacarpal	Ulnar nerve (C7, C8)	Flexes and ulnarly deviates hand
Palmaris longus	Medial epicondyle of humerus	Distal aspect of flexor retinaculum and pal-mar aponeurosis	Median nerve (C7, C8)	Flexes hand and tightens palmar aponeurosis

Continued

11

Wrist and Hand

Flexor Muscles of the Wrist and Digits—cont'd

Muscles	Proximal Attachments	Distal Attachments	Nerve and Segmental Level	Action
Flexor digitorum superficialis (humeroulnar head)	Medial epicondyle of humerus, ulnar collateral ligament, coronoid process of ulna	Bodes of middle phalanges of digits 2 to 5	Median nerve (C7, C8, T1)	Flexes digits at proximal IP joints 2 to 5 and at MCP joints 2 to 5
Flexor digitorum superficialis (radial head)	Superoanterior border of radius			
Flexor digitorum profundus (median portion)	Proximal anteromedial aspect of ulnar and interosseous membrane	Bases of distal phalanges of digits 2 to 5	Ulnar nerve (C8, T1)	Flexes digits at distal IP joints 2 to 5 and assists with flexion of hand
Flexor digitorum profundus (lateral portion)			Median nerve (C8, T1)	
Flexor pollicis longus	Anterior aspect of radius and interosseous membrane	Base of distal phalanx of thumb	Anterior interosseous nerve (C8, T1)	Flexes phalanges of first digit

Intrinsic Muscles of the Hand

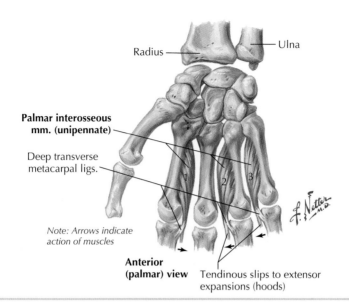

Radius

Ulna

Palmar interosseous mm. (unipennate)

Deep transverse metacarpal ligs.

1 2 3

Note: Arrows indicate action of muscles

Anterior (palmar) view

Tendinous slips to extensor expansions (hoods)

Figure 11-9
Intrinsic muscles of hand.

Muscles	Proximal Attachments	Distal Attachments	Nerve and Segmental Level	Action
Opponens pollicis	Flexor retinaculum, scaphoid, and trapezium	Lateral aspect of first metacarpal	Median nerve (C8, T1)	Opposes and medially rotates thumb
Abductor pollicis brevis		Lateral aspect of base of proximal phalanx of thumb		Abducts thumb and assists in thumb opposition
Flexor pollicis brevis				Flexes thumb
Adductor pollicis (oblique head)	Bases of metacarpals 2 and 3 and capitates	Medial aspect of base of proximal phalanx of thumb		Adducts thumb
Adductor pollicis (transverse head)	Anterior aspect of third metacarpal			
Abductor digiti minimi	Pisiform	Medial aspect of base of proximal phalanx of fifth digit	Deep branch of ulnar nerve (C8, T1)	Abducts fifth digit
Flexor digiti minimi	Hook of hamate and flexor retinaculum			Flexes proximal phalanx of fifth digit
Opponens digiti minimi		Medial aspect of fifth metacarpal		Draws fifth digit at MCP joints and extends IP joints
Lumbricals (lateral)	Tendons of flexor digitorum profundus	Lateral sides of extensor expansions 2 to 5	Median nerve (C8, T1)	Flexes digits at MCP joints and extends IP joints
Lumbricals (medial)			Deep branch of ulnar nerve (C8, T1)	
Dorsal interosseous	Adjacent sides of two metacarpals	Bases of proximal phalanges 2 to 4 and extensor expansion	Deep branch of ulnar nerve (C8, T1)	Abducts digits and assists with action of lumbricals
Palmar interosseous	Palmar aspect of metacarpals 2, 4, and 5	Bases of proximal phalanges 2, 4, and 5 and extensor expansion		Adducts digits and assists with action of lumbricals

11

Wrist and Hand

Intrinsic Muscles of the Hand—cont'd

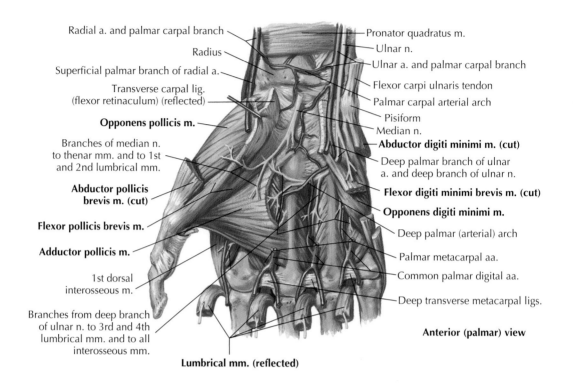

Radial a. and palmar carpal branch

Radius

Superficial palmar branch of radial a.

Transverse carpal lig. (flexor retinaculum) (reflected)

Opponens pollicis m.

Branches of median n. to thenar mm. and to 1st and 2nd lumbrical mm.

Abductor pollicis brevis m. (cut)

Flexor pollicis brevis m.

Adductor pollicis m.

1st dorsal interosseous m.

Branches from deep branch of ulnar n. to 3rd and 4th lumbrical mm. and to all interosseous mm.

Lumbrical mm. (reflected)

Pronator quadratus m.

Ulnar n.

Ulnar a. and palmar carpal branch

Flexor carpi ulnaris tendon

Palmar carpal arterial arch

Pisiform

Median n.

Abductor digiti minimi m. (cut)

Deep palmar branch of ulnar a. and deep branch of ulnar n.

Flexor digiti minimi brevis m. (cut)

Opponens digiti minimi m.

Deep palmar (arterial) arch

Palmar metacarpal aa.

Common palmar digital aa.

Deep transverse metacarpal ligs.

Anterior (palmar) view

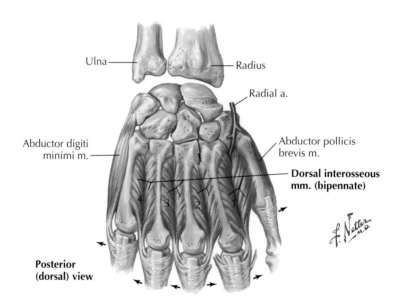

Ulna

Radius

Radial a.

Abductor digiti minimi m.

Abductor pollicis brevis m.

Dorsal interosseous mm. (bipennate)

4 3 2 1

Posterior (dorsal) view

Note: Arrows indicate action of muscles

Figure 11-10
Intrinsic muscles of hand (continued).

Median Nerve

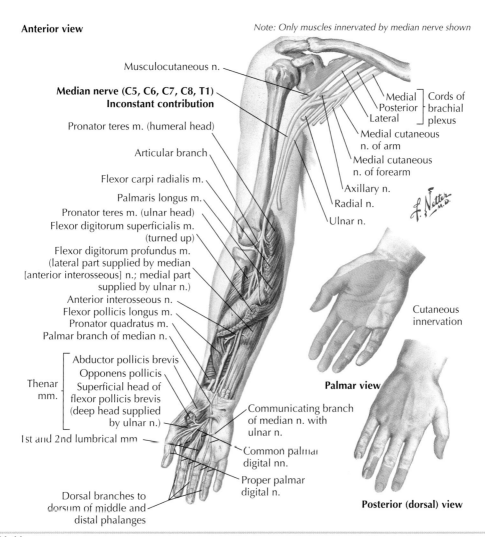

Anterior view

Note: Only muscles innervated by median nerve shown

Musculocutaneous n.

Median nerve (C5, C6, C7, C8, T1)
Inconstant contribution

Pronator teres m. (humeral head)

Articular branch

Flexor carpi radialis m.

Palmaris longus m.

Pronator teres m. (ulnar head)
Flexor digitorum superficialis m.
(turned up)

Flexor digitorum profundus m.
(lateral part supplied by median
[anterior interosseous] n.; medial part
supplied by ulnar n.)

Anterior interosseous n.
Flexor pollicis longus m.
Pronator quadratus m.
Palmar branch of median n.

Abductor pollicis brevis
Opponens pollicis
Thenar   Superficial head of
mm.   flexor pollicis brevis
(deep head supplied
by ulnar n.)

1st and 2nd lumbrical mm

Dorsal branches to
dorsum of middle and
distal phalanges

Medial ⎤ Cords of
Posterior ⎬ brachial
Lateral ⎦ plexus

Medial cutaneous
n. of arm
Medial cutaneous
n. of forearm
Axillary n.
Radial n.
Ulnar n.

Communicating branch
of median n. with
ulnar n.

Common palmar
digital nn.

Proper palmar
digital n.

Cutaneous
innervation

Palmar view

Posterior (dorsal) view

Figure 11-11
Median nerve.

Nerve	Segmental Level	Sensory	Motor
Median nerve	C6, C7, C8, T1	Palmar and distal dorsal aspects of lateral 3½ digits and lateral palm	Abductor pollicis brevis, opponens pollicis, flexor pollicis brevis, lateral lumbricals

11

Wrist and Hand

Ulnar Nerve

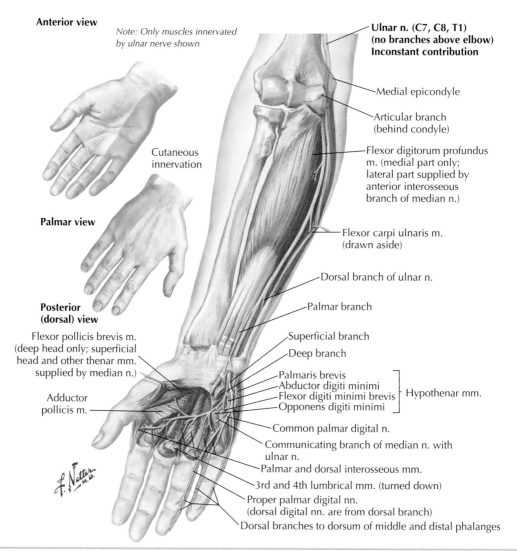

Anterior view

Note: Only muscles innervated by ulnar nerve shown

Cutaneous innervation

Palmar view

Posterior (dorsal) view

Flexor pollicis brevis m. (deep head only; superficial head and other thenar mm. supplied by median n.)

Adductor pollicis m.

Ulnar n. (C7, C8, T1) (no branches above elbow) Inconstant contribution

Medial epicondyle

Articular branch (behind condyle)

Flexor digitorum profundus m. (medial part only; lateral part supplied by anterior interosseous branch of median n.)

Flexor carpi ulnaris m. (drawn aside)

Dorsal branch of ulnar n.

Palmar branch

Superficial branch

Deep branch

Palmaris brevis
Abductor digiti minimi ⎫
Flexor digiti minimi brevis ⎬ Hypothenar mm.
Opponens digiti minimi ⎭

Common palmar digital n.

Communicating branch of median n. with ulnar n.

Palmar and dorsal interosseous mm.

3rd and 4th lumbrical mm. (turned down)

Proper palmar digital nn. (dorsal digital nn. are from dorsal branch)

Dorsal branches to dorsum of middle and distal phalanges

Figure 11-12
Ulnar nerve.

Nerve	Segmental Level	Sensory	Motor
Ulnar nerve	C7, C8, T1	Palmar and distal dorsal aspects of medial 1½ digits and medial palm	Interosseous, adductor pollicis, flexor pollicis brevis, medial lumbricals, abductor digiti minimi, flexor digiti minimi brevis, opponens digiti minimi

Radial Nerve

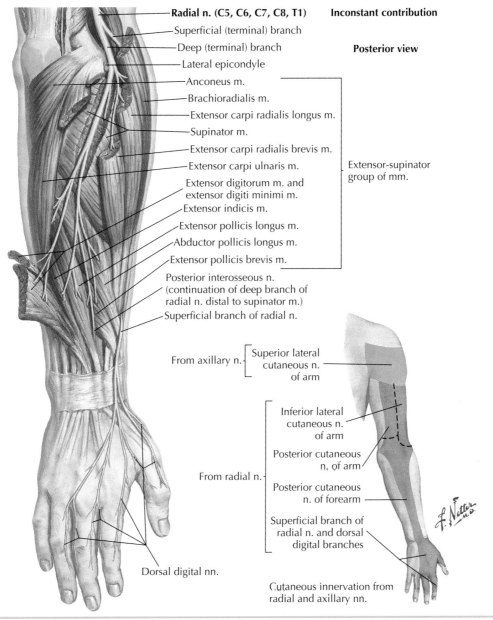

Radial n. (C5, C6, C7, C8, T1)   **Inconstant contribution**

Superficial (terminal) branch

Deep (terminal) branch   **Posterior view**

Lateral epicondyle

Anconeus m.

Brachioradialis m.

Extensor carpi radialis longus m.

Supinator m.

Extensor carpi radialis brevis m.

Extensor carpi ulnaris m.   Extensor-supinator
group of mm.

Extensor digitorum m. and
extensor digiti minimi m.

Extensor indicis m.

Extensor pollicis longus m.

Abductor pollicis longus m.

Extensor pollicis brevis m.

Posterior interosseous n.
(continuation of deep branch of
radial n. distal to supinator m.)

Superficial branch of radial n.

From axillary n. — Superior lateral
cutaneous n.
of arm

Inferior lateral
cutaneous n.
of arm

Posterior cutaneous
n, of arm

From radial n. —

Posterior cutaneous
n. of forearm

Superficial branch of
radial n. and dorsal
digital branches

Dorsal digital nn.

Cutaneous innervation from
radial and axillary nn.

Figure 11-13
Radial nerve.

Nerve	Segmental Level	Sensory	Motor
Radial nerve	C5, C6, C7, C8, T1	Dorsal aspect of lateral hand, excluding digits	No motor in hand

11

Wrist and Hand

Reliability of the Historical Examination

History	Initial Hypothesis
Pain over radial styloid process with gripping activities	Possible de Quervain syndrome[2]
Reports of an insidious onset of numbness and tingling in first three fingers; may complain that pain is worse at night	Possible carpal tunnel syndrome[3-5]
Reports of paresthesias over dorsal aspect of ulnar border of hand and fingers 4 to 5	Possible ulnar nerve compression at canal of Guyon[1,6,7]
Patient reports inability to extend MCP or IP joints	Possible Dupuytren contracture[1] Possible trigger finger[8]
Reports of falling on hand with wrist hyperextended; complains of pain with loading of wrist	Possible scaphoid fracture[9,10] Possible carpal instability[8]

History and Study Quality	Population	Interexaminer Reliability
Most bothersome symptom is pain, numbness, tingling, or loss of sensation?[11] ◆		$\kappa = .74$ (.55, .93)
Location of most bothersome symptom?[11] ◆		$\kappa = .82$ (.68, .96)
Symptoms intermittent, variable, or constant?[11] ◆		$\kappa = .57$ (.35, .79)
Hand swollen?[11] ◆	82 patients presenting to primary care clinic, orthopaedic department, or electrophysiology laboratory with suspected cervical radiculopathy or carpal tunnel syndrome	$\kappa = .85$ (.68, 1.0)
Dropping objects?[11] ◆		$\kappa = .95$ (.85, 1.0)
Entire limb goes numb?[11] ◆		$\kappa = .53$ (.26, .81)
Nocturnal symptoms wake patient?[11] ◆		$\kappa = .83$ (.60, 1.0)
Shaking the hand improves symptoms?[11] ◆		$\kappa = .90$ (.75, 1.0)
Symptoms exacerbated with activities that require gripping?[11] ◆		$\kappa = .72$ (.49, .95)

History and Study Quality	Population	Reference Standard	Sens	Spec	+LR	−LR
Age over 45 years [11] ◆	82 patients presenting to a primary care clinic, orthopaedic department, or electrophysiology laboratory with suspected cervical radiculopathy or carpal tunnel syndrome	Needle electromyography and nerve conduction studies	.64 (.47, .82)	.59 (.47, .72)	1.58 (.46, 2.4)	.60 (.35, 1.0)
Most bothersome symptom is pain, numbness, tingling, or loss of sensation[11] ◆			.04 (−.04, .11)	.91 (.83, .98)	.42 (.05, 3.4)	1.1 (.94, 1.2)
Location of most bothersome symptom[11] ◆			.35 (.16, .53)	.40 (.27, .54)	.58 (.33, 1.0)	1.6 (1.1, 2.5)
Symptoms intermittent, variable, or constant[11] ◆			.23 (.07, .39)	.89 (.81, .97)	2.1 (.74, 5.8)	.87 (.69, 1.4)
Reports of hand becoming swollen[11] ◆			.38 (.20, .57)	.63 (.50, .76)	1.0 (.57, 1.9)	.98 (.68, 1.4)
Dropping objects[11] ◆			.73 (.56, .90)	.57 (.44, .71)	1.7 (1.2, 2.5)	.47 (.24, .92)
Entire limb goes numb[11] ◆			.38 (.20, .57)	.80 (.69, .90)	1.9 (.92, 3.9)	.77 (.55, 1.1)
Nocturnal symptoms wake patient[11] ◆			.73 (.56, .90)	.31 (.19, .44)	1.1 (.79, 1.4)	.86 (.41, 1.8)
Shaking hand improves symptoms[11] ◆			.81 (.66, .96)	.57 (.43, .70)	1.9 (1.3, 2.7)	.34 (.15, .77)
Symptoms exacerbated with activities that require gripping[11] ◆			.77 (.61, .93)	.37 (.24, .50)	1.2 (.91, 1.6)	.62 (.28, 1.4)
Age 40 years or older[12] ◉	110 patients referred to laboratory for electrophysiologic examination	Nerve conduction tests	.80	.42	1.38	.48
Nocturnal symptoms[12] ◉			.77	.28	1.07	.82
Bilateral symptoms[12] ◉			.61	.58	1.45	.67

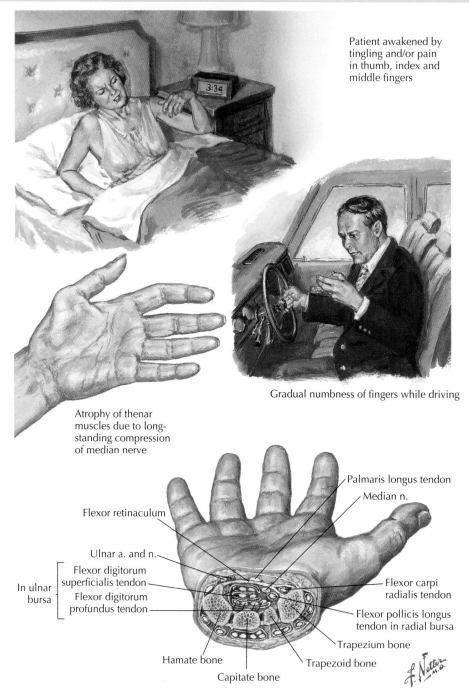

Patient awakened by tingling and/or pain in thumb, index and middle fingers

Gradual numbness of fingers while driving

Atrophy of thenar muscles due to long-standing compression of median nerve

Palmaris longus tendon

Median n.

Flexor retinaculum

Ulnar a. and n.

Flexor digitorum superficialis tendon
Flexor digitorum profundus tendon

In ulnar bursa

Flexor carpi radialis tendon

Flexor pollicis longus tendon in radial bursa

Trapezium bone

Hamate bone

Trapezoid bone

Capitate bone

Section through wrist at distal row of carpal bones shows carpal tunnel. Increase in size of tunnel structures caused by edema (trauma), inflammation (rheumatoid disease); ganglion, amyloid deposits, or diabetic neuropathy may compress median nerve

Figure 11-14
Carpal tunnel syndrome.

Test and Study Quality	Description and Positive Findings	Population	Reference Standard	Sens	Spec	+LR	−LR
Amsterdam Wrist Rules[13] ◆	Eight variables (age, sex, swelling of the wrist, swelling of the anatomical snuffbox, visible deformation, distal radius tender to palpation, pain on radial deviation, and painful axial compression of the thumb) determine the probability of a fracture. Available at http://www.amsterdamwristrules.nl/	395 consecutive adult patients presenting to emergency department with pain or tenderness secondary to acute wrist trauma		98.2 (95.1, 99.4)	21.0 (15.4, 27.9)	1.24*	.09*
Amsterdam Pediatric Wrist Rules[14] ◆	Seven variables (age, sex, swelling of the distal radius, visible deformation, distal radius tender to palpation, anatomical snuffbox tender to palpation, and supination is tender) determine the probability of a fracture. Available at http://www.amsterdamwristrules.nl/		Radiographic confirmation of wrist fracture	96.0 (92.0, 98.0)	37.0 (31.0, 44.0)	1.52*	.11*
Pershad Pediatric Wrist Rules[14] ◆	Perform radiograph if both clinical findings are present: 1. Point tenderness over the distal radius 2. Decrease of more than 20% in grip strength compared to the normal hand	379 children between 3 years and 18 years old, presenting at the emergency department with pain or tenderness secondary to acute wrist trauma		94.0 (89.0, 97.0)	26.0 (20.0, 33.0)	1.27*	.23*
Webster Pediatric Wrist Rules[14] ◆	Perform radiograph if at least one of the following clinical findings is present: 1. Radial tenderness 2. Focal swelling 3. Reduction in range of supination and pronation			99.0 (95.0, 100.0)	11.0 (7.0, 17.0)	1.11*	.09*
Rivara Pediatric Wrist Rules[14] ◆	Perform radiograph if at least one of the following clinical findings is present: 1. Gross deformity 2. Point tenderness			96.0 (91.0, 98.0)	22.0 (16.0, 28.0)	1.23*	.18*

*Values were calculated by the authors of this text.

11

Wrist and Hand

Diagnostic Utility of Tests in Identifying Scaphoid Fractures (see Fig. 11-15)

Test and Study Quality	Description and Positive Findings	Population	Reference Standard	Sens	Spec	+LR	−LR
Snuffbox tenderness[15] **2014 Meta-analysis** ◆	Examiner palpates anatomic snuffbox. Positive if pain is elicited	Statistically pooled data from 6 high-quality studies	X-ray, bone scan, or MRI confirmation of scaphoid fracture	.96 (.92, .98)	.39 (.36, .43)	1.5 (1.1, 2.1)	0.15 (0.05, 0.43)
Pain with supination against resistance[15] **2014 Meta-analysis** ◆	Examiner holds patient's hand in handshake position and directs patient to resist supination of forearm. Positive if pain is elicited	Statistically pooled data from 2 high-quality studies	X-ray, bone scan, or MRI confirmation of scaphoid fracture	.94 (.85, .98)	.73 (.63, .84)	6.1 (0.04, 10.86)	0.09 (0.00, 11.9)
Scaphoid tubercle tenderness[15] **2014 Meta-analysis** ◆	Examiner applies pressure to scaphoid tubercle. Positive if pain is elicited	Statistically pooled data from 3 high-quality studies	X-ray or bone scan confirmation of scaphoid fracture	.92 (.86, .96)	.47 (.43. .52)	1.7 (1.3, 2.1)	0.23 (0.09, 0.56)
Pain with longitudinal compression of thumb[15] **2014 Meta-analysis** ◆	Examiner holds patient's thumb and applies long-axis compression through metacarpal bone into scaphoid. Positive if pain is elicited	Statistically pooled data from 6 high-quality studies	X-ray or bone scan confirmation of scaphoid fracture	.82 (.77, .87)	.58 (.54, .62)	2.0 (1.1, 3.5)	0.24 (0.06, 0.99)
Snuffbox tenderness[16] **2014 Systematic Review** ◆	Examiner palpates anatomic snuffbox. Positive if pain is elicited	Statistically pooled data from 8 high-quality studies involving 1164 adults	X-ray, bone scan, or MRI confirmation of scaphoid fracture	.87–1.00	.03–.98	1.01–45.0	0.00–.87
Scaphoid tubercle tenderness[16] **2014 Systematic Review** ◆	Examiner applies pressure to scaphoid tubercle. Positive if pain is elicited	Statistically pooled data from 4 high-quality studies involving 879 adults	X-ray, bone scan, or MRI confirmation of scaphoid fracture	.82–1.00	.17–.57	1.20–2.01	0.00–.46
Pain with longitudinal compression of thumb[16] **2014 Systematic Review** ◆	Examiner holds patient's thumb and applies long-axis compression through metacarpal bone into scaphoid. Positive if pain is elicited	Statistically pooled data from 8 high-quality studies involving 961 adults	X-ray, bone scan, or MRI confirmation of scaphoid fracture	.48–1.00	0.22–0.97	.90–38.0	0.00–1.35

Diagnostic Utility of Hand Symptom Diagrams in Identifying Carpal Tunnel Syndrome

Test and Study Quality	Description and Positive Findings	Population	Reference Standard	Sens	Spec	+LR	−LR
Katz score[17] ◆	Subjects shaded in hand diagrams based on where they have experienced numbness, tingling, burning, or pain. Diagrams were scored based on the modified Katz system.[12] A diagram scored as "classic" or "probable" was considered positive	110 subjects who reported symptoms of burning, pain, tingling, or numbness in the hand	Nerve conduction studies	.38 (.28, .50)	.81 (.73, .87)	2.0	.77
Median nerve digit score[17] ◆	Subjects shaded in hand diagrams based on where they have experienced numbness, tingling, burning, or pain. Diagrams were scored based on the number of digits innervated by the median nerve with distal volar shading. A score of 2 or more digits was considered positive			.54 (.43, .65)	.76 (.68, .83)	2.25	.61

Diagnostic Utility of Tests in Identifying Scaphoid Fractures

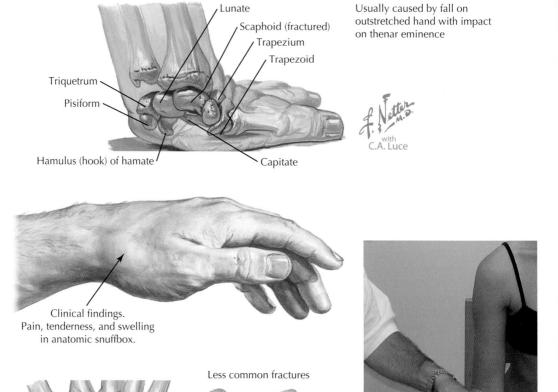

Usually caused by fall on outstretched hand with impact on thenar eminence

Lunate
Scaphoid (fractured)
Trapezium
Trapezoid
Triquetrum
Pisiform
Hamulus (hook) of hamate
Capitate

Clinical findings.
Pain, tenderness, and swelling in anatomic snuffbox.

Less common fractures

Tubercle   Distal pole

Vertical shear   Proximal pole

Fracture of middle third (waist) of scaphoid (most common)

Testing for tenderness of anatomic snuffbox

Figure 11-15
Testing for tenderness of anatomic snuffbox.

Reliability of Hand Symptom Diagrams in Identifying Carpal Tunnel Syndrome

Test and Measure and Study Quality	Description	Population	Reliability	
			Intraexaminer	**Interexaminer**
Katz score[17] ●	Subjects shaded in hand diagrams based on where they have experienced numbness, tingling, burning, or pain	110 subjects who reported symptoms of burning, pain, tingling, or numbness in the hand	κ = .86 (.49, .95)	ICC = .87 (.84, .90)
Median nerve digit score[17] ●			κ = .97 (.49, .95)	ICC = .96 (.95, .97)

Acute Pediatric Wrist Fractures: Clinical Prediction Rule

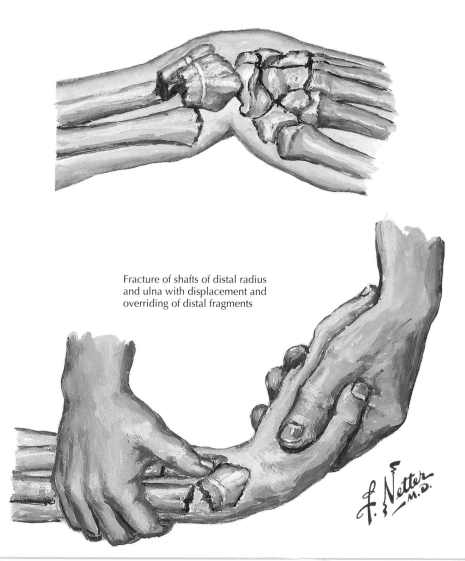

Fracture of shafts of distal radius
and ulna with displacement and
overriding of distal fragments

Figure 11-16
Fracture of forearm bones in children.

Reliability of Wrist Range-of-Motion Measurements

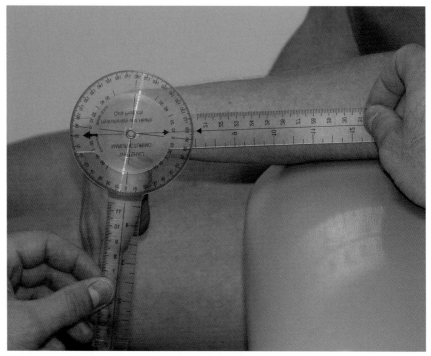

Measurement of wrist flexion

Figure 11-17
Wrist range of motion.

Test and Measure and Study Quality	Instrumentation	Population	Reliability			
			Intraexaminer	ICC	Interexaminer	ICC
PROM[19] ◆	Alignment of plastic 6 in goniometer	140 patients where PROM of wrist would be included in standard evaluation	Radial flexion	.86	Radial flexion	.88
			Ulnar flexion	.87	Ulnar flexion	.89
			Dorsal flexion	.92	Dorsal flexion	.93
			Radial extension	.80	Radial extension	.80
			Ulnar extension	.80	Ulnar extension	.80
			Dorsal extension	.84	Dorsal extension	.84
Active range of motion (AROM)[18] ●	8 in plastic goniometer	48 patients where measurements of the wrist would normally be included in examination	Wrist flexion	.96	Wrist flexion	.90
			Wrist extension	.96	Wrist extension	.85
			Radial deviation	.90	Radial deviation	.86
			Ulnar deviation	.92	Ulnar deviation	.78
Passive range of motion (PROM)[18] ●			Wrist flexion	.96	Wrist flexion	.86
			Wrist extension	.96	Wrist extension	.84
			Radial deviation	.91	Radial deviation	.66
			Ulnar deviation	.94	Ulnar deviation	.83

Reliability of Wrist Range-of-Motion Measurements—cont'd

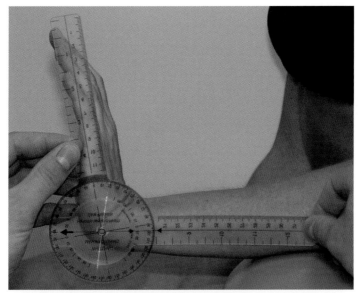

Measurement of wrist extension

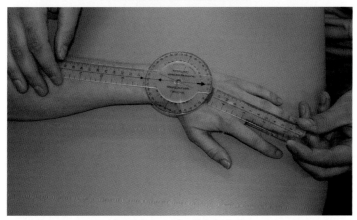

Measurement of radial deviation

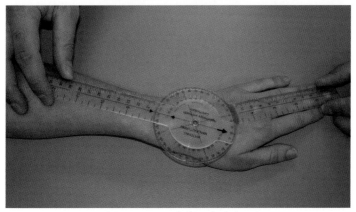

Measurement of ulnar deviation

Figure 11-18
Wrist range of motion.

11

Wrist and Hand

Reliability of Finger and Thumb Range-of-Motion Measurements

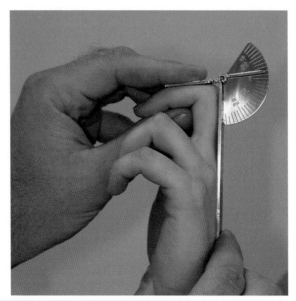

Figure 11-19
Measurement of proximal interphalangeal joint flexion.

Test and Measure and Study Quality	Instrumentation	Population	Test-Retest Reliability ICC			
Total active range of motion (AROM) of IP flexion and extension[3] ●	Finger goniometer	30 patients with hand injuries	Intraexaminer = .97 to .98 Interexaminer = .97			
Palmar abduction[7] ●			**Intraexaminer**		**Interexaminer**	
			Active	Passive	Active	Passive
	● Goniometer		.55 (.34, .87)	.76 (.69, .94)	.31 (−.18, .77)	.37 (−.42, .79)
	● Pollexograph-thumb		.71 (.62, .93)	.82 (.78, .96)	.66 (.53, .91)	.59 (.42, .89)
	● Pollexograph-metacarpal	25 healthy subjects	.82 (.78, .96)	.81 (.76, .95)	.57 (.38, .88)	.61 (.45, .89)
	● American Medical Association method		.72 (.63, .92)	.65 (.51, .90)	.24 (−.40, .73)	.52 (.28, .86)
	● American Society of Hand Therapists method		.78 (.72, .94)	.72 (.63, .93)	.55 (.34, .87)	.52 (.29, .86)
	● Intermetacarpal distance		.95 (.95, .99)	.92 (.90, .98)	.82 (.79, .96)	.79 (.78, .96)

Intraexaminer Reliability of Assessing Strength

Test and Study Quality	Instrumentation	Population	Test-Retest Reliability (ICC)	
Grip Tripod Key pinch[24] ◆	Dynamometer and pinch gauge	38 patients receiving physical therapy for hand impairments	Symptomatic .93 (.86, .96) .88 (.78, .96) .94 (.88, .97)	Asymptomatic .94 (.89, .97) .87 (.74, .93) .93 (.86, .96)
Abductor pollicis muscle strength[11] ◆	Examiner performs manual muscle testing of abductor pollicis muscle. Graded as markedly reduced, reduced, or normal compared with contralateral extremity	82 patients with suspected cervical radiculopathy or carpal tunnel syndrome	κ = .39 (.00, .80)	
Wrist extensors (mean of two efforts)[20] ◉	Dynamometer	40 patients with suspected myopathy	Dominant side = .88 (.79, .94) Nondominant side = .94 (.90, .97)	
Wrist extensors (maximum of two efforts)[20] ◉		40 patients with suspected myopathy	Dominant side = .87 (.76, .93) Nondominant side = .94 (.88, .97)	
Grip[2] ◉		21 healthy elder volunteers	Left = .95 (.89, .98) Right = .91 (.78, .96)	
Grip[4] ◉		22 asymptomatic subjects	One trial: .95 (.89, .98) Mean of three trials: .85 (.67, .94) Highest of three trials: .95 (.89, .98)	
		22 patients after carpal tunnel decompression	One trial: .97 (.94, .99) Mean of three trials: .94 (.80, .98) Highest of three trials: .97 (.92, .99)	
		22 patients after carpal tunnel decompression	One trial: .96 (.91, .98) Mean of three trials: .98 (.96, .99) Highest of three trials: .97 (.90, .99)	
Grip[21] ◉		104 healthy primary school children	Dominant side = .97 (.95, .98) Nondominant side = .95 (.92, .96)	
	Vigorimeter		Dominant side = .84 (.77, .89) Nondominant side = .86 (.80, .90)	
Grip Palmar pinch Key pinch Tip pinch[22] ◉	Pinch gauge	27 healthy volunteers	Right .99 .98 .99 .99	Left .99 .99 .98 .99
Grip Tip pinch Key pinch[23] ◉	Hand and pinch grip dynamometers	33 patients with a unilateral hand injury	Injured .93 to .97 .89 .94	Noninjured .92 to .94 .84 .86
Grip Tip pinch Jaw pinch[3] ◉	Grip dynamometer and pinch gauge	30 patients with hand injuries	Intraexaminer .96 .86 to .94 .88 to .93	Interexaminer .95 .91 .89
Wrist extensors[25] ◉	Dynamometer	30 patients presenting to a physical therapy clinic	.94	
Wrist flexion Wrist extension[26] ◉	Dynamometer	20 healthy subjects	Wrist flexion .85 Wrist extension .91	

11

Wrist and Hand

Intraexaminer Reliability of Assessing Strength—cont'd

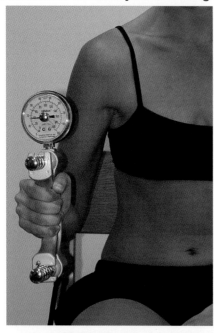

Figure 11-20
Measurement of grip strength.

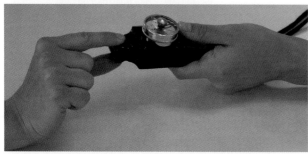

Measurement of tip
pinch strength

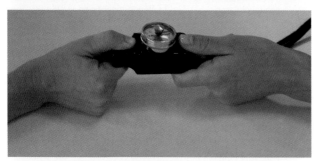

Measurement of key
pinch strength

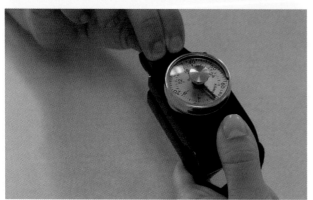

Measurement of tripod
pinch strength

Figure 11-21
Measurement of pinch
strength.

Diagnostic Utility of Weakness in Identifying Carpal Tunnel Syndrome

Test and Study Quality	Description and Positive Findings	Population	Reference Standard	Sens	Spec	+LR	−LR
Abductor pollicis brevis muscle strength[11] ◆	Strength is tested by placing thumb in a position of abduction and applying a force in direction of adduction at proximal phalanx. Positive if strength is reduced or markedly reduced compared with contralateral extremity	82 patients with suspected cervical radiculopathy or carpal tunnel syndrome	Needle electromyography and nerve conduction studies	.19 (.04, .34)	.89 (.81, .90)	1.7 (.58, 5.2)	.91 (.74, 1.1)
Abductor pollicis brevis muscle weakness[27] ◆	Patient is instructed to touch pad of thumb and pad of fifth digit together. Examiner applies posteriorly directed force over thumb IP joint toward palm. Positive if weakness is detected	228 hands referred for electrodiagnostic consultation with suspected carpal tunnel syndrome	Nerve conduction studies	.66	.66	1.94	.52

Reliability of Measuring Wrist Anthropometry

Test and Measure and Study Quality	Description	Population	Interexaminer Reliability
Wrist anteroposterior width[11] ◆	Width of wrist is measured in centimeters with pair of calipers	82 patients with suspected cervical radiculopathy or carpal tunnel syndrome	ICC = .77 (.62, .87)
Wrist mediolateral width[11] ◆			ICC = .86 (.75, .92)

Diagnostic Utility of Wrist Anthropometry in Identifying Carpal Tunnel Syndrome

Test and Study Quality	Description and Positive Findings	Population	Reference Standard	Sens	Spec	+LR	−LR
Wrist ratio index greater than .67[11] ◆	Anteroposterior width of wrist is measured and divided by mediolateral width. Positive if ratio is greater than .67	82 patients with suspected cervical radiculopathy or carpal tunnel syndrome	Needle electromyography and nerve conduction studies	.93 (.83, 1.0)	.26 (.14, .38)	1.3 (1.0, 1.5)	.29 (.07, 1.2)
T-square-shaped wrist test[27] ◆	Anteroposterior and mediolateral dimensions of wrist are measured at distal flexor wrist crease using pair of standard calipers. Positive if wrist ratio (anteroposterior dimension divided by mediolateral dimension) is .70 or more	228 hands referred for electrodiagnostic consultation with suspected carpal tunnel syndrome	Nerve conduction studies	.69	.73	2.56	.42

Reliability of Assessing Swelling

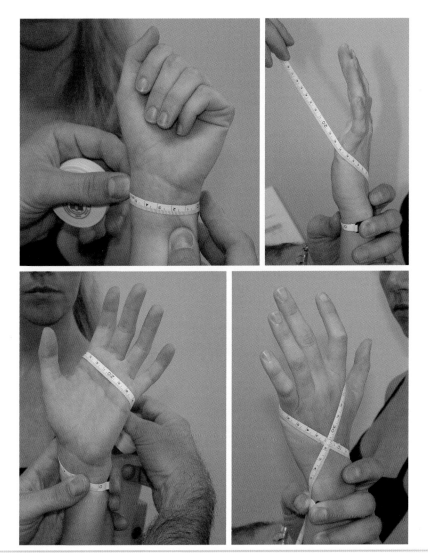

Figure 11-22
Figure-of-eight measurement.

Test and Measure and Study Quality	Description	Population	Reliability ICC	
			Intraexaminer	**Interexaminer**
Figure-of-eight test[28] ◆	Examiner places zero mark on distal aspect of ulnar styloid process. Tape measure is then brought across ventral surface of wrist to most distal aspect of radial styloid process. Next, tape is brought diagonally across dorsum of hand and over fifth MCP joint line, brought over ventral surface of MCP joints, and wrapped diagonally across dorsum to meet start of tape measure	24 individuals (33 hands) with pathologic conditions affecting hand	ICC = .99	ICC =.99
Volumetric test[28] ◆	Hand is placed vertically in standard volumeter		ICC = .99	Not reported

11

Wrist and Hand

Reliability of Sensory Testing

Test and Measure and Study Quality	Description and Positive Findings	Population	Interexaminer Reliability
Semmes-Weinstein monofilament test[24] ◆	Sensory test is performed on pulp of thumb, index finger, and long and small fingertips	36 hands with carpal tunnel syndrome	κ = .22 (.26, .42)
Median sensory field deficit of thumb pad[11] ◆	Sensation is tested with straight end of paper clip. Graded as absent, reduced, or normal sensation or hyperesthetic condition	82 patients presenting to a primary care clinic, orthopaedic department, or electrophysiology laboratory with suspected cervical radiculopathy or carpal tunnel syndrome	κ = .48 (.23, .73)
Median sensory field deficit of index finger pad[11] ◆			κ = .50 (.25, .75)
Median sensory field deficit[11] ◆			κ = .40 (.12, .68)

Diagnostic Utility of Diminished Sensation in Identifying Carpal Tunnel Syndrome

Test and Study Quality	Description and Positive Findings	Population	Reference Standard	Sens	Spec	+LR	−LR
Sensory loss at pad of thumb[11] ◆	Sensation is tested with straight end of paper clip. Positive if sensation is absent or reduced	82 patients presenting to a primary care clinic, orthopaedic department, or electrophysiology laboratory with suspected cervical radiculopathy or carpal tunnel syndrome	Needle electromyography and nerve conduction studies	.65 (.47, .84)	.70 (.47, .84)	2.2 (1.3, 3.6)	.49 (.28, .46)
Sensory loss at pad of index finger[11] ◆				.52 (.32, .72)	.67 (.32, .72)	1.6 (.92, 2.7)	.72 (.86, 1.1)
Sensory loss at pad of medial finger[11] ◆				.44 (.26, .63)	.74 (.26, .63)	1.7 (.58, .52)	.75 (.86, 1.1)
Moving two-point discrimination test[12] ◉	Examiner strokes the tip of the index finger, fifth finger, or both fingers five times with either one or two caliper tips. Positive if patient is unable to identify number of fingertips that have been stroked at least one of the five times	110 patients referred to laboratory for electrophysiologic examination	Nerve conduction tests	.32	.81	1.68	.84

Diagnostic Utility of Diminished Sensation in Identifying Carpal Tunnel Syndrome—cont'd

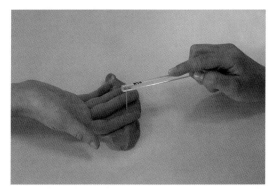

Semmes-Weinstein monofilament testing

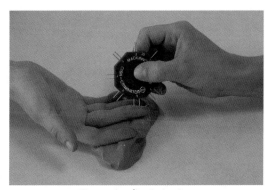

Two-point discrimination

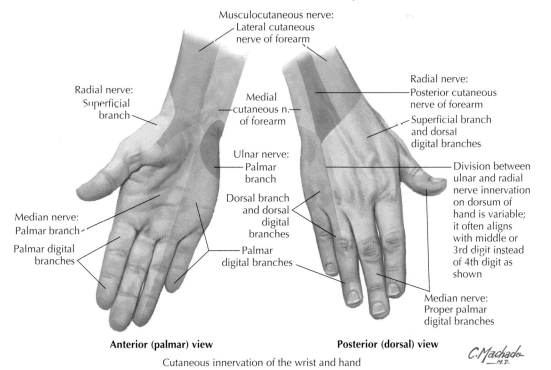

Musculocutaneous nerve:
Lateral cutaneous
nerve of forearm

Radial nerve:
Superficial
branch

Medial
cutaneous n.
of forearm

Radial nerve:
Posterior cutaneous
nerve of forearm

Superficial branch
and dorsal
digital branches

Ulnar nerve:
Palmar
branch

Division between
ulnar and radial
nerve innervation
on dorsum of
hand is variable;
it often aligns
with middle or
3rd digit instead
of 4th digit as
shown

Median nerve:
Palmar branch

Palmar digital
branches

Dorsal branch
and dorsal
digital
branches

Palmar
digital branches

Median nerve:
Proper palmar
digital branches

Anterior (palmar) view　　　**Posterior (dorsal) view**

C. Machado
_M.D.

Cutaneous innervation of the wrist and hand

Figure 11-23
Testing sensation.

11

Wrist and Hand

Reliability of the Tinel Sign

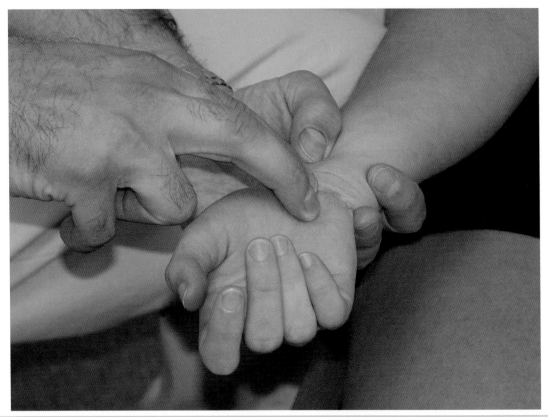

Figure 11-24
Tinel sign.

Test and Measure and Study Quality	Description and Positive Findings	Population	Reliability
Tinel A sign[11] ◆	Patient is seated with elbow flexed 30 degrees, forearm supinated, and wrist in neutral position. Examiner allows a reflex hammer to fall from a height of 6 inches along median nerve between the tendons at proximal wrist crease. Positive if patient reports a nonpainful tingling sensation along course of median nerve	82 patients with suspected cervical radiculopathy or carpal tunnel syndrome	$\kappa = .47$ (.21, .72)
Tinel B sign[11] ◆	Performed as the Tinel A sign test, above, except examiner attempts to elicit symptoms using mild-to-moderate force with reflex hammer. Positive if pain is exacerbated along course of median nerve		$\kappa = .35$ (.10, .60)
Tinel sign[24] ◆	Examiner percusses over palm from proximal palmar crease to distal wrist crease. Positive if symptoms are elicited in distribution of median nerve	36 hands with carpal tunnel syndrome	$\kappa = .81$ (.66, .98)

Diagnostic Utility of the Tinel Sign in Identifying Carpal Tunnel Syndrome

Test and Study Quality	Description and Positive Findings	Population	Reference Standard	Sens	Spec	+LR	−LR
Tinel sign[29] ◆	Examiner taps median nerve at wrist with fingers. Positive if patient reports pain or paresthesias in distribution of median nerve	142 patients referred for electrodiagnostic testing	Electrodiagnostic testing	.27 (.18, .36)	.91 (.84, 1.0)	3.0	.80
Tinel sign[27] ◆		228 hands referred for electrodiagnostic consultation regarding suspected carpal tunnel syndrome	Nerve conduction studies	.23	.87	1.77	.89
Tinel A test[11] ◆	Patient seated with elbow flexed 30 degrees, forearm supinated, and wrist in neutral position. Examiner allows reflex hammer to fall from height of 6 inches along median nerve between tendons at proximal wrist crease. Positive if patient reports nonpainful tingling sensation along course of median nerve	82 patients with suspected cervical radiculopathy or carpal tunnel syndrome	Needle electromyography and nerve conduction studies	.41 (.22, .59)	.58 (.45, .72)	.98 (.56, 1.7)	1.0 (.69, 1.5)
Tinel B test[11] ◆	Performed as the Tinel A sign test, above, except examiner attempts to elicit symptoms using mild-to-moderate force with reflex hammer. Positive if pain is exacerbated along course of median nerve			.48 (.29, .67)	.67 (.54, .79)	1.4 (.84, 2.5)	.78 (.52, 1.2)

Continued

11

Wrist and Hand

Diagnostic Utility of the Tinel Sign in Identifying Carpal Tunnel Syndrome—cont'd

Test and Study Quality	Description and Positive Findings	Population	Reference Standard	Sens	Spec	+LR	−LR
Tinel test[30] ◉	Positive if percussion of the median nerve at the wrist causes tingling in the median nerve distribution	162 hands from 81 patients seeking treatment for carpal tunnel syndrome	Electrodiagnostic testing*	.90	.81	4.7	.12
Tinel test[1] ◉	Percussion of the median nerve at the wrist (no other details)	232 patients with carpal tunnel syndrome manifestations and 182 controls	Carpal tunnel syndrome diagnosed via clinical examination	.30 (.24, .36)	.65 (.58, .71)	0.9	1.10
			Tenosynovitis via ultrasonography	.46 (.41, .53)	.85 (.80, .89)	3.1	.64
Tinel sign[12] ◉	Examiner drops square end of reflex hammer on distal wrist crease from height of 12 cm. Positive if patient reports pain or paresthesias in at least one finger innervated by median nerve	110 patients referred to laboratory for electrophysiologic examination	Nerve conduction tests	.60	.67	1.82	.60

*Also used latent class analysis to define reference standard diagnosis of carpal tunnel syndrome, but doing so resulted in study being excluded for poor quality because the reference standard was then not independent of index tests.

Reliability of the Phalen Test

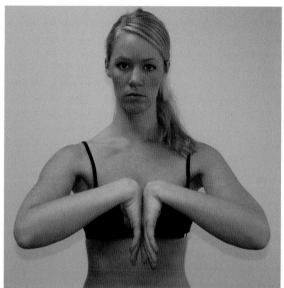

Phalen test

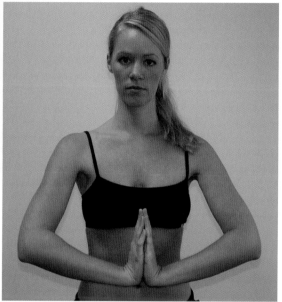

Reverse Phalen test

Figure 11-25
Phalen test.

Test and Measure and Study Quality	Description and Positive Findings	Population	Interexaminer Reliability
Phalen test[24] ◆	Patient places dorsal aspects of hands together, maintaining maximal wrist flexion for 60 seconds. Positive if symptoms are elicited in distribution of median nerve	36 hands with carpal tunnel syndrome	$\kappa = .88$ (.77, .98)
Phalen test[11] ◆	With patient seated with elbow flexed 30 degrees and forearm supinated, examiner places the wrist in maximal flexion for 60 seconds. Positive if patient experiences exacerbation of symptoms in median nerve distribution	82 patients with suspected cervical radiculopathy or carpal tunnel syndrome	$\kappa = .79$ (.59, 1.0)
Wrist extension test[24] ◆	Patient places palmar aspects of hands together, maintaining maximal wrist extension for 60 seconds. Positive if symptoms are elicited in distribution of median nerve	36 hands with carpal tunnel syndrome	$\kappa = .72$ (.55, .88)

11

Wrist and Hand

Diagnostic Utility of the Phalen Test in Identifying Carpal Tunnel Syndrome

Test and Study Quality	Description and Positive Findings	Population	Reference Standard	Sens	Spec	+LR	−LR
Phalen test[11] ◆	With patient seated with elbow flexed 30 degrees and forearm supinated, examiner places wrist in maximal flexion for 60 seconds. Positive if patient experiences an exacerbation of symptoms in median nerve distribution	82 patients with suspected cervical radiculopathy or carpal tunnel syndrome	Needle electromyography and nerve conduction studies	.77 (.61, .93)	.40 (.26, .53)	1.3 (.94, 1.7)	.58 (.27, 1.3)
Phalen test[29] ◆		142 patients referred for electrodiagnostic testing	Electrodiagnostic testing	.34 (.24, .43)	.74 (.62, .87)	1.31	.89
Phalen test[27] ◆	Patient is instructed to maximally flex wrist and hold position for 60 seconds. Positive if symptoms are produced	228 hands referred for electrodiagnostic consultation regarding suspected carpal tunnel syndrome	Nerve conduction studies	.51	.76	2.13	.64
Phalen test[30] ◐		162 hands from 81 patients seeking treatment for carpal tunnel syndrome	Electrodiagnostic testing*	.85	.79	4.0	.19
Phalen test[1] ◐	Complete wrist flexion for 60 seconds (no other details)	232 patients with carpal tunnel syndrome manifestations and 182 controls	Carpal tunnel syndrome diagnosed via clinical examination	.47 (.41, .54)	.17 (.13, .23)	0.6	3.12
			Tenosynovitis diagnosed via ultrasonography	.92 (.36, .49)	.87 (.82, .91)	7.1	.09
Reverse Phalen test[1] ◐	Complete wrist extension for 60 seconds (no other details)		Carpal tunnel syndrome diagnosed via clinical examination	.42 (.36, .49)	.35 (.29, .42)	0.6	1.66
			Tenosynovitis diagnosed via ultrasonography	.75 (.69, .80)	.85 (.80, .89)	5.0	.29

Diagnostic Utility of the Phalen Test in Identifying Carpal Tunnel Syndrome—cont'd

Test and Study Quality	Description and Positive Findings	Population	Reference Standard	Sens	Spec	+LR	−LR
Phalen test[12] ◗	Examiner instructs patient to flex both wrists to 90 degrees with dorsal aspects of hands held in opposition for 60 seconds. Positive if patient reports pain or paresthesias in at least one finger innervated by median nerve	110 patients referred to laboratory for electrophysiologic examination	Nerve conduction tests	.74	.47	1.4	.55
Phalen test[10] ◗	Patient holds forearms in pronation with elbows resting on examination table, forearms vertical and wrists in gravity-assisted flexion. Positive if symptoms are produccd	132 patients with pain of upper limb	Electrophysiologic confirmation	.79	.92	9.88	.23

*Also used latent class analysis to define reference standard diagnosis of carpal tunnel syndrome, but doing so resulted in study being excluded for poor quality because the reference standard was then not independent of index tests.

11

Wrist and Hand

Reliability of the Carpal Compression Test

Test and Measure and Study Quality	Description and Positive Findings	Population	Reliability
Carpal compression test[11] ◆	With patient seated with elbow flexed 30 degrees, forearm supinated, and wrist in neutral position, examiner places both thumbs over transverse carpal ligament and applies 6 pounds of pressure for 30 seconds maximum. Positive if patient experiences exacerbation of symptoms in median nerve distribution	36 hands with carpal tunnel syndrome	$\kappa = .77$ (.58, .96)

Diagnostic Utility of the Carpal Compression Test in Identifying Carpal Tunnel Syndrome

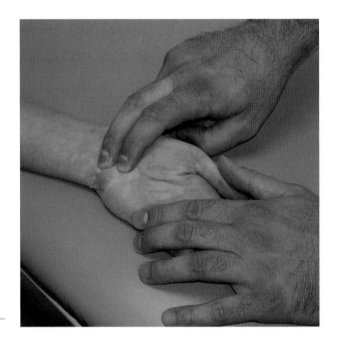

Figure 11-26
Carpal compression test.

Test and Study Quality	Description and Positive Findings	Population	Reference Standard	Sens	Spec	+LR	−LR
Carpal compression test[11] ◆	With patient seated with elbow flexed 30 degrees, forearm supinated, and wrist in neutral position, examiner places both thumbs over transverse carpal ligament and applies 6 pounds of pressure for 30 seconds maximum. Positive if patient experiences exacerbation of symptoms in median nerve distribution	82 patients presenting to a primary care clinic, orthopaedic department, or electrophysiology laboratory with suspected cervical radiculopathy or carpal tunnel syndrome	Needle electromyography and nerve conduction studies	.64 (.45, .83)	.30 (.17, .42)	.91 (.65, 1.3)	1.2 (.62, 2.4)

Diagnostic Utility of the Carpal Compression Test in Identifying Carpal Tunnel Syndrome—cont'd

Test and Study Quality	Description and Positive Findings	Population	Reference Standard	Sens	Spec	+LR	−LR
Carpal compression test[27] ◆	Examiner applies moderate pressure over median nerve just distal to distal flexor wrist crease for 5 seconds. Considered positive if pain, paresthesia, or numbness is reproduced	228 hands referred for electrodiagnostic consultation regarding suspected carpal tunnel syndrome	Nerve conduction studies	.28	.74	1.08	.97
Carpal tunnel compression test[1] ◉	Examiner exerts even pressure on the space between thenar eminence and the hypothenar eminence for 30 seconds while arm is supinated. Patient is questioned regarding symptoms every 15 seconds	232 patients with carpal tunnel syndrome manifestations and 182 controls	Carpal tunnel syndrome diagnosed via clinical examination	.46 (.40, .53)	.25 (.20, .31)	0.6	2.16
Carpal compression test[10] ◉	The examiner applies moderate pressure with thumbs over transverse carpal ligament with wrist in neutral for 30 seconds. Considered positive if pain, paresthesia or numbness is reproduced	132 patients with pain of upper limb	Electrophysiologic confirmation	.83	.92	10.38	.18

Diagnostic Utility of the Hand Elevation Test in Identifying Carpal Tunnel Syndrome

Test and Study Quality	Description and Positive Findings	Population	Reference Standard	Sens	Spec	+LR	−LR
Hand elevation test [31] ◉	Patient is asked to elevate both hands above the head for 1 minute. Positive if symptoms are reproduced	70 patients with symptoms of carpal tunnel syndrome and positive nerve conduction studies	Electrodiagnostic testing	.99	.91	11.0	.01

Diagnostic Utility of the Hand Elevation Test in Identifying Carpal Tunnel Syndrome—cont'd

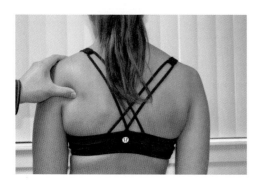

Figure 11-27
Infraspinatus test.

Test and Study Quality	Description and Positive Findings	Population	Reference Standard	Sens	Spec	+LR	−LR
Infraspinatus test [32] ●	2.5 kg of pressure is exerted for 30 seconds on the lateral edge of the infraspinatus muscle between the tip of the inferior angle of the scapula and the dorsal tip of the acromial angle. Positive if carpal tunnel syndrome symptoms appear or disagreeable local pressure is felt	34 patients with symptoms of carpal tunnel syndrome	Electrodiagnostic testing	.70	.87	5.4	.34

Reliability of Upper Limb Tension Tests

Test and Measure and Study Quality	Description and Positive Findings	Population	Interexaminer Reliability
Upper limb tension test A [11] ◆	See below	82 patients with suspected cervical radiculopathy or carpal tunnel syndrome	κ = .76 (.51, 1.0)
Upper limb tension test B [11] ◆			κ = .83 (.65, 1.0)

Diagnostic Utility of Upper Limb Tension Tests in Identifying Carpal Tunnel Syndrome

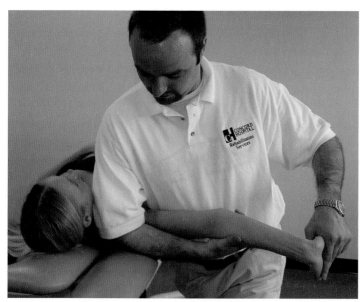

Figure 11-28
Upper limb tension test A.

Test and Study Quality	Description and Positive Findings	Population	Reference Standard	Sens	Spec	+LR	−LR
Upper limb tension test A[33] ◆	With patient supine, examiner performs scapular depression, shoulder abduction, forearm supination, wrist and finger extension, shoulder lateral rotation, elbow extension, and contralateral/ipsilateral cervical side-bending to end range or until symptom reproduction. Positive if symptoms are reproduced and changed during structural differentiation (passive contralateral/ipsilateral side bending of the neck with distal symptoms and passive wrist flexion and extension with proximal symptoms	95 hands from 58 patients with suspected carpal tunnel syndrome referred for nerve conduction studies	Needle electromyography and nerve conduction studies	.58 (.45, .71)	.84 (.72, .96)	3.67 (1.70, 7.89)	.50 (.36, .70)
Upper limb tension test A[34] ◆	Same as below	230 hands from 118 patients with a clinical diagnosis of carpal tunnel syndrome	Needle electromyography and nerve conduction studies	.93 (.88, .97)	.67 (0.0, .34)	1.00	1.05

Continued

11

Wrist and Hand

Diagnostic Utility of Upper Limb Tension Tests in Identifying Carpal Tunnel Syndrome—cont'd

Test and Study Quality	Description and Positive Findings	Population	Reference Standard	Sens	Spec	+LR	−LR
Upper limb tension test A[11] ◆ (see Video 11-1)	With patient supine, examiner performs scapular depression, shoulder abduction, forearm supination, wrist and finger extension, shoulder lateral rotation, elbow extension, and contralateral/ipsilateral cervical side-bending. Positive if symptoms are reproduced, side-to-side difference in elbow extension is greater than 10 degrees, contralateral neck side-bending increases symptoms, or ipsilateral side-bending decreases symptoms	82 patients with suspected cervical radiculopathy or carpal tunnel syndrome	Needle electromyography and nerve conduction studies	.75 (.58, .92)	.13 (.04, .22)	.86 (.67, 1.1)	1.9 (.72, 5.1)
Upper limb tension test B[11] ◆ (see Video 11-2)	With patient supine with shoulder abducted 30 degrees, examiner performs scapular depression, shoulder medial rotation, full elbow extension, wrist and finger flexion, and contralateral/ipsilateral cervical side-bending. Positive if symptoms are reproduced, side-to-side difference in wrist flexion is more than 10 degrees, contralateral neck side-bending increases symptoms, or ipsilateral side-bending decreases symptoms			.64 (.45, .83)	.30 (.17, .42)	.91 (.65, 1.3)	1.2 (.62, 2.4)

Diagnostic Utility of Scratch Collapse Test in Identifying Carpal Tunnel Syndrome

Test and Study Quality	Description and Positive Findings	Population	Reference Standard	Sens	Spec	+LR	−LR
Scratch collapse test A[35] **2018 Meta-analysis ◆**	The patient faces the examiner with elbows flexed to 90 degrees and hands facing each other while providing resistance as the examiner pushes the patient's forearms together. Next, the examiner "scratches" the skin over the carpal tunnel, and repeats the first step. A positive response is a temporary loss of external resistance with arm collapse. Immediate repetition of the first step will show strength recovery	Statistically pooled data from 3 high-quality studies involving 265 patients	Needle electro-myography and nerve conduction studies	.32 (.24, .41)	.62 (.45, .78)	.75 (.33, 1.67)	1.03 (.61, 1.74)

Diagnostic Utility of Special Tests in Identifying Carpal Instability

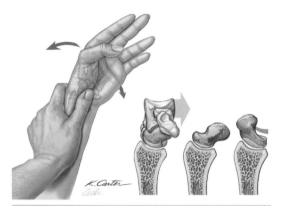

Figure 11-29
Scaphoid shift test.

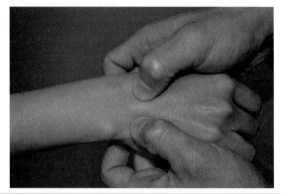

Figure 11-30
Ballottement test.

Test and Measure and Study Quality	Description	Positive Findings	Population	Reference Standard	Sens	Spec	+LR	−LR
Scaphoid shift test[36] ◐	Patient's elbow is stabilized on table with forearm in slight pronation. With one hand, examiner grasps radial side of patient's wrist with thumb on the palmar prominence of scaphoid. With the other hand, examiner grasps patient's hand at metacarpal level to stabilize wrist. Examiner maintains pressure on scaphoid tubercle and moves patient's wrist into ulnar deviation with slight extension and then radial deviation with slight flexion. Examiner releases pressure on scaphoid while wrist is in radial deviation and flexion	Positive for instability of scaphoid if scaphoid shifts, test elicits a "thunk," or symptoms are reproduced when scaphoid is released	50 painful wrists undergoing arthroscopy	Arthroscopic visualization	.69	.66	2.03	.47

Diagnostic Utility of Special Tests in Identifying Carpal Instability—cont'd

Test and Measure and Study Quality	Description	Positive Findings	Population	Reference Standard	Sens	Spec	+LR	−LR
Ballottement test[36] ⊕	Examiner stabilizes patient's lunate bone between thumb and index finger of one hand while other hand moves pisotriquetral complex in a palmar and dorsal direction	Positive for instability of lunotriquetral joint if patient's symptoms are reproduced or excessive laxity of joint is revealed			.64	.44	1.14	.82
Ulnomeniscotriquetral dorsal glide[36] ⊕	With patient seated with elbow on table and forearm in neutral, examiner places thumb over head of distal ulna. Examiner then places radial side of index proximal IP joint over palmar surface of patient's pisotriquetral complex. Examiner squeezes thumb and index finger together, creating a dorsal glide of pisotriquetral complex	Considered positive for ulnomeniscotriquetral complex instability if the patient's symptoms are reproduced or excessive laxity of the joint is revealed			.66	.64	1.69	.56

Wrist and Hand 11

Diagnostic Utility of Special Tests in Identifying de Quervain Tenosynovitis

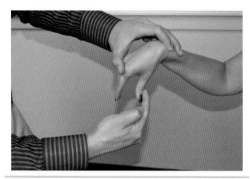

Figure 11-31
Wrist hyperflexion and abduction of the thumb test.

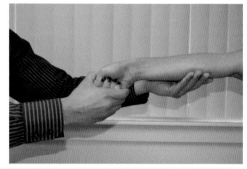

Figure 11-32
Eichhoff test.

Test and Study Quality	Description and Positive Findings	Population	Reference Standard	Sens	Spec	+LR	−LR
Wrist hyperflexion and abduction of the thumb test[37] ◐ (see Video 11-3)	Patient's wrist is hyperflexed with thumb abducted in full MCP and IP extension, resisted against the examiner's index finger. Positive with symptom exacerbation	104 patients who presented clinically with the symptoms of de Quervain disease	X-ray and ultrasonography confirmation	.99 (.96, 1.02)	.29 (−.14, .71)	1.39	.04
Eichhoff test[37] ◐	Patient performs ulnar deviation of the clenched wrist while holding the opposed thumb. Positive with symptom exacerbation			.89 (.81, .97)	.14 (−.19, .47)	1.04	.75

Reliability of Special Tests for First Carpometacarpal (CMC) Osteoarthritis

Test and Measure and Study Quality	Description and Positive Findings	Population	Interexaminer Reliability
Thumb adduction maneuver[38] ◆	Patient places the affected hand on the examination table with the elbow flexed 90 degrees and the forearm in neutral rotation. The examiner places his or her ipsilateral hand such that the examiner's thumb rests dorsally over the head of the thumb metacarpal. The examiner's contralateral hand supports the ulnar side of the patient's hand to maintain the patient's wrist in neutral position to prevent ulnar deviation of the patient's wrist. The examiner firmly directs an adduction force downward onto the patient's metacarpal head until the patient's thumb metacarpal lies parallel to the midaxis of the index metacarpal or until a firm endpoint is reached. Positive if trapeziometacarpal pain is reproduced	129 consecutive patients undergoing radiographic examination of their wrist(s) for an atraumatic complaint	$\kappa = .79$
Thumb extension maneuver[38] ◆	From the same starting position as above, examiner places his or her ipsilateral thumb along the radial aspect of the distal thumb metacarpal, 5 to 10 mm proximal to the thumb metacarpophalangeal joint, and extends the thumb until the thumb metacarpal comes to lie in a plane parallel to the palm or until a firm endpoint is reached. Positive if trapeziometacarpal pain is reproduced	129 consecutive patients undergoing radiographic examination of their wrist(s) for an atraumatic complaint	$\kappa = .84$

Diagnostic Utility of Special Tests in Identifying First Carpometacarpal (CMC) Osteoarthritis

Test and Study Quality	Description and Positive Findings	Population	Reference Standard	Sens	Spec	+LR	−LR
Grind test[39] ◆	Examiner applies axial compression along the plane of the thumb metacarpal and simultaneously rotates the thumb metacarpal base. Positive if pain reproduced in the joint	121 hands (100 symptomatic, 21 asymptomatic) from 62 consecutive patients with suspected first CMC osteoarthritis	History of pain localized to the first CMC joint and radiographic reading of osteoarthritis	.41	1.00	Undefined	.59*
Grind test[38] ◆	Examiner applies axial compression along the plane of the thumb metacarpal and simultaneously rotates the thumb metacarpal base. Positive if pain reproduced in the joint	129 consecutive patients undergoing radiographic examination of their wrist(s) for an atraumatic complaint	Attending hand surgeon's assessment combining the patient's history, physical examination, and radiographic examination	.44 (.30, .59)	.92 (.84, .97)	5.5*	.61*

Continued

11

Wrist and Hand

Diagnostic Utility of Special Tests in Identifying First Carpometacarpal (CMC) Osteoarthritis—cont'd

Test and Study Quality	Description and Positive Findings	Population	Reference Standard	Sens	Spec	+LR	−LR
Lever test[39] ◆	Examiner puts his or her thumb and index finger on both sides of the thumb basal joint and levers the first metacarpal joint radially and ulnarly to their endpoints at the basal joint. Positive if pain reproduced in the joint	121 hands (100 symptomatic, 21 asymptomatic) from 62 consecutive patients with suspected first CMC osteoarthritis	History of pain localized to the first CMC joint and radiographic reading of osteoarthritis	.81	.82	4.5*	.23*
Metacarpophalangeal (MP) extension test[39] ◆	The patient tries to extend the thumb while the examiner provides resistance against extension by placing 1 finger on the thumb interphalangeal joint. Positive if pain reproduced in the joint	121 hands (100 symptomatic, 21 asymptomatic) from 62 consecutive patients with suspected first CMC osteoarthritis	History of pain localized to the first CMC joint and radiographic reading of osteoarthritis	.65	.95	13*	.37*
Grind test[40] ◉	Axial compression is applied to the thumb, while simultaneously moving the thumb into flexion, extension, and circumduction. Positive if test elicits pain at the base of the thumb	60 patients (30 with osteoarthritis of first CMC, 30 controls with asymptomatic thumb joints but who required wrist or thumb radiographs)	Radiographic examination and positive responsiveness to intraarticular steroid injections	.30	.97	10*	.72*

Diagnostic Utility of Special Tests in Identifying First Carpometacarpal (CMC) Osteoarthritis—cont'd

Test and Study Quality	Description and Positive Findings	Population	Reference Standard	Sens	Spec	+LR	−LR
Thumb adduction maneuver[38] ◆	Patient places the affected hand on the examination table with the elbow flexed 90 degrees and the forearm in neutral rotation. The examiner places his or her ipsilateral hand such that the examiner's thumb rests dorsally over the head of the thumb metacarpal. The examiner's contralateral hand supports the ulnar side of the patient's hand to maintain the patient's wrist in neutral position to prevent ulnar deviation of the patient's wrist. The examiner firmly directs an adduction force downward onto the patient's metacarpal head until the patient's thumb metacarpal lies parallel to the midaxis of the index metacarpal or until a firm endpoint is reached. Positive if trapeziometacarpal pain is reproduced	129 consecutive patients undergoing radiographic examination of their wrist(s) for an atraumatic complaint	Attending hand surgeon's assessment combining the patient's history, physical examination, and radiographic examination	0.94 (0.82, 0.98)	0.93 (0.86, 0.97)	13.43*	0.06*
Thumb extension maneuver[38] ◆	From the same starting position as above, examiner places his or her ipsilateral thumb along the radial aspect of the distal thumb metacarpal, 5 to 10 mm proximal to the thumb metacarpophalangeal joint, and extends the thumb until the thumb metacarpal comes to lie in a plane parallel to the palm or until a firm endpoint is reached. Positive if trapeziometacarpal pain is reproduced	129 consecutive patients undergoing radiographic examination of their wrist(s) for an atraumatic complaint	Attending hand surgeon's assessment combining the patient's history, physical examination, and radiographic examination	0.94 (0.82, 0.98)	0.95 (0.87, 0.98)	18.8*	.06*

Continued

11

Wrist and Hand

Diagnostic Utility of Special Tests in Identifying First Carpometacarpal (CMC) Osteoarthritis—cont'd

Test and Study Quality	Description and Positive Findings	Population	Reference Standard	Sens	Spec	+LR	−LR
Traction-shift test[40] ●	Using a single-handed technique, the examiner applies longitudinal traction to the thumb while simultaneously applying alternate dorsal and palmar pressure over the base of the metacarpal provoke subluxation and then relocation of the joint. The test is positive if it elicits pain within the joint	60 patients (30 with osteoarthritis of first CMC, 30 controls with asymptomatic thumb joints but who required wrist or thumb radiographs)	Radiographic examination and positive responsiveness to intraarticular steroid injections	.67	1.0	Undefined	.33*

*Values were calculated by the authors of this text.

Reliability of Miscellaneous Special Tests

Test and Measure and Study Quality	Description and Positive Findings	Population	Interexaminer Reliability
Tethered median nerve test[24] ◆	Examiner passively extends patient's index finger while forearm is in supination and wrist is in full extension. Position is maintained for 15 seconds. Positive if symptoms are elicited in distribution of median nerve	36 hands with carpal tunnel syndrome	$\kappa = .49$ (.26, .71)
Pinch test[24] ◆	Patient actively pinches a piece of paper between the tip of the thumb, the index finger, and the long fingers using MCP flexion and IP extension. Positive if symptoms are elicited in distribution of median nerve	36 hands with carpal tunnel syndrome	$\kappa = .76$ (.62, .91)

Diagnostic Utility of Miscellaneous Special Tests

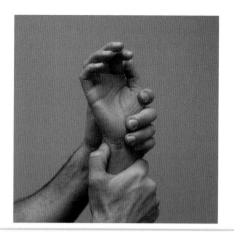

Figure 11-33
Ulnar fovea sign.

Test and Study Quality	Description and Positive Findings	Population	Reference Standard	Sens	Spec	+LR	−LR
Flick maneuver[29] ◆	Patient is instructed to demonstrate hand motions or positions the patient uses when pain is most severe. Positive if patient demonstrates a flicking down of hands similar to shaking a thermometer	142 patients referred for electrodiagnostic testing	Carpal tunnel syndrome diagnosed via electrodiagnostic testing	.37 (.27, .46)	.74 (.62, .87)	1.42	.85
Lumbrical provocation test[16] ◐	Patient is instructed to make a fist for 60 seconds. Considered positive if the patient reports paresthesia in the distribution of the median nerve	96 consecutive patients referred for electrodiagnostic testing		.37	.71	1.28	.89
Ulnar fovea sign[42] ◐	Examiner presses thumb distally and deep into the "soft spot" between the patient's ulnar styloid process and flexor carpi ulnaris tendon. Positive if patient feels exquisite tenderness similar to experienced wrist pain	272 consecutive patients undergoing wrist arthroscopy	Foveal disruption of the distal radioulnar ligaments and ulnotriquetral ligament injuries observed during arthroscopy	.95 (.90, .98)	.87 (.79, .92)	7.1 (4.5, 11.0)	.06 (.03, .11)

11

Wrist and Hand

Carpal Tunnel Syndrome: Clinical Prediction Rule

Wainner and colleagues[11] developed a clinical prediction rule for detecting carpal tunnel syndrome. The result of their study demonstrated that if five variables (a Brigham and Women's Hospital Hand Severity Scale score of more than 1.9, a wrist ratio index of more than .67, a patient report of shaking the hand for symptom relief, diminished sensation on the thumb pad, and age over 45 years) were present, the +LR was 18.3 (95% CI: 1.0, 328.3). This clinical prediction rule results in a posttest probability of 90% that the patient has carpal tunnel syndrome.

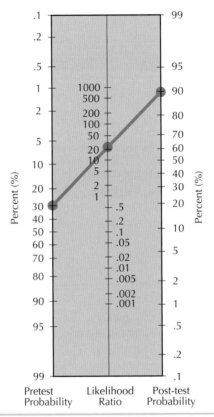

Figure 11-34
Nomogram representing the change in pretest (34% in this study) to posttest probability given the clinical prediction rule. (From Fagan TJ. Letter: Nomogram for Bayes theorem. *N Engl J Med*. 1975;293:257. Copyright 2005, Massachusetts Medical Society.)

Scaphoid Fracture: Clinical Prediction Rule

Duckworth and colleagues[43] developed a clinical prediction rule that incorporates demographic and clinical factors predictive of a scaphoid fracture. In the study, 260 patients with a clinically suspected or radiologically confirmed scaphoid fracture were evaluated within 72 hours of injury and at approximately 2 and 6 weeks after injury using clinical assessment and standard radiographs. A logistic regression model identified four variables (male gender, sports injury, anatomic snuffbox pain on ulnar deviation of the wrist within 72 hours of injury, scaphoid tubercle tenderness at 2 weeks) as independent predictors of fracture. The risk of fracture was 91% with these four positive factors. All patients who did not have pain at the anatomic snuffbox on ulnar deviation of the wrist within 72 hours of injury did not have a fracture.

Outcome Measure	Scoring and Interpretation	Test-Retest Reliability and Study Quality	MCID
Upper Extremity Functional Index	Users are asked to rate the difficulty of performing 20 functional tasks on a Likert-type scale ranging from 0 (extremely difficult or unable to perform activity) to 4 (no difficulty). A total score out of 80 is calculated by summing each score. The answers provide a score between 0 and 80, with lower scores representing more disability	ICC = .95[44] ●	Unknown (MDC = 9.1)[44]
Disabilities of the Arm, Shoulder, and Hand (DASH) **2009 Metaanalysis**	Users are asked to rate the difficulty of performing 30 functional tasks on a Likert-type scale. Of the items, 21 items relate to physical function, 5 items relate to pain symptoms, and 4 items relate to emotional and social functioning. A total score out of 100 is calculated, with higher scores representing more disability	ICC = .90[45]	10.2[45]
Michigan Hand Outcomes Questionnaire (MHQ)	Consists of 37 items on 6 scales: (1) overall hand function, (2) activities of daily living (ADLs), (3) work performance, (4) pain, (5) aesthetics, and (6) satisfaction with hand function. Users rate each item on a 5-point Likert-type scale. Answers provide a total score between 0 and 100, with higher scores indicating better hand performance	ICC = .95[46] ●	Pain = 23 Function = 13 ADL = 11 Work = 8[47]
Numeric Pain Rating Scale (NPRS)	Users rate their level of pain on an 11-point scale ranging from 0 to 10, with high scores representing more pain. Often asked as "current pain" and "least," "worst," and "average pain" in the past 24 hours	ICC = .72[48] ●	2[8,9]

ICC, Intraclass correlation coefficient; MCID, minimum clinically important difference; MDC, minimal detectable change.

Wrist and Hand

11

References

1. El Miedany Y, Ashour S, Youssef S, et al. Clinical diagnosis of carpal tunnel syndrome: old tests—new concepts. *Joint Bone Spine*. 2008;75:451–457.
2. Bohannon RW, Schaubert KL. Test-retest reliability of grip-strength measures obtained over a 12-week interval from community-dwelling elders. *J Hand Ther*. 2005;18:426–427. quiz 428.
3. Brown A, Cramer LD, Eckhaus D, et al. Validity and reliability of the Dexter hand evaluation and therapy system in hand-injured patients. *J Hand Ther*. 2000;13:37–45.
4. Coldham F, Lewis J, Lee H. The reliability of one vs. three grip trials in symptomatic and asymptomatic subjects. *J Hand Ther*. 2006;19:318–326. quiz 327.
5. Cole IC. *Fractures and ligament injuries of the wrist and hand. The Wrist and Hand. La Crosse, Wisconsin: Orthopaedic Section*. American Physical Therapy Association; 1995.
6. D'Arcy CA, McGee S. The rational clinical examination. Does this patient have carpal tunnel syndrome? *JAMA*. 2000;283:3110–3117.
7. de Kraker M, Selles RW, Schreuders TA, et al. Palmar abduction: reliability of 6 measurement methods in healthy adults. *J Hand Surg [Am]*. 2009;34:523–530.
8. Farrar JT, Berlin JA, Strom BL. Clinically important changes in acute pain outcome measures: a validation study. *J Pain Symptom Manage*. 2003;25:406–411.
9. Farrar JT, Portenoy RK, Berlin JA, et al. Defining the clinically important difference in pain outcome measures. *Pain*. 2000;88:287–294.
10. Fertl E, Wober C, Zeitlhofer J. The serial use of two provocative tests in the clinical diagnosis of carpal tunnel syndrome. *Acta Neurol Scand*. 1998;98:328–332.
11. Wainner RS, Fritz JM, Irrgang JJ, et al. Development of a clinical prediction rule for the diagnosis of carpal tunnel syndrome. *Arch Phys Med Rehabil*. 2005;86:609–618.
12. Katz JN, Larson MG, Sabra A, et al. The carpal tunnel syndrome: diagnostic utility of the history and physical examination findings. *Ann Intern Med*. 1990;112:321–327.
13. Walenkamp MMJ, Bentohami A, Slaar A, et al. The Amsterdam wrist rules: the multicenter prospective derivation and external validation of a clinical decision rule for the use of radiography in acute wrist trauma. *BMC Musculoskelet Disord*. 2015;16:389.
14. Mulders MAM, Walenkamp MMJ, Dubois BFH, et al. External validation of clinical decision rules for children with wrist trauma. *Pediatr Radiol*. 2017;47(5):590–598.
15. Carpenter CR, Pines JM, Schuur JD, et al. Adult scaphoid fracture. *Acad Emerg Med*. 2014;21(2):101–121.
16. Mallee WH, Henny EP, van Dijk CN, et al. Clinical diagnostic evaluation for scaphoid fractures: a systematic review and meta-analysis. *J Hand Surg Am*. 2014;39(9):1683–1691.e2.
17. Calfee RP, Dale AM, Ryan D, et al. Performance of simplified scoring systems for hand diagrams in carpal tunnel syndrome screening. *J Hand Surg [Am]*. 2012;37(1):10–17.
18. Horger MM. The reliability of goniometric measurements of active and passive wrist motions. *Am J Occup Ther*. 1990;44:342–348.
19. LaStayo PC, Wheeler DL. Reliability of passive wrist flexion and extension goniometric measurements: a multicenter study. *Phys Ther*. 1994;74:162–174. discussion 174-176.
20. van den Beld WA, van der Sanden GA, Sengers RC, et al. Validity and reproducibility of hand-held dynamometry in children aged 4-11 years. *J Rehabil Med*. 2006;38:57–64.
21. Molenaar HM, Zuidam JM, Selles RW, et al. Age-specific reliability of two grip-strength dynamometers when used by children. *J Bone Joint Surg Am*. 2008;90:1053–1059.
22. Mathiowetz V, Weber K, Volland G, Kashman N. Reliability and validity of grip and pinch strength evaluations. *J Hand Surg [Am]*. 1984;9:222–226.
23. Schreuders TA, Roebroeck ME, Goumans J, et al. Measurement error in grip and pinch force measurements in patients with hand injuries. *Phys Ther*. 2003;83:806–815.
24. MacDermid JC, Kramer JF, Woodbury MG, et al. Interrater reliability of pinch and grip strength measurements in patients with cumulative trauma disorders. *J Hand Ther*. 1994;7:10–14.
25. Bohannon RW, Andrews AW. Interrater reliability of hand-held dynamometry. *Phys Ther*. 1987;67:931–933.
26. Rheault W, Beal JL, Kubik KR, et al. Intertester reliability of the hand-held dynamometer for wrist flexion and extension. *Arch Phys Med Rehabil*. 1989;70:907–910.
27. Kuhlman KA, Hennessey WJ. Sensitivity and specificity of carpal tunnel syndrome signs. *Am J Phys Med Rehabil*. 1997;76:451–457.
28. Leard JS, Breglio L, Fraga L, et al. Reliability and concurrent validity of the figure-of-eight method of measuring hand size in patients with hand pathology. *J Orthop Sports Phys Ther*. 2004;34:335–340.
29. Hansen PA, Micklesen P, Robinson LR. Clinical utility of the flick maneuver in diagnosing carpal tunnel syndrome. *Am J Phys Med Rehabil*. 2004;83:363–367.
30. LaJoie AS, McCabe SJ, Thomas B, Edgell SE. Determining the sensitivity and specificity of common diagnostic tests for carpal tunnel syndrome using latent class analysis. *Plast Reconstr Surg*. 2005;116:502–507.
31. Amirfeyz R, Clark D, Parsons B, et al. Clinical tests for carpal tunnel syndrome in contemporary practice. *Arch Orthop Trauma Surg*. 2011;131(4):471–474.
32. Meder MA, Lange R, Amtage F, Rijntjes M. Proximal stimulus confirms carpal tunnel syndrome—a new test? A clinical and electrophysiologic, multiple-blind, controlled study. *J Clin Neurophysiol*. 2012;29(1):89–95.

33. Bueno-Gracia E, Tricás-Moreno JM, Fanlo-Mazas P, et al. Validity of the upper limb neurodynamic test 1 for the diagnosis of carpal tunnel syndrome. The role of structural differentiation. *Man Ther*. 2016;22:190–195.

34. Trillos M-C, Soto F, Briceno-Ayala L. Upper limb neurodynamic test 1 in patients with clinical diagnosis of carpal tunnel syndrome: A diagnostic accuracy study. *J Hand Ther*. 2018;31(3):333–338.

35. Huynh MNQ, Karir A, Bennett A. YES scratch collapse test for carpal tunnel syndrome: A systematic review and meta-analysis. *Plast Reconstr Surg Glob Open*. 2018;6(9):e1933.

36. LaStayo P, Howell J. Clinical provocative tests used in evaluating wrist pain: a descriptive study. *J Hand Ther*. 1995;8:10–17.

37. Goubau JF, Goubau L, Van Tongel A, et al. The wrist hyperflexion and abduction of the thumb (WHAT) test: a more specific and sensitive test to diagnose de Quervain tenosynovitis than the Eichhoff's test. *J Hand Surg Eur*. 2014;39(3):286–292.

38. Gelberman RH, Boone S, Osei DA, et al. Trapeziometacarpal arthritis: A prospective clinical evaluation of the thumb adduction and extension provocative tests. *J Hand Surg Am*. 2015;40(7):1285–1291.

39. Model Z, Liu AY, Kang L, et al. Evaluation of physical examination tests for thumb basal joint osteoarthritis. *Hand (N Y)*. 2016;11(1):108–112.

40. Choa RM, Parvizi N, Giele HP. A prospective case-control study to compare the sensitivity and specificity of the grind and traction-shift (subluxation-relocation) clinical tests in osteoarthritis of the thumb carpometacarpal joint. *J Hand Surg Eur Vol*. 2014;39(3):282–285.

41. Karl AI, Carney ML, Kaul MP. The lumbrical provocation test in subjects with median inclusive paresthesia. *Arch Phys Med Rehabil*. 2001;82:935–937.

42. Tay SC, Tomita K, Berger RA. The "ulnar fovea sign" for defining ulnar wrist pain: an analysis of sensitivity and specificity. *J Hand Surg [Am]*. 2007;32:438–444.

43. Duckworth AD, Buijze GA, Moran M, et al. Predictors of fracture following suspected injury to the scaphoid. *J Bone Joint Surg Br*. 2012;94(7):961–968.

44. Stratford PW, Binkley JM, Stratford DM. Development and initial validation of the upper extremity functional index. *Physiotherapy Canada*. 2001;53(4):259–267.

45. Roy JS, MacDermid JC, Woodhouse LJ. Measuring shoulder function: a systematic review of four questionnaires. *Arthritis Rheum*. 2009;61:623–632.

46. Massy-Westropp N, Krishnan J, Ahern M. Comparing the AUSCAN Osteoarthritis Hand Index, Michigan Hand Outcomes Questionnaire, and Sequential Occupational Dexterity Assessment for patients with rheumatoid arthritis. *J Rheumatol*. 2004;31:1996–2001.

47. Shauver MJ, Chung KC. The minimal clinically important difference of the Michigan hand outcomes questionnaire. *J Hand Surg [Am]*. 2009;34:509–514.

48. Li L, Liu X, Herr K. Postoperative pain intensity assessment: a comparison of four scales in Chinese adults. *Pain Med*. 2007;8:223–234.

11

Wrist and Hand

Index

Page numbers followed by "*f*" indicate figures, and "*t*" indicate tables.

Index

Index

Cervical spine *(Continued)*
  palpation assessment of pain, 106, 106t–107t
  passive mobility, 103, 103t
  patient history in, 82t
  postural assessment, 108, 108f, 109t
  range of motion measurements, 94–95, 94t
  sensation testing, 85–86, 85f
  shoulder abduction test, 114, 114f
  Spurling's A and B tests, 109t
  Spurling's to the right and left tests, 109t
  strength and endurance testing, 97f, 97t–98t
  traction test, 112, 112f, 112t
Cervical thrust manipulation, clinical prediction rule for, 127
Cervical traction, for cervical radiculopathy
  after three weeks, 130–131, 130t–131t
  cluster of findings in, 132, 132f, 132t
Cervical vertebrae
  articular facet of, 68f
    anterior, 68f
    inferior, 68f
    posterior, 68f–69f
    superior, 68f
  articular process of, 69f
    inferior, 68f
  spinous process of, 68f–69f, 71f, 145f–147f
    palpation of, 106t–107t
  tubercles of
    anterior, 68f, 71f
    posterior, 68f, 146f–147f
Cervical zygapophyseal pain syndromes, 80–82, 80f
Chemical factors, of lumbar pain, 190f
Chest expansion, in ankylosing spondylitis, 159f, 202t
Children, wrist fractures in, 563, 563f
Chin, neck distraction test and, 112t
Chin tuck neck flexion test, 97t–98t
Choanae, 21f, 67f
Chorda tympani nerve, 24f
CI. *See* Confidence interval
Circumflex artery(ies)
  deep, iliac, 271f
  femoral
    lateral, 271f
      ascending, transverse, and descending branches of, 271f
    medial, 271f
  humeral, anterior *vs.* posterior, 446f
  scapular, 446f
    groove on scapula for, 438f
Clavicle, 72f, 74f, 140f
  acromial end of, 437f
  acromial facet of, 437f
  conoid tubercle of, 437f

Clavicle *(Continued)*
  impression for costoclavicular ligament on, 437f
  ligaments of, 440f
  muscles of, 443f–444f
  in shoulder joint, 437f–438f, 446f
  sternal end of, 437f
  sternal facet of, 437f
  subclavian groove of, 437f
  surfaces of
    inferior *vs.* superior, 437f
    posterior and anterior, 437f
  trapezoid line of, 437f
Clavicular branch, of thoracoacromial artery, 446f
Clavicular tilt angle, 458t
Click-clack test, of sacroiliac joint, 250t
Clicking, in shoulder, 448t
Clinical examination
  reliability and diagnostic utility of, 1–12
    assessment of study quality, 9–10
    diagnostic accuracy, 2–8, 11t
      2×2 contingency table, 3–8, 11t
      likelihood ratios in, 6–9, 7f, 7t, 11t
      overall accuracy in, 4
      positive and negative predictive values in, 4, 4t, 11t
      pretest and posttest probability, 8
    reliability, 2–3
    sensitivity, in, 4–5, 5f, 11t
    specificity, 5–6, 5f–6f, 11t
    statistics related to, 11, 11t
    summary of, 11, 11t
Clinical prediction rule
  for carpal tunnel syndrome, 540t, 594, 594f
  for cervical thrust manipulation, 127
  for epicondylalgia, 535, 535t
  for patellofemoral pain, 372, 372f–373f
  for scaphoid fracture, 594
  of spinal manipulation, 256, 257f
  for symptomatic knee osteoarthritis, 373, 374f
  for symptomatic meniscal tear, 375, 375f–376f
  for wrist fractures, in children, 563
Clivus, of basilar part of occipital bone, 70f
Clonus, cervical myelopathy and, 121t–124t
Cluneal nerve, inferior, 270f, 270t, 323f
Coccygeal cornu (horn), 216f
Coccygeal nerve, 223t, 224f
  herniated lumbar nucleus pulposus and, 161f
Coccygeal plexus, 152f
Coccygeus muscle (ischio-), 224f
  nerve to, 152f, 223t, 224f
Coccyx
  nerves of, 152f, 223t
  osteology of, 215f–216f, 264f

Coccyx *(Continued)*
  superior articular process of, 216f
  surfaces of, dorsal *vs.* pelvic, 216f
  tip of, in female, 218f
  transverse process of, 216f
Collateral ligaments
  of elbow, 517f, 517t
    tear of, 514t
  of knee, tears of, 312t, 324t
    patient history in, 324t, 328f, 328t
    valgus stress test for, 360t
  lateral, 316f, 391f, 391t, 393f
  medial, tears of, detection of, 531, 531f, 531t
  metacarpophalangeal and interphalangeal, 546f, 546t
  plantar foot, 393t
  of radius, 517f, 517t, 544f, 544t
  of ulna, 517f, 517t, 544f–545f, 544t
Comminuted fracture, of femur, 303t into shaft, 329f
Common extensor tendon
  of forearm, 519f
  of hand, 547f
Common fibular nerve, 224f, 321t
Common flexor tendon, of hand, 549f
Complete distal biceps tendon rupture, detection of, 532–533, 532t–533t, 534f
Compression
  of cervical cord, 120, 120f, 120t
  of hand, longitudinal, for scaphoid fractures, 560t
  of nerve root, with herniated disc, 83f
  of spinal cord, with cervical fracture, 90f
  of spinal nerve roots
    degenerative disc disease, 197f
    detection of, with slump knee bend test, 193–195, 193t
    with lumbar disc herniation, 190f
Compression fracture, of cervical spine, 90f
Compression tests
  of brachial plexus, for cervical cord compression, 120, 120f, 120t
  of cervical spine, 109, 109f, 109t
  of foot and ankle, for trauma screening, 407t–408t
    direct *vs.* indirect, 409t–410t
  for glenoid labral tears
    active, 471–472, 471f, 471t–472t
      rotation with, 471f, 472t
      combined with other tests, 507t
    combinations of tests, 506t
    passive, 475t
    rotation, 469, 469f, 469t
  for pelvic pain, 277t
  of sacroiliac region, 214t, 235–236, 235f, 235t
    combined with other tests, 252t–253t, 255
  of temporomandibular joint, bilateral, 55, 55f, 55t

Index

Index

Index

Index

Index

Index

T

Index